Instructional
Course Lectures

Volume 56 2007

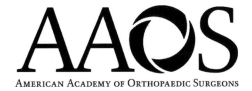

Instructional
Course Lectures

Volume 56 2007

Edited by
J. Lawrence Marsh, MD
Professor of Orthopaedic Surgery
Department of Orthopaedics and Rehabilitation
University of Iowa Hospitals and Clinics
Iowa City, Iowa

Paul J. Duwelius, MD
Adjunct Associate Professor of Orthopaedics, OHSU
Clinical Attending, St. Vincent Hospital and Medical Center
Portland, Oregon

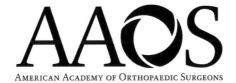

Published 2007 by the

American Academy
of Orthopaedic Surgeons
6300 North River Road
Rosemont, IL 60018

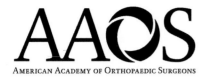

AMERICAN ACADEMY OF ORTHOPAEDIC SURGEONS

Instructional Course Lectures Volume 56
American Academy of Orthopaedic Surgeons

The material presented in the Instructional Course Lectures 56 has been made available by the American Academy of Orthopaedic Surgeons for educational purposes only. This material is not intended to present the only, or necessarily best, methods or procedures for the medical situations discussed, but rather is intended to represent an approach, view, statement, or opinion of the author(s) or producer(s), which may be helpful to others who face similar situations.

Some drugs or medical devices demonstrated in Academy courses or described in Academy print or electronic publications have not been cleared by the Food and Drug Administration (FDA) or have been cleared for specific uses only. The FDA has stated that it is the responsibility of the physician to determine the FDA clearance status of each drug or device he or she wishes to use in clinical practice.

Furthermore, any statements about commercial products are solely the opinion(s) of the author(s) and do not represent an Academy endorsement or evaluation of these products. These statements may not be used in advertising or for any commercial purpose.

Some of the authors or the departments with which they are affiliated have received something of value from a commercial or other party related directly or indirectly to the subject of their chapter.

First Edition

Copyright ©2007 by the American Academy of Orthopaedic Surgeons

ISBN 10: 0-89203-393-2
ISBN 13: 978-0-89203-393-5

Printed in the USA

Library of Congress Cataloging-in-Publication Data

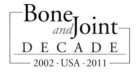

Contributors

William A. Abdu, MD, MS, Associate Professor of Orthopaedic Surgery, Dartmouth-Hitchcock Medical Center, Lebanon, New Hampshire

Kenneth J. Accousti, MD, Clinical Shoulder Fellow, Department of Orthopaedic Surgery, Mount Sinai Medical Center, New York, New York

A. Herbert Alexander, MD, Professor of Surgery, Uniformed Services University of the Health Sciences, Ketchum, Idaho

Harlan C. Amstutz, MD, Medical Director, Joint Replacement Institute, Los Angeles Orthopaedic Hospital, Los Angeles, California

Paul A. Anderson, MD, Associate Professor, Department of Orthopedics and Rehabilitation, University of Wisconsin, Madison, Wisconsin

Elizabeth A. Arendt, MD, Associate Professor, Department of Orthopaedic Surgery, University of Minnesota, Minneapolis, Minnesota

Diane Back, MBBS, BSc, FRCS Ed (Tr & Orth), Consultant Orthopaedic Surgeon, Department of Trauma and Orthopaedics, Guy's and St. Thomas' Hospital, London, United Kingdom

Roald Bahr, MD, PhD, Professor, Oslo Sports Trauma Research Center, Norwegian School of Sport Sciences, Oslo, Norway

Paul E. Beaulé, MD, FRCSC, Associate Professor, Head of Adult Reconstruction, Orthopedics, University of Ottawa, Ottawa, Ontario, Canada

J. Sybil Biermann, MD, Associate Professor, Department of Orthopaedic Surgery, Director, Musculoskeletal Oncology, University of Michigan Medical School, Ann Arbor, Michigan

Barry P. Boden, MD, The Orthopaedic Center, Rockville, Maryland

Pascal Boileau, MD, Professor, Department of Orthopaedic Surgery and Sports Traumatology, Archet 2 Hospital, Nice, France

Joseph Borrelli, Jr, MD, Associate Professor, Chief, Orthopaedic Trauma, Department of Orthopaedic Surgery, Washington University School of Medicine, St. Louis, Missouri

Martin I. Boyer, MD, MSc, FRCSC, Associate Professor, Director, Orthopaedic Hand Surgery, Washington University School of Medicine at Barnes-Jewish Hospital, St. Louis, Missouri

Ingeborg Hoff Braekken, Msci, PT, Manual Therapist, Department of Sports Medicine, Norwegian School of Sport Sciences, Oslo, Norway

Andrew K. Brown, MD, Orthopaedic Spine Research, Rothman Institute, Philadelphia, Pennsylvania

William D. Bugbee, MD, Associate Professor, Department of Orthopaedic Surgery, University of California, San Diego, La Jolla, California

Pat Campbell, PhD, Director, Implant Retrieval Laboratory, Associate Adjunct Professor, UCLA Orthopaedics, Department of Orthopaedics, University of California at Los Angeles, Los Angeles, California

Caroline M. Chebli, MD, Shoulder and Elbow Fellow, Department of Orthopaedics, University of Washington, Seattle, Washington

Christopher Chuinard, MD, MPH, Great Lakes Orthopaedic Center, Traverse City, Michigan

J.F. Myles Clough, MD, Kamloops, British Columbia, Canada

Charles H. Crawford III, MD, Resident, Department of Orthopaedic Surgery, University of Louisville, Louisville, Kentucky

Quanjun Cui, MD, MS, Department of Orthopaedic Surgery, University of Virginia School of Medicine, Charlottesville, Virginia

Frances Cuomo, MD, Chief, Shoulder Service, Department of Orthopaedic Surgery, Beth Israel Medical Center, New York, New York

Nickolaos A. Darlis, MD, PhD, Upper Extremity Fellow, Department of Orthopaedic Surgery, Allegheny General Hospital, Pittsburgh, Pennsylvania

Michael D. Daubs, MD, FACS, Instructor, Department of Orthopaedic Surgery, Washington University, St. Louis, Missouri

Ronald E. Delanois, MD, Attending, Rubin Institute for Advanced Orthopedics, Sinai Hospital, Baltimore, Maryland

David M. Dines, MD, Chairman, Professor of Orthopedic Surgery, Department of Orthopedic Surgery, Albert Einstein College of Medicine at Long Island Jewish Medical Center, New Hyde Park, New York

Joshua S. Dines, MD, Fellow, Sports Medicine, Kerlan Jobe Orthopaedic Clinic, Los Angeles, California

Douglas R. Dirschl, MD, Frank C. Wilson Distinguished Professor and Chair, UNC Department of Orthopaedics, University of North Carolina, Chapel Hill, North Carolina

Lars Engebretsen, MD, PhD, Professor and Chair, Orthopedic Center, Ullevaal University Hospital, Oslo, Norway

Evan L. Flatow, MD, Lasker Professor and Chair, Department of Orthopaedic Surgery, Mount Sinai Medical Center, New York, New York

Kevin R. Ford, MS, Research Biomechanist, Sports Medicine Biodynamics Center, Cincinnati Children's Hospital Medical Center, Cincinnati, Ohio

Robert J. Goitz, MD, Associate Professor, Chief, Division of Hand and Upper Extremity Surgery, Department of Orthopaedic Surgery, University of Pittsburgh Medical Center, Pittsburgh, Pennsylvania

Charles A. Goldfarb, MD, Assistant Professor, Department of Orthopaedic Surgery, Washington University School of Medicine, St. Louis, Missouri

Gregory J. Golladay, MD, Grand Rapids, Michigan

Simon Görtz, MD, Research Fellow, Department of Orthopaedic Surgery, University of California, San Diego, La Jolla, California

Robert A. Hart, MD, MA, Associate Professor, Department of Orthopaedics and Rehabilitation, Oregon Health and Sciences University, Portland, Oregon

J. Mi Lee Haisman, MD, Hand Surgeon, Orthopaedic Surgeon, Dartmouth, Massachusetts

Heather W. Harnly, MD, Fellow, Sports Medicine and Shoulder Service, Hospital for Special Surgery, New York, New York

Richard J. Hawkins, MD, FRCSC, Principal, Steadman Hawkins Clinic of the Carolinas, Spartanburg, South Carolina, Clinical Professor, University of Colorado, Clinical Professor, University of Texas Southwestern, Team Physician, Denver Broncos and Colorado Rockies

Ralph Hertel, MD, Department of Orthopaedic Surgery, Linden Hospital, Bern, Switzerland

Timothy E. Hewett, PhD, Director, Sports Medicine Biodynamic Center, Cincinnati Children's Medical Center, Cincinnati, Ohio

J. David Hill, MD, Clinical Fellow, Shoulder and Elbow Surgery, Department of Orthopaedic Surgery, Beth Israel Medical Center, New York, New York

Caroline Hing, BSc, MSc, MD, FRCS (Tr & Orth), Orthopaedic Fellow, Melbourne Orthopaedic Group, Melbourne, Australia

David S. Hungerford, MD, Professor, Department of Orthopaedic Surgery, Johns Hopkins University School of Medicine, Baltimore, Maryland

Deryk G. Jones, MD, Chief, Section of Sports Medicine and Cartilage Restoration, Department of Orthopaedic Surgery, Ochsner Clinic Foundation, New Orleans, Louisiana

Lynne C. Jones, PhD, Associate Professor, Director, Center for Osteonecrosis Research and Education, Department of Orthopaedic Surgery, Johns Hopkins University School of Medicine, Baltimore, Maryland

Jesse B. Jupiter, MD, Department of Orthopaedic Surgery, Massachusetts General Hospital, Boston, Massachusetts

Yongjung J. Kim, MD, Visiting Scholar, Department of Orthopaedic Surgery, Washington University, St. Louis, Missouri

Graham J. King, MD, MSc, FRCSC, Professor, Division of Orthopaedic Surgery, University of Western Ontario, St. Joseph's Health Centre, London, Ontario, Canada

Philip Kregor, MD, Nashville, Tennessee

Michel J. Le Duff, MA, Clinical Research Coordinator, Joint Replacement Institute, Los Angeles Orthopaedic Hospital, Los Angeles, California

Ronald A. Lehman, Jr, MD, Assistant Professor, Department of Orthopaedic Surgery, Walter Reed Army Medical Center, Washington, DC

Lawrence G. Lenke, MD, Jerome J. Gilden Professor of Orthopaedic Surgery, Department of Orthopaedic Surgery, Washington University, St. Louis, Missouri

Steven B. Lippitt, MD, Associate Professor, Northeastern Ohio Universities College of Medicine, Department of Orthopaedics, Akron General Medical Center, Akron, Ohio

Arthur L. Malkani, MD, Associate Professor, Chief, Adult Reconstruction, Department of Orthopaedic Surgery, University of Louisville School of Medicine, Louisville, Kentucky

Bert Mandelbaum, MD, Fellowship Director, Santa Monica Orthopaedic and Sports Medicine Group, Santa Monica, California

Neil A. Manson, MD, FRCSC, Spine Fellow, Midwest Orthopaedics at Rush, Rush University Medical Center, Chicago, Illinois

J. Lawrence Marsh, MD, Professor of Orthopaedic Surgery, Department of Orthopaedics and Rehabilitation, University of Iowa Hospitals and Clinics, Iowa City, Iowa

Paul A. Martineau, MD, FRCSC, Fellow, Section of Sports Medicine, Cleveland Clinic Sports Health, Cleveland Clinic, Cleveland, Ohio

German A. Marulanda, MD, Fellow, Rubin Institute for Advanced Orthopedics, Sinai Hospital of Baltimore, Baltimore, Maryland

Frederick A. Matsen III, Chair, Department of Orthopaedics, University of Washington, Seattle, Washington

Peter McCann, MD, Chair, Department of Orthopaedic Surgery, Beth Israel Medical Center, New York, New York

William M. Mihalko, MD, PhD, Associate Professor, University of Virginia, Department of Orthopaedic Surgery, Charlottesville, Virginia

Anthony Miniaci, MD, FRCSC, Executive Director, Head Section of Sports Medicine, Cleveland Clinic Sports Health, Cleveland Clinic, Cleveland, Ohio

Kai Mithoefer, MD, Harvard Vanguard Orthopedics and Sports Medicine, Brigham and Women's Hospital, Harvard Medical School, Boston, Massachusetts

Michael A. Mont, MD, Director, Rubin Institute for Advanced Orthopaedics, Sinai Hospital of Baltimore, Baltimore, Maryland

Daniel P. Moynihan, MD, Department of Orthopedic Surgery, Long Island Jewish Medical Center, New Hyde Park, New York

Gregory D. Myer, MS, CSCS, Sports Biomechanist, Sports Medicine Biodynamics Center, Cincinnati Children's Hospital Medical Center, Cincinnati, Ohio

Grethe Myklebust, PT, PhD, Senior Researcher, Oslo Sport Trauma Research Center, Norwegian School of Sport Sciences, Oslo, Norway

Ladislav Nagy, MD, PD, Surgery of the Hand and Peripheral Nerves, University Clinic Balgrist, Zurich, Switzerland

Odd-Egil Olsen, PT, PhD, Senior Researcher, Oslo Sports Trauma Research Center, Norwegian School of Sport Sciences, Oslo, Norway

Alvin Ong, MD, Department of Orthopaedic Surgery, Rothman Institute, Philadelphia, Pennsylvania

Fabio Orozco, MD, Department of Orthopaedic Surgery, Rothman Institute, Philadelphia, Pennsylvania

Hari K. Parvataneni, MD, Resident, Orthopaedic Surgery, Lenox Hill Hospital, New York, New York

Javad Parvizi, MD, FRCS, Director of Research, Associate Professor of Orthopaedics, Rothman Institute of Orthopaedics, Thomas Jefferson University, Philadelphia, Pennsylvania

Lars Peterson, MD, PhD, Gothenburg Medical Center, Department of Orthopaedics, University of Göteborg, Gothenburg, Sweden

Frank M. Phillips, Professor, Orthopaedic Surgery, Rush University Medical Center, Chicago, Illinois

Johanes F. Plate, BS, Rubin Institute for Advanced Orthopedics, Sinai Hospital, Baltimore, Maryland

Philippe Poitras, BASc, Research Associate, Orthopaedic Biomechanics Laboratory, University of Ottawa, Ottawa, Ontario, Canada

Michael A. Prendergast, BA, Department of Orthopaedics, Robert Wood Johnson Medical School, New Brunswick, New Jersey

James J. Purtill, MD, Assistant Professor, Department of Orthopedic Surgery, Thomas Jefferson University, Philadelphia, Pennsylvania

Arun J. Ramappa, MD, Clinical Instructor at Harvard Medical School, Department of Orthopaedic Surgery, Beth Israel Deaconess Medical Center, Boston, Massachusetts

Amar S. Ranawat, MD, Department of Orthopaedic Surgery, Lenox Hill Hospital, New York, New York

Chitranjan S. Ranawat, MD, The James A. Nicholas Chairman, Department of Orthopaedic Surgery, Lenox Hill Hospital, New York, New York

Ghazi M. Rayan, MD, Clinical Professor of Orthopaedic Surgery, Oklahoma University, Director, Oklahoma Hand Fellowship Program, Oklahoma City, Oklahoma

John M. Rhee, MD, Assistant Professor, Department of Orthopaedic Surgery, Emory University, Atlanta, Georgia

William M. Ricci, MD, Associate Professor, Department of Orthopaedic Surgery, Washington University School of Medicine, St. Louis, Missouri

K. Daniel Riew, MD, Professor, Chief, Cervical Spine Surgery, Department of Orthopaedic Surgery, Washington University School of Medicine, St. Louis, Missouri

Rachel S. Rohde, MD, Orthopaedic Surgeon, Department of Orthopaedic Surgery, William Beaumont Hospital, Royal Oak, Michigan

Richard H. Rothman, MD, PhD, Department of Orthopaedic Surgery, Rothman Institute, Philadelphia, Pennsylvania

Khaled J. Saleh, MD, MSc, FRCSC, FACS, Associate Professor and Division Head, Adult Reconstruction, Department of Orthopaedic Surgery, University of Virginia, Charlottesville, Virginia

Rick C. Sasso, MD, Assistant Professor, Clinical Orthopaedic Surgery, Indiana University School of Medicine, Indiana Spine Group, Indianapolis, Indiana

Michael K. Schaufele, MD, Assistant Professor, Departments of Orthopedics and Rehabilitation Medicine, Emory University, Atlanta, Georgia

Steven R. Schelkun, MD, San Diego, California

Jason M. Scopp, MD, Director, Center for Cartilage Repair, Peninsula Orthopaedic Associates, P.A., Salisbury, Maryland

Thorsten M. Seyler, MD, Fellow, Rubin Institute for Advanced Orthopedics, Sinai Hospital, Baltimore, Maryland

Andrew Shimmin, FAOrthA, FRACS, Dip Anat, Consultant Orthopaedic Surgeon, Melbourne Orthopaedic Group, Melbourne, Australia

Judith A. Siegel, MD, Resident, Department of Orthopaedic Surgery, Boston University Medical Center, Boston, Massachusetts

Michael S. Sirkin, MD, Assistant Professor, Chief, Orthopaedic Trauma Service, Orthopaedics, New Jersey Medical School, Newark, New Jersey

Arnhilo Skjølberg, Physiotherapist, Orkanger Fysikalske Institiuti, Orkanger, Norway

James R. Slauterbeck, Orthopedic Surgery and Rehabilitation, University of Vermont, Burlington, Vermont

Dean G. Sotereanos, MD, Professor, Vice Chair, Department of Orthopaedics, Drexel University, Allegheny General Hospital, Pittsburgh, Pennsylvania

John W. Sperling, MD, Department of Orthopedic Surgery, Mayo Clinic, Rochester, Minnesota

Gordon H. Stock, MD, Orthopaedic Research Fellow, Department of Orthopaedics, Thomas Jefferson University, Rothman Institute, Philadelphia, Pennsylvania

Misty Suri, MD, Fellow, Reconstructive Knee and Shoulder Surgery and Sports Medicine, Steadman Hawkins Clinic of the Carolinas, Spartanburg, South Carolina

Robert M. Szabo, MD, MPH, Professor of Orthopaedic Surgery, Orthopaedics, University of California Davis, Davis, California

T. David Tarity, BS, Research Fellow, Rothman Institute Orthopaedics, Thomas Jefferson University, Philadelphia, Pennsylvania

Paul Tornetta III, MD, Professor and Vice Chairman, Director, Orthopaedic Trauma, Department of Orthopaedic Surgery, Boston University Medical Center, Boston University School of Medicine, Boston, Massachusetts

Alexander R. Vaccaro, MD, Professor of Orthopaedics and Neurosurgery, Department of Orthopaedics, Thomas Jefferson University, Rothman Institute, Philadelphia, Pennsylvania

Eugene R. Viscusi, MD, Director, Acute Pain Management, Department of Anesthesiology, Thomas Jefferson University, Philadelphia, Pennsylvania

Andrew J. Weiland, MD, Department of Orthopaedics, Hospital for Special Surgery, New York, New York

Riley J. Williams III, MD, Associate Professor of Orthopedic Surgery, Sports Medicine and Shoulder Service, Hospital for Special Surgery, Weill Cornell Medical College, New York, New York

Thomas W. Wright, MD, Professor, UF Orthopaedic and Sports Medicine Institute, Gainesville, Florida

Preface

First presented at the AAOS annual meeting in 1942, the Instructional Course Lecture program continues to be a cornerstone of the educational offerings at the annual meeting of the American Academy of Orthopaedic Surgeons. At the 2006 meeting in Chicago, 178 courses were taught by 844 faculty members and were attended by more than 11,000 participants. As always these courses provide the most up-to-date synthesized information on topics of orthopaedic science, clinical knowledge, and surgical techniques. All lectures are accompanied by detailed outlines and all courses provide abundant time for questions, discussion, and interaction with faculty members. In an effort to evolve and continue to offer courses of maximal interest, for the first time surgical skills courses were part of the 2006 curriculum. Courses were selected by committee members Terry Light, MD; Vincent Pellegrini, Jr, MD; Paul Duwelius, MD; Frederick Azar, MD; Dempsey Springfield, MD; James Heckman, MD, and myself. The program would not have occurred without the able guidance of Kathie Niesen, education manager, who pulls it all together.

The ICL volume, in this its 56th edition, represents the enduring legacy of the ICL lecture series program. It occurs primarily because of the efforts of the chapter authors to commit their lectures and outlines to a written and illustrated text with a turnaround time that allows this volume to be offered at the annual meeting 1 year later. This volume contains the work of more than 100 authors complied in 45 chapters. The topics span a wide spectrum of orthopaedic knowledge and cover some of the most relevant and popular subjects in current orthopaedics. Along with the book is 119 minutes of video recorded on DVD emphasizing surgical techniques.

For the editor, identifying the potential chapters from among the more than 170 courses, most with three or more lectures, that best represent the most relevant information possible that are least redundant to previous volumes is a major challenge. To facilitate optimal choices, we have begun a process whereby the upcoming ICL chair will serve as assistant editor to the volume. This will provide important experience and continuity and allow the chapter authors to be selected earlier in their course cycle. I am grateful to Paul Duwelius for serving in this role for this volume and for his skillful and timely editing of the chapters on adult reconstruction.

This project could not happen without the efforts of many contributors on the path to publication, including Marilyn L. Fox, PhD, director of the AAOS publications department, Lisa Claxton Moore, managing editor of the Instructional Course Lecture series, and Kathleen Anderson, associate senior editor. Reid L. Stanton, Manager of Electronic Media at AAOS, organized and edited the DVD material. My assistant, Jennifer Kirschling, kept manuscripts moving in and out of the office and as always made my job possible. I am grateful to Stuart Weinstein, MD, not only for affording me the honor of participating in the Academy's Instructional Course Lecture Committee, but for his leadership in orthopaedic surgery.

On behalf of all of the contributors to this volume and to those who provided the background support, I hope that you, the readers, find the 56th edition to be a worthy continuation of this long-lasting series. It represents another edition to a series that provides a yearly cross-sectional snapshot of the widening and evolving and endlessly fascinating field of orthopaedic surgery. I hope you enjoy it and find it to be educational.

J. L. Marsh, MD
Iowa City, Iowa

Table of Contents

Section 3 Adult Reconstruction: Pain Management in Joint Arthroplasty

Section 4 Adult Reconstruction: Hip

Section 7 Sports Medicine

Section 8 Practice Management

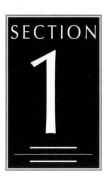

SECTION 1

Shoulder

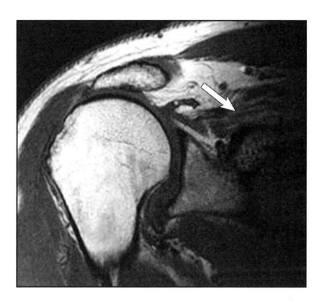

Technical Pearls on How to Maximize Healing of the Rotator Cuff

Kenneth J. Accousti, MD

Evan L. Flatow, MD

Abstract

Rotator cuff tears are common in today's aging population. Repair of the torn rotator cuff tendon can be performed by a variety of methods including open, mini-open, and arthroscopic techniques. Many surgical and nonsurgical factors affect whether a tendon will successfully heal to the tuberosity after repair. A high rate of failure of healing of the tendon to the tuberosity occurs even in procedures performed by experienced surgeons. Patients who have retears after rotator cuff repair still have improvement in pain and function; however, outcomes are not as favorable compared with those of patients who have intact cuffs after surgery.

Patient age, size and chronicity of the tear, and muscle degeneration and atrophy are major factors that affect successful healing of the rotator cuff. Surgical factors include proper surgical technique, tear pattern recognition, adequate subacromial decompression, cuff mobilization, preparation of the tuberosity, suture and knot tying technique, anchor placement, and surgeon experience. A proper postoperative rehabilitation regimen is also important to protect the repair during the first 12 weeks of tendon healing.

Progress continues in developing grafts and growth factors to stimulate and enhance the patient's intrinsic healing potential and to reinforce the surgical repair. The future of rotator cuff repair may also involve gene therapy and supplementation with growth factors to improve the healing rates of surgically repaired rotator cuff tendons.

Instr Course Lect 2007;56:1-10.

Rotator cuff disorders are the most common source of shoulder pain reported by patients. A large percentage of the population who are older than 50 years of age have a tear in the rotator cuff; however, many of these tears are asymptomatic. In one study, 33% of the shoulders of 50- to 60-year old cadavers had a full-thickness rotator cuff tear and 100% of cadavers 70 years or older

had a full-thickness rotator cuff tear.[1] Proposed etiologies for rotator cuff tears and degeneration include direct mechanical trauma secondary to impingement from subacromial spurs, acute trauma from injury, and intrinsic tendon degeneration secondary to decreased vascularity and compromised tissue healing properties associated with aging. The true etiology of rotator cuff tears is prob-

ably a combination of all three factors.

With the advent of arthroscopic rotator cuff repair in the early 1990s, considerable progress has been made in minimally invasive surgery of the shoulder. Although open rotator cuff repair is often considered the gold standard, recent advances in arthroscopic surgical techniques including anchor fixation and double-row suturing, as well as improved surgeon familiarity and comfort with arthroscopic repair, has produced results similar to those obtained using open and mini-open rotator cuff repair.[2-8]

In the recent literature, failure rates as high as 90% have been reported for repairs of rotator cuff tears.[9] The generally accepted retear rate is 25% to 40%.[3-8] Many factors are involved in healing the rotator cuff tendon to the tuberosity; therefore, many weak links in the healing chain contribute to the high rate of failure. Factors that the surgeon cannot control include muscle atrophy and fatty degeneration (leading to fibrosis and increased stiffness creating high tensile loads at the repair site), large tear size, poor tendon quality secondary to aging and de-

Table 1
Long-Term Results in Patients With Large or Massive Rotator Cuff Tears

Study	No. of Patients	Follow-up	Tear Size	Repair Method	Retear Rate (%)	Preoperative UCLA Score	Postoperative UCLA Score	Preoperative Constant Score	Postoperative Constant Score	Preoperative ASES Shoulder Score	Postoperative ASES Shoulder Score
Galatz et al[9] (2004)	18	36 months	> 2 cm	Arthroscopic	94	NA	NA	NA	NA	48	80
Bishop et al[16] (2006)	32 (Open)	12 months	All	Open	31	NA	NA	53	80	40	85
	40 (Arthroscopic)	12 months	All	Arthroscopic	47	NA	NA	53	75	46	84
Boileau et al[17] (2005)	65	26 months	All	Arthroscopic	29	12	32.3	52	84	NA	NA
Tauro[4] (1998)	53	21 months	All	Arthroscopic	NA	17	41/45	NA	NA	NA	NA
Gerber et al[11] (2000)	27	37 months	Massive	Open	37	NA	NA	49	85	NA	NA
Rokito et al[14] (1999)	30	65 months	> 3 cm	Open	NA	12	31	NA	NA	NA	NA
Galatz et al[18] (2001)	33	10 years	All	Open	NA	NA	NA	NA	81	NA	NA

UCLA = University of California, Los Angeles; ASES = American Shoulder and Elbow Surgeons; NA = not applicable

creased vascularity, and repetitive trauma from impingement. The surgeon can control factors related to surgical technique and postoperative rehabilitation regimens.

Harryman and associates[10] evaluated postoperative patient satisfaction and function in 122 patients who had surgery for repair of the rotator cuff. Ultrasound was used to assess rotator cuff integrity. Patients with intact repairs had better postoperative strength and function, whereas those with persistent defects had decreased range of motion and decreased function when performing activities of daily living. Of 122 patients, 105 had persistent defects; however, 90% of these patients were satisfied with pain relief even though their functional results were inferior to those of the group of patients with intact repairs. Gerber and associates[11] also reported excellent outcomes for patients with structurally intact repairs for massive rotator cuff tears fixed with an open repair.

Postoperative strength correlated with the integrity of the repair, and continued weakness was related to the size of rerupture.[10,12] Although better functional results are achieved in patients with intact repairs, patients with retearing can still have relief of pain and improvement in function.[13] Satisfactory long-term results in pain relief and increased range of motion can be achieved in patients with large and massive tears, even if a retear occurs[14] (Table 1).

Major factors that contribute to the failure of rotator cuff repairs are incomplete or incorrect diagnosis, postoperative complications, poor surgical technique, and an inappropriate or incorrect postoperative rehabilitation regimen.[15] Factors that result in continued postoperative pain include axillary or suprascapular nerve palsies, cervical stenosis or radiculopathy, thoracic outlet syndrome, pathology of the long head of the biceps, acromioclavicular joint osteoarthritis, glenohumeral

instability, glenohumeral osteoarthritis, and labral tears (superior labrum anterior posterior or Bankart tears).

Uncontrollable Factors Associated With Rotator Cuff Healing

Some factors that affect healing of the rotator cuff are beyond the surgeon's control. Patient age, chronicity of the tear, large tear size, muscle atrophy, and fatty degeneration are all associated with inferior postoperative outcome. The surgeon should inform the patient of the expected outcome and function before surgery. The duration of rehabilitation after either arthroscopic or open surgery is the same; patients must be informed that they may not have maximum improvement in pain relief and function until 1 year after surgery.[14]

In a retrospective study of patients with chronic rotator cuff tears with an average follow-up of 13 years, Cofield and associates[19] reported that preoperative tear size was the most significant factor affecting long-term outcome with regard to patient satisfaction, range of motion, strength, and the need for resurgery. More advanced patient age and decreased preoperative motion and strength were associated with a larger tear. Delayed repair also has been shown to lead to a decreased rate of tendon healing secondary to increased muscle stiffness (from muscle atrophy) and decreased bone mineral density of the proximal humerus.[20,21] Although no study has yet been performed to quantify the rate of tear size progression, it appears that this rate varies from patient to patient. It is important to inform patients of the risks of nonsurgical intervention, including increasing tear size and progression of muscle atrophy, which is irreversible.

Surgical Factors

Surgical technique and postoperative rehabilitation are the two aspects of rotator cuff repair that the surgeon can control. Surgical factors include surgical technique (open, mini-open, or arthroscopic repair), tear pattern recognition, adequate subacromial decompression, cuff mobilization, preparation of the tuberosity, suture and knot tying technique, anchor placement, and surgeon experience. Postoperative rehabilitation, although not performed under the direct supervision of the surgeon, is controlled by the surgeon (including postoperative immobilization). An emerging field in tendon healing technology involves the use of biologic factors and grafts to promote tendon healing. Although many improvements have been made in surgical technique, the future of rotator cuff surgery will

depend on improvements in the biology of rotator cuff healing.

Methods of repair include all-arthroscopic repair, arthroscopically assisted mini-open repair, and open repair. The advantages of arthroscopic repair compared with any open repair technique include decreased deltoid morbidity, easier mobilization of the tendons, improved visualization and treatment of any intra-articular pathology, improved recognition of tear configuration, and less postoperative pain and stiffness.[22] The major advantage of open and mini-open repairs is the ability to "feel" the quality of the tendon, to obtain good suture purchase in the tendon via a Mason-Allen stitch, and to use grafting techniques and tendon transfers. With current arthroscopic techniques, the results of all-arthroscopic repairs are comparable to those of open and mini-open repairs.[2-8]

Pattern recognition and definition of the tear is an important factor in planning the proper releases and repair of rotator cuff tears. Most tears involve the supraspinatus tendon alone, but can progress to include the infraspinatus and subscapularis tendons. If the anterior portion of the supraspinatus is torn, the posterior corner of the tendon will remain tethered to the infraspinatus and posterior aspect of the greater tuberosity, creating an L-shaped tear. The converse is true with a posterior supraspinatus tear—the anterior supraspinatus tethered to the rotator interval and greater tuberosity produces a reverse L-shaped tear. Crescent tears are smaller, more mobile tears involving the supraspinatus tendon, whereas U-shaped tears are large retracted tears that may extend into the infraspinatus and subscapularis (Fig-

ure 1). A large L-shaped tear may appear as a U-shaped tear; however, it is important to determine the tear shape, because the repair and releases will be different for each tear configuration (Figure 2). Adequate bursectomy is crucial for recognition of the tear configuration and postoperative pain relief, as well as to ease the passing and retrieval of sutures when performing an arthroscopic repair. Removing bursa and unhealthy cuff tissue also decreases the likelihood of "repairing" the bursa to the tuberosity.

Another important facet of rotator cuff repair involves adequate decompression of the subacromial space.[23-26] In one study, 90% of failed large and massive rotator cuff repairs were linked to continued impingement and inadequate decompression.[23] Another study reported that more than 50% of failed rotator cuff repairs did not include acromioplasty.[24] Care must be taken not to remove too much of the acromion, which could cause deltoid detachment (a devastating complication that will lead to cuff repair failure). The amount of bony resection is determined after evaluation of preoperative imaging studies to assess the size of the acromial spur. Usually, 4 to 6 mm (the width of the burr) of bone resection is adequate to decompress the subacromial space. Aggressive subacromial débridement and release of the coracoacromial ligament can lead to anterosuperior humeral escape for patients with large or massive irreparable rotator cuff tears.[27]

Proper cuff mobilization is an important aspect of rotator cuff repair. Repairs made with undue tension are likely to fail secondary to tension overload at the repair site.[23,28-31] The tendon must be released to prevent excessive tension when the arm is ad-

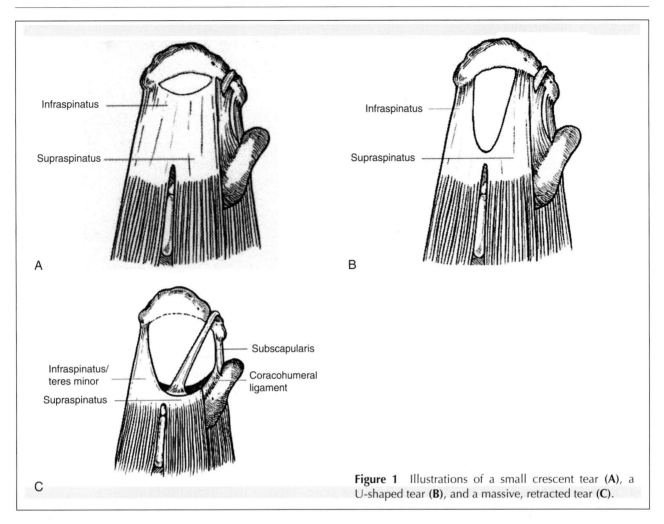

Figure 1 Illustrations of a small crescent tear (**A**), a U-shaped tear (**B**), and a massive, retracted tear (**C**).

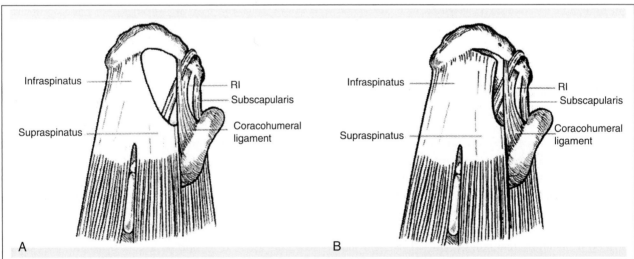

Figure 2 **A,** Illustration of an L-shaped tear prior to reduction. If this tear is large, it can be mistaken for a U-shaped tear. **B,** Reduction of an L-shaped tear is achieved with an anterior laterally directed pull, reducing the corner of the tear to the anterior lateral tuberosity. RI = rotator interval.

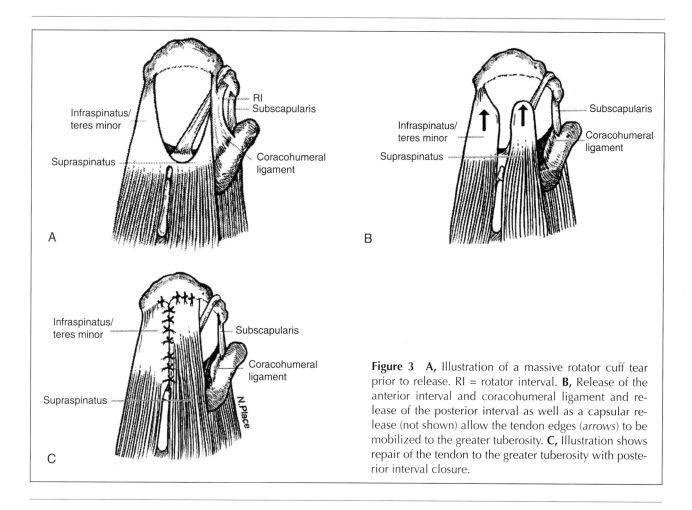

Figure 3   **A,** Illustration of a massive rotator cuff tear prior to release. RI = rotator interval. **B,** Release of the anterior interval and coracohumeral ligament and release of the posterior interval as well as a capsular release (not shown) allow the tendon edges (*arrows*) to be mobilized to the greater tuberosity. **C,** Illustration shows repair of the tendon to the greater tuberosity with posterior interval closure.

ducted at the side (Figure 3). Cuff mobilization techniques were first developed with open cuff repair and later modified for arthroscopic surgery. Arthroscopic release provides a more controlled environment with better visualization of the cuff for mobilization. Aggressive release greater than 2 cm medial to the superior glenoid rim will risk injury to the suprascapular nerve. Care must be taken not to transect the suprascapular nerve at the spinoglenoid notch during a posterior interval slide.[32] Release of the subscapularis also risks injury to the musculocutaneous and axillary nerve on its anterior and inferior borders, respectively. An interval slide is used when differential retraction is present (for example, supraspinatus retracted, but subscapu-laris intact). Mobilization in continuity maintains the attachment of the lateral aspect of the rotator interval between the anterior supraspinatus and superior subscapularis. This release in continuity is used for tears of both the supraspinatus and subscapularis. By preserving this lateral bridge "comma," the hoop stresses of the intact lateral band help to maintain the reduction of the supraspinatus laterally on the greater tuberosity[33] (Figure 4).

After the tendon edges have been mobilized sufficiently for a repair without undue tension (the tear edge easily reduces to the tuberosity), the edges of the tendon and tuberosity must be prepared to allow for maximal ingrowth potential. Any frayed or devitalized cuff edge should be débrided. It is important to remove any tough bursa that may be confused with cuff tendon. The tuberosity is cleaned of all soft tissue using a mechanical shaver and curette. Large excrescences on the greater tuberosity should be smoothed down with a burr to prevent mechanical impingement between the repaired cuff and the acromion; however, frank decortication of the footprint is avoided because it could weaken the bone fixation. In a study by St. Pierre and associates,[34] no significant improvement in tendon healing to a cancellous trough occurred compared with healing to a cortical bone.

The weakest link in the chain of rotator cuff repair is the tendon. Most tears occur through unhealthy,

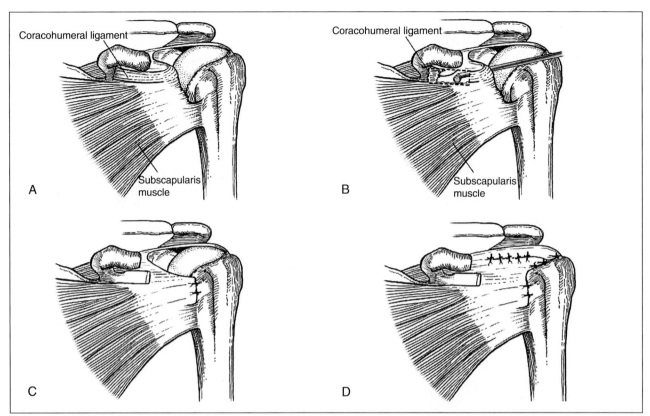

Figure 4 **A,** Illustration of a subscapularis and supraspinatus tear with retraction. **B,** Release of the coracohumeral ligament and rotator interval (*dotted lines*) leaving the lateral connection between the upper subscapularis and anterior supraspinatus. **C,** Repair of the subscapularis. The connection that is maintained between the supraspinatus and subscapularis helps to hold the anterior supraspinatus laterally. **D,** Repair of the supraspinatus after a posterior interval release and closure. By maintaining the lateral connection between the subscapularis and the supraspinatus, the subscapularis repair helps to anchor the supraspinatus over the greater tuberosity.

degenerated tissue that has poor suture-holding properties. Rotator cuff tears are extremely rare in young patients, even with the occurrence of traumatic glenohumeral dislocations. For some tendons, rotator cuff repair is similar to repairing an old, worn sock with "rotten fibers." In a study of modes of failure of revision surgery, Cummins and Murrell[35] found that 19 of 22 failures were secondary to suture pullout through the tendon. Tissue-grasping stitches such as the Mason-Allen stitch are superior to simple or mattress sutures. Gerber and associates[36] reported a twofold increase in ultimate tensile strength for the modified Mason-Allen suture com-

pared with the use of a simple suture configuration. The modified Mason-Allen stitch did not produce histologic evidence of tissue necrosis in vivo.[37] The massive cuff stitch was shown to be equal to the modified Mason-Allen stitch with respect to ultimate tensile strength (233 N versus 246 N, respectively). These two stitches were superior to simple and horizontal suture configurations (72 N and 77 N, respectively).[38] The massive cuff stitch (Mac stitch) can be thrown arthroscopically and involves placing a tissue-grasping stitch into the tendon perpendicular and lateral to a second simple throw used to secure the tendon to the anchor.

Tendon fixation to bone is also a critical process for cuff healing. Bone anchors provide stronger fixation than bone tunnels in cadaveric studies.[39,40] Studies on cyclic loading for failure models also show that properly placed bone anchors are superior to bone tunnels.[28] Proper technique involves placing bone anchors at the correct depth (Figure 5). Inserting an anchor too deep will cause chafing of the suture on the bone, which leads to failure at the suture-bone interface. Placing the anchor too superficially will cause impingement and failure of the suture at the proud eyelet. Suture anchors should be placed at least 45° away from the pull of the

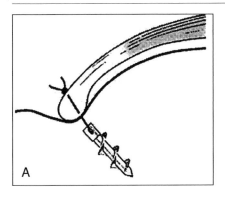
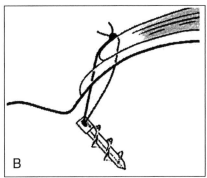
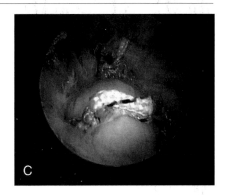

Figure 5 **A,** Illustration of a tight suture loop holds the tendon edge to the footprint and anchor. Note the inclination of the anchor, which is directed away from the pull of the tendon. **B,** A loose suture loop will allow the tendon to pull away from the footprint. **C,** Arthroscopic photograph shows that proper tension in the suture loop will produce dimpling of the tendon tissue down toward the anchor.

tendon. This "deadman" angle provides the best mechanical advantage for the suture-anchor construct to resist pullout of the anchor and lengthening of the suture by equilibrating the pull of the tendon away from the anchor and suture toward the anchor.[41] Bone quality varies within the tuberosity itself. Most rotator cuff repairs will be made in elderly patients who have some degree of osteoporosis of the proximal humerus. The degree of osteoporosis is directly correlated with pullout strength.[42] Preoperative radiographs and MRIs should be examined for the presence of bone cysts that will interfere with sound fixation in the tuberosity. The proximal portion of the greater tuberosity has higher pullout strength than the distal portion. The anterior and middle thirds of the greater tuberosity have a higher average pullout strength (68%) compared with the posterior aspect of the greater tuberosity. The lesser tuberosity provides the strongest fixation and is 32% stronger than the greater tuberosity.[42]

Bioabsorbable anchors are commonly used for fixation of rotator cuff tears and for Bankart and superior labrum anterior and posterior tears. Advantages of bioabsorbable anchors over metal anchors include gradual load transfer to healing tissue, reduced need for hardware removal, radiolucency, and no signal interference with postoperative MRI. Complications associated with bioabsorbable anchors include osteolysis, synovitis, sterile sinus tracts, and hypertrophic fibrous encapsulation.[43] Metal anchors allow assessment of anchor migration or pullout. Polymers of polylactic acid are primarily used because they reabsorb slower and produce less synovitis than polyglycolic acid anchors. Bioabsorbable anchors have comparable pullout strength and modes of failure compared with metallic anchors.[28,44,45]

The experience of the surgeon is also important for success in rotator cuff repair, especially for arthroscopic repairs. Arthroscopic repair of a large, retracted tear should only be attempted by a surgeon with adequate experience with these types of tears. After approximately 2 hours, the bursa and soft tissues in the subacromial space become engorged and swollen, making arthroscopic knot tying and visualization difficult. Surgeons should choose repair methods with which they are comfortable. If tears are not repairable by either open or arthroscopic techniques, débridement, gentle acromioplasty, and a partial repair may provide relief of pain and improvement in function. Revision rotator cuff repair is challenging because of scarring and adhesions in the subacromial and subdeltoid space. A previous failed repair may be an indicator of poor tendon quality and healing capacity. Djurasovic and associates[46] determined that positive indicators for successful revision surgery included an intact deltoid, good tendon quality, preoperative elevation above horizontal, and only one prior surgery.

Postoperative treatment can be as crucial as surgical technique for successful healing of the rotator cuff. The repair must be protected from active or active-assisted range of motion for the first 6 weeks after surgery to allow for ingrowth of the tendon to the bone surface. Failure to protect the repair resulted in a high failure rate in an experimental model.[37] One study showed that 5 of 31 failed rotator cuff repairs was caused by aggressive physical therapy.[47] The early use of weights and resistive exercises also has been shown to contribute to the failure of rotator cuff repair.[48] Rehabilitation therapy can be tailored to the size of the tear. Smaller, stable tears can be mobilized earlier than large, retracted tears that should be protected with an abduction pillow for 6 weeks after repair. The senior author recommends that most patients who have undergone rotator cuff repair should have the arm immobilized in a sling for 6 weeks with no physical therapy during this period. After 6 weeks, passive and active assisted range-of-motion exercises are performed under the supervision of a physical therapist. Light resistive exercises are not begun until 3 months postoperatively. Stiffness is rare after arthroscopic rotator cuff repair.

The Future of Rotator Cuff Healing: The Biologic Factor

The future of rotator cuff surgery will involve the addition of biologic factors and grafts to promote healing and ingrowth of the repaired tendon into the bone. The healing potential of degenerated tendons decreases with advancing patient age. The goal of biologic agents would be to repair or replace tissue by delivering cells, providing a scaffold for cellular ingrowth, and using proteins, protein fragments, and DNA to impart growth and healing.[49,50] Biologic grafts include autografts, allografts, and xenografts. Growth factors include bone morphogenetic proteins, transforming growth factor-β, platelet-derived growth factor, and fibroblast growth factor.

Autografts used to reinforce repairs include tensor fascia lata, coracoacromial ligament, central quadriceps tendon, and long head of biceps brachii. Allografts include cadaveric human rotator cuff tendon and human dermis (Graft Jacket, Wright Medical, Arlington, TN). Xenografts are the most com-

monly used grafts because of their increased availability, and are used to reinforce repairs and fill in residual defects. Xenografts include bovine dermis (Orthomend, Stryker, Mahwah, NJ), chemically cross-linked porcine dermis (Permacol, Zimmer, Warsaw IN), and porcine small intestine submucosa (Restore patch, DePuy Orthopaedics, Warsaw, IN). These grafts all act as a primary resorbable scaffold for native cells to populate and lay down matrix for tendon growth. The most important component of the extracellular matrix is type I collagen, which is the primary collagen responsible for the mechanical strength of tendons.[51] The tensile strengths of these xenografts do not match that of a healthy human rotator cuff and are not meant to add mechanical strength to the repair site. Extracellular matrix scaffolds have a much lower modulus and load-to-failure properties than native tendon; therefore, they are not intended to be load-sharing devices secondary to their increased compliance. In a study by Dejardin and associates,[52] porcine small intestine submucosa grafts were used in canine rotator cuff defects. Results showed gross and histologic continuity of the grafted tendon and a mode of repair failure the same as that of native infraspinatus tendon. The porcine small intestine submucosa graft was ultimately resorbed from the graft site, leaving only native tissue.

Complications associated with tissue grafts include the inability to achieve the desired functional result, graft rupture, formation of adhesions, failure of incorporation with native tissue, foreign body reaction, infection, necrosis, and delayed healing. Donor site morbidity is associated with autografts. In

a controlled, prospective randomized study, preliminary results comparing the Restore patch with no patch for chronic, large to massive (two-tendon) tears showed no statistical difference; however, a trend toward less favorable results was found with the Restore patch compared to repairs without the patch.[53]

Cell-based growth factor and gene therapies have not yet been applied to human trials for tendon repair. A mixture of bone morphogenetic protein-2 through -7, transforming growth factor-β1, -β2, and β3, and fibroblast growth factor was used to augment sheep infraspinatus tendon repair. Results showed a significantly stronger attachment between the tendon and the bone.[16,18] The future of rotator cuff grafting will most likely involve a mixture of a soft-tissue scaffold such as a cross-linked type I collagen graft, xenograft imbedded with growth factors, or DNA carrying viral vectors to increase and promote the healing potential of the patient.

Summary

Rotator cuff tears are common in today's aging population. The challenging aspect of tendon repair is the high rate of failure at the bone-tendon interface. Many factors affect the surgical outcome, including surgical technique, postoperative rehabilitation regimens, patient age, tendon quality, degree of muscle atrophy, and medical comorbidities. Tendon and muscle quality are the two most important factors affecting the ease and success of rotator cuff repair. With time, tears progress in size, although the exact rate of progression is variable. Patients with few or no symptoms and small- to moderate-sized tears must be informed of the risks associated with nonsurgical treatment. Smaller, one-tendon tears are much more likely to heal than larger, retracted, two-tendon tears.

Key surgical factors include proper visualization of the tear, an understanding of the tear pattern, adequate decompression, solid fixation through the tendon and bone, and secure knots. Other sources of pain such as the biceps tendon, acromioclavicular joint, labral pathology, and glenohumeral arthritis should also be treated. If tendons are too degenerated to repair, partial repair and decompression may relieve pain and slow the process of cuff-tear arthropathy. Important preoperative steps include strengthening the deltoid and scapular stabilizers and improving range of motion. Stiffness should be treated before the rotator cuff repair.

Postoperative satisfaction and function is usually improved, even in the absence of complete healing of the repaired tendon. Although patients with intact rotator cuffs have higher postoperative functional scores, patients with defects in the repair still have pain relief and improved function compared with their preoperative level.

References

1. Depalma AF, Gallery G, Bennett GA: Variational anatomy in degenerative lesions of the shoulder joint. *Instr Course Lect* 1949;6:225-281.

2. Gartsman GM, Khan M, Hammerman SM: Arthroscopic repair of full-thickness tears of the rotator cuff. *J Bone Joint Surg Am* 1998;80:832-840.

3. Burkhart S: Arthroscopic repair of massive rotator cuff tears: Concept of margin convergence. *Tech Shoulder Elbow Surg* 2000;1:232-239.

4. Tauro JC: Arthroscopic rotator cuff repair: Analysis of technique and results at 2- and 3-year follow-up. *Arthroscopy* 1998;14:45-51.

5. Wolf EM, Pennington WT, Agrawal V: Arthroscopic rotator cuff repair: 4- to 10-year results. *Arthroscopy* 2004;20(1):5-12.

6. Severud EL, Ruotolo C, Abbott DD, Nottage WM: All arthroscopic versus mini-open rotator cuff repair. *Arthroscopy* 2003;19:234-238.

7. Weber S: Comparison of all arthroscopic and mini-open rotator cuff repairs, *Proceedings of the 2001 Annual Meeting.* Rosemont, IL, Arthroscopic Association of North America, 2001.

8. Gleyze P, Thomazeau H, Flurin P, Lafosse L, Gazielly DF, Allard M: Arthroscopic rotator cuff repair: A multicentric retrospective study of 87 cases with anatomical assessment. *Rev Chir Orthop Reparatrice Appar Mot* 2000;86:566-574.

9. Galatz LM, Ball CM, Teefey SA, Middleton WD, Yamaguchi K: The outcome and repair integrity of completely arthroscopically repaired large and massive rotator cuff tears. *J Bone Joint Surg Am* 2004;86:219-224.

10. Harryman DT, Mack LA, Wang KY, Jackins SE, Richardson ML, Matsen FA: Repairs of the rotator cuff: Correlation of functional results with integrity of the cuff. *J Bone Joint Surg Am* 1991;73:982-989.

11. Gerber C, Fuchs B, Hoder J: The results of repair of massive tears of the rotator cuff. *J Bone Joint Surg Am* 2000;82:505-515.

12. Rokito AS, Zuckerman JD, Gallagher MA, Cuomo F: Strength after repair of the rotator cuff. *J Shoulder Elbow Surg* 1996;5:12-17.

13. Jost B, Pfirrmann CW, Gerber C: Clinical outcome after structural failure of rotator cuff repairs. *J Bone Joint Surg Am* 2000;82:304-314.

14. Rokito AS, Cuomo F, Gallagher M, Zuckerman JD: Long-term functional outcome of repair of large and massive chronic tears of the rotator cuff. *J Bone Joint Surg Am* 1999;81:991-997.

15. Karas EH, Iannotti JP: Failed repair of the rotator cuff: Evaluation and treatment of complications. *Instr Course Lect* 1998;47:87-95.

16. Bishop J, Klepps S, Lo IK, Bird J, Gladstone JN, Flatow EL: Cuff integrity after arthroscopic versus open rotator cuff repair: A prospective study. *J Shoulder Elbow Surg* 2006;15:290-299.

17. Boileau P, Brassart N, Watkinson DJ, Carles M, Hatzidakis AM, Krishnan SG: Arthroscopic repair of full-thickness tears of the supraspinatus: Does the tendon really heal? *J Bone Joint Surg Am* 2005;87:1229-1240.

18. Galatz LM, Griggs S, Cameron BD, Iannotti JP: Prospective longitudinal analysis of postoperative shoulder function: A ten-year follow-up study of full-thickness rotator cuff tears. *J Bone Joint Surg Am* 2001;83:1052-1056.

19. Cofield RH, Parvizi J, Hoffmeyer PJ, Lanzer WL, Ilstrup DM, Rowland CM: Surgical repair of chronic rotator cuff tears: A prospective long-term study. *J Bone Joint Surg Am* 2001;83:71-77.

20. Galatz LM, Rothermich SY, Zaegel M, Silva MJ, Havlioglu N, Thomopoulos S: Delayed repair of tendon to bone injuries leads to decreased biomechanical properties and bone loss. *J Orthop Res* 2005;23:1441-1447.

21. Hersche O, Gerber C: Passive tension in the supraspinatus musculotendinous unit after long-standing rupture of its tendon: A preliminary report. *J Shoulder Elbow Surg* 1998;7:393-396.

22. Yamaguchi K, Levine WN, Marra G, Galatz LM, Klepps S, Flatow EL: Transitioning to arthroscopic rotator cuff repair: The pros and cons. *Instr Course Lect* 2003;52:81-92.

23. Bigliani LU, Cordasco FA, McIlveen SJ, Musso ES: Operative treatment of failed repairs of the rotator cuff. *J Bone Joint Surg Am* 1992;74:1505-1515.

24. DeOrio JK, Cofield RH: Results of a second attempt at surgical repair of a failed intial rotator cuff repair. *J Bone Joint Surg Am* 1984;66:563-567.

25. Flugstad D, Matsen FA, Larry I, Jackins SE: Failed acromioplasty: Etiology and prevention. *Orthop Trans* 1986;10:229.

26. Hawkins RJ, Chris AD, Kiefer GN: Failed anterior acromioplasties. *Orthop Trans* 1987;11:223.

27. Flatow EL, Pollock RG, Bigliani LU: Coracoacromial ligament preservation in rotator cuff surgery. *Tech Orthop* 1994;9:97-98.

28. Burkhart SS, Diaz-Pagan JL, Wirth MA, Athanasiou KA: Cyclic loading of anchor based rotator cuff repairs: Confirmation of the tension overload phenomenon and comparison of suture anchor fixation with transosseous fixation. *Arthroscopy* 1997;13:720-724.

29. Burkhart SS, Johnson TC, Wirth MA, Athanasiou KA: Cyclic loading of transosseous rotator cuff repairs: Tension overload as a possible cause of failure. *Arthroscopy* 1997;13:172-176.

30. Tauro JC: Arthroscopic "interval slide" in the repair of large rotator cuff tears. *Arthroscopy* 1999;15:527-530.

31. Tauro JC: Arthroscopic repair of large rotator cuff tears using the interval slide technique. *Arthroscopy* 2004;20:13-21.

32. Miller SL, Gladstone JN, Cleeman E, Klein MJ, Chiang AS, Flatow EL: Anatomy of the posterior rotator interval: Implications for cuff mobilization. *Clin Orthop Relat Res* 2003;408:152-156.

33. Lo I, Burkart SS: The interval slide in continuity: A method of mobilizing the anterosuperior rotator cuff without disrupting the tear margins. *Arthroscopy* 2004;20:435-441.

34. St Pierre P, Olson EJ, Elliott JJ, O'Hair KC, McKinney LA, Ryan J: Tendon-healing to cortical bone compared with healing to a cancellous trough: A biomechanical and histological evaluation in goats. *J Bone Joint Surg Am* 1995;77:1858-1866.

35. Cummins CA, Murrell GA: Mode of failure for rotator cuff repair with suture anchors identified at revision surgery. *J Shoulder Elbow Surg* 2003;12:128-133.

36. Gerber C, Schneeberger AG, Beck M, Schlegel U: Mechanical strength of repairs of the rotator cuff. *J Bone Joint Surg Br* 1994;76:371-380.

37. Gerber C, Schneeberger AG, Perren SM, Nyffeler RW: Experimental rotator cuff repair: A preliminary study. *J Bone Joint Surg Am* 1999;81:1281-1290.

38. Ma CB, MacGillivray JD, Clabeaux J, Lee S, Otis JC: Biomechanical evaluation of arthroscopic rotator cuff stitches. *J Bone Joint Surg Am* 2004;86:1211-1216.

39. Reed SC, Glossop N, Ogilvie-Harris DJ: Full-thickness rotator cuff tears: A biomechanical comparison of suture vs. bone anchor techniques. *Am J Sports Med* 1996;24:46-48.

40. Hecker AT, Shea M, Hayhurst JO, Myers ER, Meeks LW, Hayes WC: Pull-out strength of suture anchors for rotator cuff and Bankart lesion repairs. *Am J Sports Med* 1993;21:874-879.

41. Burkhart SS: The deadman theory of suture anchors: Observations along a south Texas fence line. *Arthroscopy* 1995;11:119-123.

42. Tingart MJ, Apreleva M, Zurakowski D, Warner JJP: Pullout strength of suture anchors used in rotator cuff repair. *J Bone Joint Surg Am* 2003;85:2190-2198.

43. Ciccone WJ, Motz C, Bently C, Tasto JP: Bioabsorbable implants in orthopaedics: New developments and clinical applications. *J Am Acad Orthop Surg* 2001;9:280-288.

44. Barber FA, Herbert MA: Suture anchors: Update 1999. *Arthroscopy* 1999;15:719-725.

45. Warme WJ, Arciero RA, DAvoie FH III, Uhorchak JM, Walton M: Nonabsorbable versus absorbable suture anchors for open Bankart repair: A prospective, random-ized comparison. *Am J Sports Med* 1999; 27:742-746.

46. Djurasovic M, Marra G, Arroyo JS: Revison rotator cuff repair: Factors influencing results. *J Bone Joint Surg Am* 2001;83:1849-1855.

47. Bigliani LU, Cordasco FA, McIlveen SJ, Musso ES: Operative treatment of failed repairs of the rotator cuff. *J Bone Joint Surg Am* 1992;74:1505-1515.

48. Nevaiser RJ, Neviaser TJ: Reoperation for failed RCR: Analysis of 46 cases. *Orthop Trans* 1989;13:509.

49. DeFranco MJ, Derwin K, Ionnotti JP: New therapies in tendon reconstruction. *J Am Acad Orthop Surg* 2004;12:298-304.

50. Butler DL, Goldstein SA, Guilak F: Functional tissue engineering: The role of biomechanics. *J Biomech Eng* 2000;122:570-575.

51. Tauro JC, Parsons JR, Ricci J, Alexander H: Comparison of bovine collagen xenografts to autografts in the rabbit. *Clin Orthop Relat Res* 1991;266:271-284.

52. Dejardin LM, Arnoczky SP, Ewers BJ, Haut RC, Clarke RB: Tissue-engineered rotator cuff tendon using porcine small intestine submucosa: Histologic and mechanical evaluation in dogs. *Am J Sports Med* 2001;29:175-184.

53. Iannotti JP, Codsi MS, Kwon YW, Derwin K, Ciccone J, Brems JJ: Porcine small intestine submucosa augmentation of surgical repair of chronic two-tendon cuff tears: A randomized, controlled trial. *J Bone Joint Surg Am* 2006;88:1238-1244.

Irreparable Rotator Cuff Tears: What to Do and When to Do It; The Surgeon's Dilemma

David M. Dines, MD

Daniel P. Moynihan, MD

Joshua S. Dines, MD

Peter McCann, MD

Abstract

Irreparable rotator cuff tears have been defined as those tears that because of their size and retraction cannot be repaired primarily. Patients with an irreparable tear present with a variety of symptoms and physical findings, and their management depends on the clinical situation and the specific location of the tear. Most of these tears occur in the older, less active patient and many of these patients are best treated without surgery. For those in whom surgery is indicated, the best procedure should be tailored to the tear.

Instr Course Lect 2007;56:13-22.

Irreparable rotator cuff tears are infrequent but well-defined lesions consisting of massive rotator cuff tears that are not repairable by conventional means. Rockwood and others[1-3] defined irreparable tears as those that, because of their size and retraction, cannot be repaired primarily to their insertion onto the tuberosities despite conventional techniques of mobilization and soft-tissue releases. Goutallier and associates[4] classified rotator cuff tears on the basis of the amount of muscle atrophy and fatty infiltration of the affected rotator cuff muscles demonstrated by CT scans. Often, these tears are associated with concomitant arthritis of the glenohumeral joint, making treatment options even more complex.[5]

Patients with irreparable rotator cuff tears can present with a variety of manifestations. They may have no symptoms or mild symptoms, or they may be completely disabled and in severe pain. The true incidence of irreparable rotator cuff tears is not known; however, anatomic studies on cadavera and imaging studies of asymptomatic patients have demonstrated rotator cuff tears in 30% to 50% of older patients, especially those older than 70 years of age.[6-8] Tempelhof and associates[9] studied 411 asymptomatic individuals and found that 38% of those older than the age of 70 years had full-thickness rotator cuff tears. Rotator cuff tears with an increased degree of fatty infiltration and muscle atrophy in association with a high-riding humeral head to the acromion are at high risk for irreparability. Goutallier and associates[4] used CT scans to evaluate fatty infiltration, but MRI is probably more sensitive.

Massive irreparable rotator cuff tears occur in two physiologically distinct patient groups, but they can present in all age and activity groups. Most often, these tears occur in physiologically older, lower-demand patients (who are older than 70 years and usually female) who have been asymptomatic until minor trauma created symptoms. The second group consists of physiologically younger, more active patients, often in the sixth decade of life, who present with dramatic symptoms of pain and disability after an acute event or with a history of rotator cuff surgery or of chronic rotator cuff injury.

In addition to different clinical presentations, irreparable rotator

One or more of the authors or the departments with which they are affiliated have received something of value from a commercial or other party related directly or indirectly to the subject of this chapter.

cuff tears also occur in two distinct anatomic patterns. Complete tears of the supraspinatus, infraspinatus, and teres minor tendons are posterosuperior failures and are more common. Complete tears of the supraspinatus and subscapularis tendons, sometimes with damage or disruption of the long head of the biceps tendon, are anterosuperior failures. Both anatomic patterns often result in severe disability and poor function. Loss of the coracoacromial arch combined with anterosuperior instability may lead to escape of the humeral head, a potentially devastating clinical situation.

Pathomechanics

The rotator cuff comprises four muscles whose tendons form a histologically confluent sleeve of tissue around the humeral head that inserts into the tuberosities of the proximal part of the humerus. This anatomic arrangement allows the cuff to provide a wide range of active motion as well as stability by concavity compression at the glenohumeral joint.[10] In this way, the rotator cuff acts as a dynamic stabilizer, resisting upward motion of the humeral head during contraction of the deltoid muscle. When there is an irreparable rotator cuff tear, the stabilizing force couple is lost, allowing the humeral head to displace superiorly during contraction of the deltoid. This displacement is associated with a loss of elevation and, in some instances, with superior shoulder instability.[11]

Patient Presentation
Clinical Findings

The presenting history, chief symptom, and results of physical examination of a patient with an irreparable rotator cuff tear can be a confusing picture. Patients can have variable amounts of pain, unpredictable deficits in both the active and the passive range of motion, and inconsistent levels of disability. The physical examination reveals atrophy of the scapular muscles in patients who have had long-standing lesions. In more severe cases, crepitus and hemarthrosis also may be evident. Patients can have varying degrees of weakness and loss of motion, ranging from little or no deficit to a complete loss of active motion.

Patients with posterosuperior disruption of the rotator cuff often have decreased abduction, forward flexion, and active external rotation, giving rise to two classic physical findings. One is a positive external rotation lag sign, which is the inability to externally rotate the arm against resistance or to hold the arm in external rotation against resistance. With complete loss of external rotation power, the patient may have the second classic finding: a positive hornblower's sign (Figure 1). The hornblower's sign has been shown to have 100% sensitivity and 93% specificity with regard to indicating irreparable tears of the teres minor.[12]

Patients who have an anterosuperior failure often have decreased abduction and forward flexion. They can have increased passive external rotation as well as positive bellypress and lift-off signs. The lift-off sign was described by Gerber and Krushell.[13] The patient places the dorsum of the hand against the lumbar spine. If he or she can lift the hand off the back, the subscapularis is functioning. When the patient cannot internally rotate the shoulder enough to place the hand behind the back, a belly-press test can be used. A belly-press test is considered to be positive (also indicating loss of sub-

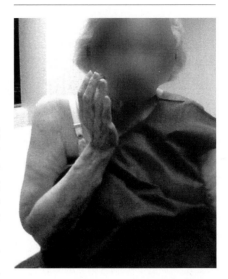

Figure 1   Positive hornblower's sign.

scapularis function) when the patient cannot keep the wrist straight and the elbow away from the side when he or she presses the palm against the abdomen. Patients with complete loss of rotator cuff function may only be able to shrug the shoulder.

Radiographic Findings

Imaging studies including plain radiographs, CT, and MRI can help to guide both the diagnosis and the treatment of irreparable rotator cuff tears. The position of the humeral head, evidence of degenerative arthritis of the glenohumeral joint, and disorders of the acromioclavicular joint are seen on plain radiographs. CT scans have been used to assess rotator cuff muscle atrophy and fatty infiltration. Goutallier and associates[4] classified the quantity of fatty infiltration as 0 (no fat within the muscle), 1 (minimal fatty infiltration), 2 (more muscle than fat), 3 (fat content equal to muscle content), or 4 (more fat than muscle). MRI is the most effective modality used to assess the involved shoulder, and it has replaced CT as the imaging modality of choice for the assessment of rotator cuff lesions. MRI can demonstrate rotator cuff tears with 100% sensitivity and can be used to estimate the width of a tear (with up to 77% accuracy) and retraction (within 5 mm) 63% of the time.[14] More importantly, MRI can be used to assess fatty infiltration more effectively, as described previously (Figure 2).

The amount of fatty infiltration of the rotator cuff muscles is directly related to the likelihood of a retear and to the functional outcome.[15,16] When the muscle has type 3 or 4 fatty infiltration, it is of poor quality and will not improve after surgical repair. The extent of fatty infiltration of the rotator cuff muscles has proven to be a valuable preoperative guide for assessment of the potential reparability of a massive rotator cuff tear.[15,16]

Management
Treatment of symptomatic irreparable rotator cuff tears is extremely challenging because, at present, there are no perfect solutions to this complex and sometimes disabling problem. Treatment depends on the presenting symptoms (pain and/or disability), age, and functional level. Other issues such as medical comorbidities, the presence of an intact coracoacromial arch, and possible concomitant glenohumeral arthritis are also factors that must be considered in the treatment plan. The treatment options range from conservative (nonsurgical) to surgical intervention. Surgical options include débridement with or without partial rotator cuff repair, tendon transfer, muscle tendon slide procedures, the use of rotator cuff allografts and synthetic grafts, arthrodesis, and shoulder arthroplasty, including the use of reverse ball prostheses.

No one treatment is best for all irreparable rotator cuff tears. The

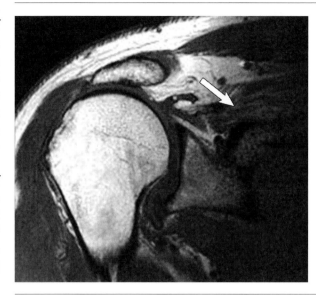

Figure 2 T1-weighted MRI scan demonstrating severe fatty deposition (arrow) and muscle atrophy in an irreparable rotator cuff tear. (Image used with permission from Theodore Miller, MD, North Shore-Long Island Jewish Health System.)

surgeon needs to select the type of procedure that will provide the best outcome as dictated by the specific patient's needs. Unfortunately, there have been no evidence-based, prospective, matched-patient studies comparing the different nonsurgical and surgical options, to our knowledge.

Nonsurgical Management
Many chronic irreparable rotator cuff tears can be treated successfully without surgery. A nonsurgical approach to relieve pain and create "biomechanically compensated" function by muscle substitution with use of the remaining rotator cuff, deltoid, and periscapular muscles is often the best method of initial treatment.

Nonsurgical treatment includes nonsteroidal anti-inflammatory medications, steroid injections, and local therapeutic modalities to relieve pain. Early restoration of the passive range of motion and activity modification are imperative initially. Once pain relief has been obtained and the range of motion has been restored, specific strengthening exercises for the remaining rotator cuff, deltoid, and scapular muscles can be started

to recreate a stable fulcrum for deltoid function. Strengthening exercises for the internal and external rotators of the shoulder should include resistive exercises below chest level initially. Deltoid strengthening exercises begin with the patient supine and are then progressed to antigravity positions such as sitting and standing. It may take more than 3 months for conservative treatment to be successful.

There have been few specific reports on the outcomes of conservative treatment of irreparable tears. In one study on the nonsurgical management of 53 patients, Bokor and associates[17] found that 39 patients had no to slight pain at the time of follow-up. The success rate correlated directly with the duration of symptoms before treatment. Patients with symptoms for less than 3 months did better than those who had had symptoms for longer than 6 months. The final result was usually evident after 6 months of nonsurgical management.

Surgical Management
The surgical management of irreparable rotator cuff tears includes sev-

eral procedures of varying degrees of complexity. These procedures include subacromial débridement and acromioplasty with or without partial repairs, tendon transfers, and the use of conventional or reverse prostheses. The choice of procedure depends on the patient's age, activity level, joint stability, and concomitant arthritic changes.

Subacromial Débridement, Partial Repair, Cuff Débridement, and Biceps Tenotomy: Open and Arthroscopic In some instances, subacromial decompression and rotator cuff débridement alone may relieve symptoms in patients with a massive irreparable tear of the rotator cuff.[1,18-23] Subacromial débridement is indicated in healthy, lower-demand patients whose primary symptom is pain. The best results are in patients who have active elevation and control of the descent of the shoulder as well as glenohumeral stability. Patients in whom a subacromial injection relieves symptoms and improves function are good candidates for this procedure.

These procedures have been performed both arthroscopically and through open techniques. An arthroscopic débridement has the advantage of not violating the deltoid insertion. The procedures can include all or any of the following: limited, nondestabilizing acromioplasty (smoothing the acromion without release of the coracoacromial ligament); bursectomy; débridement of the rotator cuff edge; and release of a damaged long head of the biceps tendon. A tuberoplasty of the greater tuberosity and acromioclavicular joint resection also may be indicated depending on the presenting symptoms.

Burkhart and associates[24] described the advantage of a partial repair of the posterior and anterior portions of the tear without transposition or transfer in selected patients. They described a "suspension bridge model" whereby continuity between the anterior and posterior tendons resulted in a fibrous frame reconstruction close to the equator of the humeral head, creating a force to stabilize the humeral head against the glenoid and enabling the deltoid to raise the arm.[11] Burkhart and associates[24] reported that 13 of 14 patients had pain relief and improvement of function after such a partial repair. According to the UCLA Shoulder Rating Scale, which assigns a maximum of 10 points for pain, 10 points for function, and 5 points each for the range of motion, strength of forward flexion, and overall patient satisfaction,[25] the mean score improved from 9.8 to 27.6 points.

Reports of the clinical experience with débridement have been anecdotal and retrospective. In 1995, Rockwood and associates[1] reported decreased pain and improved function in 44 of 53 shoulders at an average of 6.5 years after open acromioplasty, decompression, and rotator cuff débridement. Gartsman[18] reported that 26 of 33 patients had decreased pain and an improved range of motion but decreased strength at an average of 5 years after an open repair. In a study by Ellman and associates,[19] arthroscopic débridement resulted in pain relief in 19 of 22 shoulders with an irreparable tear but there was no significant increase in strength or range of motion. Burkhart[26] described good pain relief and function in 10 of 11 patients who had undergone arthroscopic débridement alone for treatment of a biomechanically stable irreparable rotator cuff tear. In later reviews, however, Zvijac and associates[22] and Kempf and associates[23] noted sub-

stantial deterioration in pain relief, strength, and functional outcome in short periods of time after arthroscopic débridement procedures.

Walch and associates[27] reported relief of pain in 74 of 87 patients who had undergone a tenotomy of the long head of the biceps tendon for the treatment of an irreparable rotator cuff tear, but there was no effect on the range of motion or strength. One third of these patients also had an arthroscopic acromioplasty, which clouded the true results of the tenotomy.

Fenlin and associates[28] described tuberoplasty in 20 patients, 19 of whom had a successful result. They performed the procedure through open surgery, but it could be done arthroscopically, and it included shaving and reshaping of the overhang on the greater tuberosity to create a recontoured subacromial space that would articulate smoothly with the undersurface of the acromion.

From this review of the literature, certain principles emerge. Débridement is best performed in elderly low-demand patients with irreparable rotator cuff tear for which other muscles have compensated. There are no real differences between the results of open and arthroscopic procedures; however, arthroscopic techniques are less invasive and do not violate the deltoid insertion. Loss of the coracoacromial arch is associated with severe failures;[29] therefore, decompression should include flattening and shaping of the acromion as opposed to a true release of the coracoacromial ligament in this patient population. Débridement does not consistently improve function in patients with pain and poor function. In such instances, other surgical reconstructive options should be considered, especially in younger, more active patients.

Rotator Cuff Reconstructive Procedures: Tendon Transfers and Graft Procedures The approaches used to reconstruct irreparable massive rotator cuff tears include transfers of the existing rotator cuff tendons, tendon transfers from other periscapular muscles, and repair of tissue with grafts or synthetic substitutions. In the past, the upper third of the subscapularis tendon was transferred to repair a residual anterosuperior defect in the rotator cuff.[30] Unfortunately, transfer of the subscapularis tendon risks loss of power of internal rotation and creation of a possible internal rotation contracture. For this reason, the procedure is no longer advocated.

Tendon transfers from other periscapular muscle groups are useful in young, active patients with an irreparable rotator cuff tear and profound functional weakness as the primary symptom. These patients must have good deltoid function. The tendons that have most commonly been transferred include the latissimus dorsi for posterosuperior rotator cuff tears[3,31,32] and the pectoralis major for irreparable anterosuperior tears.[33-35]

In 1992, Gerber[31] reported the early results of latissimus dorsi transfer for treatment of massive rotator cuff tears. The latissimus dorsi muscle is used to restore external rotation and head depression forces that were lost as a result of the massive tear. Gerber found good to excellent results in 13 of 16 patients, and the results were stable for more than 10 years. He noted that the results were better when the subscapularis tendon was intact (Figure 3).

Miniaci and MacLeod[36] reported satisfactory results in 14 of 17 patients who had undergone a latissimus dorsi transfer after a failure of a previous surgical repair of a massive rotator cuff tear. In their series, primary latissimus dorsi transfer was rarely indicated for irreparable massive rotator cuff tears, and they recommended primary repair, débridement, or partial repair as the initial surgical procedure.

Iannotti and associates[37] described improvements with regard to pain relief and function in 9 of 14 patients who had been treated with a latissimus dorsi transfer. All patients had active electromyographic activity within the transferred latissimus dorsi with adduction of the arm or with resisted isometric external rotation with the arm at the side. No patient had electromyographic activity of the transfer with active forward elevation, and no patient had electromyographic activity with external rotation in more than one plane of motion. Twelve of the 14 patients had a clear demonstration of the tendon transfer on MRI. This study supports the concept of a tenodesis effect with some active functional role of the latissimus dorsi transfer.

Subcoracoid pectoralis major transfer has been reported at several centers.[33-35] In each series, the upper portion of the pectoralis major was passed under the conjoined tendon and sutured to the lesser tuberosity (Figure 4). Resch and associates[33] reported on a series of 12 patients, 6 of whom had a negative belly-press test postoperatively; all 4 patients with preoperative instability had resolution of that symptom. Overall, the improvement was good to excellent in 8 of the 12 patients. Wirth and Rockwood[35] reported satisfactory results in 10 of 13 patients who had undergone a pectoralis major transfer.

Warner and Gerber[38] reported the use of a split pectoralis major tendon transfer or split pectoralis major-teres major transfer in complicated cases of unstable anterosuperior rotator cuff deficiency. Twenty patients underwent these procedures, and in 11 of them the split pectoralis tendon transfer alone was used. All patients in the series were evaluated with the system described by Constant and Murley,[39] which consists of individual scores for pain (15 points), activity (20 points), active mobility (40 points), and strength (25 points). The mean improvement in the Constant score was from 42 to 61 points, with the nine patients treated with a combination of a split pectoralis major and teres major transfer having a mean improvement from 34 to 55 points. These results were in patients who had complicated disorders with limited functional goals. Tests for subscapularis insufficiency remained positive after the surgery for all patients.

Aldridge and associates[40] reported the use of a pectoralis major and latissimus dorsi tendon transfer to treat massive cuff defects in 11 patients with minimal pain and a limited range of motion and function. On the average, active elevation increased from 42° to 86°; active external rotation, from 0° to 13°; strength in elevation, from 2.3 to 3.1 lb (1.0 to 1.4 kg); and strength in external rotation, from 2.1. to 2.7 lb (0.95 to 1.2 kg). Four patients reported feeling no better, two had slight improvement, and five had substantial improvement.

Tendon transfers are complex surgical procedures that require a long period of rehabilitation. They are not indicated for older, more debilitated patients because the amount of muscle reeducation determines, to some degree, the amount of success. For this reason, patients who are not willing to sub-

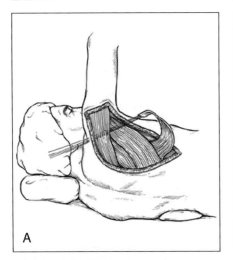
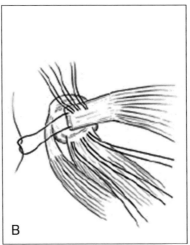
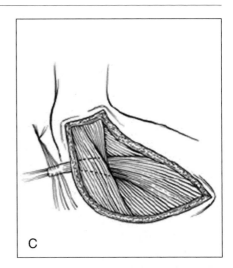
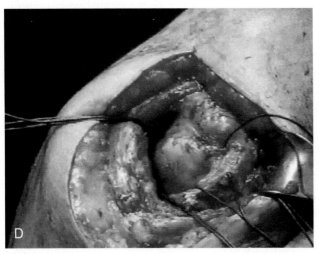
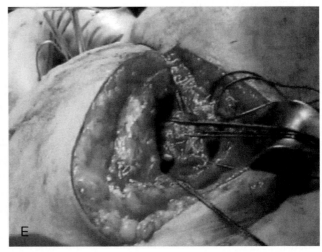

Figure 3 Latissimus dorsi tendon transfer technique. **A,** The tagged latissimus dorsi tendon is passed under the deltoid. **B** and **D,** The tendon is prepared for fixation. **C** and **E,** The latissimus tendon covering the posterosuperior defect. (Illustrations reprinted with permission from Warner JJP, Iannotti JP, Gerber C (eds): *Complex and Revision Problems in Shoulder Surgery*. Philadelphia, PA, Lippincott-Raven, 1997, pp 195-196. Photographs used with permission from Russell F. Warren, MD, The Hospital for Special Surgery.)

mit to extensive long rehabilitation programs should not undergo these procedures.

Tissue substitution with synthetic materials and with autogenous and allograft tissue implants has been attempted, but there are limited published data on these procedures. Neviaser and associates[41] reported good to excellent results in 14 of 16 patients treated with a freeze-dried allograft for a massive, but probably not irreparable, tear. Synthetic allograft patches have been used to augment rotator cuff repairs. Unfortunately, these tendon substitutes can create foreign body reactions leading to rejection and then cannot replace the atrophic or weakened rotator cuff muscle. These muscles must function if functional improvement is to be expected.

Glenohumeral Arthrodesis Glenohumeral arthrodesis is usually used when the deltoid and rotator cuff muscles are not functional. Arthrodesis is the best treatment of some high-demand patients disabled by a irreparable cuff tear who require a strong, stable shoulder girdle for function. Patients treated with a glenohumeral arthrodesis can expect a strong shoulder girdle but limited rotation. As with any arthrodesis, nonunion as well as postoperative limitations of motion and function are substantial concerns following a glenohumeral arthrodesis.

Conventional and Reverse Arthroplasty An arthroplasty may be the best treatment for some patients

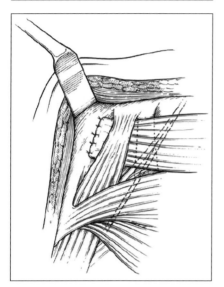

Figure 4 Subcoracoid pectoralis major transfer technique. The upper portion of the pectoralis major is passed under the conjoined tendon, filling an anterosuperior defect. (Reprinted from: Resch H, Povacz P, Ritter E, Matschi W. Transfer of the pectoralis major muscle for the treatment of irreparable rupture of the subscapularis tendon. *J Bone Joint Surg Am* 2000;82:375.)

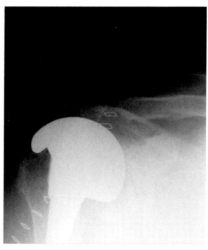

Figure 5 A shoulder hemiarthroplasty with an extended-coverage head used to treat an irreparable rotator cuff tear and glenohumeral arthritis in a patient with a competent coracoacromial arch.

with an irreparable rotator cuff tear and concomitant arthritis or anterosuperior instability. Patients with an irreparable rotator cuff tear and glenohumeral arthritis but a competent coracoacromial arch have had successful results following hemiarthroplasty with or without an extended-coverage humeral head component[42-44] (Figure 5). These patients can expect pain relief with a reasonable return of function. Field and associates[44] reported on the use of hemiarthroplasty for the treatment of cuff tear arthropathy and an irreparable rotator cuff tear in 16 patients. Twelve patients had a good to excellent return of function and pain relief, but the procedure was unsuccessful in four patients. All patients with an unsuccessful result had had a previous acromioplasty and an unstable shoulder. Hemiar-

throplasty should not be done in patients who have had previous surgery, including acromioplasty, or in those with anterosuperior shoulder instability.

Arntz and associates[45] reported on 23 patients with disabling pain associated with an irreparable rotator cuff tear. Twelve patients were treated with a hemiarthroplasty and 11 patients with an arthrodesis. The authors concluded that hemiarthroplasty was the better method for managing complex irreparable tears of the rotator cuff in shoulders in which the articular surface had been destroyed but only when the deltoid was functional. In their series, arthrodesis was better for patients who had both an irreparable rotator cuff tear and irreparable deficiencies of the deltoid muscle.

In a study by Williams and Rockwood,[43] 21 shoulders underwent a hemiarthroplasty for cuff tear arthropathy. At the time of follow-up, 18 of the 21 had mild or no pain and 3 had moderate pain. All patients had improved function and were satisfied

with the result.

Hemiarthroplasty is not indicated for patients who have an irreparable tear with anterosuperior instability and glenohumeral arthritis. For such patients and those with pseudoparalysis of the shoulder, a reverse ball prosthesis is now recommended. This is a new prosthesis, and long-term results are not yet known. Initially described by Grammont and Baulot,[46] the reverse ball prosthesis is based on a biomechanical design in which the center of rotation is located within the glenoid component, medializing the center of rotation and increasing the deltoid lever arm. The sheer force of the deltoid is converted into a compressive force, increasing the deltoid advantage (Figure 6). The reverse ball prosthesis has been used extensively in Europe. It has recently been approved for use in the United States for patients with rotator cuff arthropathy.

Reports from Europe have indicated that the reverse ball prosthesis provides better results than hemiarthroplasty in patients with an irreparable rotator cuff tear. Improvements in pain relief, anterior elevation, and function have been substantial in some midterm follow-up studies;[47-50] however, these procedures are not without complications. Long-term glenoid loosening remains a concern, and increased rates of hematoma, infection, and instability have been reported.[50-52]

Summary
Chronic irreparable rotator cuff tears can cause substantial shoulder pain and disability. As a result of the complex pathology in shoulders with irreparable rotator cuff tears, there are many different clinical scenarios and many available treatment

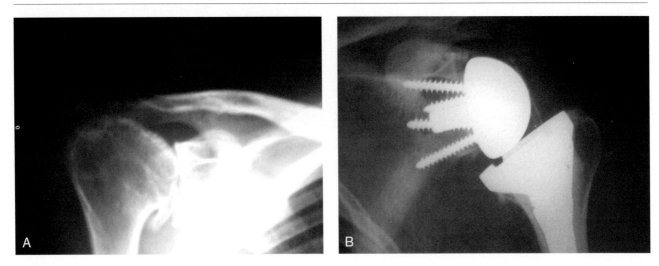

Figure 6 **A,** Preoperative radiograph demonstrating advanced osteoarthritis. **B,** Postoperative radiograph demonstrating the reverse ball prosthesis.

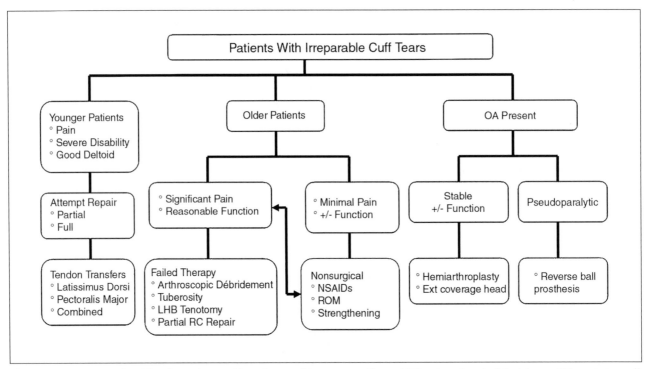

Figure 7 Treatment algorithm for patients with an irreparable rotator cuff tear. LHB = long head of the biceps, RC = rotator cuff, NSAIDs = nonsteroidal anti-inflammatory drugs, ROM = range of motion, and OA = osteoarthritis.

options (Figure 7). For this reason, careful patient evaluation and treatment selection are critical to ensure a good result. Many chronic irreparable rotator cuff tears can be treated nonsurgically, especially when the shoulder has reasonably good func-

tion. The goals of surgical reconstruction must be considered in terms of the patient's individual needs, medical condition, and functional abilities.

Débridement and partial repair can be considered for some patients,

whereas reconstruction of the rotator cuff is most useful in young, active patients for whom functional restoration is important. Latissimus dorsi muscle transfer is the preferred treatment of active disabled patients with a posterosuperior irreparable cuff defect and good deltoid function. Anterosuperior irreparable defects can be treated with pectoralis and teres major tendon transfers but with less predictable results. A hemiarthroplasty can be considered for patients with severe disability, arthritis, and glenohumeral stability; however, in patients with unstable glenohumeral arthritis, the reverse ball prosthesis will provide more predictable pain relief and return of function, at least in the short term.

References

1. Rockwood CA Jr, Williams GR Jr, Burkhead WZ Jr: Débridement of degenerative irreparable lesions of the rotator cuff. *J Bone Joint Surg Am* 1995;77:857-866.

2. Cofield RH: Rotator cuff disease of the shoulder. *J Bone Joint Surg Am* 1985;67:974-979.

3. Warner JJ: Management of massive irreparable rotator cuff tears: the role of tendon transfer. *Instr Course Lect* 2001;50:63-71.

4. Goutallier D, Postel JM, Bernageau J, Lavau L, Voisin MC: Fatty muscle degeneration in cuff ruptures. Pre- and postoperative evaluation by CT scan. *Clin Orthop Relat Res* 1994;304:78-83.

5. Sugihara T, Nakagawa T, Tsuchiya M, Ishizuki M: Prediction of primary reparability of massive tears of the rotator cuff on preoperative magnetic resonance imaging. *J Shoulder Elbow Surg* 2003;12:222-225.

6. Depalma AF, Callery G, Bennett GA: Variational anatomy and degenerative lesions of the shoulder joint. *Instr Course Lect* 1949;6:255-281.

7. Codman EA: Rupture of the supraspinatus. *Am J Surg* 1938;42:603-606.

8. Sher JS, Uribe JW, Posada A, Murphy BJ, Zlatkin MB: Abnormal findings on magnetic resonance images of asymptomatic shoulders. *J Bone Joint Surg Am* 1995;77:10-15.

9. Tempelhof S, Rupp S, Seil R: Age-related prevalence of rotator cuff tears in asymptomatic shoulders. *J Shoulder Elbow Surg* 1999;8:296-299.

10. Lippitt S, Matsen F: Mechanisms of glenohumeral joint stability. *Clin Orthop Relat Res* 1993;291:20-28.

11. Burkhart SS, Danaceau SM, Pearce CE: Arthroscopic rotator cuff repair: analysis of results by tear size and by repair technique-margin convergence versus direct tendon-to-bone repair. *Arthroscopy* 2001;17:905-912.

12. Walch G, Boulahia A, Calderone S, Robinson AH: The 'dropping' and 'hornblower's' signs in elevation of rotator cuff tears. *J Bone Joint Surg Br* 1998;80:624-628.

13. Gerber C, Krushell RJ: Isolated rupture of the tendon of the subscapularis muscle. Clinical features in 16 cases. *J Bone Joint Surg Br* 1991;73:389-394.

14. Iannotti JP, Zlatkin MB, Esterhai JL, Kressel HY, Dalinka MK, Spindler KP: Magnetic resonance imaging of the shoulder. Sensitivity, specificity, and predictive value. *J Bone Joint Surg Am* 1991;73:17-29.

15. Gerber C, Fuchs B, Hodler J: The results of repair of massive tears of the rotator cuff. *J Bone Joint Surg Am* 2000;82:505-515.

16. Goutallier D, Postel JM, Gleyze P, Leguilloux P, Van Driessche S: Influence of cuff muscle fatty degeneration on anatomic and functional outcomes after simple suture of the full-thickness tears. *J Shoulder Elbow Surg* 2003;12:550-554.

17. Bokor DJ, Hawkins RJ, Huckell GH, Angelo RL, Schickendantz MS: Results of nonoperative management of full-thickness tears of the rotator cuff. *Clin Orthop Relat Res* 1993;294:103-110.

18. Gartsman GM: Massive, irreparable tears of the rotator cuff. Results of operative débridement and subacromial decompression. *J Bone Joint Surg Am* 1997;79:715-721.

19. Ellman H, Kay SP, Wirth MA: Arthroscopic treatment of full-thickness rotator cuff tears: 2- to 7-year follow up study. *Arthroscopy* 1993;9:195-200.

20. Burkhart SS: Arthroscopic treatment of massive rotator cuff tears. Clinical results and biomechanical rationale. *Clin Orthop Relat Res* 1991;267:45-56.

21. Levy HJ, Gardner RD, Lemak LJ: Arthroscopic subacromial decompression in the treatment of full-thickness rotator cuff tears. *Arthroscopy* 1991;7:8-13.

22. Zvijac JE, Levy HJ, Lemak LJ. Arthroscopic subacromial decompression in the treatment of full thickness rotator cuff tears: a 3- to 6-year follow-up. Arthroscopy. 1994;l0:518-23.

23. Kempf JF, Gleyze P, Bonnomet F, et al: A multicenter study of 210 rotator cuff tears treated by arthroscopic acromioplasty. *Arthroscopy* 1999;15:56-66.

24. Burkhart SS, Nottage WM, Ogilvie-Harris DJ, Kohn HS, Pachelli A: Partial repair of irreparable rotator cuff tears. *Arthroscopy* 1994;10:363-370.

25. Ellman H, Hanker G, Bayer M: Repair of the rotator cuff. End-result study of factors influencing reconstruction. *J Bone Joint Surg Am* 1986;68:1136-1144.

26. Burkhart SS: Arthroscopic débridement and decompression for selected rotator cuff tears. Clinical results, pathomechanics, and patient selection based on biomechanical parameters. *Orthop Clin North Am* 1993;24:111-123.

27. Walch G, Edwards TB, Boulahia A, Nove-Josserand L, Neyton L, Szabo I: Arthroscopic tenotomy of the long head of the biceps in the treatment of rotator cuff tears: clinical and radiographic results of 307 cases. *J Shoulder Elbow Surg* 2005;14:238-246.

28. Fenlin JM Jr, Chase JM, Rushton SA, Frieman BG: Tuberoplasty: creation of an acromiohumeral articulation—a treatment option for massive, irreparable rotator cuff tears. *J Shoulder Elbow Surg* 2002;11:136-142.

29. Flatow EL: Coracoacromial ligament preservation in rotator cuff surgery. *J Shoulder Elbow Surg* 1994;3:573.

30. Cofield R: Subscapular muscle transposition for repair of chronic rotator cuff tears. *Surg Gynecol Obstet* 1982;154:667-672.

31. Gerber C: Latissimus dorsi transfer for the treatment of irreparable tears of the rotator cuff. *Clin Orthop Relat Res* 1992;275:152-160.

32. Warner JJ, Parsons IM IV: Latissimus dorsi tendon transfer: a comparable analysis of primary and salvage reconstruction of massive, irreparable rotator cuff tears. *J Shoulder Elbow Surg* 2001;10:514-521.

33. Resch H, Povacz P, Ritter E, Matschi W: Transfer of the pectoralis major muscle for the treatment of irreparable rupture of the subscapularis tendon. *J Bone Joint Surg Am* 2000;82:372-382.

34. Galatz LM, Connor PM, Calfee RP, Hsu JC, Yamaguchi K: Pectoralis major transfer for anterior-superior subluxation in massive rotator cuff insufficiency. *J Shoulder Elbow Surg* 2003;12:1-5.

35. Wirth MA, Rockwood CA Jr: Operative treatment of irreparable rupture of the

subscapularis. *J Bone Joint Surg Am* 1997;79:722-731.

36. Miniaci A, MacLeod M: Transfer of the latissimus dorsi muscle after failed repair of a massive tear of the rotator cuff. A two to five-year review. *J Bone Joint Surg Am* 1999;81:1120-1127.

37. Iannotti JP, Hennigan S, Herzog R, et al: Latissimus dorsi tendon transfer for irreparable posterosuperior rotator cuff tears. Factors affecting outcome. *J Bone Joint Surg Am* 2006;88:342-348.

38. Warner JJP, Gerber C: Treatment of massive rotator cuff tears: posterior-superior and anterior- superior, in Iannotti JP (ed): *The Rotator Cuff: Current Concepts and Complex Problems.* Rosemont, IL, American Academy of Orthopaedic Surgeons, 1998, pp 59-94.

39. Constant CR, Murley AH: A clinical method of functional assessment of the shoulder. *Clin Orthop Relat Res* 1987;214: 160-164.

40. Aldridge JM III, Atkinson TS, Mallon WJ: Combined pectoralis major and latissimus dorsi tendon transfer for massive rotator cuff deficiency. *J Shoulder Elbow Surg* 2004;13:621-629.

41. Neviaser JS, Neviaser RJ, Neviaser TJ: The repair of chronic massive ruptures of the rotator cuff of the shoulder by the use of a freeze-dried rotator cuff. *J Bone Joint Surg Am* 1978;60:681-684.

42. Zuckerman JD, Scott AJ, Gallagher MA: Hemiarthroplasty for cuff tear arthropathy. *J Shoulder Elbow Surg* 2000;9:169-172.

43. Williams GR Jr, Rockwood CA Jr: Hemiarthroplasty and rotator cuff-deficient shoulders. *J Shoulder Elbow Surg* 1996;5:362-367.

44. Field LD, Dines DM, Zabinski SJ, Warren RF: Hemiarthroplasty of the shoulder for rotator cuff arthropathy. *J Shoulder Elbow Surg* 1997;6:18-23.

45. Arntz CT, Matsen FA III, Jackins S: Surgical management of complex irreparable rotator cuff deficiency. *J Arthroplasty* 1991;6:363-370.

46. Grammont PM, Baulot E: Delta shoulder prosthesis for rotator cuff rupture. *Orthopedics* 1993;16:65-68.

47. Baulot E, Chabernaud D, Grammont PM: [Results of Grammont's inverted prosthesis and omarthritis associated with major cuff destruction. Apropos of 16 cases]. *Acta Orthop Belg* 1995;61(Suppl 1):112-119.

48. Boulahia A, Edwards TB, Walch G, Baratta RV: Early results of a reverse design prosthesis in the treatment of arthritis of the shoulder in elderly patients with a large rotator cuff tear. *Orthopedics* 2002;25:129-133.

49. Rittmeister M, Kerschbaumer F: Grammont reverse total shoulder arthroplasty in patients with rheumatoid arthritis and nonreconstructible rotator cuff lesions. *J Shoulder Elbow Surg* 2001;10:17-22.

50. Sirveaux F, Favard L, Oudet D, Huguet D, Lautman S: Grammont inverted total shoulder arthroplasty in the treatment of glenohumeral arthritis with massive and non repairable cuff rupture, in Walch G, Boileau P. Molé D (eds): *2000 Shoulder Prosthesis: Two to Ten Year Follow Up.* Paris, France, Sauramps Médical, 2001, pp 247-52.

51. Gilbart M, Steinmann P, Gerber C: The Delta III reverse ball-and-socket shoulder prosthesis: Clinical results. Presented at the Annual Meeting of the American Academy of Orthopaedic Surgeons, 2004 Mar 10-14; San Francisco, CA.

52. Gilbart M, Pirkl C, Gerber C: Complications associated with the Delta-III reverse ball-and-socket shoulder prosthesis. Presented at the Annual Meeting of the American Academy of Orthopaedic Surgeons; 2004 Mar 10-14; San Francisco, CA.

Principles for the Evaluation and Management of Shoulder Instability

Frederick A. Matsen III, MD
Caroline M. Chebli, MD
Steven B. Lippitt, MD

Abstract

During use of the normal shoulder, the humeral head is centered within the glenoid and the coracoacromial arch. When the shoulder cannot maintain this centered position during use, it is unstable. An unstable shoulder prevents normal function of the upper extremity. Shoulder instability is not the same as joint laxity. Joint laxity is a property of normal joints and allows the shoulder to attain its full range of functional positions.

The concavity of the glenoid and the coracoacromial arch along with the passive and active forces that press the humeral head into the glenoid and the coracoacromial arch maintain the head in its centered position. This concavity-compression mechanism is dependent on the integrity of the glenoid and the coracoacromial arch, muscular compression, and restraining ligaments of the shoulder. Loss of any of these elements due to developmental, degenerative, traumatic, or iatrogenic factors may compromise the ability of the shoulder to center the humeral head in the glenoid.

Instr Course Lect 2007;56:23-34.

The questions to answer during an evaluation of a patient with suspected instability are: (1) Is the problem in the glenohumeral joint? (2) Is the problem one of failure to maintain the humeral head in its centered position? (3) What mechanical factors are contributing to this instability? (4) Are the identified mechanical factors amenable to surgical repair or reconstruction? This evaluation is based primarily on a carefully elicited history, a physical examination of the stability mechanics, and plain radiographs. If more complex imaging methods are needed to discover subtle or "occult" instability, the condition is often not responsive to surgical correction.

For surgical treatment of glenohumeral instability to be appropriate, the instability must be attributable to mechanical factors that can be modified by surgery. The causes may be deficiencies of the glenoid concavity, deficiencies in the muscles that compress the head into the socket, and/or deficiencies in the capsule and ligaments.

Instability is one of the most commonly diagnosed and treated conditions of the shoulder. Diverse and admittedly confusing approaches to this problem have been proposed, making it difficult to understand how best to evaluate and manage affected patients. This chapter offers a practical foundation to aid in the understanding of clinical shoulder stability and instability.[1,2]

Glenohumeral stability requires that the humeral head remain centered in the glenoid fossa. When the humeral head does not remain centered, the patient has glenohumeral instability.

The glenohumeral joint is a balance between mobility and stability.[3] Its mobility is limited by the joint capsule, which prevents the humeral head from rotating into excessive positions. The joint capsule and associated ligaments act as checkreins to rotation and function only at the extremes of motion, when they

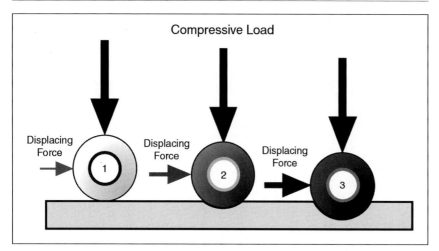

Figure 1 Concavity-compression. The deeper the concavity, the greater the displacing force that can be resisted for a given compressive load. (Reproduced with permission from Matsen FA III, Lippitt SB. Principles of glenohumeral stability, in Matsen FA III, Lippitt SB, DeBartolo SE (eds): *Shoulder Surgery: Principles and Procedures*. Philadelphia, PA, WB Saunders, 2004, p 83.)

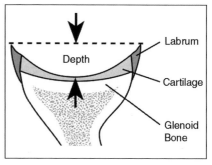

Figure 2 The glenoid concavity. The socket is deepened by the thicker cartilage on its periphery and by the glenoid labrum. (Reproduced with permission from Matsen FA III, Lippitt SB: Principles of glenoid concavity, in Matsen FA III, Lippitt SB, DeBartolo SE (eds): *Shoulder Surgery: Principles and Procedures*. Philadelphia, PA, WB Saunders, 2004, p 88.)

come under tension. Although they also limit translation of the humeral head on the glenoid, restraint of translation alone cannot keep the head centered (just as a dog's leash cannot keep the dog in the center of the yard unless it severely limits the dog's motion). During the midrange of motion, the capsule and ligaments are lax and, therefore, allow the humeral head to be passively translated during physical assessments such as the sulcus and drawer tests. Despite the capsuloligamentous laxity, which is required for normal shoulder mobility, the humeral head remains precisely centered in the glenoid fossa during active motion of the normal shoulder.[4] This centering is necessary in order for the hand to be precisely and securely positioned in space. If the relative position of the humeral head and glenoid fossa were not secure and precise, the hand could not write, paint, throw, lift, hit, or operate with accuracy. The fact that the humeral head remains precisely centered, even in the shoulders of a gymnast with extreme joint laxity

who is performing a vault or holding the iron-cross position, demonstrates the remarkable ability of the shoulder to be stabilized by concavity-compression.[5]

Stability of the glenohumeral joint is critical for precise and strong function of the upper extremity. In the past, the mechanisms providing stability have been categorized as "static" and "dynamic" or as "active" and "passive." It is now recognized that the entire system functions as an integrated whole. For example, in the past it was stated that the antero-inferior glenohumeral ligament is the primary static stabilizer of the shoulder. This is patently not the case because when a person sleeps or rests in a chair, the inferior glenohumeral ligament is not under tension (and thus is not functional) and, although the muscles around the shoulder are relaxed, the glenohumeral joint is not unstable. Similarly, the rotator cuff muscles have been called "dynamic stabilizers" of the shoulder, but, even in an anesthetized shoulder, the passive tension in these muscles provides suffi-

cient compression to stabilize the ball in the socket (as observed in the operating room when the shoulder muscles are paralyzed).

The glenohumeral stabilizing system has several key elements. The concavity of the glenoid, the muscles that compress the humeral head into the glenoid, the coracoacromial arch, the capsuloligamentous restraints, and adhesion-cohesion of the articular surfaces all contribute to stability. Deficiencies or defects in any of these structures can lead to instability. **(DVD 3.1)**

Glenoid Concavity

A ball sitting on a flat table has no tendency to center itself. Even a slight displacing force causes it to slide or roll. If the table has a concavity, the ball will sit at the base of the concavity. The deeper the concavity, the more force it takes to move the ball out of it. The stability is increased if a greater force presses the ball into the concavity (Figure 1). This mechanism is known as concavity-compression.[6]

The glenoid concavity has three

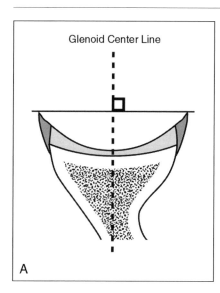

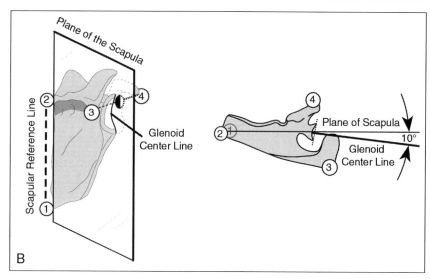

Figure 3 **A,** The glenoid center line is perpendicular to the center of the glenoid concavity. **B,** The glenoid center line is close to perpendicular to the medial border of the scapula (left) and points slightly posterior to the plane of the scapula (right). (Reproduced with permission from Matsen FA III, Lippitt SB: Principles of glenoid concavity, in Matsen FA III, Lippitt SB, DeBartolo SE (eds): *Shoulder Surgery: Principles and Procedures*. Philadelphia, PA, WB Saunders, 2004, p 89.)

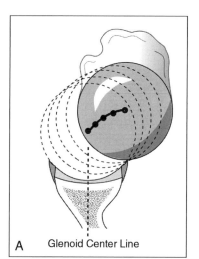

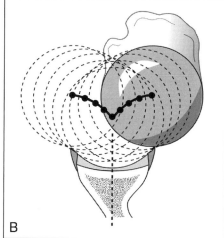

Figure 4 The glenoidogram. **A,** The glenoidogram is the path taken by the center of the humeral head as it translates across the face of the glenoid. **B,** Translation anteriorly and posteriorly across a normally concave glenoid traces a gull wing-shaped path. (Reproduced with permission from Matsen FA III, Lippitt SB: Principles of glenoid concavity, in Matsen FA III, Lippitt SB, DeBartolo SE (eds): *Shoulder Surgery: Principles and Procedures*. Philadelphia, PA, WB Saunders, 2004, pp 100-101.)

humerus. This flexible periphery enables small deviations from fixed ball-and-socket kinematics without compromising the intrinsic stability of the articulation. The glenoid center line is perpendicular to the glenoid articular surface and points slightly posterior to the plane of the scapula (Figure 3).

The adequacy of the glenoid concavity in different directions can be assessed with use of three related measures. The term glenoidogram is used to describe the path taken by the center of the humeral head as it is translated over the surface of the glenoid in a given direction. It normally has a gull-wing shape with a medially pointing apex at the glenoid center line (Figure 4). This shape results from the fact that when the humeral head moves away from the center of the glenoid concavity, its center displaces laterally. A glenoid lacking a lip has a flattened glenoidogram: when the head moves toward the flattened part of the glenoid lip, it does not move lat-

components: the osseous glenoid, which is slightly concave; the articular cartilage, which is thicker at the periphery and thinner in the center and thus makes the concavity deeper; and the glenoid labrum, which

further deepens the glenoid concavity[7] (Figure 2). Because of its increased compliance, the glenoid labrum optimizes the surface area of glenohumeral contact and creates a conforming seal with the head of the

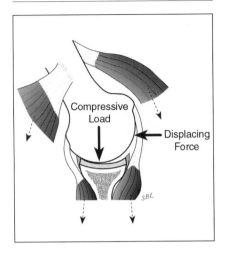

Figure 5 The stability ratio is the force necessary to displace the humeral head from the glenoid center divided by the load compressing the humeral head into the glenoid. (Reproduced with permission from Matsen FA III, Lippitt SB: Principles of glenoid concavity, in Matsen FA III, Lippitt SB, DeBartolo SE (eds): *Shoulder Surgery: Principles and Procedures*. Philadelphia, PA, WB Saunders, 2004, p 105.)

erally. The lateral movement of the humeral head as it is translated across the face of the glenoid can be noted on physical examination of the normal shoulder.

The stability ratio is the force necessary to displace the head from the glenoid divided by the load compressing the head into the concavity (Figure 5). The stability ratio is greatest when the head is at the center of the glenoid fossa because that is where the concavity is deepest. The stability ratio is lower when the humeral head is not centered in the glenoid. The stability ratio is calculated from the slope of the glenoidogram. The so-called load-and-shift test is a clinical analog of the stability ratio. The load-and-shift test is performed by pressing the humeral head into the glenoid fossa and, while the compression is maintained, noting the resistance to translation of the head toward the

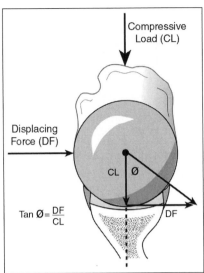

Figure 6 The balance stability angle is the maximal angle that the net force on the humeral head forms with the glenoid center line before dislocation occurs. The net humeral joint-reaction force is the vector sum of the displacing force and the compressive load. The tangent of the balance stability angle is the stability ratio. (Reproduced with permission from Matsen FA III, Lippitt SB: Principles of glenoid concavity, in Matsen FA III, Lippitt SB, DeBartolo SE (eds): *Shoulder Surgery: Principles and Procedures*. Philadelphia, PA, WB Saunders, 2004, p 108.)

lip in different directions.

The balance stability angle is the maximal angle between the glenoid center line and the net humeral joint-reaction force before the humeral head dislocates from the glenoid (Figure 6). Experimentally, the contribution of the glenoid shape to glenohumeral stability can be measured by orienting the glenoid with the center line pointing vertically upward and then tipping it until an unconstrained ball rolls out. In this instance, the net force on the ball is the vertically oriented force of gravity, so the angle of tip at the moment of dislocation is the balance stability angle. The so-called jerk test, in which the humeral head slips out the back of the glenoid with cross-

body adduction, is a clinical analogue of the laboratory measurement of the balance stability angle.

Scapular Factors in Instability
The Glenoid
The glenoid faces slightly posteriorly. A line perpendicular to the glenoid concavity is the glenoid center line. This line normally is approximately 10° from the plane of the scapula (Figure 3). Anterior deviation of this line laterally is referred to as anteversion; posterior deviation of this line laterally is retroversion. When maximal shoulder stability is needed—for example, when performing a bench press—the scapula and glenoid rotate forward to ensure that all forces remain aligned with the glenoid center line.

A scapula that is malaligned because of poor shoulder kinematics may increase the angle between the glenoid center line and the net humeral joint-reaction force to a point where the centering of the humeral head is compromised. Clinically, problems of scapular misalignment are suggested when the scapulothoracic muscles fail to position the glenoid to best align it with the net humeral joint-reaction forces.

An anteverted or retroverted glenoid is less effective in centering the humeral head in the glenoid because the glenoid center line is no longer aligned with the forces generated by the scapulohumeral muscles. Glenoid version can be estimated clinically from standardized axillary radiographs or from CT scans.

A flattened glenoid may not provide sufficient concavity for effective concavity-compression. The glenoid may be flattened in a given direction because it is dysplastic, because the glenoid labrum and peripheral cartilage are excessively small or compliant, because the glenoid labrum and peripheral cartilage are worn, because the labrum is avulsed from the glenoid lip, or because the glenoid lip is fractured.[8] A flattened glenoid is suggested when the humeral head translates without a feeling of going over a lip, when there is diminished resistance to the load-and-shift test, or when there is a positive jerk test.

The Muscles

The humeral head is compressed into the glenoid by the muscles of the rotator cuff and other scapulo-humeral and thoracohumeral muscles. The line of action of each of these muscles is not, as is often described, one of depression of the humeral head away from the acromion; rather, it is one of compression of the humeral head into the glenoid concavity (Figure 5).

The subscapularis muscle is the primary anterior compressor. Its effective strength is assessed by positioning the arm in maximal internal rotation (with the elbow flexed to a right angle and the hand behind the back) to minimize the contribution of other internal rotators, such as the pectoralis major, the latissimus dorsi, and the teres major, and then noting the amount of isometric internal rotation torque that can be generated. This is known as the lumbar push-off test.

The supraspinatus muscle is the primary superior compressor. Its effective strength is assessed by positioning the arm in 90° of elevation in the plane of the scapula and in internal rotation (so that the supraspinatus lies over the top of the humeral head) and then noting the amount of isometric elevation torque that can be generated. This is known as the supraspinatus test.

The infraspinatus is the primary posterior compressor (assisted to a degree by the teres minor). Its effective strength is assessed by positioning the arm in neutral rotation and slight elevation in the plane of the scapula with the elbow bent to a right angle and then noting the amount of isometric external rotation torque that can be generated. This is known as the infraspinatus test.

The important characteristic of the muscles of the rotator cuff is that they can function as head compressors in almost any position of the glenohumeral joint. Other muscles, such as the deltoid, long head of the biceps, pectoralis, latissimus, teres major, and pectoralis major, can contribute to humeroglenoid compression in certain glenohumeral positions. For example, when the arm is elevated 90° in the plane of the scapula, the deltoid becomes a strong compressor of the head into the glenoid.

The effectiveness of concavity-compression can be dramatically demonstrated by first performing an anterior-posterior drawer test on the relaxed shoulder and noting the ability of the head to translate on the glenoid. The same drawer test is then repeated while the arm is held in abduction by the patient, increasing the net humeral joint force vector pressing the humeral head into the glenoid fossa in the normal shoulder. Even with the minimal compressive force generated by gentle active abduction, the humeral head can no longer be translated by the examiner.

Paralysis, detachment, or dysfunction of the subscapularis, supraspinatus, and/or infraspinatus result in loss of humeral head compression. Instability in the direction of the affected tendon may result. As an example, supraspinatus deficiency is commonly associated with superior displacement of the humeral head relative to the glenoid.

The Coracoacromial Arch

As Codman recognized in the 1920s, the glenohumeral joint is not the only important articulation between the humerus and the scapula.[9] Of comparable importance is the articulation between the coracoacromial arch and the proximal humeral convexity (the spherical contour provided by the external surface of the tuberosities and the rotator cuff).

The principle of concavity-compression applies to the ball-and-socket joint between the proximal humeral convexity and the coracohumeral arch. The primary compressor of this articulation is the deltoid. Compression into the arch also results when the arm presses down, such as when the arms are used to rise from an armchair, during walking with a cane or crutches, and when an athlete performs bar dips, activities in which stability of the shoulder is essential. The marvel of the design of the shoulder is that the centers of rotation for the humeral head, the proximal humeral convexity, the glenoid fossa, and the coracoacromial arch are all superimposed in the normal stable shoulder (Figure 7).

The critically important stabilizing effect of the articulation between the coracoacromial arch and the proximal humeral convexity is demonstrated by the devastating antero-superior instability that results when an acromioplasty is performed in the presence of rotator cuff deficiency. Even when the rotator cuff is intact, disruption of the coracoacromial arch may compromise the ability of the joint to remain centered in the presence of a superiorly directed force.

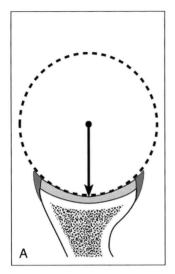
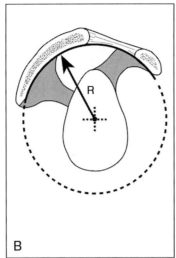
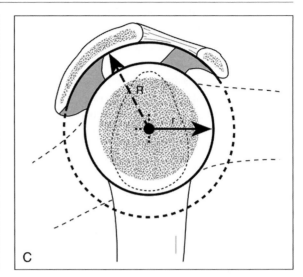

Figure 7 Centers of rotation. **A** and **B**, In the stable and normally aligned shoulder, the centers of rotation of the humeral articular surface and the glenoid concavity and the proximal humeral convexity and the coracoacromial arch all are superimposed. **C,** The difference in the radius of the humeral head (r) and that of the proximal humeral convexity (R) is made up by the rotator cuff and the tuberosities. (Reproduced with permission from Matsen FA III, Lippitt SB: Principles of glenohumeral stability, in Matsen FA III, Lippitt SB, DeBartolo SE (eds): *Shoulder Surgery: Principles and Procedures*. Philadelphia, PA, WB Saunders, 2004, p 82.)

The Glenohumeral Ligaments and Capsule

In mid-range positions, the glenohumeral capsule and its associated ligaments are lax and do not exert a centering effect. At the extremes of motion, however, these structures become important contributors to humeral centering.[10] First, they prevent humeral rotation beyond the point where the muscles are effective. As is the case for muscles in general, the rotator cuff muscles are able to generate the most force when they are in midexcursion. They become less effective when they are maximally extended. It is the job of the capsule and ligaments to prevent the rotator cuff muscles from becoming overstretched. Second, the ligaments come under progressively greater tension at the extremes of motion. This tension creates a compressive force that is essentially collinear with the force that would otherwise be exerted by the muscle overlying it. This force takes over in positions where the muscle force

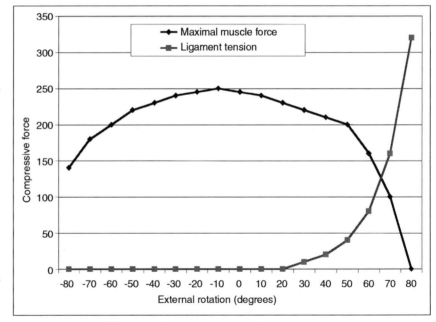

Figure 8 Hypothetical graph showing the interplay between muscular and capsular tension. As the humerus is passively externally rotated, the force that the subscapularis can generate drops off, while the force generated by the anterior capsular ligaments increases in a complementary manner.

drops off (Figure 8).

Third, the ligaments substitute for muscle forces in positions where no muscle is present. For example, the coracohumeral ligament and ro-

tator interval capsule that lie between the supraspinatus and subscapularis tendons provide a compressive force when the arm is in adduction.[11] Another example is the inferior glenohumeral ligament complex that lies in the tendon-free zone beneath the glenohumeral joint and provides a compressive force when the arm is abducted. These capsuloligamentous effects are energy-efficient. For example, the compressive effect of the tension in the coracohumeral ligament and the rotator interval capsule centers the humeral head when the arm is at rest by the side without consuming muscular energy. Similarly, the compressive effect of the inferior glenohumeral ligament helps to center the humeral head when the arm is in the cocking and early acceleration phases of the throw without consuming additional energy.

When the capsuloligamentous restraints are deficient, the joint can overrotate into positions in which the muscles are less able to provide adequate compression. As a result, patients with a substantial avulsion of the capsule from the glenoid often describe weakness of the arm when it is abducted and externally rotated. Similarly, patients with a deficiency of the inferior glenohumeral ligament have difficulty throwing because muscular contraction cannot substitute for the compressive forces provided by the intact ligament.

Adhesion-Cohesion and the Suction Cup

There are two other centering mechanisms that do not require energy. One is adhesion-cohesion, a process in which the wettable surfaces of the humeral and glenoid cartilage and the wettable surfaces of the coracoacromial arch and the proximal humeral convexity adhere to each other because of the adhesive and cohesive properties of water molecules. These properties enable the two sets of surfaces to glide easily on each other while simulta-

neously preventing them from separating. The power of adhesion-cohesion can be demonstrated by placing a drop of water between two microscope slides and noting the ease with which they slide and the difficulty of distracting them. The second mechanism is the glenohumeral suction cup.[12] The center of a suction cup is noncompliant while the periphery is flexible. This is exactly the structure of the glenoid surface: thin cartilage overlies bone in the center, and compliant capsule, labrum, and thicker cartilage are at the periphery (Figure 2). As a result, the glenoid can stick to the humeral head, like a child's suction-cup arrow can stick to a glass window. The suction-cup mechanism is enhanced by the slightly negative intra-articular pressure within the joint.

Neither the adhesion-cohesion nor the suction-cup mechanism consumes energy, and both provide so-called low-cost centering when the arm is at rest. These mechanisms also have the convenient property of working in any position of the shoulder.

When the conforming glenoid lip is lacking or when the joint surfaces are no longer covered with smooth wettable hyaline cartilage, the shoulder will often feel "out of place." For example, in a total shoulder replacement, the polyethylene glenoid component neither conforms to the humeral head, to allow a suction-cup effect, nor is wettable, to allow adhesion-cohesion. As a result, patients treated with total shoulder arthroplasty may experience less secure centering of the humeral head on the glenoid than do those with a normal shoulder. The adhesion-cohesion and suction-cup mechanisms may also be disrupted when there is a joint effusion or hemarthrosis. **(DVD 3.2)**

Evaluation of the Shoulder for Instability
History

Shoulder stability is the ability to keep the ball centered in the socket. The diagnosis of instability is based on a carefully elicited history and on direct observation of the shoulder's centering capability.[1]

When one obtains the patient's history, it is useful to start with an open-ended question such as "How does your arm bother you?" and then give the patient plenty of opportunity to reply while one listens for descriptions suggestive of mechanical symptoms, such as "slip," "goes out," or "gives way." The history is more indicative of instability if these symptoms are episodic with interspersed periods of relatively normal function. It is helpful to have the patient describe or show the arm positions in which these episodes of instability occur. Instability in abduction, extension, and external rotation is usually anteroinferior, whereas instability in flexion, internal rotation, and adduction is usually posterior. The severity of the instability is indicated by the frequency of these episodes, the functional disruption that they cause, and whether the patient can recenter the humerus without help. A description of the initial episode can also indicate the likelihood of traumatic injury to the stabilizing structures. Here, a little understanding of basic mechanics is helpful (Figure 9). When a 33-lb (147-N) force is applied to the hand of the abducted, externally rotated upper extremity, its lever arm to the center of the humeral head is about 30 inches (76 cm). In opposition to this torque is the tension in the anterior-inferior glenohumeral ligament that works through a lever arm of 1 inch (2.5 cm). The torque equilibrium equation indicates that essentially

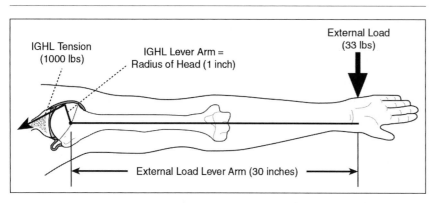

IGHL Tension (1000 lbs)

IGHL Lever Arm = Radius of Head (1 inch)

External Load (33 lbs)

External Load Lever Arm (30 inches)

Figure 9 Mechanics of the Bankart lesion. When a 33-lb (147-N) load is applied to the hand of the outstretched arm, the resulting torque can produce a tension in the inferior glenohumeral ligament (IGHL) of 1000 lb (4448 N). This is due to the difference between the external load lever arm (30 inches [76 cm]) and the IGHL lever arm (1 inch [2.5 cm]). (Reproduced with permission from Matsen FA III, Lippitt SB: Principles of glenohumeral ligaments and capsule, in Matsen FA III, Lippitt SB, DeBartolo SE (eds): *Shoulder Surgery: Principles and Procedures.* Philadelphia, PA, WB Saunders, 2004, p 122.)

1000 lb (4448 N) of tension in the inferior glenohumeral ligament would result from the 33-lb force exerted on the outstretched arm, clearly enough to avulse the capsulolabral complex from the anterior-inferior aspect of the glenoid, producing a Bankart lesion. In contrast, a rear-end motor-vehicle collision, even with a relative velocity of 30 mi/hr (48.2 km/hr), would not be expected to produce a Bankart lesion in the driver whose hands were on the steering wheel. Similarly, a hard fall on the outstretched hand might apply enough force to avulse the posterior aspect of the labrum, whereas lifting a moderately sized box might not. The clinician needs to visualize what the suggested mechanism might produce at the tissue level.

If there is a substantial tissue injury, surgical intervention may be needed to achieve strong anatomic healing. If there is no reason to suspect a tissue injury, rehabilitation of the strength and coordination of the stabilizing musculature rather than surgery is likely to be the treatment of first choice.

Although there are many other critical elements of the history, three key questions need to be answered: (1) Is the humeral head really becoming uncentered during the symptomatic episodes or is something else going on? (2) In which direction is the head moving when it leaves the glenoid center? (3) Is the instability the result of a substantial tear or detachment and, if so, what tissues are likely to be involved? It is often easier to sort out these questions by carefully obtaining a history than by any other means.

Physical Examination

The physical examination should try to answer these same three questions. An easy way to start is to have the patient demonstrate the position of the shoulder when the initial injury occurred and the mechanism of the initial injury as well as the subsequent episodes. It is most useful if the patient can say, "My shoulder goes out when I do this." Close observation prevents one from making a misdiagnosis of glenohumeral instability when, in fact, the problem is scapu-

lothoracic snapping, for example. This "no touch" part of the examination is nonthreatening for the patient and informative for the physician.

When the "no touch" examination is inconclusive, the examiner can then look for apprehension and statements of recognition when the shoulder is placed in positions characteristic of common instability patterns. The examiner should start with the contralateral shoulder so that the patient will know what to expect during the examination of the involved shoulder. The anterior apprehension test is conducted by placing the arm in abduction, extension, and external rotation. The posterior apprehension test is conducted by placing the arm in adduction, midflexion, and internal rotation. Instability or a sensation of impending instability in one of these positions can help confirm whether the instability is anterior or posterior. Tests for instability are most conclusive when the patient volunteers, "That's how my shoulder feels when it's ready to go out." Pain alone on these tests is insufficient evidence of instability.

A second important element of the physical examination for stability is to determine the status of the glenoid concavity, particularly in the direction of the instability. This is conveniently accomplished by having the seated patient relax with the forearm resting on the thigh. First, the anterior and posterior translatability of the humeral head is determined as a measure of joint laxity. Next, the humeral head is pressed into the glenoid fossa while anterior and then posterior translation is attempted (the load-and-shift test). Easy translation of the head while it is being pressed into the glenoid center suggests that the lip of the glenoid concavity is deficient in that direction. Anterior deficiency of the glenoid lip is most commonly the result of a Bankart lesion or a glenoid lip fracture. Posterior lip deficiency may result from deficiency or detachment of the posterior aspect of the labrum or a posterior glenoid fracture. In traumatic instability, translation of the humeral head over the edge of the glenoid lip may be accompanied by a grinding sensation as the head moves over the area from which the labrum has been avulsed or the osseous lip has been fractured. If the patient recognizes this sensation as what he or she feels when the shoulder goes out of place, the diagnosis is reinforced.

A third important element of the physical examination for stability is the assessment of the muscles that compress the humeral head into the glenoid. These evaluations include tests for the isometric strength of the subscapularis, supraspinatus, and infraspinatus.

Other elements of the physical examination may include tests of laxity, such as assessments for the drawer and sulcus signs. It must be recognized, however, that the ability of the examiner to demonstrate that the joint is translatable (lax) does not mean that the shoulder is unstable. It is important to recall that lax yet stable joints are essential for gymnasts.

Imaging of the Shoulder

The primary purpose of the radiographic examination is to determine, on standardized views, (1) whether the humeral head is seated well in the glenoid, (2) if there is a major glenoid osseous defect inferiorly or posteriorly, and if there is a major humeral head defect posteriorly or anteriorly (3) (Figure 10).

It is tempting to perform a CT scan for every patient with an unstable shoulder. However, often the

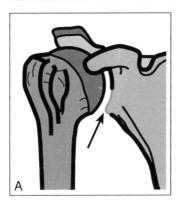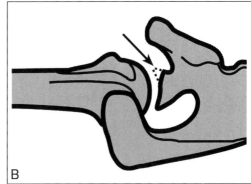

Figure 10 Radiographic views of the glenohumeral joint. The anteroposterior view in the plane of the scapula shows loss of the glenoid surface line inferiorly (arrow) (**A**), and the axillary view shows an anterior defect of the glenoid rim (arrow) (**B**). (Reproduced with permission from Matsen FA III, Lippitt SB: Principles of glenoid concavity, in Matsen FA III, Lippitt SB, DeBartolo SE (eds): *Shoulder Surgery: Principles and Procedures*. Philadelphia, PA, WB Saunders, 2004, p 117.)

relevant osseous anatomy can be assessed adequately on a plain anteroposterior radiograph in the plane of the scapula, which shows humeral head centering and the integrity of the anterior glenoid lip line; an apical oblique radiograph, which shows defects in the posterolateral aspect of the humeral head and anteroinferior aspect of the glenoid lip; and a true axillary radiograph, which shows humeral centering along with anterior humeral head defects and anterior or posterior glenoid bone defects. If these studies do not show the bone anatomy adequately, a CT scan is indicated.

Under certain circumstances, additional information may be desired regarding the capsular and labral tissues, the bone, the rotator cuff, or the neurologic status of the muscles. In such instances, additional tests such as MRI, CT, electromyography, or diagnostic arthroscopy may be helpful. These additional examinations are not commonly needed because most of the information required for clinical decision-making when glenohumeral instability is suspected can be acquired by care-

fully obtaining a history, performing a physical examination, and making plain radiographs.

Treatment of Instability
Defining the Problem

Before considering a surgical solution, the surgeon needs to be confident that the problem is glenohumeral instability (ie, the humeral head is not remaining centered in the glenoid) and a mechanical problem that can best be treated by surgical intervention (rather than by rehabilitation or activity modification) has been clearly identified.[1,2] It is recognized that anteroposterior drawer tests, sulcus signs, MRI of labral and capsular abnormalities, translatability on examination of the patient under anesthesia, and "drive-through" signs on arthroscopy are not diagnostic of glenohumeral instability or predictive of the success of surgical management. It is also apparent that recurrent instability associated with uncontrolled epilepsy, inferior subluxation of the humeral head in a patient who has had a stroke, multidirectional instability associated with generalized ligament laxity, and vol-

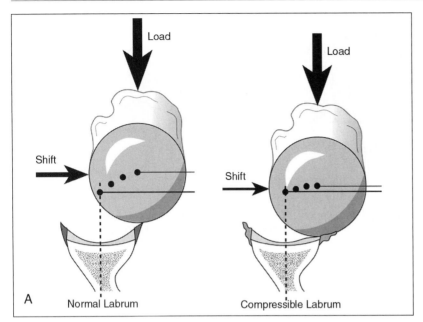
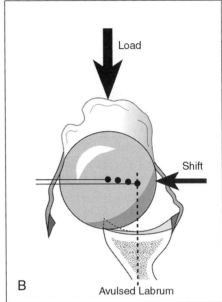
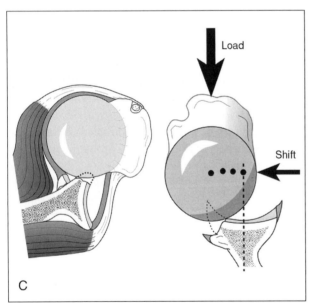
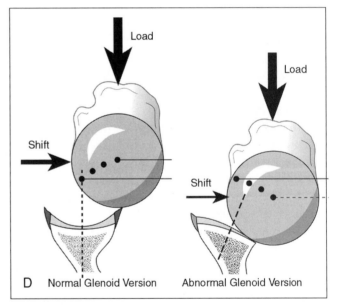

Figure 11   Deficiencies of the glenoid rim. **A,** Compressible labrum. **B,** Avulsed labrum. **C,** Fractured glenoid lip. **D,** Glenoid dysplasia. (Reproduced with permission from Matsen FA III, Lippitt SB: Principles of glenoid concavity, in Matsen FA III, Lippitt SB, DeBartolo SE (eds): *Shoulder Surgery: Principles and Procedures*. Philadelphia, PA, WB Saunders, 2004, pp 109-111.)

untary instability may not be best treated with shoulder surgery.

The primary decision regarding whether to perform the surgical procedure in an open fashion or arthroscopically depends on whether the treatment is directed at deepening the fossa, reorienting a maloriented fossa, repairing or tightening the ligaments, reattaching torn tendons, or restoring osseous defects. Until the anatomic/ mechanical objective is determined, discussion of the surgical approach is secondary.

Treatment Principles

Rather than describing the surgical techniques in detail, which has been done elsewhere,[13,14] the principles that can be applied to the treatment of specific mechanical problems will be outlined.

When the concavity is deficient, many of the stabilizing mechanisms are compromised (Figure 11). When the instability is secondary to glenoid deficiency, this deficiency must

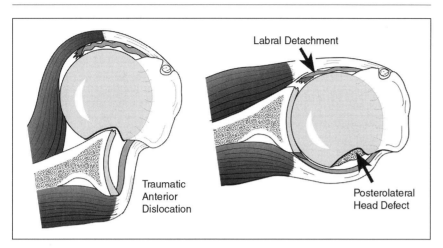

Figure 12 Typical pathology of traumatic anterior glenohumeral instability. **A**, A traumatic dislocation. **B**, Anatomic defects persisting after reduction. (Reproduced with permission from Matsen FA III, Lippitt SB: Principles of glenohumeral ligaments and capsule, in Matsen FA III, Lippitt SB, DeBartolo SE (eds): *Shoulder Surgery: Principles and Procedures*. Philadelphia, PA, WB Saunders, 2004, p 121.)

be addressed. Soft-tissue repairs or reconstructions may be sufficient when the soft-tissue elements of the concavity are compromised. However, it is difficult to compensate for a substantial osseous defect with a soft-tissue repair because soft tissue cannot withstand the compressive loads as well as bone can. When the osseous lip of the glenoid is flat but ample, it can be built up with use of a glenoid osteoplasty in which the bone beneath the lip is cut, lifted up, and held up with a wedge-shaped bone graft.[15] Major bone loss at the glenoid periphery can be addressed with a bone graft placed so that the graft reestablishes the extent of the glenoid fossa.[16] When the acromion and the coracoacromial ligament have been sacrificed, allowing anterosuperior escape of the proximal part of the humerus, no anatomic reconstruction has proved satisfactory, and a reverse shoulder prosthesis needs to be considered.

When the cartilage of the glenoid lip is eroded, the resulting loss of depth of the glenoid can be restored by repairing the labrum and capsule upon the surface of the glenoid at its lip. A labrum that is intact but not as high and stabilizing as desired can be augmented with capsulolabral plication and/or injection augmentation. When the glenoid labrum is avulsed from the osseous glenoid lip, the fossa-deepening effect of the labrum can be restored by securely reattaching it to the face of the glenoid (not the neck).[17] When the capsule and the glenohumeral ligaments have been torn or avulsed from the glenoid, their integrity can be restored with a direct repair (Figure 12). Reconstruction to address capsular or ligamentous deficiencies resulting from previous surgery or from chronic or recurrent injury may require the use of a tendon graft from the humerus to the glenoid.

When the tendon of an otherwise intact subscapularis is deficient, a hamstring tendon graft may enable secure reattachment of the muscle to the bone. In selected circumstances, muscle transfers such as a pectoralis major transfer to the lesser tuberosity

or other more complex procedures may be considered.

When instability is caused by denervation or irreparable detachment of the muscles that normally compress the humeral head into the glenoid fossa, surgical treatment other than glenohumeral arthrodesis may not be effective.

Summary

Effective surgical reconstruction of the unstable shoulder requires assurance that humeroscapular instability is the problem, that the mechanical cause of the instability is discernable, and that the mechanical cause of the instability is surgically treatable.

References

1. Lippitt S, Matsen FA III: Mechanisms of glenohumeral joint stability. *Clin Orthop Relat Res* 1993;291:20-28.

2. Matsen FA III, Titelman RM, Lippitt SB, Rockwood CA Jr, Wirth MA: Glenohumeral instability, in Rockwood CA Jr, Matsen FA 3rd, Wirth MA, Lippitt SB (eds): *The Shoulder*, ed 3. Philadelphia, PA, Saunders, 2004, vol 2, pp 655-794.

3. Matsen FA III, Fu FH, Hawkins RJ (eds): *The Shoulder: A Balance of Mobility and Stability*. Rosemont, IL, American Academy of Orthopaedic Surgeons, 1993.

4. Schiffern SC, Rozencwaig R, Antoniou J, Richardson ML, Matsen FA III: Anteroposterior centering of the humeral head on the glenoid in vivo. *Am J Sports Med* 2002;30:382-387.

5. Lippitt SB, Harris SL, Harryman DT II, Sidles J, Matsen FA III: In vivo quantification of the laxity of normal and unstable glenohumeral joints. *J Shoulder Elbow Surg* 1994;3:215-223.

6. Lippitt SB, Vanderhooft EP, Harris SL, Sidles JA, Harryman DT II, Matsen FA III: Glenohumeral stability from concavity-compression: A quantitative analysis. *J Shoulder Elbow Surg* 1993;2:27-35.

7. Fehringer EV, Schmidt GR, Boorman RS, et al: The anteroinferior labrum helps center the humeral head on the glenoid. *J Shoulder Elbow Surg* 2003;12:53-58.

8. Lazarus MD, Sidles JA, Harryman DT II, Matsen FA III: Effect of a chondral-labral

defect on glenoid concavity and glenohumeral stability: A cadaveric model. *J Bone Joint Surg Am* 1996;78:94-102.

9. Codman EA: *The Shoulder, Rupture of the Supraspinatus Tendon and Other Lesions in or About the Subacromial Bursa.* Malabar, FL, Robert E Kreiger, 1984.

10. Harryman DT II, Sidles JA, Clark JM, McQuade KJ, Gibb TD, Matsen FA III: Translation of the humeral head on the glenoid with passive glenohumeral motion. *J Bone Joint Surg Am* 1990;72:1334-1343.

11. Harryman DT II, Sidles JA, Harris SL, Matsen FA III: The role of the rotator interval capsule in passive motion and stability of the shoulder. *J Bone Joint Surg Am* 1992;74:53-66.

12. Gibb TD, Sidles JA, Harryman DT II, McQuade KJ, Matsen FA III: The effect of capsular venting on glenohumeral laxity. *Clin Orthop Relat Res* 1991;268:120-127.

13. Matsen FA III, Lippitt SB, Sidles JA, Harryman DT II: *Practical Evaluation and Management of the Shoulder.* Philadelphia, PA, WB Saunders, 1994.

14. Matsen FA III, Lippitt SB, De Bartolo SE (eds): *Shoulder Surgery: Principles and Procedures.* Philadelphia, PA, WB Saunders, 2004.

15. Metcalf MH, Duckworth DG, Lee SB, et al: Posteroinferior glenoplasty can change glenoid shape and increase the mechanical stability of the shoulder. *J Shoulder Elbow Surg* 1999;8:205-213.

16. Churchill SR, Moskal M, Lippitt SB, Matsen FA III: Extracapsular anatomically contoured anterior glenoid bone grafting for complex glenohumeral instability. *Tech Shoulder Elbow Surg.* 2001;2:210-218.

17. Thomas SC, Matsen FA III: An approach to the repair of avulsion of the glenohumeral ligaments in the management of traumatic anterior glenohumeral instability. *J Bone Joint Surg Am* 1989;71:506-513.

Shoulder Disorders in the Overhead Athlete

Arun J. Ramappa, MD

Richard J. Hawkins, MD, FRCS(C)

Misty Suri, MD

Abstract

Overhead athletes place enormous loads on shoulder structures during the throwing cycle. These extraordinary stresses can result in a variety of injuries. Many of these injuries can coexist and are often associated with excessive anterior shoulder laxity, sometimes referred to as instability, thereby making the diagnosis and treatment of the athlete's shoulder extremely challenging. Although elite throwers represent a small percentage of individuals with shoulder disorders, the evaluation of this subgroup can provide insight for the treatment of the general patient with a shoulder disorder.

Instr Course Lect 2007;56:35-43.

The understanding of the athlete's shoulder has grown tremendously over the previous 30 years. Overhead athletes place enormous loads on the capsular, labral, and tendinous structures of the shoulder during the acceleration and deceleration phases of the throwing cycle.[1] These forces actually remodel the bone into retrotorsion during throwing in the young athlete. The extraordinary stresses placed on the overhead athlete's shoulder can result in a variety of injuries, many of which can simultaneously exist. The presence of multiple pathologies can make

the diagnosis and treatment of the athlete's shoulder extremely challenging.

Evolving knowledge of the overhead athlete's shoulder has resulted in an awareness of the association between laxity, instability, and associated pathology. One difficulty of investigating this association is the ill-defined use of the term "instability" in the literature concerning the throwing athlete's shoulder. Instability is often used interchangeably with the term "laxity." However, glenohumeral instability generally should be defined as excessive translation of the humeral head on the glenoid that results in symptoms interpreted as instability. Typically, throwers sustain injuries secondary to repetitive use rather than from acute trauma. The purpose of this chapter is to introduce the reader to

the challenge of diagnosing and treating the often multiple pathologies that can occur in the throwing shoulder. The relationship of both laxity and atraumatic instability to the throwing shoulder is also discussed.

Historical Perspective

In the 1970s, the interest of orthopaedists in the painful shoulder of overhead athletes increased.[2] Following Neer's[3] support of outlet impingement as a source of shoulder pain, this disorder was diagnosed in many overhead athletes. Open subacromial decompression was performed on many athletes, with limited success.[4,5] With the advent of shoulder arthroscopy, it was hoped that this new tool would provide improved outcomes for the throwing athlete. However, arthroscopic techniques did not improve the rate of return to competition after subacromial decompression.[6] The low rate of return to pretreatment levels of performance after surgery for outlet impingement prompted further studies.

Jobe and others advocated underlying capsular laxity as a primary cause of the painful throwing shoulder. Anterior capsular laxity was

One or more of the authors or the departments with which they are affiliated have received something of value from a commercial or other party related directly or indirectly to the subject of this chapter.

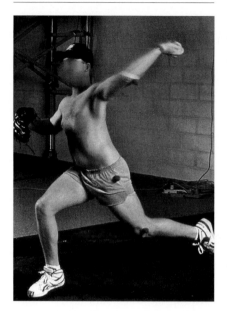

Figure 1   The cocking phase of throwing with maximum external rotation.

proposed as the source of the increased external rotation seen in overhead athletes. Advocates of this theory suggested that repetitive microtrauma occurred when the arm was placed in the cocking position and resulted in stretching of the anterior capsule. Although this plastic deformation of the capsule permitted increased external rotation in some patients, it sometimes led to increased anterior glenohumeral laxity and, often, shoulder disability.[7-10] The relationship of instability to impingement was described: anterior capsular laxity permitted anterior translation of the humerus, resulting in secondary subacromial impingement.[10] Various surgical procedures were developed to treat this cause of the painful throwing shoulder and primarily involved capsulolabral reconstruction.[11-13] The rates of success for such procedures improved compared with procedures for subacromial decompression, but remained lower than desirable for this high-demand patient population.[11]

In the early 1990s, a new location of impingement was recognized. Walch and associates[14] and others described impingement of the undersurface of the rotator cuff on the posterosuperior labrum and glenoid rim, or internal impingement.[15] The contributory role of internal impingement to the painful throwing shoulder gained importance in the orthopaedic literature. Many authors have proposed that anterior capsular laxity initiates or exacerbates internal impingement and that correction of the underlying laxity would eliminate this form of rotator cuff impingement.

Superior labrum anterior posterior (SLAP) lesions are another cause of disability in the throwing shoulder.[16,17] Since the initial description by Andrews and associates[18] and the formal classification by Snyder and associates,[19] this pathology has been recognized in the throwing shoulder. Repair of SLAP lesions has led to high rates of return to play in professional baseball pitchers.[20] SLAP lesions also have been associated with instability.[21-24] SLAP lesions introduce a different pathologic concept than internal impingement, keeping in mind some overlap in etiology, and these two conditions are frequently present at the same time.

Biomechanics

The throwing cycle comprises four primary phases: wind-up, cocking, acceleration, and follow-through.[25-27] The cocking and follow-through phases have been subdivided into early and late cocking phases and deceleration and follow-through, respectively.[28-30] Windup is defined as the initiation of movement until stride foot contact. The cocking phase begins with stride foot contact and ends

with maximum external rotation (Figure 1). The portion of the throwing cycle between maximum external rotation and ball release comprises the acceleration phase. The follow-through phase ensues.

During the throwing cycle, the arm is placed in extreme positions. Maximum external rotation is nearly 180° during the cocking phase. From this position, the arm internally rotates to a position of 105° of external rotation at ball release.[1,29] The shoulder is abducted approximately 100° (between 90° and 110°) during the cocking and acceleration phases. The arm rotates from a position of horizontal abduction of 30°, to a position of 14° of adduction during the acceleration phase, and returns to a position of 0° of abduction at ball release.[29]

The glenohumeral joint experiences dramatic forces and torques during the throwing cycle. Internal rotation and abduction torques of approximately 110 N have been described during the late cocking phase.[1] Anterior shoulder forces have been estimated at 380 N during the cocking phase. During the acceleration phase, peak angular velocity approaches 7,000°/s.[29] Distraction forces acting on the shoulder average approximately 950 N at ball release.[1] During arm deceleration, a compressive force of 1,090 N and a posterior shear force of 400 N act on the glenohumeral joint.[30]

Electromyographic studies have characterized the pattern of muscle firing during the throwing cycle. Biceps activity is relatively low throughout the cycle except for the deceleration phase.[25,28] The rotator cuff musculature is most active during the late cocking phase and relatively quiet during the acceleration phase. The upper subscapularis, however, remains highly active during acceleration.[28,31] Scapular stabilizers and humeral internal rotators also provide coordinated muscle movement to generate the throwing motion.[28,31]

Pathophysiology

It is unclear whether anterior laxity exists in the throwing shoulder. Bigliani and associates[32] have shown that in a group of professional baseball players, pitchers had a higher prevalence of a sulcus sign than position players. However, in the same study, no difference was found in inferior laxity when comparing dominant to nondominant shoulders. Studies comparing anterior glenohumeral laxity in the throwing and nonthrowing shoulders of professional pitchers have found contradictory results. Two studies that used manual testing and stress radiography showed no significant differences.[33,34] One study using cutaneous markers demonstrated increased translation between a thrower's dominant and nondominant shoulder.[35]

Controversy also persists regarding the relationship of anterior laxity and internal impingement. Many authors believe that impingement of the posterosuperior rotator cuff in the abducted, externally rotated (ABER) position is a physiologic phenomenon. These authors suggest that repetitive placement of the arm in this position results in attrition of the cuff.[14,36] Arthroscopic and MRI studies support this theory and suggest that contact of the cuff in the ABER position is not unique to athletes.[37,38] Others have proposed that internal impingement is particularly prevalent in throwing shoulders because anterior capsular laxity initiates and exacerbates the internal impingement lesion.[39] It is believed that encroachment of the

posterosuperior cuff occurs as the humeral head translates anteriorly as the arm is placed in the ABER position. In accordance with this theory, correction of the underlying laxity should eliminate this form of internal impingement.

Experimental and clinical studies suggest that SLAP lesions are associated with increased anterior glenohumeral translation and instability. Further classification of SLAP lesions includes descriptions of superior labral lesions that extend either to the anterior glenoid margin, posterior glenoid rim, or both.[17,40] Experimentally produced SLAP lesions have been shown to decrease the shoulder's resistance to torsion in the ABER position and to place increased strain on the inferior glenohumeral ligament.[22] Cadaveric studies also have shown increased anterior and inferior glenohumeral translation after the creation of SLAP lesions.[23] Clinical studies have also shown a high association of Bankart lesions with SLAP lesions (especially for high-grade SLAP lesions).[21,24]

Burkhart and Morgan, strong advocates of the central role that SLAP lesions play in the painful throwing shoulder, propose that intrinsic anterior laxity does not exist in such shoulders. They suggest that a contracted posterior capsule results in a posterosuperior shifting of the glenohumeral contact point. This shifting, in turn, accentuates the torsional stress placed on the biceps anchor when the arm is placed in the ABER position and results in the "peel-back" phenomenon producing a SLAP lesion. These authors believe that a "pseudolaxity," not a true laxity, is present secondary to disruption of the labral ring. A corollary to this theory is that repair of the SLAP lesions eliminates the "pseudolaxity." It has

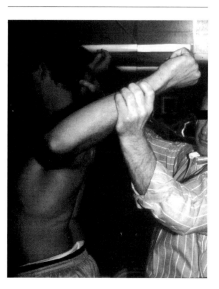

Figure 2 An overhead athlete with increased external rotation.

been suggested that surgical procedures intended to decrease capsular laxity may be successful because they reciprocally tighten the anterior capsule, thereby balancing the contracted posterior capsule.[16-20,41-43] According to Morgan and Burkhart and others, [16-20,41-43] tight posterior structures exacerbate this peel-back phenomenon. Therefore, in the overhead athlete, posterior stretching is important. Occasionally, in refractory cases, posterior capsule release may be indicated. Previous work by Harryman and associates[44] showed that posterior capsular tightening leads to anterior and superior translation of the humerus with arm flexion rather than posterior translation. However, a recent cadaveric study demonstrated that posterior capsular tightening resulted in posterosuperior migration of the humeral head when the arm was abducted and externally rotated.[45]

The throwing shoulders of overhead athletes show increased external rotation in abduction when compared with the shoulders of nonthrowing individuals[34,46,47] (Figure 2). This increase in external rotation has been attributed to anterior capsular laxity.[8,42,43] Recently, humeral retrotorsion has been identified as a potential factor contributing to this increase in external rotation and especially to the loss of internal rotation.[34,46-48] It has been suggested that during growth, osseous adaptation occurs at the proximal humeral physis in response to repetitive throwing, resulting in increased humeral retrotorsion. In a study of overhead throwing athletes, Pieper[48] has shown that humeral retrotorsion correlated with shoulder disability; specifically, patients who had asymptomatic shoulders had significantly higher humeral retrotorsion compared with athletes with disabled shoulders. Humeral retrotorsion is adaptive, which can be protective, and little or no retrotorsion can lead to increased internal impingement. In Europe, with patients who have recalcitrant symptoms related to internal impingement, a proximal humeral rotational osteotomy has been performed to produce increased humeral retrotorsion, thereby eliminating the impingement; however, the results of such extensive surgery are marginal in elite overhead athletes.[36]

Clinical Evaluation
An accurate patient history is important in the evaluation of the painful throwing shoulder. Pain is typically reported and is associated with loss of performance. Mechanical or instability symptoms also may be present. Symptoms should be further characterized by information on onset, location, and timing of occurrence. For example, if an athlete's pain is located posteriorly rather than anteriorly, the clinician may focus on posterosuperior cuff pathology instead of anterior labral pathology. Maneuvers that precipitate,

exacerbate, or ameliorate the symptoms provide insight for determining the diagnosis. The timing of the symptoms during the throwing cycle has significant diagnostic implications. For example, pain that occurs when the arm is forcefully abducted and externally rotated may suggest an injury to the posterosuperior cuff or labrum. It is also vital to obtain a detailed account of previous treatment. If a patient has received a diagnostic or therapeutic injection or has undergone a surgical procedure, it is important to determine and quantify any immediate or long-term benefit from the intervention.

A thorough physical examination will help determine the diagnosis. First, cervical motion should be assessed along with use of the Spurling maneuver to detect cervical pathology. The posterior shoulder girdle should be evaluated for atrophy because suprascapular nerve palsy can be present with shoulder dysfunction. Scapular motion should be checked for synchrony and winging, a condition often present in the painful throwing shoulder. The scapula should be observed from the back during forward elevation for dyskinesia, protraction, retraction, and winging. Often, resistance to forward elevation accentuates scapular abnormalities, especially winging. Scapular winging can be most evident at 30° resisted forward elevation, during push-ups or wall push, or when rising from a chair with the use of the patient's arms. Glenohumeral range of motion should be carefully observed with particular attention to external and internal rotation and total arc of motion, both at the side and particularly at 90° of abduction. Care should be taken to stabilize the scapula to isolate glenohumeral mo-

tion. The presence and amount of the internal rotation deficit relative to the uninjured shoulder should be noted. Strength testing should be documented. Palpation to locate crepitus and elicit tenderness provides evidence of specific shoulder pathology.

Stability testing includes both an assessment of glenohumeral translation and provocative maneuvers. With the patient seated, the load and shift test is performed to evaluate anterior and posterior translation; inferior traction is applied to evaluate the sulcus sign.[49] The degree of translation of the humeral head relative to the glenoid is quantified as: grade 1 (< 1 cm), up the glenoid face to the rim; grade 2 (1 to 2 cm), perched on the glenoid rim; or grade 3 (> 2 cm), over the glenoid rim. The inferior sulcus sign, if present, is reported in millimeters and can be measured from the inferior aspect of the acromion to the superior aspect of the humeral head. The normal shoulder sits 7 or 8 mm from the inferior acromion; that is, the normal distance from the inferior acromion to the superior humeral head is 7 or 8 mm. A measurement of distance from the inferior acromion to the superior humeral head of < 1 cm is rated as grade 1. The normal 7 to 8 mm distance between the inferior acromion and the superior humeral head is included in the sulcus sign measurement. For example, a sulcus sign measurement of 17 mm (normal 7 to 8 mm plus 10 mm more with the downward force of the test) is grade 2. It is imperative to compare both shoulders. The newly defined rotator interval lesion might be present with a sulcus sign that does not disappear in 25° to 30° of external rotation. The apprehension test, described by Rowe and Zarins,[50] is a cornerstone of testing for anterior instability but is rarely present in a thrower.

Various provocative maneuvers are vital aspects to the examination. Impingement maneuvers, such as the Neer and Hawkins sign for outlet impingement and the cross-arm adduction maneuver for acromioclavicular impingement, are helpful.[4] Internal impingement can be investigated by palpating along the posterior glenoid margin to detect the presence of tenderness. Jobe's relocation test, when performed to assess for posterior shoulder pain, is useful for evaluating posterosuperior cuff injury and especially internal impingement.[49] When the maneuver eliminates the posterior pain associated with placing the arm in abduction and external rotation, it suggests internal impingement. The relocation test was initially described for assessing anterior glenohumeral instability by eliminating apprehension produced when the arm is placed in an abducted and externally rotated position and posterior stress applied to the upper arm.[7] When the maneuver eliminates the posterior pain associated with placing the arm in abduction and external rotation, it suggests internal impingement. This relocation test (for pain) must be differentiated from the apprehension sign (for instability). Both examinations are done with the patient supine and the arm stressed in maximum abduction and external rotation. The presence of posterior pain that is relieved by a posterior directed force on the humerus signifies a positive relocation test. This is not to be confused with the feeling of instability or coming out of joint that indicates a positive apprehension sign.

Various maneuvers have been described for SLAP assessment. The authors prefer O'Brien's active compression test and the moving valgus test described by O'Driscoll to detect a SLAP lesion.[51] O'Brien's active compression test is performed with the athlete's arm in 90° of forward elevation and 10° of adduction with the thumb pointing down to the floor (internal rotation). A resistance force is placed downward by the examiner with enough force to break down the athlete's contradicting upward force. If pain is less with repeated thumb up/external rotation, this indicates a positive test. Different pathologies are indicated based on the location of the pain. If the pain is deep, this indicates a SLAP lesion. If the pain is superficial and on top of the shoulder and there is tenderness to palpation at the acromioclavicular joint, a cross-body test should be performed. If this test is positive, this indicates acromioclavicular pathology. O'Driscoll's moving valgus test is done with the patient in the sitting position with the shoulder in maximum abduction and external rotation. A moving valgus force is applied. Shoulder pain indicates a positive test. Biceps signs should also be elicited from a positive Speed's test.

Because multiple areas of injury may coexist, it is often difficult to establish one diagnosis. However, the examination should help to determine the effects of each component of the shoulder disability. Anesthetic injections in the subacromial and acromioclavicular joints, biceps tendon sheath, and intra-articular glenohumeral spaces can be effective diagnostic tools. MRI can help identify shoulder pathology and may aid in diagnosis.

If an anesthetic injection is placed into an area causing pain, pain will be temporarily relieved in that area. After the injection and adequate time for the anesthetic to take effect, the provocative maneuvers specific to the patient's symptoms are repeated, with notation of relief of symptoms as well as subjective notation of the patient's relief.

Nonsurgical Treatment

Rehabilitation is the initial treatment regimen for athletes with shoulder disability from suspected anterior laxity and its associated pathologies. Emphasis is placed on stretching the posterior capsule and strengthening the glenohumeral rotators and scapular stabilizers. Scapular exercises include push-ups plus bear hugs, seated rows, shrugs, and upright rows.[52,53] The goals of these exercises are to keep the humeral head centered in the glenoid cavity and to prevent migration in the superior or anterior directions. The exercises are intended to promote control of the glenohumeral joint rather than to provide gains in power. These exercises are useful components of an injury prevention program for asymptomatic overhead athletes. Nonsurgical management can include the use of nonsteroidal anti-inflammatory drugs and occasionally includes the use of corticosteroid injections. These pathologies are common during the playing season and can range in severity. Conservative treatment as described, including selective rest, is usually successful.

Surgical Treatment

Surgical treatment should only be considered after unsuccessful nonsurgical treatment. Typically, a 3-month rehabilitation program that results in no improvement or a 6-month program that does not achieve a preinjury level of performance may be considered indications for surgery.[54] There will frequently be a period of total cessation of all throwing activity for the athlete. The success of surgical treatment is dependent on the accuracy of the diagnosis. Foregoing conservative treatment may be considered in the thrower with a large SLAP lesion, which will not improve with nonsurgical treatment. Unfortunately, many diagnoses and pathologies concomitantly exist. In some instances, the diagnosis is made by exclusion when the surgeon is influenced by pathologic findings. For example, the diagnosis may be confusing until arthroscopy clearly shows an isolated SLAP lesion. The challenge is to surgically correct the appropriate pathology; however, the surgeon should be wary of doing too much.

Surgical evaluation involves examination of both shoulders for range of motion and translation with the patient under general anesthesia. Comparing the translation of both shoulders, especially in the anterior direction, can be meaningful.[55] Following this examination, arthroscopic examination of the shoulder is performed with particular attention focused on the anterior labrum and capsule, the superior labrum and biceps anchor, the undersurface of the supraspinatus and infraspinatus, the biceps tendon, and the subacromial space.

By evaluating findings from the patient history, physical examination, radiography, MRI, diagnostic injections, and arthroscopy, the primary pathology can usually be determined. If the posterior capsule remains tight, a capsular release may be indicated.[42,43] For isolated internal impingement, débridement of the posterosuperior rotator cuff and posterosuperior labrum should be performed.[56]

SLAP lesions are characterized as follows: type I SLAP lesions exhibit a torn labrum with an intact biceps anchor, whereas in type II lesions

the biceps anchor is unstable. Type III lesions are characterized by a tear of the labrum in a bucket-handle configuration with a stable biceps anchor; in type IV lesions, the geometry of the tear is similar to type III but the biceps anchor is unstable and there is splitting into the biceps. SLAP lesions should be treated appropriately: type I lesions are arthroscopically débrided; type II lesions are repaired using suture anchor fixation; in type III lesions, the bucket-handle portion is excised and the remaining biceps anchor is débrided or fixed if necessary; and type IV lesions are treated with excision of the bucket handle or fixation of the remaining labral anchor if necessary and the biceps is either repaired, released, or tenodesis is performed.[57] Biceps degeneration has been recognized as a source of pain in the shoulder and tenotomy of a diseased tendon has been shown to relieve pain.[58-60] If it is the initial episode of surgical alteration of the biceps in a professional thrower, most surgeons will try to repair a split in the biceps tendon with a suture. Unfortunately, throwers may return with biceps pain. The authors have little experience with success of biceps tenotomy or tenodesis in a professional thrower but have had good success in position players, especially with the nondominant shoulder. If the SLAP lesion is significant enough, fixation of the SLAP lesion itself may address anterior capsular laxity if it was present preoperatively. In the overhead athlete, biceps tenotomy and tenodesis remain controversial treatments. The surgeon should be cautious in accepting outlet impingement as the primary diagnosis; if a spur is present, subacromial smoothing may be appropriate, particularly in the absence of all other

pathology and with 100% relief with subacromial anesthetic injection to impingement sites.[4,5]

When anterior capsular laxity is present, it is often treated in addition to concomitant pathology such as partial articular-sided cuff tears and posterosuperior labral pathology. It has been shown that overhead athletes with internal impingement have a higher rate of return to competitive play when thermal capsulorrhaphy is used in addition to treatment of cuff or labral injuries.[61,62] The authors reserve the use of capsulorrhaphy to patients with increased glenohumeral translation compared with the uninjured shoulder, especially in the presence of internal impingement and/or SLAP pathology. Thermal capsular shrinkage has been helpful; suture capsulorrhaphy can also be used.

With an interval lesion with a positive sulcus sign in external rotation, and examination of the shoulder joint reveals slight increased anterior translation, no evidence of SLAP lesion, no internal impingement, and no subacromial pathology, suture closure of the rotator interval may be appropriate. The addition of anterior capsulorrhaphy is controversial.

A thrower with excessive anterior translation, a clean subacromial space, no interval lesion, no SLAP lesion, no internal impingement, and with a redundant anterior capsule and labral degeneration, the only option may be an anterior capsule labral reconstruction that now can be done arthroscopically.

Appropriate surgery may consist of several procedures such as SLAP fixation, labral débridement, thermal capsulorrhaphy, resection of the subacromial scar, and smoothing of the undersurface of the acromion.

Summary

The role of anterior glenohumeral laxity or instability in the disabled shoulder of the overhead athlete is yet unresolved. Many authors believe that the increased external rotation commonly found in overhead throwers is caused by anterior capsular laxity.[7,8,10,61] This theory states that anterior capsular laxity can become excessive and is the primary cause of disability in the throwing shoulder. Laxity can result in excessive anterior glenohumeral translation and can cause outlet impingement and posterosuperior rotator cuff and labral impingement.

Clinical studies have shown no differences in laxity in the throwing and nonthrowing shoulders of asymptomatic overhead athletes.[32-34] Posterosuperior rotator cuff and labral impingement, or internal impingement, has been shown both arthroscopically and radiographically in nonthrowing shoulders.[37,38]

Recently, humeral retrotorsion has been identified as a potential factor that influences the durability of the throwing shoulder.[46-48] Increased humeral retrotorsion appears to be an adaptive phenomenon and may be protective. In Europe, rotational osteotomy of the proximal humerus has been performed on some patients with posterosuperior cuff and labral impingement who have not responded to arthroscopic treatment.[36] The increase in external rotation and decrease in internal rotation in overhead athletes has been attributed to this increase in retrotorsion. The increased retrotorsion has not been associated with an increased arc of motion, but rather a shift of the arc of total motion. No study has explored the relationship between humeral retrotorsion,

anterior capsular laxity, and posterior capsular contracture in overhead athletes with symptomatic throwing shoulders.

The evaluation of the disabled throwing shoulder remains a diagnostic challenge because pathologies can coexist. However, a careful patient history, thorough physical examination, radiographic studies, selective diagnostic injections, MRI, examination under anesthesia, and arthroscopic evaluation can usually result in a diagnosis. Anterior capsular laxity may exist but is usually not the primary disorder. The authors recommend treating the primary pathology; if laxity is also apparent, thermal capsular shrinkage or suture plication of the anterior capsule can be performed.

References

1. Werner SL, Gill TJ, Murray TA, Cook TD, Hawkins RJ: Relationships between throwing mechanics and shoulder distraction in professional baseball pitchers. *Am J Sports Med* 2001;29:354-358.

2. Tullos HS, King JW: Throwing mechanism in sports. *Orthop Clin North Am* 1973;4:709-720.

3. Neer CS II: Anterior acromioplasty for the chronic impingement syndrome in the shoulder: A preliminary report. *J Bone Joint Surg Am* 1972;54:41-50.

4. Hawkins RJ, Kennedy JC: Impingement syndrome in athletes. *Am J Sports Med* 1980;8:151-158.

5. Tibone JE, Jobe FW, Kerlan RK, et al: Shoulder impingement syndrome in athletes treated by an anterior acromioplasty. *Clin Orthop Relat Res* 1985;198:134-140.

6. Roye RP, Grana WA, Yates CK: Arthroscopic subacromial decompression: Two- to seven-year follow-up. *Arthroscopy* 1995;11:301-306.

7. Jobe FW: Impingement problems in the athlete. *Instr Course Lect* 1989;38:205-209.

8. Jobe FW, Kvitne RS, Giangarra CE: Shoulder pain in the overhand or throwing athlete: The relationship of

anterior instability and rotator cuff impingement. *Orthop Rev* 1989;18:963-975.

9. Jobe FW, Giangarra CE, Kvitne RS, Glousman RE: Anterior capsulolabral reconstruction of the shoulder in athletes in overhand sports. *Am J Sports Med* 1991;19:428-434.

10. Kvitne RS, Jobe FW: The diagnosis and treatment of anterior instability in the throwing athlete. *Clin Orthop Relat Res* 1993;291:107-123.

11. Montgomery WH, Jobe FW III: Functional outcomes in athletes after modified anterior capsulolabral reconstruction. *Am J Sports Med* 1994;22:352-358.

12. Bigliani LU, Kurzweil PR, Schwartzback CC, Wolfe IN, Flatow EL: Inferior capsular shift procedure for anterior-inferior shoulder instability in athletes. *Am J Sports Med* 1994;22:578-584.

13. Altchek DW, Dines DM: Shoulder injuries in the throwing athlete. *J Am Acad Orthop Surg* 1995;3:159-165.

14. Walch G, Boileau P, Noel E, Donell ST: Impingement of the deep surface of the supraspinatus tendon on the posterosuperior glenoid rim: An arthroscopic study. *J Shoulder Elbow Surg* 1992;1:238-245.

15. Davidson PA, Elattrache NS, Jobe CM, Jobe FW: Rotator cuff and posterior-superior glenoid labrum injury associated with increased glenohumeral motion: A new site of impingement. *J Shoulder Elbow Surg* 1995;4:384-390.

16. Burkhart SS, Morgan CD: The peel-back mechanism: Its role in producing and extending posterior type II SLAP lesions and its effect on SLAP repair rehabilitation. *Arthroscopy* 1998;14:637-640.

17. Morgan CD, Burkhart SS, Palmeri M, Gillespie M: Type II SLAP lesions: Three subtypes and their relationships to superior instability and rotator cuff tears. *Arthroscopy* 1998;14:553-565.

18. Andrews JR: Broussard TS, Carson WG: Arthroscopy of the shoulder in the management of partial tears of the rotator cuff: a preliminary report. *Arthroscopy* 1985;1:117-122.

19. Snyder SJ, Karzel RP, Del Pizzo W, Ferkel RD, Friedman MJ: SLAP lesions of the shoulder. *Arthroscopy* 1990;6:274-279.

20. Burkhart SS, Morgan C: SLAP lesions in the overhead athlete. *Orthop Clin North Am* 2001;32:431-441.

21. Cordasco FA, Steinmann S, Flatow EL, Bigliani LU: Arthroscopic treatment of glenoid labral tears. *Am J Sports Med* 1993;21:425-430.

22. Rodosky MW, Harner CW, Fu FH: The role of the long head of the biceps muscle and superior glenoid labrum in anterior stability of the shoulder. *Am J Sports Med* 1994;22:121-130.

23. Pagnani MJ, Deng XH, Warren RF, Torzilli PA, Altchek DW: Effect of lesions of the superior portion of the glenoid labrum on glenohumeral translation. *J Bone Joint Surg Am* 1995;77:1003-1010.

24. Kim TK, Queale WS, Cosgarea AJ, McFarland EG: Clinical features of the different types of SLAP lesions: An analysis of one hundred and thirty-nine cases: Superior labrum anterior posterior. *J Bone Joint Surg Am* 2003;85:66-71.

25. Jobe FW, Moynes DR, Tibone JE, Perry J: An EMG analysis of the shoulder in pitching: A second report. *Am J Sports Med* 1984;12:218-220.

26. Gowan ID, Jobe FW, Tibone JE, Perry J, Moyney DR: A comparative electromyographic analysis of the shoulder during pitching: Professional versus amateur pitchers. *Am J Sports Med* 1987;15:586-590.

27. Kelly BT, Backus SI, Warren RF, Williams RF: Electromyographic analysis and phase definition of the overhead football throw. *Am J Sports Med* 2002;30:837-844.

28. DiGiovine NM, Jobe FW, Pink M, Perry J: An electromyographic analysis of the upper extremity in pitching. *J Shoulder Elbow Surg* 1992;1:15-25.

29. Dillman CJ, Fleisig GS, Andrews JR: Biomechanics of pitching with emphasis upon shoulder kinematics. *J Orthop Sports Phys Ther* 1993;18:402-408.

30. Fleisig GS, Andrews JR, Dillman CJ, Escamilla RF: Kinetics of baseball pitching with implications about injury mechanisms. *Am J Sports Med* 1995;23:233-239.

31. Jobe FW, Tibone JE, Perry J, Mpynes D: An EMG analysis of the shoulder in throwing and pitching: A preliminary report. *Am J Sports Med* 1983;11:3-5.

32. Bigliani LU, Codd TP, Connor PM, Levine WN, Littlefield MA, Hershon SJ: Shoulder motion and laxity in the professional baseball player. *Am J Sports Med* 1997;25:609-613.

33. Ellenbecker TS, Mattalino AJ, Elam E, Caplinger R: Quantification of anterior translation of the humeral head in the throwing shoulder: Manual assessment versus stress radiography. *Am J Sports Med* 2000;28:161-167.

34. Crockett HC, Gross LB, Wilk KE, et al: Osseous adaptation and range of motion at the glenohumeral joint in professional baseball pitchers. *Am J Sports Med* 2002;30:20-26.

35. 35.Sethi PM, Tibone JE, Lee TQ: Quantitative assessment of glenohumeral translation in baseball players. *Am J Sports Med* 2004;32:1711-1715.

36. Riand N, Levigne C, Renaud E, Walch G: Results of derotational humeral osteotomy in posterosuperior glenoid impingement. *Am J Sports Med* 1998;26:453-459.

37. Halbrecht JL, Tirman P, Atkin D: Internal impingement of the shoulder: Comparison of findings between the throwing and nonthrowing shoulders of college baseball players. *Arthroscopy* 1999;15:253-258.

38. McFarland EG, Hsu CY, Neira C, O'Neil O: Internal impingement of the shoulder: A clinical and arthroscopic analysis. *J Shoulder Elbow Surg* 1999;8:458-460.

39. Paley KJ, Jobe FW, Pink MM, Kvitne RS, ElAttrache NS: Arthroscopic findings in the overhand throwing athlete: Evidence for posterior internal impingement of the rotator cuff. *Arthroscopy* 2000;16:35-40.

40. Maffet MW, Gartsman GM, Moseley B: Superior labrum-biceps tendon complex lesions of the shoulder. *Am J Sports Med* 1995;23:93-98.

41. Barber FA, Morgan CD, Burkhart SS, Jobe CM: Current Controversies: Point counterpoint: Labrum/biceps/cuff dysfunction in the throwing athlete. *Arthroscopy* 1999;15:852-857.

42. Burkhart SS, Morgan CD, Kibler WB: The disabled throwing shoulder: Spectrum of pathology: Part I. Pathoanatomy and biomechanics. *Arthroscopy* 2003;19:404-420.

43. Burkhart SS, Morgan CD, Kibler WB: The disabled throwing shoulder: Spectrum of pathology. Part II. Evaluation and treatment of SLAP lesions in throwers. *Arthroscopy* 2003;19:531-539.

44. Harryman DT II, Sidles JA, Clark JM, McQuade KJ, Gibb TD, Matsen FA III: Translation of the humeral head on the glenoid with passive glenohumeral motion. *J Bone Joint Surg Am* 1990;72:1334-1343.

45. 45.Grossman MG, Tibone JE, McGarry MH, Schneider DJ, Veneziani S, Lee TQ: A cadaveric model of the throwing shoulder: A possible etiology of superior labrum anterior-to-posterior lesions. *J Bone Joint Surg Am* 2005;87:824-831.

46. Osbahr DC, Cannon DL, Speer KP: Retroversion of the humerus in the throwing shoulder of college baseball pitchers. *Am J Sports Med* 2002;30:347-353.

47. Reagan KM, Meister K, Horodyski MB, Werner DW, Carruthers C, Wilk K: Humeral retroversion and its relationship to glenohumeral rotation in the shoulder of college baseball players. *Am J Sports Med* 2002;30:354-360.

48. Pieper HG: Humeral torsion in the throwing arm of handball players. *Am J Sports Med* 1998;26:247-253.

49. Silliman JF, Hawkins RJ: Classification and physical diagnosis of instability of the shoulder. *Clin Orthop Relat Res* 1993;291:7-19.

50. Rowe CR, Zarins B: Recurrent transient subluxation of the shoulder. *J Bone Joint Surg Am* 1981;63:863-872.

51. O'Brien SJ, Pagnani MJ, Fealy S, McGlynn SR, Wilson JB: The active compression test: A new and effective test for diagnosing labral tears and acromioclavicular joint abnormality. *Am J Sports Med* 1998;26:610-613.

52. Moseley JB Jr, Jobe FW, Pink M, Perry J, Tibone J: EMG analysis of the scapular muscles during a shoulder rehabilitation program. *Am J Sports Med* 1992;20:128-134.

53. Decker MJ, Hintermeister RA, Faber KJ, Hawkins RJ: Serratus anterior muscle activity during selected rehabilitation exercises. *Am J Sports Med* 1999;27:784-791.

54. Meister K: Injuries to the shoulder in the throwing athlete: Part two. Evaluation/treatment. *Am J Sports Med* 2000;28:587-601.

55. Faber KJ, Homa K, Hawkins RJ: Translation of the glenohumeral joint in patients with anterior instability: Awake examination versus examination with the patient under anesthesia. *J Shoulder Elbow Surg* 1999;8:320-323.

56. Sonnery-Cottet B, Edwards TB, Noel E, Walch G: Results of arthroscopic treatment of posterosuperior glenoid impingement in tennis players. *Am J Sports Med* 2002;30:227-232.

57. Nam EK, Snyder SJ: The diagnosis and treatment of superior labrum, anterior and posterior (SLAP) lesions. *Am J Sports Med* 2003;31:798-810.

58. Walch G, Madonia G: Arthroscopic tenotomy of the long head of the biceps in rotator cuff ruptures, in Gazielly DF, Gleyze P, Thomas T (eds): *The Cuff*. Paris, France, Elsevier, 1997, pp 350-355.

59. Sethi N, Wright R, Yamaguchi K: Disorders of the long head of the biceps tendon. *J Shoulder Elbow Surg* 1999;8:644-654.

60. Gill TJ, McIrvin E, Mair SD, Hawkins RJ: Results of biceps tenotomy for treatment of pathology of the long head of the biceps brachii. *J Shoulder Elbow Surg* 2001;10:247-249.

61. Levitz CL, Dugas J, Andrews JR: The use of arthroscopic thermal capsulorrhaphy to treat internal impingement in baseball players. *Arthroscopy* 2001;17:573-577.

62. Reinold MM, Wilk KE, Hooks TR, Dugas JR, Andrews JR: Thermal-assisted capsular shrinkage of the glenohumeral joint in overhead athletes: A 15- to 47-month follow-up. *J Orthop Sports Phys Ther* 2003;33:455-467.

The Difficult Proximal Humerus Fracture: Tips and Techniques to Avoid Complications and Improve Results

John W. Sperling, MD
Frances Cuomo, MD
J. David Hill, MD
Ralph Hertel, MD
Christopher Chuinard, MD, MPH
Pascal Boileau, MD

Abstract

The indications and techniques for surgical management of fractures of the proximal humerus remain controversial, and the results of treatment are often disappointing, with a relatively high complication rate. Anatomic reduction can be difficult, and loss of fixation because of poor bone quality may lead to fracture displacement and malunion. Hemiarthroplasty has a high rate of shoulder stiffness, tuberosity resorption, and glenohumeral instability. There is a wide variety of surgical techniques and implants to treat these fractures, but there is little guidance in the literature on specific indications for their use. Therefore, it is important for orthopaedic surgeons to be familiar with techniques to avoid complications and improve results when treating proximal humerus fractures.

Instr Course Lect 2007;56:45-57.

Treatment of proximal humerus fractures remains highly controversial, with results that are frequently poor. The classification systems that are currently used have been shown to have poor interobserver and intraobserver reliability.[1-6] In addition, the outcomes of surgery for displaced proximal humerus fractures have been mixed, with some reports demonstrating that surgical outcomes were similar to those for patients treated nonsurgically.[7-9]

Anatomic reconstruction of proximal humerus fractures can be challenging. Fracture displacement and subsequent malunion frequently occur in the elderly patient population because of osteoporotic bone.[7,10]

Among younger patients, proximal humerus fractures are associated with high-energy injuries, and associated soft-tissue injuries can be a significant cause of continued disability despite fracture treatment.[11-13] In the highly comminuted or humeral head-splitting fracture, hemiarthroplasty has been reported to have a significant rate of tuberosity resorption, limitation of motion, and instability.[10,14-17]

Therefore, to minimize complications and improve outcomes, orthopaedic surgeons who treat patients with proximal humerus fractures should be familiar with the indications for using specific surgical techniques.

Surgical Techniques

Most proximal humerus fractures may be treated nonsurgically. For those requiring surgery, the goals of surgical intervention are to obtain an anatomic reduction, to maintain reduction with rigid fixation, and to

One or more of the authors or the departments with which they are affiliated have received something of value from a commercial or other party related directly or indirectly to the subject of this chapter.

maximize functional outcome and pain relief. Several options for proximal humerus fixation exist, including osteosuture, tension band techniques, intramedullary fixation using flexible or rigid nails, percutaneous fixation, use of plates, and hemiarthroplasty.

The choice of fixation technique depends on the fracture type and the bone quality of the patient. Traditionally, tuberosity fractures have been successfully treated with osteosutures or tension bands. Surgical neck fractures can be treated surgically with percutaneous or open techniques. Three- and four-part fractures in younger patients with good bone quality are typically treated with either percutaneous or open fixation; older patients are typically treated with hemiarthroplasty. The exception to this general guideline is a valgus-impacted, four-part proximal humerus fracture, which, even in elderly patients, is more amenable to fixation than a true four-part displaced fracture.

Osteosuture and Tension Band Techniques
Background
The most reliable method of fixation for many proximal humerus fractures involves incorporation of the rotator cuff tendons because of comminution of the tuberosity fragments or presence of osteoporotic bone. Heavy, nonabsorbable suture or wires passed through the tendon at the bone-tendon interface may be used to reduce and secure the tuberosity fragments. The wires or sutures are placed in figure-of-8 patterns from the tuberosities to the humeral shaft. The addition of flexible intramedullary nails adds stability to surgical neck fractures. Biomechanical data have revealed that the addition of Enders nails increases

the stability of osteosuture constructs in surgical neck fractures.[18,19] Osteosuture is applicable to all fractures types. In isolated tuberosity fractures, osteosuture alone may be sufficient to obtain and maintain a satisfactory reduction.[20] In more complex fracture patterns, osteosuture is an excellent adjunct to other forms of fixation.[21-23]

Surgical Technique
The patient is placed in the beach-chair position. A lateral deltoid splitting approach is recommended for patients with isolated greater tuberosity fractures, whereas a standard deltopectoral approach is recommended for those with lesser tuberosity fractures and fractures involving the surgical neck. Once mobilized, the tuberosity fragments are reduced. Drill holes are placed around the periphery of the fracture bed in the humeral head and shaft. Passing and tying the heavy suture through these drill holes in figure-of-8 fashion secures the tuberosities and humeral head together as a single fragment (Figure 1). When the surgical neck is involved, small longitudinal incisions placed slightly lateral to the articular margin are made in line with the rotator cuff fibers over the greater or lesser tuberosities for Enders nail insertion (Figure 2). An awl is used to penetrate the bone for nail insertion. If the greater tuberosity is intact, it is large enough to accept two Enders nails, whereas the lesser tuberosity is large enough for only one nail. The presence of a fracture in a tuberosity precludes the placement of a nail in that tuberosity because of insecure fixation. When placing two greater tuberosity nails, posterior and anterior insertion sites are used. It is helpful to place the posterior nail first because once it is partially inserted, it

can be used to lever the proximal fragment and aid in maintaining the reduction and preventing the humeral head from falling posteriorly.

The second nail is inserted approximately 1.0 to 1.5 cm anterior to the first. Placing nails of two different lengths helps to prevent a stress riser in the humeral shaft near the distal tip of the nails. Nails between 22 and 27 cm in length are generally adequate. Drill holes are made in the humeral shaft lateral to the biceps tendon. Sutures are placed through the proximal eyelets of the nails, passed deep to the rotator cuff tendon between the nails, and are then crossed in a figure-of-8 fashion. The sutures are then passed through the predrilled holes in the humeral shaft. The nails are impacted well below the cuff, and fracture reduction is evaluated before tightening the tension band. The stability of the fixation is assessed intraoperatively to establish safe parameters for postoperative rehabilitation and to prevent subsequent stress on the repair.

Isolated tuberosity fractures are treated in a similar manner. In addition to figure-of-8 fixation to the humeral head and shaft through predrilled holes, the rotator cuff is repaired. A tear will be found most often in the rotator interval. Repair of the rotator cuff tear before the tuberosity fixation will relieve tension on the figure-of-8 fixation.

Results of Treatment
Flatow and associates[20] demonstrated good or excellent outcomes in 100% of patients treated with osteosuturing of two-part greater tuberosity fractures at 4.5-year follow-up. Satisfactory outcomes were also demonstrated in 14 healthy, active patients with three-part fractures treated with tension band wiring of the tuberosities at 54-month follow-

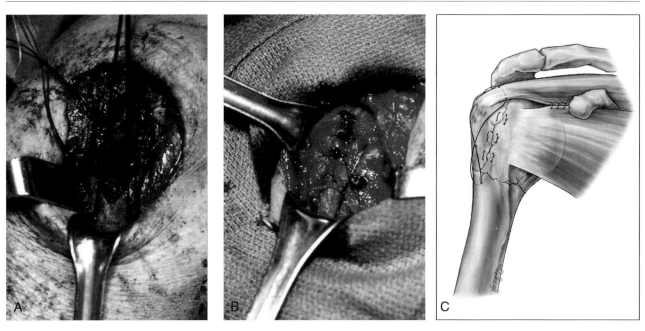

Figure 1 **A,** Intraoperative photograph of a greater tuberosity two-part fracture in which nonabsorbable suture is passed through the tuberosity fragment and the rotator cuff tendon and through drill holes in the shaft. **B,** Intraoperative photograph shows the fracture is reduced and the sutures are tied in figure-of-8 fashion. **C,** Illustration of a three-part fracture shows that the tuberosity is first repaired to the humeral head fragment as in A and B. The humeral head/tuberosity fragment is then secured to the shaft. Closing the rotator cuff reduces tension on the repair.

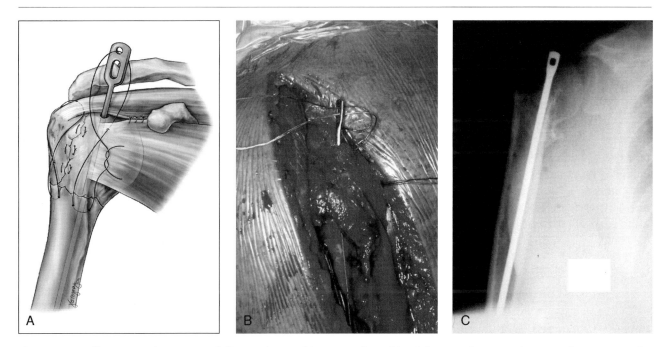

Figure 2 **A,** Illustration of an intramedullary Enders nail being used to add stability to a three-part fracture; after repairing the tuberosity fracture, an Enders nail is placed into the tuberosity/head fragment and into the shaft. **B,** Intraoperative photograph shows the suture (or wire) placed through the Enders nail eyelet. **C,** Radiograph shows the Enders nail properly impacted beneath the surface of the head to prevent impingement.

up.[24] In a more recent study, Flatow and associates[25] observed good or excellent outcomes in 82% of patients treated with osteosuturing of the tuberosities supplemented with intramedullary Enders nails for two- and three-part fractures. Others have used a novel method of intramedullary Kirschner wire fixation supplemented with tension band wiring in four-part displaced fractures and observed satisfactory outcomes in 63% of patients.[26] Thus, the use of the osteosuture technique using nonabsorbable heavy suture or wire with or without the addition of intramedullary Enders nails for the fixation of proximal humerus fractures is supported by clinical data.

Percutaneous Fixation
Background
To decrease the risk of devascularization of the humeral head, less invasive techniques such as percutaneous fixation have been developed. Percutaneous fixation may result in less stiffness by avoiding extensive dissection. Disadvantages associated with this type of fixation are less rigid fracture fixation,[27,28] pin complications such as loosening and infection,[29,30] the risk to anatomic structures,[23] and pin migration.[30] Furthermore, several authors have noted that the percutaneous technique is technically demanding.[18,29,31]

Fractures amenable to closed reduction and percutaneous pinning include two- and three-part fractures in patients with good bone quality and without comminution as well as valgus-impacted, four-part fractures.[18,30] As a prerequisite, a closed reduction must be possible. The inability to perform closed reduction of a displaced fracture may be the result of the biceps tendon or other interposed soft tissue in the fracture site. Patient compliance with postoperative care is a must for this technique. Alternate forms of fixation are recommended for patients who will be noncompliant with postoperative care.

Surgical Technique
The patient is positioned supine or in the beach-chair position with the involved extremity draped free to allow full manipulation of the arm. Fluoroscopy is used to obtain both AP and axillary views, which is accomplished through a combination of arm movement and angulation of the fluoroscopic arm. The reduction maneuver is then performed. The humeral shaft fragment tends to be displaced anteriorly because of the pull of the pectoralis major; thus, the recommended reduction maneuver uses posteriorly directed pressure, traction, and forward flexion of the arm. It is necessary to recreate the native humeral anteversion. Pins or Kirschner wires may be used as joysticks, or other percutaneously applied reduction aids may be used to manipulate the fragments into the desired reduction.[32] The use of terminally threaded pins and 4.0-mm cannulated screws are recommended for fixation.

Once the fracture is reduced, the threaded pins are introduced through stab incisions at the lateral aspect of the deltoid. The first two pins are introduced inferiorly and directed superomedially into the humeral head fragment. A third pin is directed in a similar manner, but with a more anterior starting point. Finally, to maximize stability and hold a greater tuberosity fragment reduced, a greater tuberosity pin is inserted from a superolateral starting point and directed infero-medially to capture the medial cortex of the humeral shaft. The locations of the axillary nerve and cephalic vein should be carefully noted during pin placement to avoid injury. The pins are trimmed beneath the skin surface. The arm is placed in a sling for 6 weeks. After 3 weeks, the patient is permitted gentle passive range of motion, including pendulum exercises. Serial radiographs and clinical examinations are performed to check for loss of reduction, pin migration, and infection. Once evidence of healing is present, the pins are removed. At this point, active range of motion is instituted.

Results of Treatment
Jaberg and associates[29] reported good or excellent results in 70% of 48 patients at an average 3-year follow-up after percutaneous fixation of unstable proximal humerus fractures. Resch and associates[33] reported on 27 patients with three- and four-part fractures, most of which were valgus-impacted, that were treated with percutaneous methods. At an average 24-month follow-up, all of the patients were satisfied with the results of treatment. The Constant score for the three-part fractures averaged 91% compared with the opposite uninjured extremity, whereas the score for the four-part fractures averaged 87% compared with the opposite uninjured extremity. Similarly, good or excellent results were observed in 12 of 14 patients treated with percutaneous cannulated screw fixation of two- and three-part proximal humerus fractures.[32] Percutaneous fixation of proximal humerus fractures may lead to satisfactory outcomes when the patients are properly selected and the technical challenges of the technique are mastered.

Rigid Intramedullary Nailing

Background

Intramedullary nailing of proximal humerus fractures combines the strength of open fixation techniques with the minimal dissection of percutaneous techniques. Intramedullary nails may be inserted through deltoid-splitting approaches. Because the nail is intramedullary, the lever arm of the screws into the humeral head is shorter than that used with plate fixation techniques; thus, the incidence of fixation failure caused by screw pullout would be expected to be lower with intramedullary nailing than with plating techniques. The use of a deltoid-splitting approach allows the incorporation of osteosuture as a supplement to fixation.[22] A well-recognized disadvantage is the violation of the rotator cuff for the starting point of the nail. The indications for the use of intramedullary nails are two-part humeral neck fractures that require surgical treatment and three- and four-part fractures of the proximal humerus with minimal comminution.

Surgical Technique

Although various humeral intramedullary nails are available, the general concepts of the surgical technique for insertion are similar with all types. Patients are placed in the beach-chair position. The involved upper extremity is draped free to allow manipulation of the arm. A fluoroscope is placed at the head of the table and positioned to allow AP and axillary views to be obtained. A lateral deltoid-splitting approach is used and care is taken to avoid injury to the axillary nerve at the most inferior limit of the dissection. In patients with three- and four-part fractures, it may be necessary to use Kirschner wires, Stein-

mann pins, or an elevator to adequately reduce the fragments.[22] Additionally, it may be helpful to place osteosutures in the rotator cuff and tuberosity fragments to achieve and maintain reduction.[22] Once a satisfactory reduction is achieved, the intramedullary nail entry point is identified. An incision in the supraspinatus tendon is made in line with the muscle fibers. The nail should smoothly enter the intramedullary canal. The starting point is 1 to 1.5 cm posterior to the biceps tendon and 5 to 8 mm medial to the middle facet of the greater tuberosity sulcus. A starting point that is too lateral will cause the fracture to assume a varus position on nail insertion. After confirming the correct starting point position with two 90° fluoroscopic views, the medullary canal is reamed using either a motorized or handheld reamer. The nail is then gently advanced into the medullary canal to a depth that will avoid subacromial impingement, usually at least 3 to 4 mm below the greater tuberosity surface (Figure 3). Interlocking screws are placed through stab incisions using the targeting device. By using multiple screws at several different angles, the tuberosity fragments may be fixed with one or more screws. Distal interlocking screws are placed using the freehand technique and fluoroscopic imaging. Passive and active-assisted exercises are started as tolerated in the immediate postoperative period. Radiographs are obtained at postoperative weeks 2 and 6 to confirm the maintenance of reduction.

Results of Treatment

Rajasekhar and associates[34] reported on the use of intramedullary nail fixation on 25 two- and three-part fractures of the proximal humerus. At an average 18-month follow-up, 20

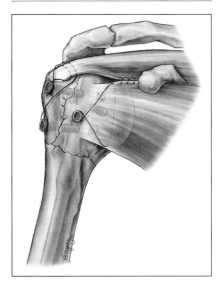

Figure 3 Illustration shows nonabsorbable sutures used to reduce the tuberosity and head fragments during the placement of a rigid intramedullary humeral nail. The sutures may then be secured through drill holes in the humeral shaft or around the screw heads as shown. These osteosutures reinforce the proximal humeral fixation by using the strength of the rotator cuff tendon. The distal locking screws that add stability to the nail are not shown.

of 25 patients had a good or excellent outcome as measured by the Constant score. The age-adjusted scores for patients older than 60 years were similar to those of patients younger than 60 years. One nonunion and one instance of osteonecrosis accounted for two of the five poor outcomes. Other complications included stiffness requiring arthroscopic release and loosening of a screw after fracture healing requiring removal. In another study of intramedullary nails to repair two-, three-, and four-part fractures, fixation was supplemented with osteosuture in the presence of comminution. Of the original 221 patients in this study, 64 patients had 1-year data available for analysis. The Constant score at 12-month follow-up for all fractures was 86% of the opposite unaffected extremity. In general, function declined with the severity of the fracture pattern. The complication rate was high and consisted mostly of screws backing out. Other complications included osteonecrosis, deep infection, stiffness, pseudarthrosis, implant failure, and dislocation.[22]

Flexible Plate Osteosynthesis

The aim of flexible plate osteosynthesis is to achieve reduction and fixation without additional devascularization of the humeral head and provide an optimal environment for osseous repair and revascularization. This is achieved by using a thin implant functioning as a load-sharing and not as a load-bearing device. Provided that a medial buttress can be restored, angular stability of the implant is not required and may indeed be detrimental (keeping the fragments apart and impeding secondary impaction). Anatomic reduction of the greater to the lesser tuberosity is the key to providing immediate- and medium-term stability; it essentially provides a stable circular platform on which the humeral head can rest, transforming a four-part fracture into a simple humeral neck fracture (Figure 4). Joint reaction forces created by the resting tone of the rotator cuff muscles will stabilize the humeral head. Therefore, it may not be absolutely necessary to introduce a screw or blade into the humeral head, which is of great advantage, especially in patients with osteoporotic bone in whom minimal or no hardware purchase can be obtained in the humeral head.[35,36]

Surgical Approach

The beach-chair position is used with a deltopectoral approach. A vertical skin incision in the direction

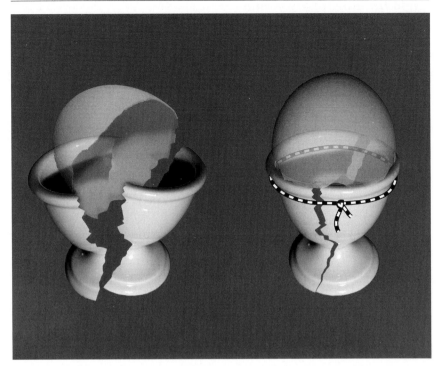

Figure 4 Illustration of the eggshell model to depict a four-part fracture (*left*) and stable reconstruction of the epiphyseal segment as obtained by simple reduction of the tuberosities (*right*).

of Langer's lines is recommended. The cephalic vein is retracted laterally, and the interval is fully developed without detachment of the deltoid muscle. Image intensification is used after preliminary reduction (using a plate with one screw) and at the end of the procedure. The second view (lateral view of the humerus) is obtained by internal rotation of the arm, which is only possible after preliminary fixation of the fracture.

Technique of Reduction and Internal Fixation

Before proceeding with reduction and internal fixation (Figure 5), care must be taken to ensure that the medial hinge is not disrupted. When it is, it must be reduced first (Figure 6). A No. 2 braided suture is passed through the infraspinatus tendon. A 2.5-mm hole is drilled a few mil-

limeters distal to the tip of the greater tuberosity landmark (a V-shaped fracture line that almost always occurs just lateral to the bicipital groove). A straight, proximally slightly overbent, 3.5-mm, one-third tubular steel plate is positioned in the appropriate position. The humeral head is gently reduced (lifted up) using a laminar spreader. The goal is an incomplete reduction rather than an overreduction. Fine reduction is obtained by additional gentle lifting of the humeral head and by pulling on the suture in an anterior and slightly inferior direction. Preliminary fixation of the greater tuberosity to the humeral head is obtained using a thin and flexible (1 mm) Kirschner wire. Reduction and preliminary flexible Kirschner wire fixation of the lesser tuberosity to the humeral head is followed by an indirect reduction maneuver. Automatic

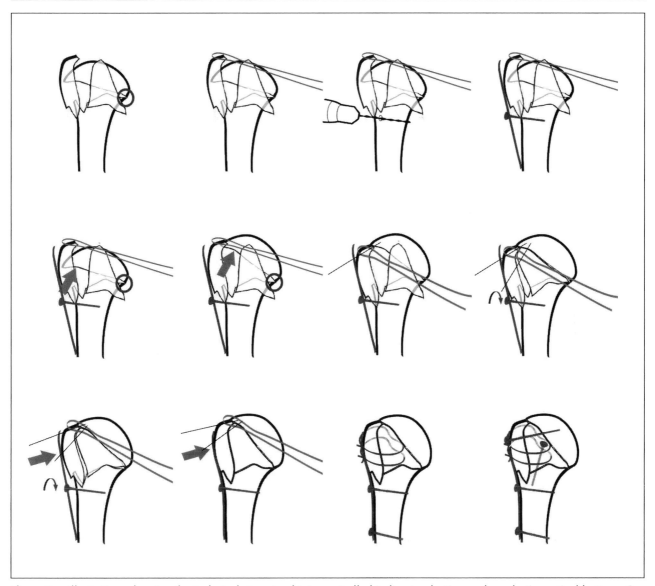

Figure 5   Illustrations showing the technical steps to obtain controlled indirect reduction and an elastic cortical buttress. See text for details.

reduction is obtained by placing a screw through the plate. The plate pushes the fragments into position. Because of its elasticity, the plate snugly conforms to the shape of the proximal humerus. The elastic recoil force stabilizes the entire construct. Two or more No. 2 sutures are used to pull the tuberosities together to provide enough stability for passive rehabilitation exercises. Now the hu-meral head cannot escape, but guided settling of the fracture can still occur. A proximal screw can be optionally inserted, although it may not secure enough holding strength, especially in osteoporotic bone. Finally, an an-teroposterior screw (a cannulated screw is recommended) can be used to stabilize the lesser tuberosity against the humeral shaft. Use of this screw is optional, and it does not always hold well in osteoporotic bone.

Although use of the first screw is critical, all other screws are optional. If the critical screw does not hold, a small amount of bone cement can be used to increase its purchase. Should the medial hinge be disrupt-ed, reconstruction of the hinge is re-quired as a first step (Figure 6). The construct should be stable enough for patients to perform pendulum exercises.

Technical Difficulties and Complications

Inability to obtain adequate reduction of the tuberosities will result in inherent instability of the construct because a stable platform for the head has not been restored. Al- though the general alignment might seem acceptable at fist glance on the postoperative radiograph, when the tuberosities are not correctly re- duced there is a high risk of second- ary displacement.

Early complications are related to the loss of reduction. Late complica- tions include stiffness, impaired healing, and in the long term, partial or total osteonecrosis. The inci- dence of several of these complica- tions depends (among other factors) on the accuracy with which the ini- tial reduction-fixation was obtained.

Results

Although it is still unclear which is the optimal treatment, adequate functional results can be obtained when reduction and stabilization are performed in the described manner. Selection of a balanced osteosynthe- sis adapted to the weak bone is nec- essary. Bulky, stiff implants may cause additional damage without providing the necessary stability. Obtaining metaphyseal buttressing appears to be the key to achieving the necessary load-sharing fixation to create a stable interface between the perfused tuberosities and the ex- posed cancellous bone of the hu- meral head (Figure 7). Additional studies are necessary to better un- derstand and define the subtle re- quirements to optimize this type of fixation by identifying the right bal- ance between bone and implant as

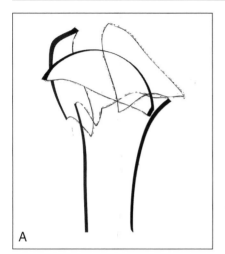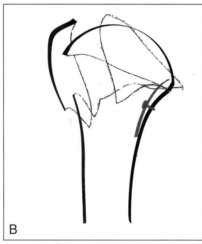

Figure 6   Illustration showing a disrupted medial hinge (**A**), which is reconstructed with a preliminary Kirschner wire or by using an intramedullary 2.0-mm plate aimed at preliminary restoration (**B**). All subsequent steps are shown in Figure 5.

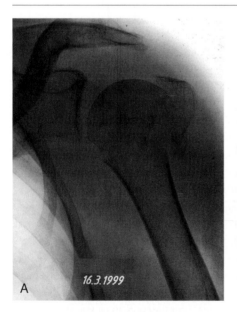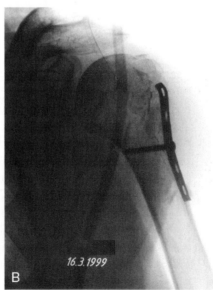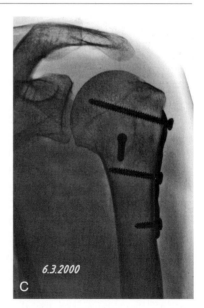

Figure 7   Preoperative (**A**), postoperative (**B**), and 1-year postoperative (**C**) radiographs showing the desired anatomic recon- struction in a patient who underwent flexible plate osteosynthesis to treat a proximal humerus fracture.

well as to determine the long-term results of this technique.

Shoulder Arthroplasty for Complex Proximal Humerus Fractures

Prosthetic replacement is a well-accepted method of treatment of selected three- and four-part proximal humerus fractures; however, to be successful it must replicate anatomy and function in the most hostile of biologic environments.[37] The bony and soft-tissue destruction distorts anatomic landmarks, the bone is often of poor quality, and it may be difficult to identify common landmarks such as the bicipital groove.[38-43] In addition, the available implants are often unsuited for the dual tasks of osteosynthesis and arthroplasty. Because the goal of shoulder arthroplasty is to restore pain-free function, the surgeon must choose an implant that accounts for the hostile biologic environment and pair this with a technique that is reliable, reproducible, and easy to perform to give each patient the opportunity for a good outcome.

The main complication resulting in a poor outcome after hemiarthroplasty for humeral fracture is loss of fixation of the greater tuberosity.[44] There are several factors under the surgeon's control that can lead to this complication, including poor prosthesis design (bulky prosthetic neck that prevents adequate bone grafting or good tuberosity-shaft contact), prosthesis malpositioning (too high and/or too retroverted), tuberosity malpositioning (too high, too low, and/or too posterior), inadequate tuberosity fixation (lack of cerclage and tension band fixation and sole use of prosthetic holes), and overaggressive rehabilitation.

Every effort must be made to use

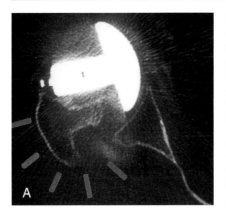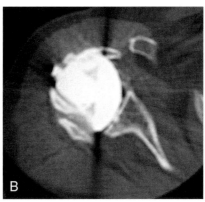

Figure 8   **A,** CT scan showing poor reduction of tuberosity. **B,** CT scan showing migration of the lesser tuberosity and a posterior greater tuberosity.

principles designed specifically for the treatment of humeral fractures because patients who are candidates for shoulder arthroplasty tend to be older, female, and less active than those receiving a prosthesis for osteoarthritis.[45,46] Anatomic tuberosity positioning is critical for restoration of function.[47-52] Therefore, the greater and lesser tuberosities must be returned to their native positions, with respect to both height and rotation; moreover, they must be united to the shaft if they are to function at all. In patients with humeral fractures, the prosthesis must adapt to the patient's anatomy and not the anatomy to the prosthesis.

Poor Prosthesis Design

The design and shape of the prosthesis should not obstruct anatomic reconstruction. Many proximal humeral prostheses are too bulky to allow anatomic placement of the tuberosities; with such implants, either the greater tuberosity remains too posterior or the cancellous bone must be excavated from it to allow it to rotate anteriorly. Good contact between the tuberosities and the shaft is necessary to achieve union. A prosthesis should allow bone graft from the discarded humeral head to

be placed where it can benefit reconstruction of the tuberosities. The surgeon must remember that this is first and foremost fracture treatment—not arthritis treatment.

The surgeon should choose a fracture stem that has a low profile so anatomic reduction of the unaltered tuberosities can be performed with ample bone grafting from the humeral head. A low-profile body with less metal allows more bone to be placed around the stem. Fins or other projections from the prosthesis should help and not hinder the reconstruction or block tuberosity placement (Figure 8).

Prosthesis Malpositioning

A proud prosthesis may lead to poor function. Overtensioning the superior cuff may lead to pain and limited overhead mobility by stretching or tearing the supraspinatus (because of impingement of the supraspinatus between the prosthetic head and the acromial arch). Overlengthening may also place excessive tension on the tuberosity repair, resulting in loss of fixation with migration and nonunion. Excessive retroversion of the prosthesis may lead to poor function by increasing traction forces on the tuberosity fixation sutures, especially when the arm is in internal rotation, leading to posterior detachment and migration of the greater tuberosity and a poor clinical result.

Specialized fracture instrumentation may result in positioning the prosthesis more accurately and, therefore, create a more anatomic reconstruction of the proximal humerus. Before surgery, a full-length radiograph of the contralateral humerus may be obtained to measure the distance from the epicondylar axis to the top of the humeral head. A jig can then be used to measure this distance and to control retroversion. The principles are simple: to restore appropriate length (humeral height) a ruler is necessary, and to properly recreate an angle (humeral retroversion), a protractor is necessary.

Tuberosity Malpositioning

Restoration of the height and position of the tuberosities must then be addressed. In the horizontal plane, the key is to reposition the greater tuberosity when the arm is in neutral rotation. In the vertical plane, the top of the greater tuberosity must be located at the level of or 3 to 5 mm below the prosthetic head. Overreduction of the greater tuberosity in the vertical plane will result in rotator cuff stretching or tearing.

Even with excellent planning and advanced instrumentation, it is possible to misjudge the position of the tuberosities after initial fixation. A reduction that is thought to be excellent at the time of surgery can be unsatisfactory on postoperative radiographs. For this reason, an intraoperative AP radiograph should be obtained before final tuberosity fixation to ensure correct positioning of the tuberosities.

Inadequate Tuberosity Fixation

Tuberosity fixation should not rely solely on sutures placed through fin holes because they do not hold the tuberosities to the prosthetic neck, and, with motion, the holes can cut the sutures. Furthermore, fixation through the fins is unnecessary provided there is a means by which to place multiple cerclage sutures around the neck of the prosthesis. In a biomechanical study, Frankle and associates[47] demonstrated that the addition of cerclage sutures to the construct improves stability, especially when the reduction is anatomic. Solid fixation of the tuberosities can be obtained with four horizontal cerclage sutures and six vertical tension band sutures that keep the tuberosities opposed to the bone graft and humerus.[53,54]

Overaggressive Rehabilitation

In a large multicenter investigation of hemiarthroplasty for patients with proximal humerus fractures, Boileau and associates[55] found that early passive mobilization led to twice the rate of tuberosity migration compared with patients whose shoulders were immobilized. The patients who were immobilized regained motion with time, and they had significantly better active elevation than those who had tuberosity complications. For this reason, it is recommended that the arm be immobilized in a position of neutral rotation until tuberosity union occurs.

Patients may spend at minimum 4 to 6 weeks in a sling in neutral rotation to allow union of the tuberosities. Only pendulum exercises are allowed during this period; after the first 6 weeks, gentle, active, patient-directed physical therapy is allowed, provided it is below the patient's pain threshold. Strengthening does

not begin until motion has been regained and bony consolidation is achieved. Maximum benefit will likely not be achieved until 1 year postoperatively. It is much easier to manage stiffness than it is to manage complications from improper tuberosity position or nonunion.

Surgical Technique

The patient should be placed in the beach-chair position with the arm draped free to allow access to the humeral shaft. A long deltopectoral approach (from the clavicle, directly over the coracoid process, to the pectoralis insertion) will allow access to the humerus with minimal trauma to the deltoid. Hohmann retractors placed above the coracoacromial ligament and the acromion facilitate the proximal exposure. Recession of the superior 1 to 2 cm of the pectoralis insertion aids distal exposure. The long head of the biceps tendon should be followed into the rotator interval and the interval to the coracoid process opened. Based on the surgeon's preference, the intra-articular portion of the biceps may be resected and a tenodesis to the pectoralis tendon performed.

The tuberosities can then be retracted and prepared. Care should be taken to minimize dissection and preserve any periosteal attachments. Traction sutures, placed with the arm in abduction and internal rotation, are used to "open the book" to allow removal of the humeral head fragments and inspection of the glenoid. Four sutures are placed around the greater tuberosity at the bone-tendon junction (two sutures in the infraspinatus and two sutures in the teres minor). One temporary suture is placed around the lesser tuberosity and also at the bone-tendon junction. The humeral head size is then selected, with selection biased

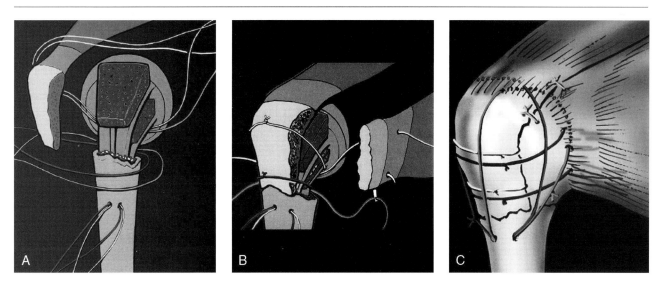

Figure 9 **A,** Illustration showing sutures placed around the humeral neck. **B,** Illustration showing the greater tuberosity fixed with two sutures with the arm in neutral rotation; the lesser tuberosity is fixed with the remaining two sutures. **C,** Illustration showing the final construct with the tuberosities sutured; two tension-band sutures from the diaphysis through the tendons complete the repair.

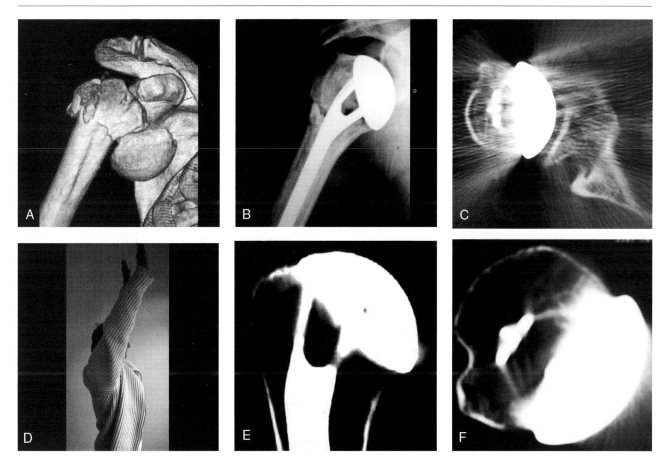

Figure 10 **A,** Preoperative three-dimensional CT reconstruction shows a four-part fracture. **B,** Radiograph showing good healing of tuberosities in the proper position. **C,** CT scan showing proper tuberosity placement. **D,** Photograph showing active elevation. **E,** CT scan showing bone healing. **F,** CT scan showing tuberosity position.

toward a smaller head if two sizes are available.

The arm is placed in adduction and extension for preparation of the humeral canal. Reaming is done by hand. A trial implant is attached to the jig and inserted into the humeral shaft with the arm in extension and external rotation. The arm is then placed in flexion, and the construct is reduced to determine both the final height and retroversion. The greater tuberosity should be positioned level 5 mm below the top of the prosthetic head, overhanging the fin, anteriorly. The head should face the glenoid, and the bicipital groove should not zigzag. When this is done, two heavy sutures are placed through drill holes in the proximal shaft (to be used later as the vertical tension band sutures), and the final prosthesis is cemented into place while the jig holds the position for the surgeon.

Once the final implant has been cemented, the prosthesis is reduced and placed in neutral rotation and reconstruction of the tuberosities begins. The four heavy cerclage sutures are passed around the neck of the prosthesis to control the tuberosities: two for both tuberosities. The arm is placed in neutral rotation, and the greater tuberosity is secured to the lateral aspect of the prosthesis over bone graft with two of the sutures. Next, the two remaining horizontal sutures are placed through the tendon of the subscapularis in an inside-out fashion (adjacent to the bone of the lesser tuberosity) and tied. The construct is completed by passing the diaphyseal sutures vertically through the tendons, biasing one posteriorly (through infraspinatus and supraspinatus) for the greater tuberosity, and biasing one anteriorly (through the subscapularis and supraspinatus) for the lesser tuberosity (Figure 9). The rotator interval is then closed. Shoulder motion should be tested to assess both the fixation and the anteroposterior stability. Results should show approximately 50% of posterior drawer, a minimum of 40° of external rotation, and full internal rotation (forearm parallel to the trunk with the arm in abduction) (Figure 10). **(DVD 5.1)**

Summary

The principles of fracture fixation of the proximal humerus are the same regardless of the technique and include accurate diagnosis, anatomic reduction, appropriate fixation selection, rigid fixation, incorporation of the soft tissue to augment fixation, and physician-supervised rehabilitation. When these principles are followed, surgeons and patients afford themselves the best opportunity to maximize results.

References

1. Bernstein J, Adler LM, Blank JE, Dalsey RM, Williams GR, Iannotti JP: Evaluation of the Neer system of classification of proximal humeral fractures with computerized tomographic scans and plain radiographs. *J Bone Joint Surg Am* 1996;78:1371-1375.

2. Brorson S, Bagger J, Sylvest A, Hrobjartsson A: Low agreement among 24 doctors using the Neer-classification: Only moderate agreement on displacement, even between specialists. *Int Orthop* 2002;26:271-273.

3. Neer CS II: Displaced proximal humeral fractures: Part I. Classification and evaluation. *J Bone Joint Surg Am* 1970;52:1077-1089.

4. Neer CS II: Displaced proximal humeral fractures: Part 2. Treatment of three-part and four-part displacement. *J Bone Joint Surg Am* 1970;52:1090-1103.

5. Neer CS II: Four-segment classification of proximal humeral fractures: Purpose and reliable use. *J Shoulder Elbow Surg* 2002;11:389-400.

6. Neer CS II: Fracture classification systems: Do they work and are they useful? *J Bone Joint Surg Am* 1994;76:789-790.

7. Court-Brown CM, Garg A, McQueen MM: The translated two-part fracture of the proximal humerus: Epidemiology and outcome in the older patient. *J Bone Joint Surg Br* 2001;83:799-804.

8. Leyshon RL: Closed treatment of fractures of the proximal humerus. *Acta Orthop Scand* 1984;55:48-51.

9. Zyto K, Ahrengart L, Sperber A, Tornkvist H: Treatment of displaced proximal humeral fractures in elderly patients. *J Bone Joint Surg Br* 1997;79:412-417.

10. Boileau P, Krishnan SG, Tinsi L, Walch G, Coste JS, Mole D: Tuberosity malposition and migration: Reasons for poor outcomes after hemiarthroplasty for displaced fractures of the proximal humerus. *J Shoulder Elbow Surg* 2002;11:401-412.

11. Blom S, Dahlback LO: Nerve injuries in dislocations of the shoulder joint and fractures of the neck of the humerus: A clinical and electromyographic study. *Acta Chir Scand* 1970;136:461-466.

12. Cofield RH: Comminuted fractures of the proximal humerus. *Clin Orthop Relat Res* 1988;230:49-57.

13. Linson MA: Axillary artery thrombosis after fracture of the humerus. *J Bone Joint Surg Am* 1980;62:1214-1215.

14. Demirhan M, Kilicoglu O, Altinel L, Eralp L, Akalin Y: Prognostic factors in prosthetic replacement for acute proximal humerus fractures. *J Orthop Trauma* 2003;17:181-189.

15. Prakash U, McGurty DW, Dent JA: Hemiarthroplasty for severe fractures of the proximal humerus. *J Shoulder Elbow Surg* 2002;11:428-430.

16. Robinson CM, Page RS, Hill RM, Sanders DL, Court-Brown CM, Wakefield AE: Primary hemiarthroplasty for treatment of proximal humeral fractures. *J Bone Joint Surg Am* 2003;85-A:1215-1223.

17. Tanner MW, Cofield RH: Prosthetic arthroplasty for fractures and fracture-dislocations of the proximal humerus. *Clin Orthop Relat Res* 1983;179:116-128.

18. Williams GR, Wong KL: Two-part and three-part fractures: Open reduction and internal fixation versus closed reduction and percutaneous pinning. *Orthop Clin North Am* 2000;31:1-21.

19. Williams GR, Lawson LA, Iannotti JP, Lisser SP: The influence of intramedul-

lary fixation on figure-of-eight wiring for surgical neck fractures of the proximal humerus: A biomechanical comparison. *J Shoulder Elbow Surg* 1997;6:423-428.

20. Flatow EL, Cuomo F, Maday MG, Miller SR, McIlveen SJ, Bigliani LU: Open reduction and internal fixation of two-part displaced fractures of the greater tuberosity of the proximal part of the humerus. *J Bone Joint Surg Am* 1991;73:1213-1318.

21. Gerber C, Werner CML, Vienne P: Internal fixation of complex fractures of the proximal humerus. *J Bone Joint Surg Br* 2004;86:848-855.

22. Mittlmeier TWF, Stedtfeld HW, Ewert A, Beck M, Frosch B, Gradl G: Stabilization of proximal humeral fractures with an angular and sliding stable antegrade locking nail (Targon PH). *J Bone Joint Surg Am* 2003;85:136-146.

23. Szyszkowitz R, Wolfgang S, Schleifer P, Cundy P: Proximal humerus fractures: Management techniques and expected results. *Clin Orthop Relat Res* 1993;292: 13-25.

24. Hawkins RJ, Bell RH, Gurr K: The three part fracture of the proximal part of the humerus: Operative treatment. *J Bone Joint Surg Am* 1986;68:1410-1414.

25. Flatow EL, Cuomo F, Maday MG, Miller SG, McIlveen SJ, Bigliani LU: Open reduction and internal fixation of two-and three-part displaced surgical neck fractures of the proximal humerus. *J Shoulder Elbow Surg* 1992;1:287-295.

26. Darder A, Darder A Jr, Sanchis V, Gastaldi E, Gomar F: Four-part displaced proximal humerus fractures: Operative treatment using Kirschner wires and a tension band. *J Orthop Trauma* 1993;7: 497-505.

27. Koval KJ, Blair B, Takei R, Kummer F, Zuckerman J: Surgical neck fractures of the proximal humerus: A laboratory evaluation of ten fixation techniques. *J Trauma* 1996;40:778-783.

28. Wheeler DL, Colville M: Biomechanical comparison of intramedullary and percutaneous pin fixation for proximal humerus fracture fixation. *J Orthop Trauma* 1997; 11:363-367.

29. Jaberg H, Warner JJP, Jakob RP: Percutaneous stabilization of unstable fractures of the humerus. *J Bone Joint Surg Am* 1992;74:508-515.

30. Rowles DJ, McGrory JE: Percutaneous pinning of the proximal part of the humerus. *J Bone Joint Surg Am* 2001;83:1695-1699.

31. Iannotti JP, Ramsey ML, Williams GR, Warner JJP: Nonprosthetic management of proximal humeral fractures. *J Bone Joint Surg Am* 2003;84:1578-1593.

32. Chen C, Chao E, Tu Y, Ueng SW, Shih C: Closed management and percutaneous fixation of unstable proximal humerus fractures. *J Trauma* 1998;45:1039-1045.

33. Resch H, Povacz P, Frohlich R, Wambacher M: Percutaneous fixation of three- and four-part fractures of the proximal humerus. *J Bone Joint Surg Br* 1997;79:295-300.

34. Rajasekhar C, Ray PS, Bhamra MS: Fixation of proximal humeral fractures with the Polarus nail. *J Shoulder Elbow Surg* 2001;10:7-10.

35. Hertel R, Hempfing A, Stiehler M, Leunig M: Predictors of humeral head ischemia after intracapsular fracture of the proximal humerus. *J Shoulder Elbow Surg* 2004;13:427-433.

36. Hertel R: Fractures of the proximal humerus in osteoporotic bone. *Osteoporos Int* 2005;16(suppl 2):S65-S72.

37. Neer CS II: Articular replacement of the humeral head. *J Bone Joint Surg Am* 1955;37:215-228.

38. Boileau P, Walch G: Three-dimensional geometry of the proximal humerus: Implications for the surgical technique and prosthetic design. *J Bone Joint Surg Br* 1997;75:857-865.

39. Boileau P, Walch G, Mazzoleni N, Urien JP: In vitro study of humeral retrotorsion. *J Shoulder Elbow Surg* 1993;2(suppl):33.

40. Iannotti JP, Gabriel JP, Schneck SL, Evans BG, Misra S: The normal glenohumeral relationships: An anatomical study of one hundred and forty shoulders. *J Bone Joint Surg Am* 1992;74:491-500.

41. Doyle AJ, Burks RT: Comparison of humeral head retrotorsion with the humeral axis/biceps groove relationship: A study in live subjects and cadavers. *J Shoulder Elbow Surg* 1998;7:453-457.

42. Kummer F, Pekins R, Zuckerman JD: The use of the bicipital groove for alignment of the humeral stem in shoulder arthroplasty. *J Shoulder Elbow Surg* 1998;7:144-146.

43. Tillet E, Smith M, Fulcher M, Shanklin J: Anatomical determination of humeral head retroversion: The relationship of the central axis of the humeral head to the bicipital groove. *J Shoulder Elbow Surg* 1993;2:255-256.

44. Boileau P, Krishnan SG, Tinsi L, Walch G, Coste JS, Mole D: Tuberosity malposition and migration: reasons for poor outcomes after hemiarthroplasty for displaced fractures of the proximal humerus. *J Shoulder Elbow Surg* 2002;11:401-412.

45. Horak J, Nilson B: Epidemiology of fractures of the upper end of the humerus. *Clin Orthop Relat Res* 1993;289:156-160.

46. Rose SH, Melton LJ III, Morrey BF, Ilstrup DM, Riggs BL: Epidemiologic features of humeral fractures. *Clin Orthop Relat Res* 1982;168:23-30.

47. Frankle MA, Greenwald DP, Markee BA, Ondrovic LE, Lee WE: Biomechanical effects of malposition of tuberosity fragments on the humeral prosthetic reconstruction for four-part proximal humerus fractures. *J Shoulder Elbow Surg* 2001;10:321-326.

48. Compito CA, Self EB, Bigliani LU: Arthroplasty and acute shoulder trauma: Reasons for success and failure. *Clin Orthop Relat Res* 1994;307:27-36.

49. Kralinger F, Schwaiger R, Wambacher M, et al: Outcome after primary hemiarthroplasty for fracture of the head of the humerus: A retrospective multicentre study of 167 patients. *J Bone Joint Surg Br* 2004;86:217-219.

50. Christoforakis JJ, Kontakis GM, Katonis PG, et al: Relevance of the restoration of humeral length and retroversion in hemiarthroplasty for humeral head fractures. *Acta Orthop Belg* 2003;69:226-232.

51. Gerber RT, Hersche O, Berberat C: The clinical relevance of posttraumatic avascular necrosis of the humeral head. *J Shoulder Elbow Surg* 1998;7:586-590.

52. Zuckerman JD, Como F, Koval KJ: Proximal humerus replacement for complex fractures: Indications and surgical technique. *Instr Course Lect* 1997;46:7-14.

53. Boileau P, Walch G: Shoulder arthroplasty for fractures: Problems and solutions, in Walch G, Boileau P (eds): *Shoulder Arthroplasty*, Heidelberg, Germany, Springer-Verlag, 1999, pp 297-314.

54. Boileau P, Walch G, Krishnan SG: Tuberosity osteosynthesis and hemiarthroplasty for four-part fractures of the humerus. *Tech Shoulder Elbow Surg* 2000;1:96-109.

55. Boileau P, Coste JS, Ahrens PM, Staccini P: Prosthetic shoulder replacement for fracture: Results of the multicentre study, in *2000 Prothèses d'Épaule Recul de 2 à 10 Ans*. Montpellier, France, Sauramps Médical, 2001, pp 561-578.

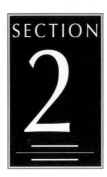

SECTION 2

Hand and Wrist

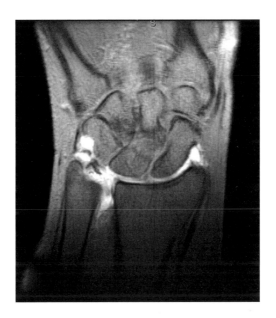

Distal Radius Fractures: What's In and What's Out

Martin I. Boyer, MD, MSc, FRCS(C)

Abstract

Sound peer-reviewed data on the surgical treatment of distal radius fractures, in terms of patients' functional outcome, ability to return to work, complications, and radiographic results, are few. At present, treatment of distal radius fractures is focused on the restoration of articular alignment, radial length, and volar inclination of the articular surface. Early diagnosis and treatment of fracture complications, such as type II complex regional pain syndrome, is encouraged based on published peer-reviewed data.

Inst Course Lect 2007;56:61-64.

Although there is a lack of sound peer-reviewed data on the surgical treatment of distal radius fractures, various approaches are available; the choice of surgical treatment and method of fixation is according to fracture type.

Patient History and Examination

Relevant elements of the patient's medical history include a history of diabetes mellitus, coronary artery disease, stroke, peripheral vascular disease, or collagen vascular disease. This information is relevant because these conditions can increase perioperative risks and have an effect on the patient's ability to cooperate with aggressive postoperative range-of-motion and strength-building therapy. The use of medications such as aspirin, warfarin, clopidogrel bisulfate, and other drugs that can affect clotting should be determined. These medications have relevance in terms of the intraoperative tourniquet management, as would a patient's history of sickle cell disease.

The degree of initial displacement of the fracture should be evaluated based on the patient's history or evaluation of initial injury radiographs. If reduction was required, it should be recorded. The progressive development of neurologic symptoms associated with acute carpal tunnel syndrome and/or acute ulnar nerve compression at Guyon's canal should be assessed. Persistent or worsening numbness or sensory dysfunction in the distribution supplied by the median nerve, including motor weakness of the thenar musculature, are indications for median nerve decompression.

On physical examination, the integrity of the overlying soft-tissue envelope should be evaluated. More severe soft-tissue injuries should be expected in patients with high-energy injuries (such as a fall from greater than standing height) compared with low-energy injuries (such as a fall from a standing position in elderly patients with osteoporosis). Associated open wounds and the degree of contamination should be assessed. Recent data have shown uniformly poor outcomes in patients with open distal radius fractures.[1]

The carpus should be examined for the presence of swelling or pain. Frequently, the presence of pain over the scapholunate interosseous ligament or lunotriquetral ligament can be directly assessed, even in patients with a displaced fracture. In patients with associated intercarpal ligament disruption, early diagnosis and treatment may affect long-term prognosis. The volar and dorsal compartments of the forearm and hand should be assessed for compartment syndrome, especially in patients with high-energy injuries.

Radiographic Evaluation

PA and lateral radiographs of the distal radius and ulna and the entire forearm should be obtained if the

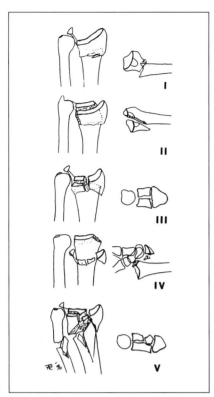

Figure 1 The Fernandez classification of distal radius fractures. Type I: Bending fracture (either a Smith or an extra-articular Colles type fracture. Type II: Shearing fracture (dorsal or volar Barton's fracture). Type III: Compression fracture (die-punch fracture). Type IV: Avulsion-type fracture (with or without associated intercarpal ligament tears). Type V: Combined fracture (components of types I, II, III, and IV). (Reproduced from Fernandez DL: Fractures of the distal radius: Operative treatment. *Instr Course Lect* 1993;42:73-88.)

patient has pain, swelling, or deformity about the elbow or proximal forearm. Additional oblique radiographs may include anatomic tilt radiographs in which a PA radiograph is obtained with the x-ray beam inclined 11° from distal to proximal to better assess the articular surface of the distal radius in the frontal plane, and a lateral radiograph in which the x-ray beam is inclined 22° distal to proximal to better assess articular congruity of the lunate fossa in the

sagittal plane.[2] Forty-five degree oblique views from the PA view may also be obtained to assess articular displacement of both radiocarpal and distal radioulnar joints as well.

Cole and associates[3] reported that CT scans are useful in the assessment of distal radius fractures. In this study, the authors found that articular gap and step displacements are better assessed on CT scans done in the frontal and sagittal planes than on plain PA and lateral radiographs.

MRI with or without intra-articular injection of contrast may be indicated in patients in the subacute and chronic stages following distal radius fracture if intercarpal ligament or triangular fibrocartilage complex injury is suspected. In the preoperative assessment of patients with acute injuries, if there is no evidence of static intercarpal deformity on plain radiographs, MRI might be relevant in the evaluation if there are positive physical examination findings in the carpus.

Initial Management and Classification

The treatment of a displaced fracture of the distal radius begins in the emergency department with appropriate closed reduction and three-point immobilization. Administration of a fracture hematoma block with 10 mL of 2% lidocaine without epinephrine is the recommended analgesia. A neurologic examination is performed before instilling local anesthetic so that neurologic changes that occur subsequent to the infiltration of the local anesthetic (before the reduction maneuver) can be recorded. After reduction, the patient's limb is immobilized either above the elbow in a sugar-tong splint or in a splint consisting of dorsal and radial slabs that begin be-

low the elbow and extend to the distal metacarpus. All fingers are left mobile, and early thumb and finger motion and edema control are prescribed. Repeat radiographs are then obtained.

After closed reduction, immobilization, and radiographic evaluation, it should be determined whether the reduction is acceptable; if the reduction is acceptable, whether the fracture is stable; and if the fracture is not stable, how the fracture can be made stable by surgical reduction and fixation. Classification of the fracture will help make these determinations. The Fernandez classification, which divides the fractures into five groups based on the mechanism of injury, is useful in this regard[4] (Figure 1). The need for surgical treatment is based on the fracture type. Results of the initial closed reduction and the surgeon's assessment of stability (defined as the ability to maintain reduction with splinting or casting) determines the specific type of fixation that will be used.

Definitive Management

When surgical treatment is chosen, the fracture type dictates the approach and the method of fixation. For type I fractures, either volar or dorsal plate fixation may be done. Percutaneous pins can also be used alone or in combination with plate fixation to increase the fracture stability during the healing period.

For type II fractures, because the mechanism of injury was shearing, a buttress plate placed either along the volar aspect of the distal radius (for volar Barton-type fractures) or along the dorsal aspect of the distal radius (for dorsal Barton-type fractures) is indicated.

Volar buttress plates are usually placed via an anterior open approach either between the flexor carpi radialis tendon and the radial artery or through the base of the flexor carpi radialis tendon sheath. This incision is not continued distally as a carpal tunnel decompression because the path of this incision would directly cross the palmar cutaneous branch of the median nerve, risking its injury. Although this exposure is excellent for extra-articular Smith or Colles fractures and is suitable for straightforward volar Barton fractures, poor visualization of the ulnar aspect of the volar extra-articular surface of the distal radius is obtained. If additional visualization of the ulnar volar aspect of the distal radius is desired, an extended carpal tunnel approach may be used. Care should be taken not to injure the median or ulnar nerve with prolonged uninterrupted retraction during this approach. Although excellent visualization of the ulnar volar extra-articular distal radius is obtained, it is more difficult to expose and fix the radial styloid via this exposure.

For open fixation of a dorsal Barton fracture, a standard dorsal approach through the third dorsal compartment is performed with radial elevation of the second dorsal compartment and ulnar elevation of the fourth dorsal compartment. Based on surgeon preference, the extensor pollicis longus tendon may or may not be replaced in its sheath before closure. The dorsal wrist capsule and subsheath of the fourth and second compartments are raised concurrently.

Compression fractures of the distal radius can be treated with limited open reduction and percutaneous pin fixation or with formal open reduction from either a volar or dorsal approach. The use of volar fixation using locked type plates to buttress die-

punch fractures is increasingly popular because it does not compromise extensor tendon function. Treatment of type IV fractures usually involves fixation of the radial styloid with screws placed through open incisions or percutaneously and open or arthroscopic treatment of the intercarpal ligament disruptions. Fixation of type V fractures is based on surgeon preference, with treatment options ranging from percutaneous pins to external fixators and dorsal and volar approaches for open reduction and internal fixation.

External fixators (either bridging or nonbridging) can be useful in treating type I, III, or V fractures. They have the greatest use in the treatment of open fractures or fractures with severe soft-tissue swelling. Noted complications include injury to the superficial radial nerve, overdistraction of the carpus, or complex regional pain syndrome.[5]

The decision to treat the fracture by open reduction and internal fixation (and not with percutaneous pinning, interfocal pinning, or external fixation) should be made before entering the operating room and is based on the surgeon's understanding of fracture mechanism, the results of the closed reduction, and the assessment of fracture stability after initial splinting and immobilization. This will allow for preoperative planning, ensure the availability of the appropriate equipment, and facilitate the execution of the surgical plan.

In addition to the surge in popularity of volar locked plate fixation, fragment-specific systems that also use locking technologies are becoming increasingly popular. These implants are especially useful when placed along the radial aspect of the distal radius or when used for fragment-specific fixation of volar ulnar or dorsal ulnar articular frag-

ments. These implants are generally thin and when placed dorsally have not had the same degree of extensor tendon dysfunction as thicker dorsally placed implants used in the past.[6]

Whether concurrent fixation of distal ulnar shaft fractures should be performed is assessed preoperatively. If the frontal stability of the ulna is compromised following radius fracture fixation, then concurrent fixation should be performed. The use of blade plates or locked plates to fix the distal ulna in normal patients and in elderly patients with osteopenic bone is now a reliable surgical option.

Complications and Results

Despite appropriate treatment of distal radius fractures, patients may develop type II complex regional pain syndrome following either nonsurgical or surgical treatment. Patients should be assessed specifically for peripheral nerve embarrassment at the cubital tunnel, pronator, or carpal tunnel. Placzek and associates[7] recently demonstrated that peripheral nerve decompression in these patients may lead to a substantial reduction in symptoms and significant subjective improvement in objective measures of wrist and hand motion and functions.

Summary

Treatment of distal radius fractures is in a state of evolution, likely because of the recent proliferation of both volar locked plates as well as dorsal low contour plate and screw systems. Future advances in care will result from careful analysis of data evaluating function and complications of fractures treated by various surgical techniques and approaches.

References

1. Rozental TD, Beredjiklian PK, Bozentka DJ: Functional outcome and complications following two types of dorsal plating for unstable fractures of the distal part of the radius. *J Bone Joint Surg Am* 2003;10:1956-1960.

2. Boyer MI, Korcek KJ, Gelberman RH, Gilula LA, Ditsios K, Evanoff B: Anatomical tilt views of the distal radius: An ex-vivo analysis of operative fixation. *J Hand Surg [Am]* 2004;29:116-122.

3. Cole RJ, Bindra RR, Evanoff BA, Gilula LA, Yamaguchi K, Gelberman RH: Radiographic evaluation of osseous displacement following intra-articular fractures of the distal radius: Reliability of plain radiography versus computed tomography. *J Hand Surg [Am]* 1997;5:792-800.

4. Fernandez DL: Fractures of the distal radius: Operative treatment. *Instr Course Lect* 1993;42:73-88.

5. Sanders RA, Keppel FL, Waldrop JI: External fixation of distal radius fractures: Results and complications. *J Hand Surg [Am]* 1991;16:385-391.

6. Axelrod TS: Complications of the AO/ASIF titanium distal radius plate system (pi plate) in internal fixation of the distal radius: A brief report. *J Hand Surg [Am]* 1998;23:737-741.

7. Placzek JD, Boyer MI, Gelberman RH, Sopp B, Goldfarb C: Nerve decompression for complex regional pain syndrome type II following upper extremity surgery. *J Hand Surg [Am]* 2005;30:69-74.

Traumatic Wrist Instability: What's In and What's Out

Charles A. Goldfarb, MD

Abstract

Traumatic wrist instability encompasses a wide spectrum of injuries from the subtle partial ligament tear to the dramatic perilunate dislocation. A timely diagnosis is based on the patient's history and physical examination together with radiographic and advanced imaging studies. Early intervention has been associated with improved patient outcomes.
Instr Course Lect 2007;56:65-68.

Traumatic wrist instability has a spectrum of clinical presentations from the subtle discomfort of a partial lunotriquetral (LT) ligament tear to the significant pain caused by an acute perilunate dislocation. Although the understanding of traumatic wrist instability has advanced in the past 5 years, current treatment recommendations continue to be based on the retrospective reporting of outcomes. A radiographic diagnosis can be made in more severe forms of wrist instability; however, the patient history and physical examination are vital components for achieving an accurate diagnosis in those with a less clear-cut injury presentation.

Preoperative Evaluation

The patient history should focus on the mechanism and duration of the wrist injury and any prior treatment. Duration of the injury is a crucial component of the treatment algorithm because timely treatment is believed to increase the likelihood of a successful outcome.[1,2] The physical examination is helpful in assessing the injury and should begin with an evaluation of point tenderness. The scapholunate (SL) ligament can be assessed for dorsal tenderness at 1 cm distal to Lister's tubercle. Localized pain at the SL ligament together with a positive scaphoid shift test is highly suggestive of SL ligament pathology.[3] The scaphoid shift test is performed by stabilizing the forearm and applying dorsal pressure on the volar tubercle of the scaphoid as the wrist is taken from ulnar to radial deviation. By preventing scaphoid flexion (with volar pressure on the scaphoid), the integrity of the SL ligament can be assessed. Symptomatic laxity is manifested as a dorsal pain and an audible clunk (as the scaphoid subluxates over the dorsal distal radius). To place the symptomatic shift test in the proper perspective, the contralateral wrist and extremity should always be assessed and the generalized ligamentous laxity should be evaluated.

The LT ligament can be assessed with palpation of the LT interval. The LT shuck test, performed by grasping the lunate (as palpated dorsally) and the triquetrum (as localized through grasping the pisiform volarly) and applying differential volar-dorsal forces, allows assessment of pain and excess motion.[4] Pain at the LT interval also can be assessed through radially directed pressure on the ulnar aspect of the triquetrum (which causes pain if the LT ligament is compromised).[5] A thorough assessment of the SL and LT articulations provides valuable information regarding dissociative wrist instability.

Plain radiographs should be obtained in all patients. Instability identified on plain radiographs is termed static, whereas stress radiographs (such as the clenched fist view) are needed to diagnose dynamic instability. In static SL instability, the scaphoid flexes and the lunate extends. This instability is manifested as an increased SL angle (> 70°) on the lateral radiograph, a ring sign caused by viewing the scaphoid tuberosity en fosse (ring to

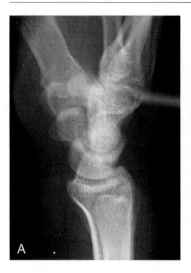 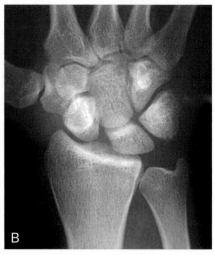 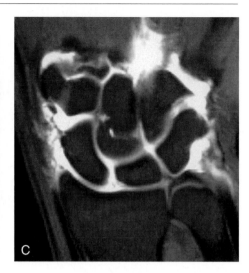

Figure 1 A, Lateral radiograph of the wrist demonstrates extension of the lunate and an SL angle greater than 70°, which suggests a complete SL ligament tear. **B,** PA radiograph of the wrist demonstrates an SL gap of more than 3 mm and a ring sign (ring to proximal pole distance < 7 mm). Both of these findings suggest a complete SL tear. **C,** MRI arthrogram demonstrates free flow of contrast between the radiocarpal and midcarpal joints, confirming a complete SL ligament tear.

proximal pole distance, < 7 mm) (Figure 1, *A*), and a widening of the SL joint (> 3 mm) on the PA radiograph (Figure 1, *B*). Isolated LT instability is rarely identified on plain radiographs but may be diagnosed by carpal arc incongruity.[6]

A patient with point tenderness at either the SL or LT ligament with negative provocative maneuvers and negative radiographs usually warrants additional evaluation. Although immobilization can be considered to help with discomfort, it may only delay a diagnosis. MRI arthrogram is recommended to evaluate the carpus to rule out a wrist ligament tear that would benefit from early repair (Figure 1, *C*). Alternatively, the evaluation can proceed directly to wrist arthroscopy that allows diagnosis and treatment. In patients with point tenderness at the SL or LT ligament, positive provocative maneuvers (different from the contralateral extremity) and negative radiographs, MRI arthrogram, or arthroscopy can be considered.

Arthroscopy

Arthroscopy has become the gold standard for the evaluation of the SL, LT, radiocarpal, and ulnocarpal ligaments.[7,8] Arthroscopy also has a role in the treatment of patients with dynamic wrist instability and those patients with partial ligament injuries. Arthroscopy does not yet have a principal role in the treatment of patients with static instability; the open approach remains the gold standard for treating these patients. The arthroscopic classification of interosseous ligament injuries by Geissler and associates[9] is helpful in guiding treatment. Grade I injuries show ligament attenuation without incongruency; grade II injuries include slight incongruency and gapping (less than a probe width); grade III injuries show incongruency and the ability to pass a probe between the two bones; and grade IV injuries show marked incongruency and allow the placement of the arthroscope between the two bones.

Treatment

Dissociative instability occurs within a carpal row and most commonly involves the SL or LT ligaments. Nondissociative instability, such as midcarpal instability, occurs between carpal rows. The SL interosseous ligament plays a key role in maintaining the normal alignment between the scaphoid and the lunate bones. Its dorsal segment is its strongest area (resistance to distraction force, 250 N).[10] However, static SL instability probably requires the injury of additional ligaments including the radioscapho-capitate, the dorsal radiocarpal, the dorsal intercarpal, and perhaps the scaphotrapezial ligament. In patients with static injuries of less than 3 weeks duration, an isolated repair of the dorsal SL ligament is performed if technically feasible. Reduction is facilitated with Kirschner wires used as joysticks to flex the lunate and extend the scaphoid.[11,12] Kirschner wires are used to stabilize the repair (for 8 weeks), and suture anchors are used to reattach the ligament. Injuries of 3 to 8 weeks duration are treated with a dorsal capsulodesis in addition to the repair (presuming the scaphoid is mobile). Capsulodesis is added to the procedure to prevent scaphoid flexion and to avoid the development of radial styloid scaphoid arthrosis, which is caused by the altered loading of the scaphoid-distal radius articulation.[13] The traditional Blatt capsulodesis and the Szabo capsulodesis may both be effective in providing a tether to prevent scaphoid flexion and to create a link to stabilize the proximal carpal row.[14,15] The data supporting the use of these treatment options are mixed. Szabo and associates[15] reported clinical results for 22 wrists in 21 patients with chronic, flexible SL instability at follow-up of more than 1 year. Results concerning maintenance of carpal row alignment and the prevention of deformity recurrence were encouraging. Lavernia and associates[16] also reported satisfactory results with capsulodesis in 24 of 27 patients with dynamic or static instability. Both the SL angle and gap were improved at the last patient follow-up. However, Wyrick and associates[2] found the results unreliable and Moran and associates[1] reported disappointing outcomes in 31 patients with either chronic dynamic or static instability at an average follow-up of 54 months. Wrist flexion was decreased, grip strength was not improved, and the SL gap and scaphoid flexion worsened over time. Pain was improved but not eliminated in most patients. These findings can be used to question the use of capsulodesis in patients with a chronic (> 3 months) SL injury.

The treatment of patients with an injury of more than 8 weeks duration, or those patients with a less flexible deformity, is controversial because the results of SL interosseous treatment are less than ideal 3 to 4 weeks after injury and uncertain between 3 and 8 weeks after injury; however, there is general consensus that neither repair nor capsulodesis is helpful after 8 weeks. Multiple treatments may be considered although none are widely accepted as uniformly efficacious. Repair and capsulodesis, proximal row carpectomy, scaphoid excision and four-corner arthrodesis (for example, fusion of the lunate, capitate, triquetrum, and hamate), a bone-ligament-bone reconstruction, and a linkage of the scaphoid and the lunate with a screw (the reduction and association of the scaphoid and lunate [RASL] procedure [MP Rosenwasser, MD, personal communication, 2000]) have all been used.[17,18]

Arthroscopy is valuable for the diagnosis and treatment of patients with a dynamic SL instability or a partial tear of the SL or LT ligaments.[19,20] In two retrospective studies, ligament débridement alone provided satisfactory outcomes at 2-year follow-up. Thirteen of 14 patients had excellent pain relief and early return to function after arthroscopic débridement of chronic, partial tears of the SL or LT ligaments.[19] At an average follow-up of 27 months, 85% of patients with a partial SL ligament tear and 100% of patients with a partial LT tear had complete or nearly complete resolution of symptoms and increased strength.[20] Ligament débridement with stabilization using Kirschner wires (for approximately 8 weeks) to provide a fibrous ankylosis also may be used for partial ligament tears; the best results (85% success) were achieved in patients with injuries of less than 3 months duration and a side to side difference of less than 3 mm.[21] Ligament repair is recommended whenever the dorsal segment is torn and reparable.

The arthroscopic grading of the ligament injury can be helpful with a treatment algorithm, but it cannot be used in isolation. The timing of the injury must be considered, and the quality of the ligament should also be evaluated. For example, a grade IV injury of less than 3 weeks duration and with a satisfactory ligament should be treated with an open ligament repair. However, a grade IV ligament injury of 6 weeks duration without satisfactory ligament substance for repair will need alternative treatment such as arthroscopic débridement and pinning or capsulodesis. The same finding at 4 months might lead to a salvage procedure such as scaphoid excision and four-corner arthrodesis.

Dynamic SL instability may be associated with the presence of an occult dorsal wrist ganglion.[22] Arthroscopy may be beneficial in assessing this pathology and in providing effective treatment through arthroscopic excision of the dorsal wrist ganglion. It is uncertain whether the ganglion is caused by the instability. It is likely that treatment of the ganglion (with excision of part of the capsule) leads to the formation of scar tissue, which minimizes symptomatic instability. Rizzo and associates[23] found excellent results after arthroscopic excision of dorsal wrist ganglion. Patients had improved strength and motion without instability. Open excision of ganglion is also efficacious with a resolution of the scapholunate shift in 20 of 21 wrists and excellent functional outcomes.[22]

Dynamic SL instability may also be effectively treated in an open fashion. Capsulodesis alone has been shown to be effective in eliminating pain. Wintman and associates[24] reported excellent results in 15 of 17 patients treated with the Blatt capsulodesis.

Static LT ligament injuries (whether acute or chronic) are much less common than SL ligament injuries; perilunate dislocation and ulnocarpal impaction must be ruled out.[25] The isolated, chronic LT ligament injury may respond to nonsurgical treatment including splinting and corticosteroid injection. For patients in whom nonsurgical treatment is unsuccessful, no one treatment option has been proven superior. Shin and associates[26] compared ligament repair, ligament reconstruction using a strip of extensor carpi ulnaris, and fusion in young patients (average age, 31 years) with nonacute injuries. The patients had an average follow-up of 9 years. Only 8 of 57 patients had ligament reconstructions, but these patients were most likely to avoid complication at 5-year follow-up (69% of these patients had no complications and did not require additional surgery). Patients who had ligament repair and those treated with fusion had markedly higher complication rates and more often needed additional surgery. Although no treatment option was found to be ideal, the group treated with fusion had the worst outcomes.

Summary

Traumatic wrist instability remains a treatment challenge, but advances have improved the ability to maximize outcomes. Early diagnosis is facilitated through the use of MRI arthrogram and wrist arthroscopy. Early treatment in the form of ligament repair or stabilization provides better outcomes.

References

1. Moran SL, Cooney WP, Berger RA, Strickland J: Capsulodesis for the treatment of chronic scapholunate instability. *J Hand Surg [Am]* 2005;30:16-23.

2. Wyrick JD, Youse BD, Kiefhaber TR: Scapholunate ligament repair and capsulodesis for the treatment of static scapholunate dissociation. *J Hand Surg [Br]* 1998;23:776-780.

3. Watson HK, Ashmead Dt, Makhlouf MV: Examination of the scaphoid. *J Hand Surg [Am]* 1988;13:657-660.

4. Reagan DS, Linscheid RL, Dobyns JH: Lunotriquetral sprains. *J Hand Surg [Am]* 1984;9:502-514.

5. Ambrose L, Posner MA: Lunate-triquetral and midcarpal joint instability. *Hand Clin* 1992;8:653-668.

6. Gilula LA, Weeks PM: Post-traumatic ligamentous instabilities of the wrist. *Radiology* 1978;129:641-651.

7. Cooney WP: Evaluation of chronic wrist pain by arthrography, arthroscopy, and arthrotomy. *J Hand Surg [Am]* 1993;18:815-822.

8. Weiss AP, Akelman E, Lambiase R: Comparison of the findings of triple-injection cinearthrography of the wrist with those of arthroscopy. *J Bone Joint Surg Am* 1996;78:348-356.

9. Geissler WB, Freeland AE, Savoie FH, McIntyre LW, Whipple TL: Intracarpal soft-tissue lesions associated with an intra-articular fracture of the distal end of the radius. *J Bone Joint Surg Am* 1996;78:357-365.

10. Berger RA, Imeada T, Berglund L, An KN: Constraint and material properties of the subregions of the scapholunate interosseous ligament. *J Hand Surg [Am]* 1999;24:953-962.

11. Elsaidi GA, Ruch DS, Kuzma GR, Smith BP: Dorsal wrist ligament insertions stabilize the scapholunate interval: Cadaver study. *Clin Orthop Relat Res* 2004;425:152-157.

12. Mitsuyasu H, Patterson RM, Shah MA, Buford WL, Iwamoto Y, Viegas SF: The role of the dorsal intercarpal ligament in dynamic and static scapholunate instability. *J Hand Surg [Am]* 2004;29:279-288.

13. Burgess RC: The effect of rotatory subluxation of the scaphoid on radio-scaphoid contact. *J Hand Surg [Am]* 1987;12:771-774.

14. Blatt G: Capsulodesis in reconstructive hand surgery: Dorsal capsulodesis for the unstable scaphoid and volar capsulodesis following excision of the distal ulna. *Hand Clin* 1987;3:81-102.

15. Szabo RM, Slater RR Jr, Palumbo CF, Gerlach T: Dorsal intercarpal ligament capsulodesis for chronic, static scapholunate dissociation: Clinical results. *J Hand Surg [Am]* 2002;27:978-984.

16. Lavernia CJ, Cohen MS, Taleisnik J: Treatment of scapholunate dissociation by ligamentous repair and capsulodesis. *J Hand Surg [Am]* 1992;17:354-359.

17. Davis CA, Culp RW, Hume EL, Osterman AL: Reconstruction of the scapholunate ligament in a cadaver model using a bone-ligament-bone autograft from the foot. *J Hand Surg [Am]* 1998;23:884-892.

18. Weiss AP: Scapholunate ligament reconstruction using a bone-retinaculum-bone autograft. *J Hand Surg [Am]* 1998;23:205-215.

19. Ruch DS, Poehling GG: Arthroscopic management of partial scapholunate and lunotriquetral injuries of the wrist. *J Hand Surg [Am]* 1996;21:412-417.

20. Weiss AP, Sachar K, Glowacki KA: Arthroscopic debridement alone for intercarpal ligament tears. *J Hand Surg [Am]* 1997;22:344-349.

21. Whipple TL: The role of arthroscopy in the treatment of scapholunate instability. *Hand Clin* 1995;11:37-40.

22. Hwang JJ, Goldfarb CA, Gelberman RH, Boyer MI: The effect of dorsal carpal ganglion excision on the scaphoid shift test. *J Hand Surg [Br]* 1999;24:106-108.

23. Rizzo M, Berger RA, Steinmann SP, Bishop AT: Arthroscopic resection in the management of dorsal wrist ganglions: Results with a minimum 2-year follow-up period. *J Hand Surg [Am]* 2004;29:59-62.

24. Wintman BI, Gelberman RH, Katz JN: Dynamic scapholunate instability: Results of operative treatment with dorsal capsulodesis. *J Hand Surg [Am]* 1995;20:971-979.

25. Palmer AK: Triangular fibrocartilage disorders: Injury patterns and treatment. *Arthroscopy* 1990;6:125-132.

26. Shin AY, Weinstein LP, Berger RA, Bishop AT: Treatment of isolated injuries of the lunotriquetral ligament: A comparison of arthrodesis, ligament reconstruction and ligament repair. *J Bone Joint Surg Br* 2001;83:1023-1028.

Acute Fractures of the Scaphoid

J. Mi Lee Haisman, MD
Rachel S. Rohde, MD
Andrew J. Weiland, MD

Abstract

Fractures of the scaphoid must be treated promptly to minimize the risk of malunion and nonunion. Although most scaphoid fractures have been reported to heal well with cast immobilization, advances in surgical techniques have greatly changed the decision-making process for treatment. It is worthwhile to review the different management options for acute fractures.

Instr Course Lect 2007;56:69-78.

The scaphoid is the most commonly fractured carpal bone, accounting for approximately 60% of carpal fractures and 11% of all hand fractures.[1,2] Often misdiagnosed as a simple wrist sprain, scaphoid fractures may go on to malunion or nonunion. Patients with one of these problems will almost always present later because of persistent wrist pain. Malunions and nonunions are especially challenging conditions to treat successfully and, if untreated, they usually produce abnormal carpal kinematics that can lead to wrist arthrosis.[3,4] Thus, early diagnosis and vigilant care of an

acute scaphoid fracture are warranted.[5,6]

Mechanism of Injury

Scaphoid fractures usually result from a fall. Most commonly, the patient lands on the hand with the wrist in extension and radial deviation.[7-9] Other mechanisms of injury can cause a scaphoid fracture.[9,10] The exact mechanism of failure is a subject of debate. Some have suggested that the scaphoid fails secondary to excessive compression along its concave medial articulation with the capitate, whereas others believe that the scaphoid fails secondary to excessive tension.[10-12]

Weber and Chao[8] created scaphoid fractures in cadavers with the wrist in only 95° to 100° of dorsiflexion and a load applied to the radial portion of the palm. The force was magnified four times at the radioscaphoid joint, and the proximal

pole appeared to be caught between the radius and capitate.

Diagnosis

Patients with a scaphoid fracture most often present with wrist pain. They almost always have tenderness and a fullness in the anatomic snuffbox. Axial compression of the thumb, which compresses the scaphoid, usually elicits pain. Sometimes there is discomfort just with percussion of the tip of an abducted thumb. Forced ulnar deviation of a pronated wrist can also elicit pain.[13]

Pain and tenderness in the anatomic snuffbox should warrant studies to rule out a scaphoid fracture. Even if initial radiographs reveal negative findings, the wrist should be immobilized in a wrist splint or short arm-thumb spica cast and the radiographs should be repeated in 1 to 2 weeks.[14] If a fracture is not seen on the repeat radiographs and a scaphoid fracture is still suspected, CT, MRI, or a bone scan should be done.[15-18] CT is fast, convenient, and the most sensitive and specific of the studies; bone scanning is the least sensitive and specific.[19,20] When the patient has sustained multiple injuries and a scaphoid fracture is suspected, CT

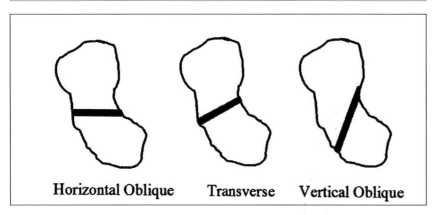

Figure 1   Russe classification of scaphoid fractures.

or MRI should be performed as soon as medically safe and possible. When immobilization will result in a great loss of patient productivity, these additional imaging modalities may be performed at the time of the initial presentation if the plain radiographs reveal negative findings. Associated injuries, including ligamentous injuries, should be considered and looked for, but that is beyond the scope of this review.

Anatomy

Derived from the Greek word *skaphe,* meaning skiff or boat, the scaphoid is named for its likeness to a boat. This is a great simplification; it is shaped more like a banana with a twist. The scaphoid serves a complex role, as is reflected in its osseous anatomy. The entire proximal, distal, and medial surfaces as well as half of the lateral side are covered with articular cartilage.

The main blood supply to the scaphoid is from the radial artery.[21] A dorsal ridge serves as the attachment point for the dorsal joint capsule, and perforating branches from the radial artery supply approximately 75% of the intraosseous blood. Through retrograde flow, the dorsal branches also supply all of the proximal pole. The distal pole appears to have its own abundant blood supply from volar branches of the radial artery. There is a less consistent blood supply through the scapholunate ligament as well.

Obletz and Halbstein[22] examined 297 scaphoids and found that 13% had no foramina proximal to the waist, 20% had only one small foramen proximal to the waist, and 67% had two or more foramina proximal to the waist. Thus, the blood supply to the proximal pole is the most tenuous.

Although the scaphoid is mostly covered with articular cartilage, there are important sites of ligamentous attachment. Along the ulnar aspect of the proximal pole, the scapholunate interosseous ligament, composed of the dorsal, proximal, and palmar regions, links the scaphoid to the lunate.[23,24] When a scaphoid fractures, the proximal fragment tends to extend with the attached lunate, and the distal fragment remains flexed, creating a "humpback" deformity.[3] Attaching directly on the scapholunate interosseous ligament is the radioscapholunate ligament, which acts as a neurovascular conduit. The radioscapholunate ligament is flanked on the radial side by the long radiolunate ligament, which passes along the palmar aspect of the proximal part of the

scaphoid as it inserts on the lunate. Even more radial is the radioscaphocapitate ligament, which has substantial insertions on the waist of the scaphoid.[24]

At the distal articulation of the scaphoid is the v-shaped scaphotrapezial ligament.[25] Just proximal to this attachment along the dorsum is the attachment for the dorsal intercarpal ligament.[26] The scaphocapitate ligament is found almost confluent with the fibro-osseous tunnel of the flexor carpi radialis tendon, which runs directly palmar to the distal pole of the scaphoid as it heads toward the trapezium.[27]

Classification of Fractures

Russe[28] classified scaphoid fractures as horizontal oblique, transverse, or vertical oblique (Figure 1). The vertical oblique type accounts for only 5% of fractures. This fracture pattern results in the most shear forces across the fracture site, thus making it the most unstable type. Horizontal oblique types have the most compressive forces across the fracture site, whereas transverse fractures have a combination of compressive and shear forces.

We prefer to use the classification system devised by Herbert, which incorporates the stability of the fracture as well as delayed unions and nonunions[29] (Figure 2). Type A fractures include fractures of the tubercle (A1) and incomplete fractures through the waist (A2), which are inherently stable patterns. Type B fractures are acute and unstable; they include distal oblique fractures (B1), complete fractures through the waist (B2), proximal pole fractures (B3), and transscaphoid perilunate fracture-dislocations of the carpus (B4). Type C fractures are delayed unions, and type D fractures are established nonunions.

Prosser and associates[30] expanded the classification of distal pole fractures (Figure 3). Type I indicates a tuberosity fracture; type II, a distal intra-articular fracture; and type III, an osteochondral fracture.

Most scaphoid fractures (approximately 75%) occur at the waist, whereas only about 20% occur in the proximal third.[10,28] The least common location is the distal third of the scaphoid, and fractures in that location are more common in children than in adults.[31]

Fracture Management

The true incidence and natural history of scaphoid fractures and the consequences of malunions and nonunions are not known because not all individuals with a scaphoid fracture present for medical attention. This selection bias should be kept in mind when specific studies are used to justify management choices.

The reported nonunion rates of scaphoid fractures range from 5% to 25%.[28,32-34] The factors associated with nonunion include fracture displacement of >1 mm, proximal fracture, osteonecrosis, vertical oblique fracture, and smoking.[35-38]

Mack and associates[39] found that wrist arthritis developed in patients with scaphoid nonunion. In the first 10 years following a scaphoid fracture, the changes were seen only in the scaphoid. In the second decade, there was radioscaphoid arthritis. Pancarpal arthritis ensued after 20 to 30 years. This process was accelerated by displacement or dorsal intercalary segment instability patterns. Mack and associates also found that the fracture location and configuration did not correlate with degenerative changes. In a study of 56 untreated nonunions, Ruby and associates[40] reported that degeneration was present in 31 of 32 patients who had been in-

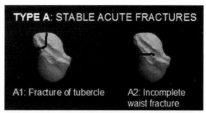

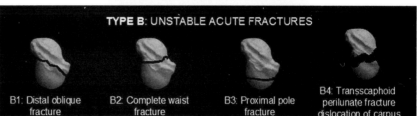

Figure 2   Herbert classification of scaphoid fractures.

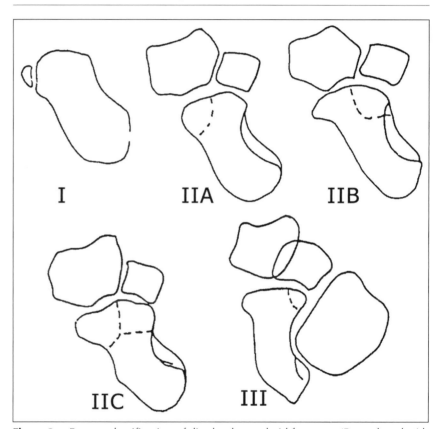

Figure 3   Prosser classification of distal pole scaphoid fractures. (Reproduced with permission from Prosser AJ, Brenkel IJ, Irvine GB: Articular fractures of the distal scaphoid. *J Hand Surg [Br]* 1988;13:87-91.)

jured at least 5 years earlier. Thus, scaphoid nonunion is not an innocuous condition.

Distal Pole Fractures

Fractures of the distal pole of the scaphoid tend to heal well. Most can be treated closed (with 4 to 8 weeks of immobilizaton) and, probably because of the rich vascularization of the distal pole, union is the rule.[30,41] However, displaced intra-articular fractures (Prosser type II) are generally thought to require surgical management to minimize the risk of degenerative arthritis.

Waist Fractures

Fractures of the scaphoid waist can be difficult to manage. Some can be treated closed whereas others should be internally stabilized.

Nondisplaced Waist Fractures It has been reported that >90% of nondisplaced waist fractures treated with immobilization alone unite.[33,42,43] The difficulty is determining which fractures are nondisplaced. A CT scan along the long axis of the scaphoid enables one to assess displacement.[20,44] Determining union is also difficult. Dias and associates[45] reported that critical examination of radiographs at 1 year revealed that the nonunion rate was higher (12.3%) than they had initially suspected. A radiographic assessment of healing at 12 weeks is probably not very reliable. Thus, some scaphoid fractures that are classified as nondisplaced actually might be displaced, and some that are considered to have healed can actually be nonunions.

The treatment options for a nondisplaced waist fracture must be discussed thoroughly with the patient. The patient's lifestyle, expectations, compliance, and demands (for return to work or sports) must all be considered. Although the fracture will most likely heal with cast immobilization, the patient must know the risks, benefits, and alternatives.

The main disadvantages of immobilization, compared with surgery, are more frequent office visits to check that the cast fits properly, more frequent radiographs to check fracture alignment, potential skin breakdown, prolonged immobilization until complete healing has occurred, stiffness of immobilized joints, and even perhaps a longer time to healing.[46] The immobilization period after surgery is shorter or even unnecessary.[46-48] If the fracture has been rigidly fixed, it is safe for the patient to perform gentle range-of-motion exercises. Additional advantages of surgical intervention are that the fracture is substantially less likely to lose its alignment and ideally is fixed with compression, which has been reported to shorten the time to healing.[46] The reduction should be anatomic, and the fixation should be stable. The disadvantages of surgery include the potential for infection; wound complications; injury to nerves, ligaments, or tendons; injury to the vascular supply to the scaphoid; hardware failure or the need for its removal; and other associated risks such as anesthesia complications. Percutaneous stabilization of nondisplaced waist fractures has become popular. The techniques have evolved such that the benefits outweigh the risks, as discussed later.

Displaced Waist Fractures Scaphoid fractures with ≥1 mm of displacement are considered unstable. Cooney and associates[35] defined displacement as a fracture gap of 1 mm seen on any plain radiographic projection, a scapholunate angle of >60°, or a radiolunate angle of >15°. It has also been shown[20] that a displaced fracture tends to have an intrascaphoid angle of >35°. The displaced scaphoid fracture should be reduced and stabilized surgically (unless there are other conditions that contraindicate surgery) because the risk of malunion or nonunion of such a fracture is unacceptable.

Proximal Pole Fractures

Unless surgery is contraindicated or the patient refuses it, acute fractures of the proximal pole of the scaphoid should be treated surgically. The proximal pole has the most tenuous blood supply, which is thought to explain the higher rates of nonunion compared with those of fractures at the distal pole or the waist.[21] Despite the lack of data, it is believed that internal fixation reduces the risk of nonunion and perhaps decreases the chances of proximal fragment collapse due to osteonecrosis.

The choice of fixation depends on the size of the proximal fragment. If the fragment is large enough, a headless compression screw can be used. The type of screw is not as important as the starting point, which should be proximal and dorsal. It is critical to obtain good, preferably central, purchase on the proximal fragment, and ideally the screw should be placed orthogonal to the line of the fracture. If the fragment is too small to accept such a screw, then temporary Kirschner wires can be used to hold the fracture reduced.

Treatment Options
Cast Immobilization

The best method of cast immobilization is controversial. The position of the wrist has not been definitively shown to affect healing.[49] There have been conflicting results associated with immobilization of the elbow and thumb.[50,51] Studies have shown that short arm-thumb spica casts provide adequate immobilization of scaphoid fractures; thus, they are used by us and are accepted widely as a treatment option.[42,52,53]

If cast immobilization is the only treatment chosen, then it should be continued until the fracture has healed. For proximal pole fractures, this can take 12 weeks or longer.[28] Although we are not aware of any data suggesting the superiority of long arm–thumb spica casts over short arm–thumb spica casts, we initially immobilize proximal fractures as well as severely comminuted or unstable fractures in a long arm–thumb spica cast.

Prolonged cast immobilization is becoming less well tolerated, especially by younger patients who want to return to work and sports as soon as possible. Patient expectations are now pushing the trend to fix even nondisplaced scaphoid fractures, although long-term outcomes do not seem to differ between open and closed treatment of such fractures.[54] Patients are more satisfied with early mobilization.[48,55]

Open Techniques
Volar Approach
The classic Russe approach to the scaphoid is through a volar exposure.[28] This yields excellent visualization with less risk of injury to the main blood supply, which is on the dorsal side. This exposure is required if an alignment instrument such as the Huene jig is used with a Herbert screw. A longitudinal incision is made just radial to the flexor carpi radialis tendon, which is retracted to the ulnar side. Distally, the incision is carried over the tubercle of the scaphoid, forming a hockey-stick incision. A longitudinal incision then is made in the volar wrist capsule, with care taken not to injure the radioscapho-capitate ligament. The nonarticular portion of the proximal part of the trapezium may need to be resected to gain central access to the distal part of the scaphoid; the capsule here may be incised horizontally to gain access to the scaphotrapezial joint. The fracture is reduced with use of a dental pick or Kirschner wire "joysticks." Anatomic reduction should be achieved before fixation.

This exposure is especially good for inspecting the entire volar surface of the scaphoid. The disadvantages of this approach are the potential for scarring, which could limit wrist extension; a risk of injury to the volar radiocarpal ligaments; and the inability to assess and address the dorsal scapholunate ligament.

With an open volar approach, fixation options are numerous. If the approach was used mainly for reduction purposes, Kirschner wires may be used to stabilize the fracture. A reduction/alignment guide can be used in preparation for a Herbert screw. Alternatively, a guidewire can be passed under fluoroscopic guidance starting at the distal or proximal aspect of the scaphoid in preparation for a cannulated screw system, as will be elaborated on later in this chapter.

Dorsal Approach
The dorsal approach to the scaphoid is centered over Lister's tubercle. A transverse skin incision is made over the proximal pole of the scaphoid. The extensor retinaculum is longitudinally incised to retract the tendons of the second and third dorsal compartments. Care must be taken not to disturb the dorsal ridge, in which the main blood supply to the scaphoid is found. The wrist capsule is incised longitudinally, without injuring the deeper scapholunate ligament. This approach provides excellent visualization of the proximal portion of the scaphoid, especially with the wrist in maximum flexion. This is the preferred open approach to proximal pole fractures. A guidewire can be placed for use with a cannulated screw system or a Herbert screw can be placed freehand.

Percutaneous Techniques
Percutaneous scaphoid fixation is becoming increasingly popular as it

becomes more apparent that many of the risks of the open techniques can be avoided with use of this method.[48] The healing time is at least the same as that associated with cast immobilization.[56] Bond and associates[46] reported that the average time to healing was 7 weeks for patients treated with percutaneous screw fixation compared with 12 weeks for those treated with a cast. In their study, the surgical group was able to return to work after only 8 weeks compared with 15 weeks for the cast immobilization group; there was no functional difference after 2 years.

The basic concept is to place a guidewire percutaneously along the central axis of the scaphoid and then use a cannulated screw system for definitive internal fixation. This approach should be reserved for fractures that are not displaced or that can be anatomically reduced by closed or arthroscopic means. A surgeon must be comfortable using both distal and proximal starting points for the percutaneous techniques.

The key to the procedure is to achieve the most centrally placed screw possible while holding the fracture in compression (W McCallister, MD, et al, unpublished data read at the Annual Meeting of the American Society for Surgery of the Hand, Baltimore, MD, 2001). Slade and Moore[57] reported that the central axis of the scaphoid can be found with fluoroscopic guidance by pronating and flexing the wrist so as to align the distal and proximal poles of the scaphoid in the radiographic beam. The center of the circle formed by the scaphoid on this view is the central axis, and this is where the screw is ideally placed.

The setup for the percutaneous technique requires the use of palpa-

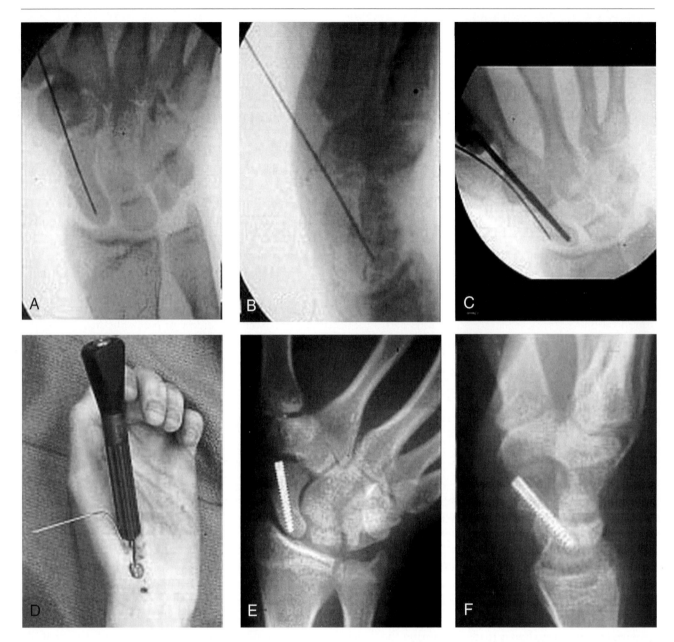

Figure 4 Volar (distal) percutaneous technique. **A** and **B**, Posteroanterior and lateral views of the guidewire. **C** and **D**, Hand-drilling over the guidewire. The derotational wire has been placed. **E** and **F**, Posteroanterior and lateral views of Acutrak Mini screw fixation.

ble osseous landmarks as well as a mini-fluoroscopy unit covered with a sterile drape. The patient is placed supine with the arm supported on a hand table. With the volar percutaneous approach, the distal aspect of the scaphoid is used as the entry point for fixation (Figure 4). Again, this is preferred for distal pole frac-tures that warrant fixation. The guidewire is started palmar at the tubercle, and the trajectory is toward the dorsum of the wrist. Achievement of a good starting point is sometimes aided by removal of overhanging trapezial bone in the area of the scaphotrapezial joint through a limited skin incision. Slade and Moore[57] even advocated starting the guidewire in the trapezium to obtain a central position in the scaphoid.

We prefer to use a 16-gauge needle to find the starting point for the guidewire. It is less likely to perforate the surgeon's gloves or the sterile drape of the mini-fluoroscopy unit than is direct manipulation of the double-cut guidewire. Once proper orientation is confirmed with fluoroscopy, the cannulated screw system of choice is used. Unlike the dorsal approach, this volar approach does not violate the proximal cartilaginous surface of the scaphoid, although studies have shown that this defect subsequently heals.[58,59]

With the dorsal percutaneous approach (Figure 5), the proximal pole of the scaphoid is used as the entry point for fixation. With the wrist in maximum flexion and slight ulnar deviation, the proximal pole of the scaphoid is presented for introduction of the 16-gauge needle through the skin of the dorsal aspect of the wrist. Once the position of the needle is confirmed radiographically, the guidewire can be driven through the needle. The surgeon can hold the needle and stabilize the wrist, making sure of the correct orientation, while the assistant drives the guidewire into the scaphoid. This approach was found to result in the most central screw placement in the distal pole in a cadaver study; however, whether this makes a difference clinically is still to be seen.[60]

Arthroscopy also has been used in conjunction with the percutaneous approach to provide visualization of the fracture site without violation of important structures as can occur with the open technique (Figure 6). If fracture reduction is required, it can be done with fluoroscopic guidance alone or with the aid of arthroscopic visualization and manipulation. A joystick technique can be used to manipulate the fractured ends of the scaphoid, with use of 0.062-inch (1.574-mm) Kirschner wires (preferred) or 0.045-inch (1.143-mm) Kirschner wires (Figure 7). If the fracture is not reducible by closed means or with arthro-

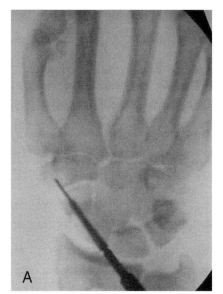 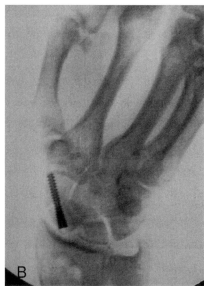

Figure 5   Fluoroscopic views of the dorsal percutaneous technique. The Acutrak Mini 2 screw is self-drilling and tapping over a 0.045-inch (1.143-mm) guidewire.

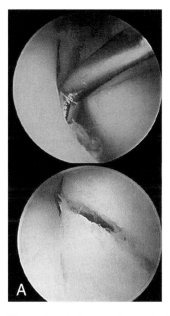 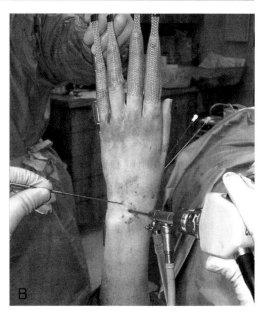

Figure 6   Arthroscopic evaluation (**A**) and clinical photograph (**B**) of scaphoid fracture reduction and ligaments through a midcarpal portal. (Courtesy of Joseph F. Slade III, MD.)

scopic assistance, then an open approach is recommended in lieu of the percutaneous approach. The arthroscopic technique also allows assessment for other associated intra-articular injuries such as ligamentous structures.

There are many choices for fixation with the percutaneous technique (Figure 8). AO screws with prominent heads have been replaced in popularity by headless compression screws. The Herbert screw (Zimmer, Warsaw, Indiana) was the original

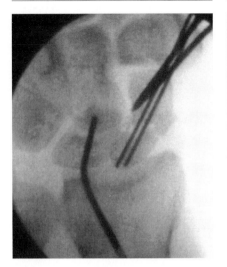

Figure 7 Percutaneous reduction of a displaced scaphoid fracture. A guidewire is passed from proximal to distal and is withdrawn volarly past the fracture site until fracture reduction has been achieved. To aid in reduction, joystick Kirschner wires can be placed dorsally into the distal pole of the scaphoid and into either the proximal pole or the lunate. A small curved hemostat also can be introduced percutaneously for difficult reductions. Once fracture reduction is obtained, the guidewire is passed retrograde through the fracture site and out the dorsum of the wrist, in preparation for a cannulated screw system. An additional stabilizing or derotational Kirschner wire is shown here. (Courtesy of Joseph F. Slade III, MD.)

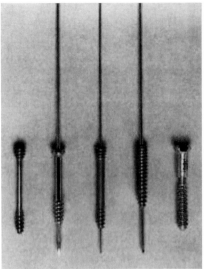

Figure 8 Fixation screws for the scaphoid. From left: Herbert screw, AO 3.5-mm cannulated screw, Herbert-Whipple screw, Acutrak cannulated screw, and Universal Compression screw. (Reproduced with permission from Toby EB, Butler TE, McCormack TJ, Jayaraman G: A comparison of fixation screws for the scaphoid during application of cyclical bending loads. *J Bone Joint Surg Am* 1997;79:1191.)

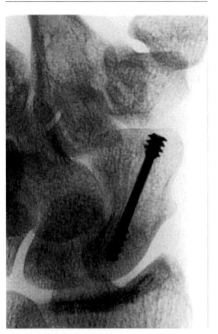

Figure 9 Herbert-Whipple screw for a scaphoid fracture.

headless compression screw introduced for use in the scaphoid, but it is not cannulated and it is practical only for use with the open technique. The Herbert-Whipple screw (Zimmer) (Figure 9) and the Acutrak screw (Acumed, Hillsboro, Oregon) are cannulated. Biomechanical studies have shown that wider screws provide better resistance to lateral displacement forces, as their resistance is proportional to the radius of the screw to the fourth power.[61] In a comparison of the screws loaded cyclically, the Acutrak screw was found to be the strongest, was the least likely to fail

catastrophically, and produced the most compression.[61,62] The Acutrak Standard screw (used with a 0.045-inch [1.143-mm] guidewire, 2-mm hex size) and the Acutrak Mini screw (used with a 0.035-inch [0.889-mm] guidewire, 1.5-mm hex size) are not self-drilling. The new Acutrak Mini 2 screw (1.5-mm hex size) is self-drilling and self-tapping, which makes it convenient to advance over a 0.045-inch (1.143-mm) guidewire. We prefer to use the Acutrak Mini 2 screw because of the smaller defect that is created in the surface of the scaphoid, the larger guidewire (less risk of breakage), and the ease of placement without having to predrill or tap.

The chosen implant should be buried below the level of the cartilage on both ends of the scaphoid to prevent the development of radio-

scaphoid or scaphotrapezial arthritis. When measuring the length of the screw according to the manufacturer's directions, one must consider that the screw length is often about 4 mm shorter than the measured guidewire, which will render it approximately 2 mm countersunk at each end. If arthroscopy is used, screw placement can be confirmed to be deep to the articular surface of the scaphoid.

Summary

We consider surgery to be indicated for all displaced scaphoid fractures, proximal pole fractures regardless of displacement, fractures associated with perilunate injuries, open fractures, and fractures in multiply injured patients. Other decision-making factors are whether there is a great potential for morbidity from prolonged immobilization, the occupation of the patient, and a lack of evidence of healing after 3 to 4 months of conservative treatment of the fracture.

References

1. Hove LM: Epidemiology of scaphoid fractures in Bergen, Norway. *Scand J Plast Reconstr Surg Hand Surg* 1999;33:423-426.

2. Sherman SB, Greenspan A, Norman A: Osteonecrosis of the distal pole of the carpal scaphoid following fracture: A rare complication. *Skeletal Radiol* 1983;9:189-191.

3. Amadio PC, Berquist TH, Smith DK, Ilstrup DM, Cooney WP III, Linscheid RL: Scaphoid malunion. *J Hand Surg [Am]* 1989;14:679-687.

4. Lindstrom G, Nystrom A: Natural history of scaphoid non-union, with special reference to "asymptomatic" cases. *J Hand Surg [Br]* 1992;17:697-700.

5. Langhoff O, Andersen JL: Consequences of late immobilization of scaphoid fractures. *J Hand Surg [Br]* 1988;13:77-79.

6. Verdan C, Narakas A: Fractures and pseudarthrosis of the scaphoid. *Surg Clin North Am* 1968;48:1083-1095.

7. Frykman G: Fracture of the distal radius including sequelae: Shoulder-hand-finger syndrome, disturbance in the distal radio-ulnar joint and impairment of nerve function. A clinical and experimental study. *Acta Orthop Scand* 1967;(suppl 108):3t.

8. Weber ER, Chao EY: An experimental approach to the mechanism of scaphoid waist fractures. *J Hand Surg [Am]* 1978;3:142-148.

9. Mayfield JK: Mechanism of carpal injuries. *Clin Orthop Relat Res* 1980;149:45-54.

10. Linscheid RL, Weber ER: Scaphoid fractures and nonunion, in Cooney WP, Linscheid RL, Dobyns JH (eds): *The Wrist: Diagnosis and Operative Treatment*. St. Louis, Mosby, 1998, pp 385-430.

11. Cobey MC, White RK: An operation for non-union of fractures of the carpal navicular. *J Bone Joint Surg* 1946;28:757-764.

12. Todd AH: Fractures of the carpal scaphoid. *Br J Surg* 1921;9:7-26.

13. Powell JM, Lloyd GJ, Rintoul RF: New clinical test for fracture of the scaphoid. *Can J Surg* 1988;31:237-238.

14. Sjolin SU, Andersen JC: Clinical fracture of the carpal scaphoid: Supportive bandage or plaster cast immobilization? *J Hand Surg [Br]* 1988;13:75-76.

15. Temple CL, Ross DC, Bennett JD, Garvin GJ, King GJ, Faber KJ: Comparison of sagittal computed tomography and plain film radiography in a scaphoid fracture model. *J Hand Surg [Am]* 2005;30:534-542.

16. Breederveld RS, Tuinebreijer WE: Investigation of computed tomographic scan concurrent criterion validity in doubtful scaphoid fracture of the wrist. *J Trauma* 2004;57:851-854.

17. Kumar S, O'Connor A, Despois M, Galloway H: Use of early magnetic resonance imaging in the diagnosis of occult scaphoid fractures: The CAST Study (Canberra Area Scaphoid Trial). *N Z Med J* 2005;118:U1296.

18. Brooks S, Cicuttini FM, Lim S, Taylor D, Stuckey SL, Wluka AE: Cost effectiveness of adding magnetic resonance imaging to the usual management of suspected scaphoid fractures. *Br J Sports Med* 2005;39:75-79.

19. Bain GI: Clinical utilisation of computed tomography of the scaphoid. *Hand Surg* 1999;4:3-9.

20. Sanders WE: Evaluation of the humpback scaphoid by computed tomography in the longitudinal axial plane of the scaphoid. *J Hand Surg [Am]* 1988;13:182-187.

21. Gelberman RH, Menon J: The vascularity of the scaphoid bone. *J Hand Surg [Am]* 1980;5:508-513.

22. Obletz BE, Halbstein BM: Non-union of fractures of the carpal navicular. *J Bone Joint Surg* 1938;20:424-428.

23. Berger RA: The gross and histologic anatomy of the scapholunate interosseous ligament. *J Hand Surg [Am]* 1996;21:170-178.

24. Berger RA, Landsmeer JM: The palmar radiocarpal ligaments: A study of adult and fetal human wrist joints. *J Hand Surg [Am]* 1990;15:847-854.

25. Bettinger PC, Linscheid RL, Berger RA, Cooney WP III, An KN: An anatomic study of the stabilizing ligaments of the trapezium and trapeziometacarpal joint. *J Hand Surg [Am]* 1999;24:786-798.

26. Viegas SF, Yamaguchi S, Boyd NL, Patterson RM: The dorsal ligaments of the wrist: anatomy, mechanical properties, and function. *J Hand Surg [Am]* 1999;24:456-468.

27. Berger RA: The anatomy of the scaphoid. *Hand Clin* 2001;17:525-532.

28. Russe O: Fracture of the carpal navicular. Diagnosis, non-operative treatment, and operative treatment. *J Bone Joint Surg Am* 1960;42:759-768.

29. Herbert TJ: *Fractured Scaphoid*. St Louis, Quality Medical, 1990.

30. Prosser AJ, Brenkel IJ, Irvine GB: Articular fractures of the distal scaphoid. *J Hand Surg [Br]* 1988;13:87-91.

31. Vahvanen V, Westerlund M: Fracture of the carpal scaphoid in children: A clinical and roentgenological study of 108 cases. *Acta Orthop Scand* 1980;51:909-913.

32. Cooney WP III, Dobyns JH, Linscheid RL: Nonunion of the scaphoid: Analysis of the results from bone grafting. *J Hand Surg [Am]* 1980;5:343-354.

33. Leslie IJ, Dickson RA: The fractured carpal scaphoid: Natural history and factors influencing outcome. *J Bone Joint Surg Br* 1981;63:225-230.

34. Linscheid RL, Dobyns JH, Beabout JW, Bryan RS: Traumatic instability of the wrist: diagnosis, classification, and pathomechanics. *J Bone Joint Surg Am* 2002;84:142.

35. Cooney WP, Dobyns JH, Linscheid RL: Fractures of the scaphoid: A rational approach to management. *Clin Orthop Relat Res* 1980;149:90-97.

36. Nolte PA, van der Krans A, Patka P, Janssen IM, Ryaby JP, Albers GH: Low-intensity pulsed ultrasound in the treatment of nonunions. *J Trauma* 2001;51:693-703.

37. Szabo RM, Manske D: Displaced fractures of the scaphoid. *Clin Orthop Relat Res* 1988;230:30-38.

38. Eddeland A, Eiken O, Hellgren E, Ohlsson NM: Fractures of the scaphoid. *Scand J Plast Reconstr Surg* 1975;9:234-239.

39. Mack GR, Bosse MJ, Gelberman RH, Yu E: The natural history of scaphoid non-union. *J Bone Joint Surg Am* 1984;66:504-509.

40. Ruby LK, Stinson J, Belsky MR: The natural history of scaphoid non-union. A review of fifty-five cases. *J Bone Joint Surg Am* 1985;67:428-432.

41. Mody BS, Belliappa PP, Dias JJ, Barton NJ: Nonunion of fractures of the scaphoid tuberosity. *J Bone Joint Surg Br* 1993;75:423-425.

42. Gellman H, Caputo RJ, Carter V, Aboulafia A, McKay M: Comparison of short and long thumb-spica casts for non-displaced fractures of the carpal scaphoid. *J Bone Joint Surg Am* 1989;71:354-357.

43. McLaughlin HL, Parkes JC II: Fracture of the carpal navicular (scaphoid) bone: Gradations in therapy based upon pathology. *J Trauma* 1969;9:311-319.

44. Nakamura R, Imaeda T, Horii E, Miura T, Hayakawa N: Analysis of scaphoid fracture displacement by three-dimensional computed tomography. *J Hand Surg [Am]* 1991;16:485-492.

45. Dias JJ, Brenkel IJ, Finlay DB: Patterns of union in fractures of the waist of the scaphoid. *J Bone Joint Surg Br* 1989;71:307-310.

46. Bond CD, Shin AY, McBride MT, Dao KD: Percutaneous screw fixation or cast immobilization for nondisplaced scaphoid fractures. *J Bone Joint Surg Am* 2001;83:483-488.

47. Herbert TJ, Fisher WE: Management of the fractured scaphoid using a new bone screw. *J Bone Joint Surg Br* 1984;66:114-123.

48. Haddad FS, Goddard NJ: Acute percutaneous scaphoid fixation: A pilot study. *J Bone Joint Surg Br* 1998;80:95-99.

49. Hambidge JE, Desai VV, Schranz PJ, Compson JP, Davis TR, Barton NJ: Acute fractures of the scaphoid: Treatment by cast immobilisation with the wrist in flexion or extension? *J Bone Joint Surg Br* 1999;81:91-92.

50. Clay NR, Dias JJ, Costigan PS, Gregg PJ, Barton NJ: Need the thumb be immobilised in scaphoid fractures? A randomised prospective trial. *J Bone Joint Surg Br* 1991;73:828-832.

51. Kaneshiro SA, Failla JM, Tashman S: Scaphoid fracture displacement with forearm rotation in a short-arm thumb spica cast. *J Hand Surg [Am]* 1999;24:984-991.

52. McAdams TR, Spisak S, Beaulieu CF, Ladd AL: The effect of pronation and supination on the minimally displaced scaphoid fracture. *Clin Orthop Relat Res* 2003;411:255-259.

53. Terkelsen CJ, Jepsen JM: Treatment of scaphoid fractures with a removable cast. *Acta Orthop Scand* 1988;59:452-453.

54. Saeden B, Tornkvist H, Ponzer S, Hoglund M: Fracture of the carpal scaphoid: A prospective, randomised 12-year follow-up comparing operative and conservative treatment. *J Bone Joint Surg Br* 2001;83:230-234.

55. Rettig AC, Kollias SC: Internal fixation of acute stable scaphoid fractures in the athlete. *Am J Sports Med* 1996;24:182-186.

56. Adolfsson L, Lindau T, Arner M: Acutrak screw fixation versus cast immobilisation for undisplaced scaphoid waist fractures. *J Hand Surg [Br]* 2001;26:192-195.

57. Slade JF, Moore AE: Dorsal percutaneous fixation of stable, unstable, and displaced scaphoid fractures and selected nonunions. *Atlas Hand Clin* 2003;8:1.

58. Slade JF III, Grauer JN, Mahoney JD: Arthroscopic reduction and percutaneous fixation of scaphoid fractures with a novel dorsal technique. *Orthop Clin North Am* 2001;32:247-261.

59. Salter RB: The physiologic basis of continuous passive motion for articular cartilage healing and regeneration. *Hand Clin* 1994;10:211-219.

60. Chan KW, McAdams TR: Central screw placement in percutaneous screw scaphoid fixation: a cadaveric comparison of proximal and distal techniques. *J Hand Surg [Am]* 2004;29:74-79.

61. Toby EB, Butler TE, McCormack TJ, Jayaraman G: A comparison of fixation screws for the scaphoid during application of cyclical bending loads. *J Bone Joint Surg Am* 1997;79:1190-1197.

62. Wheeler DL, McLoughlin SW: Biomechanical assessment of compression screws. *Clin Orthop Relat Res* 1998;350:237-245.

Distal Radioulnar Joint Instability

Robert M. Szabo, MD, MPH

Abstract

The distal radioulnar joint is inherently unstable. Pathologic instability can be acute or chronic; it can be dorsal, palmar, or multidirectional; and it can result primarily from soft-tissue injury or osseous malunion. Recognition of the type and cause of instability is fundamental to provide effective treatment.

Instr Course Lect 2007;56:79-89.

The distal radioulnar joint is a distal articulation in the biarticulate rotational arrangement of the forearm. This articulation allows only one degree of motion: pronation and supination. The sigmoid notch of the radius is concave and is shallow with a radius of curvature of 15 mm. The ulnar head is semicylindrical and has an articulate convexity of 220° with a radius of curvature of 10 mm.[1] The ulnar head is surrounded by an ulnar carpal ligament complex. This consists of the ulnolunate and ulnotriquetral ligaments, which originate from the palmar radioulnar ligament near the ulnar styloid process. When seen through an arthroscope, these ligaments appear to be continuous with the triangular fibrocartilage.

Anatomy of the Distal Radioulnar Joint

The triangular fibrocartilage is a fibrocartilaginous disk originating at the junction of the lunate fossa and the sigmoid notch and inserting at the base of the ulnar styloid. Its central portion is cartilaginous, and it is designed for weight bearing. It is also avascular. The peripheral margins are composed of thick lamellar cartilage designed for tensile loading and are called the dorsal and palmar radioulnar ligaments. The peripheral margins of the triangular fibrocartilage are well vascularized from the palmar and dorsal branches of the anterior interosseous artery and from the ulnar artery. The ulnar styloid is the continuation of the subcutaneous ridge of the ulnar shaft, and it stands as a strut on the end of the ulna to stabilize the ulnar soft tissues of the wrist. The sheath of the extensor carpi ulnaris, the ulnocarpal ligaments, and the triangular fibrocartilage help to maintain the congruency of the distal radioulnar joint with attachments at the base of the ulnar styloid; together, they are known as the triangular fibrocartilage complex.[2-6]

The radius of curvature of the ulna does not equal that of the sigmoid notch. Full congruity of two articulating surfaces is therefore not possible. The shallow sigmoid cavity and the difference between the radii of curvature of the sigmoid notch and the ulnar head cause the ulna to translate volarly in supination and dorsally in pronation. In the extremes of forearm rotation, <10% of the ulnar head may be in contact with the notch.[1] Translation is normal. In pronation, the ulna translates 2.8 mm dorsally from a neutral position; in supination, the ulna translates 5.4 mm volarly from a neutral position.[7] The stability of the distal radioulnar joint is provided by the joint surface morphology, the joint capsule, the dorsal and palmar radioulnar ligaments, the interosseous membrane, and the musculotendinous units, primarily the extensor carpi ulnaris and the pronator quadratus.[8,9] The pronator quadratus and the extensor carpi ulnaris are dynamic stabilizers of the distal part of the ulna. The pronator quadratus has a superficial head that is a prime mover in forearm pronation and a deep head that helps to stabilize the distal radioulnar joint.[10] The pronator quadratus actively stabilizes the joint by coapting the ulnar head in the sigmoid notch, particularly in pronation, and it passively stabilizes the joint by vis-

Table 1
Effects of Pronation and Supination on the Dorsal and Palmar Radioulnar Ligaments and Joint Capsule

	Pronation	Supination
Dorsal radioulnar ligament	Tight as ulna displaces dorsally. Dorsal capsule imbrication stabilizes distal radioulnar joint, preventing volar translation of radius	Lax
Palmar radioulnar ligament	Lax	Tight as ulna displaces palmarly. Palmar capsule imbrication stabilizes distal radioulnar joint, preventing dorsal translation of radius

coelastic forces in supination.[11,12] The extensor carpi ulnaris is maintained in its position over the dorsal aspect of the distal part of the ulna by a separate fibro-osseous tunnel deep to and separate from the extensor retinaculum. This separate arrangement allows unrestricted rotation of the radius and ulna. An intact extensor carpi ulnaris and fibro-osseous tunnel partially stabilize the distal radioulnar joint even after the triangular fibrocartilage and other ligaments are sectioned.[13] The important role of the distal radioulnar joint capsule as a restraint and as a contributor to stability was demonstrated by Ward and associates,[14] Watanabe and associates,[15] and Marangoz and Leblebicioglu.[16] Its complementary role in posttraumatic limitations of forearm rotation was described by Kleinman and Graham.[17]

The triangular fibrocartilage, the ulnar carpal ligaments, the infratendinous extensor retinaculum, the pronator quadratus, and the interosseous membrane provide additional key soft-tissue constraints. The triangular fibrocartilage attaches to the fovea in the ulna by way of the dorsal and palmar radioulnar ligaments. The fibers that insert into the fovea are separated from those that insert into the sty-

loid by an areolar vascular tissue known as the ligamentum subcruentum.[18] There is a debate in the literature regarding the radioulnar ligaments. According to Schuind and associates,[19] in pronation the dorsal radioulnar ligament tightens as the ulna translates dorsally and in supination the palmar radioulnar ligament tightens as the ulna translates palmarly (Table 1). In contrast, Ekenstam[20] showed that in pronation the palmar radioulnar ligament becomes taut (although the dorsal capsule tightens) as the ulna translates dorsally, and in supination the dorsal radioulnar ligament tightens (although the palmar capsule becomes tight) as the ulna translates volarly. Ekenstam believed that stability in pronation depends on the tension in the volar radioulnar ligament and compression between the contact areas of the dorsal aspect of the sigmoid notch and the ulna, whereas stability in supination depends on the tension in the dorsal radioulnar ligament and the triangular fibrocartilage articular disk as well as compression between the contact areas of the volar aspect of the sigmoid notch and the ulna.

Adams and Holley[21] measured strain on the surface of the triangular fibrocartilage articular disk and calculated the strain at the dorsal and

palmar margins of the disk. In supination, strain increased dorsally; in pronation, strain increased palmarly. In a biomechanical study of 11 fresh cadavers, Ward and associates[14] measured tension in the dorsal and palmar radioulnar ligaments, joint rotation, and radial translation after sequential excision of the disk, interosseous membrane, joint capsule, and radioulnar ligaments. This experiment confirmed that the dorsal ligament tightens during pronation while the palmar ligament becomes progressively lax, whereas the converse occurs during supination.

The preponderance of biomechanical evidence supports the findings reported by Schuind and associates,[19] and the inconsistency between their observations and those presented by Ekenstam[20] can be resolved because, in pronation, the dorsal radioulnar ligament tightens and tends to displace the ulna dorsally. Left unconstrained, this dynamic tensioning would lead to subluxation and dislocation of the joint. The palmar radioulnar ligament checks that force and keeps the joint reduced. If the interosseous membrane is disrupted and the palmar radioulnar ligament is sectioned, the distal part of the ulna dislocates dorsally in pronation. If the interosseous membrane is disrupted and the dorsal radioulnar ligament is sectioned, the distal part of the ulna dislocates palmarly in supination.

Classification
Disorders of the distal radioulnar joint can be classified into four categories: (1) impaction, (2) incongruity, (3) inflammation, and (4) instability. All of these disorders can produce pain around the distal radioulnar joint and should be considered when a patient reports symptoms at the distal radioulnar joint.

Ulnar impaction is the result of a positive ulnar variance that causes the distal part of the ulna to abut against the lunate, often leading to thinning of the triangular fibrocartilage and eventually to a central tear. Some surgeons also refer to this as ulnar abutment syndrome. Incongruity refers to the lack of a smooth interface between the ulnar head and the sigmoid notch. Incongruity can be caused by a posttraumatic condition such as a distal radial fracture into the sigmoid notch, or it can be secondary to osteoarthritis or rheumatoid arthritis. Inflammation around the distal radioulnar joint is usually caused by extensor carpi ulnaris tendinitis dorsally or flexor carpi ulnaris tendinitis palmarly, and sometimes these disorders can be of a calcific variety.

Instability of the distal radioulnar joint may be acute or chronic and may be related to osseous changes after a fracture or to soft-tissue injury. Soft-tissue injury of the triangular fibrocartilage, dorsal radioulnar ligament, palmar radioulnar ligament, interosseous membrane, joint capsule, or any combination of those structures is capable of producing instability of the distal radioulnar joint. Fractures of the distal part of the radius or distal part of the ulna alter the biomechanics of the distal radioulnar joint.[22] It is important to keep in mind that instability can occur alone or in conjunction with impaction, incongruity, or inflammation. Treatment must be directed at each component of the disease complex.

Examination of the Distal Radioulnar Joint

To examine the ulnar styloid, one should follow the superficial border of the ulnar shaft distally while the wrist is in radial deviation. The ulnar styloid can be found more volarly than anticipated. This maneuver should be done with the wrist in a pronated position. The distal radioulnar joint is the most complex structure to evaluate. The most common pathologic finding is radioulnar incongruity secondary to a malunited distal radial fracture with loss of the pronation-supination arc. With loss of the volar tilt of the radius, the distal part of the ulna appears to be more prominent. With ulnar impaction, ulnar deviation and extension are limited and can be painful. The areas of pronation, supination, and flexion-extension should be determined. To test for instability of the distal radioulnar joint, the examiner should supinate the wrist while supporting the hand, perform a ballottement maneuver of the distal part of the ulna, and compare the affected side with the normal side. During this maneuver, the examiner should feel for crepitus and ask the patient if pain occurs. To check for instability of the extensor carpi ulnaris tendon, the patient should be asked to flex the elbow and pronate and supinate the forearm with the hand in slight ulnar deviation while the examiner looks for abnormal motion of the extensor carpi ulnaris tendon. Peripheral tears of the triangular fibrocartilage complex can produce instability of the distal radioulnar joint with the wrist in supination. With the patient's forearm in supination, the examiner should hold the distal part of the ulna between the thumb and index finger and test for dorsal and volar displacement of the distal part of the ulna. The so-called press-test is a simple assessment. The patient is asked to push up from a seated position using the affected wrist. This test creates an axial ulnar load and has a high sensitivity for detecting a tear of the triangular fibrocartilage complex.[23] Pain with this maneuver suggests that there is a lesion in the triangular fibrocartilage complex.

Radiographic Tests

Standard radiographs of the distal part of the ulna should be made with comparison views of the unaffected side. The images should include a true lateral radiograph made with the forearm in neutral rotation. Any deviation of >10° from a true lateral view will greatly reduce the accuracy of the examination. Ulnar variance should be measured and compared with that on the contralateral side on radiographs made with the forearm in neutral rotation and the shoulder and elbow in 90° of flexion with the x-ray beam directed from posterior to anterior.[24] Ulnar variance changes by up to a millimeter as the forearm moves from full supination to full pronation; therefore, this standard position should be used. Ulnar variance is measured by drawing a transverse line at the level of the lunate fossa and a second transverse line at the level of the ulnar head, and determining the distance between the two lines. On the posteroanterior radiograph, one should look for a fleck fracture demonstrating an avulsion of the triangular fibrocartilage complex, an ulnar styloid nonunion, and joint widening between the radius and ulna (Figure 1). Radiographic signs of injury to the distal radioulnar joint include a fracture at the base of the ulnar styloid, widening of the distal radioulnar joint space seen on the posteroanterior radiograph, >20° of dorsal radial angulation, and >5 mm of proximal displacement of the distal part of the radius.

CT scanning is the technique of choice for evaluating congruity of the distal radioulnar joint, but the same information can be obtained

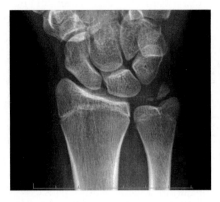

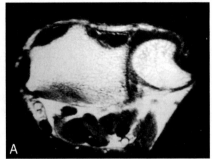

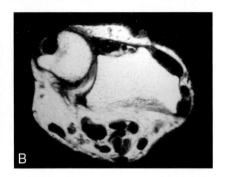

Figure 2 T1-weighted MRI of both wrists in pronation made to compare the normal wrist (**A**) with the wrist that had a dorsal distal ulnar subluxation (**B**).

Figure 1 Posteroanterior radiograph showing a distal radioulnar joint with chronic palmar instability in a 15-year-old girl who had sustained a fracture of the distal part of the radius 2 years previously. Note the large ulnar styloid nonunion fragment and a fleck fracture representing the site where the triangular fibrocartilage complex avulsed from the fovea.

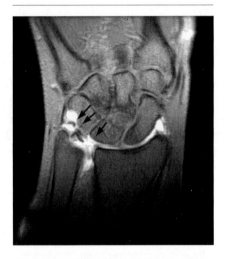

Figure 3 T2-weighted MRI showing a complex peripheral tear (double arrows) and radial tear (single arrow) of the triangular fibrocartilage complex.

with MRI (Figure 2). There are several methods for evaluating subluxation of the distal radioulnar joint, including the method described by Mino and associates,[25,26] the congruency method,[27] the epicenter method,[27] and the radioulnar ratio (RUR) method.[28] MRI is useful for identifying tears of the triangular fi-

brocartilage (Figure 3), but its specificity and sensitivity vary.[29] It is necessary to use high-resolution MRI with a dedicated wrist coil to obtain accurate scans.[30-32] Arthrography is still a valuable examination, and it is even more useful when it is combined with MRI. Arthroscopy is a sensitive method for evaluating tears of the triangular fibrocartilage complex and is considered the gold standard with which to compare the accuracy of other examinations.

Subluxation and Dislocation

By convention, the ulna is considered to dislocate with respect to the radius, but it is the radius that moves and therefore is displaced. With dorsal subluxation, the head of the ulna becomes prominent dorsally, particularly in pronation, and may snap during wrist rotation. This is usually associated with a weak and painful wrist. With complete dislocation, the ulnar head is locked in position, most commonly dorsally but on occasion palmarly. Supination is restricted with either type of dislocation because the radius cannot slip dorsally over the ulnar head.

The mechanism of action for a dorsal subluxation or dislocation of the ulna is extreme pronation and extension with the coiled and tightened extensor carpi ulnaris and ulnar carpal

ligaments acting as a sling to lift the ulnar head through the dorsal capsule. Weakening of the triangular fibrocartilage complex secondary to its avulsion (or a fracture of the ulnar styloid) and attenuation of the palmar radioulnar ligament will allow the dislocation. Sheer stress during this mechanism may produce associated chondral defects. The clinical appearance of a dorsal dislocation of the ulna is a tender prominent dorsally displaced ulna and a forearm with limited supination or locked in pronation. Direct pressure may reduce the dislocation, but the ulnar head usually springs back into a dorsal position if the forearm remains pronated. There is increased anteroposterior translation of the distal radioulnar joint with passive motion. Routine radiographs may be nondiagnostic. A posteroanterior radiograph can show the ulna overlapping the distal part of the radius. The best study with which to visualize a subluxation or dislocation is a CT examination of both wrists performed in both pronation and supination.[25,26,33-35]

Treatment of Acute Dislocations
Dorsal Subluxation and Dislocation
An acute dorsal dislocation can be reduced with digital pressure on the distal part of the ulna and forceful supination. The reduction should

be maintained for 6 weeks. Some authors[36] have advocated full supination, whereas others[37] have recommended the neutral position. Nonsurgical methods of treatment should be used only when there is congruity of the distal radioulnar joint in two planes. Open reduction with repair of the triangular fibrocartilage complex should be performed if the joint is locked and cannot be reduced, or if it is incongruous following reduction. Open repair of the triangular fibrocartilage complex is done with a dorsal incision through the fifth compartment with the extensor digiti minimi reflected radially and the extensor carpi ulnaris reflected ulnarly, thereby exposing the triangular fibrocartilage complex and visualizing the dorsal radioulnar ligament. Nonabsorbable sutures should be used to reattach the triangular fibrocartilage complex to the ulnar styloid.[38]

Ulnar styloid fractures have an important effect on the stability of the triangular fibrocartilage complex. These fractures commonly occur together with fractures of the distal part of the radius and can be a sign of instability of the triangular fibrocartilage complex. Symptomatic nonunions of the styloid can occur. Hauck and associates[2] classified these nonunions as type 1 when the distal radioulnar joint is stable and as type 2 when it is unstable. Type 1 fractures occur through the tip of the styloid, and when they become symptomatic they are often treated successfully with excision. Type 2 fractures occur through the base of the styloid, creating a much larger fragment, and usually open reduction and internal fixation and restoration of the integrity of the triangular fibrocartilage complex are recommended even if there is a nonunion.

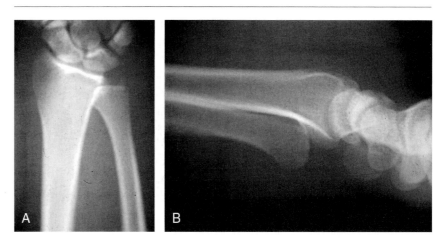

Figure 4 Standard posteroanterior (**A**) and lateral (**B**) radiographs of the wrist, demonstrating palmar dislocation of the ulna.

Palmar Dislocation The distal part of the ulna can dislocate or subluxate palmarly as a result of a fall on a supinated hand or from exertional lifting in supination, with failure of the dorsal radioulnar ligament being the critical event. Clinically, patients present with the forearm held in a supinated position. Pronation is painful and restricted.[39] The ulnar head is palpable volarly, and ulnar dysesthesias may develop from pressure on the ulnar nerve. Once again, a diagnosis can be made on the basis of good standard radiographs (Figure 4) and can be confirmed by comparing CT scans of the affected and normal wrists. A fracture or erosion of the palmar lip of the sigmoid notch may lead to persistent instability. An acute palmar dislocation can be reduced with digital pressure on the distal part of the ulna in a dorsal direction combined with forceful pronation. The treatment of an acute palmar dislocation is closed reduction with immobilization for 6 weeks in an above-the-elbow cast in a neutral or slightly pronated position. Open treatment is reserved for patients for whom closed reduction has failed. The approach is volar with careful retraction of the volar

neurovascular bundle in an ulnar direction.

Tears of the Triangular Fibrocartilage Complex
Triangular fibrocartilage tears can occur without causing instability of the distal radioulnar joint. The most common tear occurs within the articular disk of the triangular fibrocartilage, near its attachment to the radius, and is not associated with instability of the distal radioulnar joint.[40-44] The tears themselves, however, can be unstable and symptomatic. Despite the recognition of specific types of triangular fibrocartilage lesions,[45] the exact mechanisms of injury remain uncertain. Adams and associates,[40] using a laboratory model to simulate distraction of the radius and ulna through the distal radioulnar joint, postulated that such a distraction force may result from a violent axial load on the forearm. This model did not, however, produce the types of tears of the triangular fibrocartilage complex that are seen clinically. Probably, a combination of compression across the wrist trapping the disk in the ulnocarpal joint with distraction or twisting of the distal radioulnar

joint then creates enough shear forces to tear the disk.

Symptomatic instability and tears of the triangular fibrocartilage complex require surgical treatment. The peripheral rim of the triangular fibrocartilage is well vascularized and has good healing potential. Repair of these lesions with a variety of techniques can lead to healing. Historically, open repair was advocated,[38] but currently most peripheral tears can be treated arthroscopically. This arthroscopic approach repairs only the superficial fibers of the triangular fibrocartilage complex to the joint capsule and not the deep portion that inserts onto the fovea. There is much less chance that central tears of the triangular fibrocartilage complex will heal because they are in areas of hypovascularity or avascularity. Arthroscopic débridement of these lesions is recommended.[46]

Chronic Distal Radioulnar Joint Instability
Dorsal, Palmar, or Bidirectional Instability
Chronic distal radioulnar joint instability is a painful and often disabling condition. Functional bracing, which has been tested in a cadaveric model,[47] can be used for patients who do not wish to have surgery, but most patients prefer surgical treatment. It is necessary to check the osseous anatomy in patients with chronic palmar dislocation. Many patients have had a fracture of the wrist or forearm, sometimes many years before symptoms developed at the distal radioulnar joint. Bilateral radiographs of the entire wrist and forearm, made in the same position, should be compared. Osseous malalignment should be corrected. The status of the triangular fibrocartilage complex

is evaluated with either MRI or arthroscopy. If the triangular fibrocartilage complex is not repairable, a tendon reconstruction is needed and should be tightened in supination.[48,49]

Illustrative Case Report An 18-year-old, right-handed man presented with pain in the left wrist and forearm that had been increasing during the previous 2 years. He had sustained a fracture of the distal third of the left radius at the age of 12 years and had been treated nonsurgically. One month later, he fell and sustained a refracture of the radius as well as an ulnar styloid fracture. The fracture of the radius was treated with open reduction and internal fixation through a volar approach. It healed without complication, and the patient returned to full participation in volleyball, weightlifting, soccer, and snowboarding.

Three years later, he noticed swelling about the wrist and had pain at the distal part of the left ulna in association with many activities. Volar angulation of the radius could be seen on radiographs (Figure 5). The triangular fibrocartilage complex appeared normal on the MRI scan. The symptoms were attributed to malunion of the fracture and angular overgrowth of the radius resulting in palmar subluxation of the distal part of the ulna and instability of the distal radioulnar joint. The hardware was removed, and a dome osteotomy of the left radius with iliac crest bone grafting was done. A closing wedge osteotomy of the radius was not performed because of the potential that it could further destabilize the distal radioulnar joint.[50] Eight months after the surgery, the osteotomy site had healed and the patient had regained the preoperative range of wrist motion. The distal radioulnar joint was sta-

ble on examination. He resumed all of his previous activities, including volleyball and weight lifting, without any symptoms in the left upper extremity, and he was discharged from the clinic. He subsequently joined the Marine Corps and wrote to say that he had remained asymptomatic throughout all physical endeavors involved in his strenuous active training.[51]

Dorsal Subluxation and Dislocations With Fractures
Galeazzi Fractures
A Galeazzi fracture is a diaphyseal fracture of the radius associated with a dislocation of the radioulnar joint.[52] A Galeazzi fracture has also been called the "fracture of necessity" because nonsurgical treatment so often yields a poor result. The radioulnar joint may be dislocated or subluxated, and it is always affected (Figure 6). Detection of the disorder of the distal radioulnar joint in a patient with a radial shaft fracture requires a high level of suspicion. Radiographs of the contralateral side may be helpful. Rettig and Raskin[53] found that 12 of 22 fractures of the distal third of the radius (within 7.5 cm of the midarticular surface of the distal part of the radius) were associated with intraoperative instability of the distal radioulnar joint, whereas only 1 of 18 fractures in the middle third of the radial shaft (>7.5 cm from the midarticular surface of the distal part of the radius) was associated with intraoperative instability of the distal radioulnar joint. Open reduction with internal fixation of the radial fracture is the first stage of treatment of a Galeazzi fracture. If the distal radioulnar joint is stable, early motion can be initiated. If it is unstable and reducible, the wrist should be immobilized in slight supination for 4 to 6 weeks. If a sizable

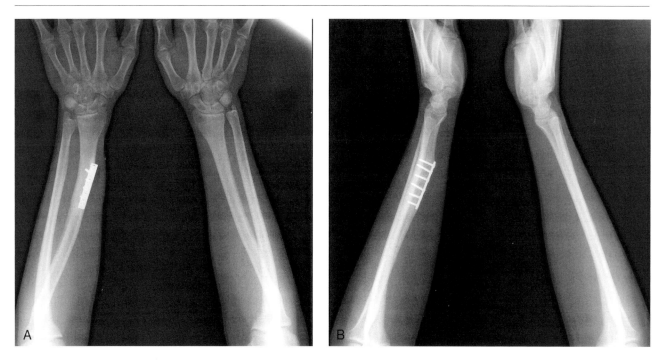

Figure 5   Posteroanterior **(A)** and lateral **(B)** radiographs made 3 years after plate fixation of a fracture of the distal part of the left radius. Note the apex volar angulation of the radius. The normal right side is shown for comparison.

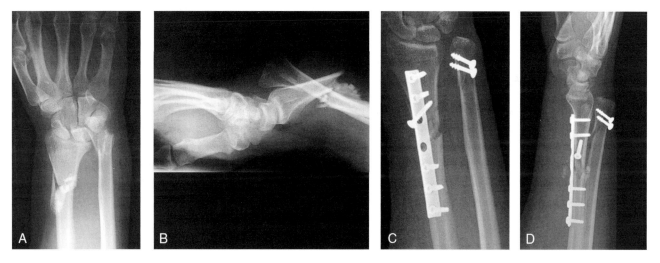

Figure 6   A 28-year-old man was seen with a Galeazzi-type fracture with an entrapped extensor carpi ulnaris tendon preventing reduction of the ulnar styloid that is attached to the triangular fibrocartilage complex. Note the disrupted distal radioulnar joint in addition to the fractures of the radius and distal part of the ulna. **A,** Posteroanterior radiograph showing the injury. **B,** Lateral radiograph showing the injury. **C,** Posteroanterior radiograph made after initial fixation of the radial and ulnar fractures. Note the widening of the distal radioulnar joint. **D,** Lateral radiograph made after initial fixation of the radial and ulnar fractures. Note the dorsal displacement of the ulna. This problem occurred because the initial surgeon did not recognize the interposition of the extensor carpi ulnaris tendon, which prevented the reduction of the ulnar styloid/triangular fibrocartilage complex. Revision was performed, and anatomic reduction and fixation was possible after the extensor carpi ulnaris tendon was repositioned dorsally.

ulnar styloid fracture is present, fixation may allow early mobilization and should be considered. If the distal radioulnar joint is irreducible, open reduction of the joint is necessary; this usually requires repair of the triangular fibrocartilage or fixation of the ulnar styloid fragment. Six weeks of immobilization in slight supination is recommended if the distal radioulnar joint requires surgical treatment. Rarely, the extensor carpi ulnaris is interposed and prevents reduction; if it is, it needs to be removed from the joint[54] (Figure 6, *C* and *D*).

Essex-Lopresti Injuries

Essex-Lopresti injuries, which are severe and disrupt the entire forearm,[55] consist of a radial head fracture with proximal migration of the radius. The migration indicates complete disruption of the interosseous ligament and the triangular fibrocartilage complex. These injuries are usually caused by a fall on the outstretched hand with axial loading. The primary stabilizer preventing proximal migration of the radius is the radial head, and the secondary stabilizers are the interosseous ligament and the triangular fibrocartilage. Diagnosing the wrist injury in this complex is important. Treatment consists of open reduction and internal fixation of the radial head if possible, with immobilization of the forearm in supination. Pinning of the distal radioulnar joint is an option, but if the pins break they can be difficult to retrieve. Comminuted radial head fractures often are not repairable and require replacement, usually with a metallic prosthesis. Silicone radial head replacements have not performed well in this situation because they fracture, causing particulate synovitis, when they are placed under load. The procedure is best done early as delayed treatment can lead to poorer results. The options for delayed surgery include radial head replacement with a prosthesis or allograft,[56] or a Sauvé-Kapandji procedure.

Multidirectional Instability

The axis of forearm motion passes through the fovea of the distal part of the ulna. The deep fibers of the distal radioulnar ligaments, the palmar radioulnar ligament, the trian-

gular fibrocartilage, the ulnolunate ligament, the ulnotriquetral ligament, and the ulnocapitate ligament all insert onto the fovea.[57] These ligamentous attachments are key to the stability of the distal radioulnar joint. The distal radioulnar joint can be stabilized surgically in one of three ways: (1) a repair of the triangular fibrocartilage complex and the distal radioulnar ligaments, (2) an extrinsic soft-tissue reconstruction either with a direct link (that is, a radioulnar tether) or an indirect link (that is, an ulnar carpal sling tenodesis), or (3) a distal radioulnar ligament reconstruction.

Procedures for Stabilization of the Distal Radioulnar Joint

The first option for stabilizing the distal radioulnar joint is to repair the triangular fibrocartilage complex to the fovea, from which it is usually found to be ruptured. When repair is not possible, reconstruction is indicated. There are several procedures for stabilization of the distal radioulnar joint, as described by Hui and Linscheid,[58] Tsai and Stilwell,[59] Breen and Jupiter,[60] Fulkerson and Watson,[61] and Ellison, Boyes, and Bunnell,[1] for example. These are all indirect stabilization procedures through an ulnocarpal sling or tenodesis, or a direct radioulnar tether extrinsic to the joint (the technique described by Fulkerson and Watson). Johnson[11] described a dynamic muscle transfer involving use of the pronator quadratus. Other distal radioulnar stabilization procedures involving reconstruction of the radioulnar ligaments were described by Scheker and associates,[62] Sanders and Hawkins,[63] and Bowers.[64] I am not aware of any long-term follow-up study of an adequate series of patients treated with such procedures. In a biomechanical cadaver model, recon-

structions of the radioulnar ligaments were found to be superior to radioulnar tethering procedures although the results of capsular repair alone most closely matched the kinematics of an intact distal radioulnar joint.[65]

I recommend the procedure described by Adams and associates[48,49] to reconstruct the ligamentous anatomy (Figure 7). Their indications and criteria for ligament reconstruction include unidirectional or bidirectional chronic instability of the distal radioulnar joint, absence of substantial arthritis, and a competent sigmoid notch rim with no residual axial instability of the forearm. Any malunion should be mild or corrected concurrently. Adams and Divelbiss[48] cautioned that, if the volar or dorsal lip of the sigmoid notch is incompetent (shallow), ligament reconstruction may not be sufficient and an opening wedge osteotomy of the distal part of the radius may be required. The procedure is done with use of a dorsal approach through the fifth extensor compartment, which provides direct access to the distal radioulnar joint. Typical findings are a triangular fibrocartilage complex that is torn from the ulna, a torn extensor carpi ulnaris sheath, concomitant carpal ligament injuries, and perhaps an ulnar styloid fracture. Adams and Berger[49] reported that, of 20 patients (12 with bidirectional instability and 8 with unidirectional instability) followed for a minimum of 1 year after the procedure, 18 recovered stability, with an 80% recovery of supination, 84% recovery of pronation, and 88% recovery of grip strength.

Salvage

If there is residual instability after a distal ulnar resection, a flexor carpi ulnaris and extensor carpi ulnaris tenodesis, as described by Breen and

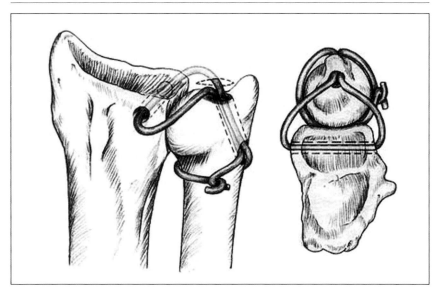

Figure 7 Dorsal and palmar ligament reconstruction, as described by Adams and Divelbiss,[48] for treatment of a chronically unstable distal radioulnar joint. (Reproduced with permission from Adams BD, Berger RA: An anatomic reconstruction of the distal radioulnar ligaments for posttraumatic distal radioulnar joint instability. *J Hand Surg Am* 2002;27:243-251.)

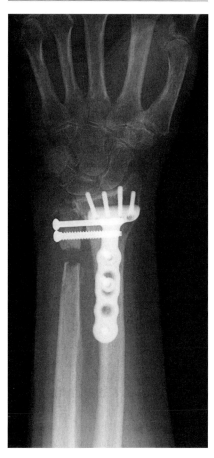

Figure 8 Open reduction and internal fixation was performed to treat a fracture of the distal part of the radius, but the dorsal subluxation of the ulna was never corrected. Arthritic changes developed in the distal radioulnar joint, with pain and limitation of pronation-supination. This problem was treated with a Sauvé-Kapandji procedure.

Jupiter,[60,66] can be considered. Wolfe and associates[67] reported that the distal part of the ulna will remain stable even after removal of more than a third of it. This may be true after a tumor resection, but it is not a reliable assumption after traumatic injuries. Wide resections of the distal part of the ulna usually require some additional form of stabilization, and tenodesis of the flexor carpi ulnaris and extensor carpi ulnaris tendons is recommended. Implantation of a metallic prosthesis to replace the distal part of the ulna can also be considered as a salvage procedure for treatment of this difficult problem.[68] The Sauvé-Kapandji procedure is a useful salvage technique when there is instability of the distal part of the ulna and arthritic changes (Figure 8). The Sauvé-Kapandji procedure involves fusion of the distal radioulnar joint and creation of a pseudarthrosis of the ulna just proximal to the arthrodesis to allow forearm rotation.[69] There can

be subluxation of the proximal ulnar stump, which can be symptomatic, after a Sauvé-Kapandji procedure, and this can be stabilized with either an extensor carpi ulnaris tenodesis, as described by Minami and associates,[70] or a flexor carpi ulnaris tenodesis, as described by Lamey and Fernandez.[71]

Summary

Acute dislocations of the distal radioulnar joint should be reduced promptly and treated with cast immobilization. If the dislocation is irreducible, open reduction is warranted. The first attempts to treat chronic instability should be directed at repairing the triangular fibrocartilage complex, but only after careful assessment for any osseous malunions along the forearm axis, which must also be corrected. If it is not possible to repair the triangular fibrocartilage complex, the osseous architecture is normal, and no arthritis is present, a ligament reconstruc-

tion can be considered, but the competency of the sigmoid notch must be evaluated carefully. If there are arthritic changes at the distal radioulnar joint, a Sauvé-Kapandji procedure should be performed, with stabilization of the proximal stump with a slip of either the flexor carpi ulnaris or the extensor carpi ulnaris.

References

1. Bowers WH: The distal radioulnar joint, in Green DP (ed): *Operative Hand Surgery*,

Vol 1, ed 3. New York, NY, Churchill Livingstone, 1993, pp 973-1019.

2. Hauck RM, Skahen J III, Palmer AK: Classification and treatment of ulnar styloid nonunion. *J Hand Surg [Am]* 1996;21:418-422.

3. Heiple KG, Freehafer AA, Van't Hof A: Isolated traumatic dislocation of the distal end of the ulna or distal radio-ulnar joint. *J Bone Joint Surg Am* 1962;44:1387-1394.

4. Linscheid RL: Biomechanics of the distal radioulnar joint. *Clin Orthop Relat Res* 1992;275:46-55.

5. Palmer AK, Werner FW: The triangular fibrocartilage complex of the wrist—anatomy and function. *J Hand Surg [Am]* 1981;6:153-162.

6. Palmer AK, Linscheid RL, Fisk GR, Taleisnik J: Symposium: Distal ulnar injuries. *Contemp Orthop* 1983;7:81-118.

7. Pirela-Cruz MA, Goll SR, Klug M, Windler D: Stress computed tomography analysis of the distal radioulnar joint: A diagnostic tool for determining translational motion. *J Hand Surg [Am]* 1991;16:75-82.

8. Gofton WT, Gordon KD, Dunning CE, Johnson JA, King GJ: Soft-tissue stabilizers of the distal radioulnar joint: an in vitro kinematic study. *J Hand Surg [Am]* 2004;29:423-431.

9. Kihara H, Short WH, Werner FW, Fortino MD, Palmer AK: The stabilizing mechanism of the distal radioulnar joint during pronation and supination. *J Hand Surg [Am]* 1995;20:930-936.

10. Stuart PR: Pronator quadratus revisited. *J Hand Surg [Br]* 1996;21:714-722.

11. Johnson RK: Stabilization of the distal ulna by transfer of the pronator quadratus origin. *Clin Orthop Relat Res* 1992;275:130-132.

12. Johnson RK, Shrewsbury MM: The pronator quadratus in motions and in stabilization of the radius and ulna at the distal radioulnar joint. *J Hand Surg [Am]* 1976;1:205-209.

13. Spinner M, Kaplan EB: Extensor carpi ulnaris: Its relationship to stability of the distal radio-ulnar joint. *Clin Orthop Relat Res* 1970;68:124-129.

14. Ward LD, Ambrose CG, Masson MV, Levaro F: The role of the distal radioulnar ligaments, interosseous membrane, and joint capsule in distal radioulnar joint stability. *J Hand Surg [Am]* 2000;25:341-351.

15. Watanabe H, Berger RA, An KN, Berglund LJ, Zobitz ME: Stability of the

distal radioulnar joint contributed by the joint capsule. *J Hand Surg [Am]* 2004;29:1114-1120.

16. Marangoz S, Leblebicioglu G: Stability of the distal radioulnar joint contributed by the joint capsule. *J Hand Surg [Am]* 2005;30:868-869.

17. Kleinman WB, Graham TJ: The distal radioulnar joint capsule: Clinical anatomy and role in posttraumatic limitation of forearm rotation. *J Hand Surg [Am]* 1998;23:588-599.

18. Kauer JM: The articular disc of the hand. *Acta Anat (Basel)* 1975;93:590-605.

19. Schuind F, An KN, Berglund L, et al: The distal radioulnar ligaments: A biomechanical study. *J Hand Surg [Am]* 1991;16:1106-1114.

20. Ekenstam F: Osseous anatomy and articular relationships about the distal ulna. *Hand Clin* 1998;14:161-164.

21. Adams BD, Holley KA: Strains in the articular disk of the triangular fibrocartilage complex: A biomechanical study. *J Hand Surg [Am]* 1993;18:919-925.

22. Kihara H, Palmer AK, Werner FW, Short WH, Fortino MD: The effect of dorsally angulated distal radius fractures on distal radioulnar joint congruency and forearm rotation. *J Hand Surg [Am]* 1996;21:40-47.

23. Lester B, Halbrecht J, Levy IM, Gaudinez R: "Press test" for office diagnosis of triangular fibrocartilage complex tears of the wrist. *Ann Plast Surg* 1995;35:41-45.

24. Epner RA, Bowers WH, Guilford WB: Ulna variance: The effect of wrist positioning and roentgen filming technique. *J Hand Surg [Am]* 1982;7:298-305.

25. Mino DE, Palmer AK, Levinsohn EM: The role of radiography and computerized tomography in the diagnosis of subluxation and dislocation of the distal radioulnar joint. *J Hand Surg [Am]* 1983;8:23-31.

26. Mino DE, Palmer AK, Levinsohn EM: Radiography and computerized tomography in the diagnosis of incongruity of the distal radio-ulnar joint: A prospective study. *J Bone Joint Surg Am* 1985;67:247-252.

27. Wechsler RJ, Wehbe MA, Rifkin MD, Edeiken J, Branch HM: Computed tomography diagnosis of distal radioulnar subluxation. *Skeletal Radiol* 1987;16:1-5.

28. Lo IK, MacDermid JC, Bennett JD, Bogoch E, King GJ: The radioulnar ratio: A new method of quantifying distal radioulnar joint subluxation. *J Hand Surg*

[Am] 2001;26:236-243.

29. Steinbach LS, Smith DK: MRI of the wrist. *Clin Imaging* 2000;24:298-322.

30. Potter HG, Asnis-Ernberg L, Weiland AJ, Hotchkiss RN, Peterson MG, McCormack RR Jr: The utility of high-resolution magnetic resonance imaging in the evaluation of the triangular fibrocartilage complex of the wrist. *J Bone Joint Surg Am* 1997;79:1675-1684.

31. Kocharian A, Adkins MC, Amrami KK, et al: Wrist: Improved MR imaging with optimized transmit-receive coil design. *Radiology* 2002;223:870-876.

32. Yoshioka H, Ueno T, Tanaka T, Shindo M, Itai Y: High-resolution MR imaging of triangular fibrocartilage complex (TFCC): Comparison of microscopy coils and a conventional small surface coil. *Skeletal Radiol* 2003;32:575-581.

33. Burk DL Jr, Karasick D, Wechsler RJ: Imaging of the distal radioulnar joint. *Hand Clin* 1991;7:263-275.

34. Cone RO, Szabo R, Resnick D, Gelberman R, Taleisnik J, Gilula LA: Computed tomography of the normal radioulnar joints. *Invest Radiol* 1983;18:541-545.

35. King GJ, McMurtry RY, Rubenstein JD, Ogston NG: Computerized tomography of the distal radioulnar joint: Correlation with ligamentous pathology in a cadaveric model. *J Hand Surg [Am]* 1986;11:711-717.

36. Linscheid RL: Disorders of the distal radioulnar joint, in Cooney WP, Dobyns JH, Linscheid RL (eds): *The Wrist: Diagnosis and Operative Treatment*. St. Louis, MO, Mosby, 1998, p 829.

37. Garcia-Elias M, Dobyns JH: Dorsal and palmar dislocations of the distal radioulnar joint, in Cooney WP, Dobyns JH, Linscheid RL (eds): *The Wrist: Diagnosis and Operative Treatment*. St. Louis, MO, Mosby, 1998, p 768.

38. Hermansdorfer JD, Kleinman WB: Management of chronic peripheral tears of the triangular fibrocartilage complex. *J Hand Surg [Am]* 1991;16:340-346.

39. Singletary EM: Volar dislocation of the distal radioulnar joint. *Ann Emerg Med* 1994;23:881-883.

40. Adams BD, Samani JE, Holley KA: Triangular fibrocartilage injury: A laboratory model. *J Hand Surg [Am]* 1996;21:189-193.

41. Adams BD: Partial excision of the triangular fibrocartilage complex articular

disk: A biomechanical study. *J Hand Surg [Am]* 1993;18:334-340.

42. Chidgey LK, Dell PC, Bittar ES, Spanier SS: Histologic anatomy of the triangular fibrocartilage. *J Hand Surg [Am]* 1991;16:1084-1100.

43. Osterman AL: Arthroscopic debridement of triangular fibrocartilage complex tears. *Arthroscopy* 1990;6:120-124.

44. Reinus WR, Hardy DC, Totty WG, Gilula LA: Arthrographic evaluation of the carpal triangular fibrocartilage complex. *J Hand Surg [Am]* 1987;12:495-503.

45. Palmer AK: Triangular fibrocartilage complex lesions: A classification. *J Hand Surg [Am]* 1989;14:594-606.

46. Minami A, Ishikawa J, Suenaga N, Kasashima T: Clinical results of treatment of triangular fibrocartilage complex tears by arthroscopic debridement. *J Hand Surg [Am]* 1996;21:406-411.

47. Millard GM, Budoff JE, Paravic V, Noble PC: Functional bracing for distal radioulnar joint instability. *J Hand Surg [Am]* 2002;27:972-977.

48. Adams BD, Divelbiss BJ: Reconstruction of the posttraumatic unstable distal radioulnar joint. *Orthop Clin North Am* 2001;32:353-363.

49. Adams BD, Berger RA: An anatomic reconstruction of the distal radioulnar ligaments for posttraumatic distal radioulnar joint instability. *J Hand Surg [Am]* 2002;27:243-251.

50. Nishiwaki M, Nakamura T, Nakao Y, Nagura T, Toyama Y: Ulnar shortening effect on distal radioulnar joint stability: A biomechanical study. *J Hand Surg [Am]* 2005;30:719-726.

51. Williams AA, Szabo RM: Case report: radial overgrowth and deformity after metaphyseal fracture fixation in a child. *Clin Orthop Relat Res* 2005;435:258-262.

52. Galeazzi R: Über ein besonderes syndrom bei verletzungen im bereich der unterarmknochen. *Arch Orthop Unfallchir* 1935;35:557-562.

53. Rettig ME, Raskin KB: Galeazzi fracture-dislocation: A new treatment-oriented classification. *J Hand Surg [Am]* 2001;26:228-235.

54. Alexander AH, Lichtman DM: Irreducible distal radioulnar joint occurring in a Galeazzi fracture—case report. *J Hand Surg [Am]* 1981;6:258-261.

55. Essex-Lopresti P: Fractures of the radial head with distal radio-ulnar dislocation; report of two cases. *J Bone Joint Surg Br* 1951;33:244-247.

56. Szabo RM, Hotchkiss RN, Slater RR Jr: The use of frozen-allograft radial head replacement for treatment of established symptomatic proximal translation of the radius: Preliminary experience in five cases. *J Hand Surg [Am]* 1997;22:269-278.

57. Nakamura T, Takayama S, Horiuchi Y, Yabe Y: Origins and insertions of the triangular fibrocartilage complex: A histological study. *J Hand Surg [Br]* 2001;26:446-454.

58. Hui FC, Linscheid RL: Ulnotriquetral augmentation tenodesis: A reconstructive procedure for dorsal subluxation of the distal radioulnar joint. *J Hand Surg [Am]* 1982;7:230-236.

59. Tsai TM, Stilwell JH: Repair of chronic subluxation of the distal radioulnar joint (ulnar dorsal) using flexor carpi ulnaris tendon. *J Hand Surg [Br]* 1984;9:289-294.

60. Breen TF, Jupiter JB: Extensor carpi ulnaris and flexor carpi ulnaris tenodesis of the unstable distal ulna. *J Hand Surg [Am]* 1989;14:612-617.

61. Fulkerson JP, Watson HK: Congenital anterior subluxation of the distal ulna. A case report. *Clin Orthop Relat Res* 1978;131:179-182.

62. Scheker LR, Belliappa PP, Acosta R, German DS: Reconstruction of the dorsal ligament of the triangular fibrocartilage complex. *J Hand Surg [Br]* 1994;19:310-318.

63. Sanders RA, Hawkins B: Reconstruction of the distal radioulnar joint for chronic volar dislocation. A case report. *Orthopedics* 1989;12:1473-1476.

64. Bowers WH: Distal radioulnar joint arthroplasty. Current concepts. *Clin Orthop Relat Res* 1992;275:104-109.

65. Gofton WT, Gordon KD, Dunning CE, Johnson JA, King GJ: Comparison of distal radioulnar joint reconstructions using an active joint motion simulator. *J Hand Surg [Am]* 2005;30:733-742.

66. Breen TF, Jupiter J: Tenodesis of the chronically unstable distal ulna. *Hand Clin* 1991;7:355-363.

67. Wolfe SW, Mih AD, Hotchkiss RN, Culp RW, Keifhaber TR, Nagle DJ: Wide excision of the distal ulna: a multicenter case study. *J Hand Surg [Am]* 1998;23:222-228.

68. Masaoka S, Longsworth SH, Werner FW, Short WH, Green JK: Biomechanical analysis of two ulnar head prostheses. *J Hand Surg [Am]* 2002;27:845-853.

69. Sauvé L, Kapandji M: Nouvelle technique de traitement chirurgical des luxations récidivantes isolées de l'extrémité inférieure du cubitus. *J Chir (Paris)* 1936;47:589-594.

70. Minami A, Suzuki K, Suenaga N, Ishikawa J: The Sauvé-Kapandji procedure for osteoarthritis of the distal radioulnar joint. *J Hand Surg [Am]* 1995;20:602-608.

71. Lamey DM, Fernandez DL: Results of the modified Sauvé-Kapandji procedure in the treatment of chronic posttraumatic derangement of the distal radioulnar joint. *J Bone Joint Surg Am* 1998;80:1758-1769.

Posttraumatic Reconstruction in the Hand

Jesse B. Jupiter, MD
Charles A. Goldfarb, MD
Ladislav Nagy, MD
Martin I. Boyer, MD, MSc, FRCS(C)

Abstract

The complex anatomy of the hand means that injuries result in substantial loss of function. The damage must be repaired to regain the lost function. Fractures need to heal in anatomic position, and the soft tissues must be supple so that the fingers can move through a useful range of motion. Evaluation and management of malunion, nonunion, bone loss, and stiff fingers are important factors in posttraumatic reconstruction of the hand.

Instr Course Lect 2007;56:91-99.

Deformity is the most common complication following fracture.[1,2] Although this chapter focuses on the indications, techniques, and outcomes of reconstructive surgery, it is clear that the optimal management of deformity is prevention. Treatment of a fracture in the hand must include a careful evaluation of rotational and angular alignment with the digits both extended and flexed.

Malunion and Nonunion of the Phalanges and Metacarpals

Deformity of the phalanges or metacarpals can be classified on the basis of the involved bone, the location of the deformity (intra-articular or extra-articular), the type of deformity (offset, angulation, rotation, or a combination), the patient's age (child or adult), and whether it is an isolated skeletal lesion or is associated with soft-tissue complications.

Phalangeal malunion may produce rotation, volar angulation, lateral angulation, and shortening, or, more often than not, a combination of these deformities.[3-6] Rotational deformities of as little as 10° can lead to scissoring of the involved digit onto an adjacent one[7] (Figure 1). Apex volar angular deformities are more likely to occur following transverse phalangeal fractures and result in a so-called pseudoclaw deformity. Lateral angular deformities may be the sequelae of more complex injuries resulting in deficient bone on one side of the diaphysis. Surgical correction of either apex volar or lateral angular malunion is achieved with either opening or closing wedge osteotomies.[1,5,8,9]

Isolated phalangeal shortening may be the sequela of spiral, long oblique, or highly comminuted fractures. On occasion, some compromise in digital flexion results from an osseous spike projecting volarly.[10,11]

Metacarpal deformity, a frequent result of fracture, is better tolerated than deformities involving the phalanges and therefore may require surgical intervention less often.[12-15] Fractures of the metacarpal neck, or so-called boxers' fractures, are frequent injuries and often result in flexion deformities at the fracture site, which usually do not cause clinical problems. Deformities involving the metacarpal neck of the index or long finger can produce functional problems such as a prominent metacarpal head in the palm, especially if the volar angulation exceeds 10°; deformities of as much as 50° may be well tolerated in the metacarpal of the little finger.[2,12-17]

Rotational deformities of <10° at the metacarpal level produce minimal functional or cosmetic problems, but >10° of rotational malalignment results in angular deviation and rotation of the involved digit.[15,18-20]

Although a volar angular malunion of the metacarpal neck may be

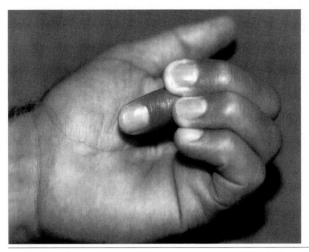

Figure 1 Rotational malunion affects the function of adjacent digits as well as the arc of digital motion. (Reproduced with permission from Faierman E, Jupiter JB: Deformity and nonunion following fractures, in Tubiana R, Gilbert A (eds): *Bone and Joint Disorders*. London, England, Martin Dunitz, 2002, pp 153-170.)

well tolerated, when this deformity lies closer to the middle of the diaphysis, the functional and cosmetic problems are substantial. Midshaft malunion of >20° in any of the four metacarpals usually requires surgical correction.[20-26]

Intra-articular malunions may result in pain, limited motion, and/or deformity. Early intervention with osteotomy and realignment, when the original fracture lines are still identifiable, may provide acceptable results.[5,27-31] Most reported cases in which intra-articular osteotomy was performed have involved the proximal interphalangeal joint.[27-30] There is limited published experience regarding intra-articular malunions of the metacarpophalangeal joints.[21,30,31] There has been more experience with intra-articular osteotomies of the base of the thumb metacarpal, with the caveat that early recognition and intervention are necessary for a successful functional result.[30-36] Alternatives to corrective osteotomy for intra-articular malunions include excision of osteocartilaginous spurs, arthroplasty, or arthrodesis.

The evaluation of a malunited fracture should include a thorough assessment of the overlying soft-tissue envelope, the neurovascular status,

the articular mobility, and the characteristics of the deformity itself. A simple deformity consists of only a skeletal injury whereas a complex malunion involves associated soft-tissue and/or articular dysfunction. Extra-articular malunions can adversely affect the function of adjacent digits, limit the overall arc of digital motion, disturb the normal muscle-tendon balance, or decrease grip strength.[5,6,22,37,38] Intra-articular malunions may result in a block to motion, capsular contracture, synovitis, or arthrosis.[5,27,29-31,38]

The radiographic evaluation must include anteroposterior, lateral, and oblique projections, with similar views of the normal side for comparison. The assessment of more complex deformities is aided by making true anteroposterior and true lateral radiographs of the involved digit proximal to the deformity and similar projections distal to the deformity. Tracings of these radiographs can be used as cutouts to be superimposed on a tracing of the contralateral, normal digit. Articular deformities may be better assessed with CT.

Several parameters influence the timing of surgical intervention: the time from the original injury, the state of the overlying soft tissue, ten-

don mobility, articular mobility, and the neurovascular status. There is concern about intervention between 4 and 8 weeks after the injury, as soft-tissue swelling may further limit the final motion and lead to a poorer outcome.[5,38] Therefore, before the corrective osteotomy is done, every effort should be made to maximize joint mobility as well as limit soft-tissue swelling. This, however, is not the case for an intra-articular malunion. The original fracture lines often can still be appreciated for up to 3 months after the fracture, and arthrosis is less likely to be present before 6 months after the injury. It is better to correct the intra-articular malunion as soon as it is recognized.

The type and location of an extra-articular osteotomy in the metacarpals or phalanges depend on several issues. Whenever soft-tissue coverage permits, the osteotomy should be performed as close as possible to the site of the deformity. The type of osteotomy is based on the location of the malunion, tendon balance, and any soft-tissue or articular contracture.

Proper exposure is crucial to gain access to the deformity, permit a sufficient length of bone for skeletal fixation, and allow access for capsulotomies or tenolysis, if needed. Before the osteotomy is performed, the accuracy of the assessment as well as the correction of the deformity is improved by using reference Kirschner wires placed perpendicular to the long axis of the bone and proximal and distal to the site of the deformity. Correction of the deformity is observed when the reference wires become parallel in the frontal, axial, and lateral planes[5,39] (Figure 2).

An incomplete osteotomy is appropriate for most purely angular deformities in the radial or ulnar plane.[4,9,10,22,26,38,40] Except when such deformities involve the middle or distal phalanges, an opening wedge osteotomy restores skeletal length and resets the tension of the extensor mechanism but requires more stable internal fixation. A closing wedge can be created with use of sequentially larger burrs, with the opposite cortex and periosteum left intact.[40] Fixation is obtained with use of small-gauge stainless-steel wire figure-of-8 loops on the tension side. Dorsal or volar apex angular deformities are corrected with an opening wedge osteotomy with an interposed bone graft, which requires stable plate fixation as a result of the more substantial deforming forces of the extrinsic muscles.[5]

Pure rotational deformities require a complete, usually transverse osteotomy. As thin a blade as possible should be used to create the osseous cut. Some authors have suggested that a pure rotational malunion of the phalanges can be corrected with a rotational osteotomy at the metacarpal level.[4,20,41-43] However, the amount of correction that can be achieved at this level is limited. Gross and Gelberman[44] found, in a cadaver study, that the deep transverse metacarpal ligament limited metacarpal rotation to 19° in the index, long, and ring fingers and to between 20° and 30° in the little finger.

Postoperative rehabilitation depends on the type of osteotomy, the security of the fixation, and whether associated capsulotomy or tenolysis was done (Figure 3). When the fixation is stable, early active motion is initiated, preferably under the supervision of a trained hand therapist.

Nonunion involving the tubular bones in the hand is extremely uncommon.[17,45] Alhough the defini-

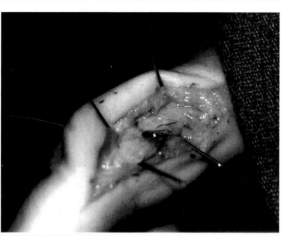

Figure 2 Intraoperative orientation of the deformity and assessment of the alignment following osteotomy are aided by observing the orientation of two sets of Kirschner wires. (Reproduced with permission from Faierman E, Jupiter JB: Deformity and nonunion following fractures, in Tubiana R, Gilbert A (eds): *Bone and Joint Disorders*. London, England, Martin Dunitz, 2002, pp 153-170.)

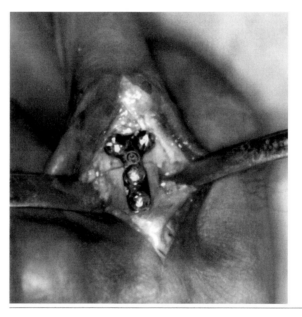

Figure 3 Intraoperative photograph showing stable internal fixation with a condylar plate. This allows immediate therapy for motion exercises. (Reprinted with permission from Jesse B. Jupiter, MD.)

tion of a nonunion depends to some degree on the time after the fracture, the definition is best a functional one in that immobilization of the hand for longer than 3 months to obtain union can lead to functional impairment.[46] Causes of nonunion include loss of bone substance, inadequate immobilization, fracture distraction, or infection. The indication for surgical treatment depends on both symptoms and functional disability. Although a variety of techniques have been described for the treatment of nonunions,[47-50] our preference has been stable internal

fixation when the involved digit has good functional potential.[46]

The Stiff Finger
Digital stiffness affects active or passive motion at the metacarpophalangeal, proximal interphalangeal, or distal interphalangeal joints. Stiffness may result from abnormal osseous or articular anatomy; decreased compliance of the periarticular soft tissues such as the palmar plate, collateral ligaments, fibrous flexor sheath, or skin; or loss of differential excursion of any of the gliding tissues such as digital nerves, ar-

teries, flexor tendons, and extensor tendons. Once the abnormality is properly identified and understood, the most efficacious treatment modalities can be instituted.[51-54]

The initial treatment must focus on the restoration of normal anatomy: the reduction and stabilization of the joints and fractures with use of pins, internal fixation, or external fixation; the repair of tendons, nerves, and blood vessels; and the provision of adequate tension-free coverage with use of local or distant flaps as required. Restoration of structure should supplant the too-early attempt at restoration of function. Restoration of as many injured parts of the finger as possible to their normal tension, length, and continuity can improve the success rate of later treatment of restoration of function.

Despite ideal treatment of the initial traumatic injury, structural problems may persist and must be addressed when identified. Osseous and articular causes of stiffness, such as arthrofibrosis and malunion (both intra-articular and extra-articular), alter considerations for therapy and the timing of surgery in the stiff finger. For example, a large osseous prominence located volarly in the subcondylar recess at the proximal interphalangeal joint will prevent the restoration of full flexion of the proximal interphalangeal joint while also limiting full tendon glide. The osseous abnormality must be corrected to allow full functional recovery. In general, severe arthrofibrosis or decreased digital flexion because of intra-articular pathology, extra-articular osseous blocks to flexion or extension, or extension-type malunion of the proximal phalanx should be treated before any intervention is performed to address the soft tissues.

Therefore, a useful principle of treatment is that arthrolysis, joint arthroplasty, osteotomy, or ostectomy be performed early to allow optimization of the postoperative rehabilitation of the soft tissues and gliding tissues.

In addition, the successful surgical correction of a chronically stiff digit requires a stable, complete, and compliant soft-tissue envelope. Split or full-thickness skin grafts may provide stable coverage of epitenon, digital sheaths, arteries, and nerves, but they form poor gliding surfaces for the restoration of easy digital motion. Replacement of such grafts with local or distant flaps may be necessary before the consideration of tenolysis and capsulectomy.

Once the structural abnormalities have been addressed, therapy should be designed to maximize the digital range of motion. Surgical intervention should be considered only after a specific therapy protocol to address each cause of the digital stiffness has been fully performed without success. Surgical decision-making hinges on accurate assessment of the active and passive ranges of motion of the proximal interphalangeal and, to a lesser extent, the metacarpophalangeal joints. Although some have ascertained that a combined arc of flexion (metacarpophalangeal, proximal interphalangeal, and distal interphalangeal motion) of >170° is required for adequate function,[1,2,4] a greater total arc of motion is often required on the ulnar side of the hand to facilitate power grasp and a lesser arc may be tolerated well on the radial side of the hand for fine thumb-index pinch activities. Likewise, full digital extension may be required on the radial side of the hand but is less important on the ulnar side, where digital flexion assumes greater importance. Each dig-

it, and indeed each patient, must be evaluated individually to determine the appropriate surgical tactics for the restoration of passive and active flexion and extension. When the patient thinks that his or her digital arc of motion is insufficient to allow daily activities of self-care, leisure, and work, surgery is indicated to improve that motion.

The correction of soft-tissue-related stiffness begins with a clinical examination of the active and passive flexion and extension of the finger. Four questions are asked during clinical examination to help in preoperative planning: (1) Can the finger be flexed passively? (2) Can the finger flex actively? (3) Can the finger be extended passively? (4) Can the finger extend actively? By definition, fingers that lack passive motion in a particular direction also lack active motion in the same direction. The answers to these questions will reliably reveal the location of the abnormal tissue as well as the surgical approach needed to address it.

Six possible permutations of finger stiffness are seen clinically, and a clearer definition of each aids in management decisions.

Type 1: Fingers that can be neither passively flexed nor passively extended have both dorsal disease (extensor tendon adhesions and/or dorsal capsular tightness and tightness of the dorsal collateral ligament) and palmar disease (A2 pulley insufficiency, palmar plate contracture, tightness of the accessory collateral ligament, checkrein contractures, or skin deficiency) preventing motion. This clinical state is often encountered in stiff fingers following replantation or penetrating trauma. The presence or absence of adhesions of the intrasynovial flexor sheath cannot be assessed directly, since the presence of dorsal disease precludes direct evaluation of active finger flexion. It is our preference to release the volar capsular proximal interphalangeal contracture and provide a stable compliant soft-tissue cover (with either local or distant flaps) as initial treatment. Following correction of the flexion deformity in these fingers, we perform a dorsal capsular and collateral ligament release and an extensor tenolysis in the initial surgical setting. We do not operate on both the dorsal and the palmar aspects of the finger at the same time, as swelling may make it impossible to maintain the surgical gains during postoperative motion therapy. We prefer to obtain passive flexion first, and then, if necessary, to address the lack of active flexion later. In addition, palmar contracture can be addressed at the time of flexor tendon lysis or reconstruction. If a dorsal release and extensor tenolysis is performed with the use of a local anesthetic, active finger flexion can be evaluated directly by asking the patient to flex the finger in the operating room. If a regional or general anesthetic is used, a traction test is performed with use of the flexor digitorum profundus tendon of the affected finger. If these tests demonstrate flexor tendon adhesions, the flexion contracture release and flexor tenolysis can be performed in the same surgical setting.

Type 2: Fingers that can be neither passively flexed nor actively extended have dorsal extensor adhesions and/or dorsal joint and collateral ligament contractures without palmar contracture. As in the type 1 finger (but more commonly encountered), the dorsal contracture prevents a preoperative assessment of the flexor mechanism. Treatment includes a dorsal extensor tenolysis and soft-tissue release followed, if necessary, by a flexor tendon tenolysis or reconstruction as a staged

procedure once full passive finger flexion has been achieved. When internal fixation implants have been used, removal of the implant with resection of the ipsilateral lateral band and transverse retinacular ligament is combined with extensor tenolysis to restore passive digital flexion.

Type 3: These fingers can be neither actively flexed nor passively extended, but unlike the first two groups they can be passively flexed. Passive flexion demonstrates that there are no clinically important extensor adhesions, dorsal capsular tightness, or tightness of the dorsal collateral ligament. Surgical treatment, therefore, focuses on the volar aspect of the finger. A palmar contracture prevents finger extension; all potential etiologies, as mentioned above, need to be considered in the preoperative planning. With a palmar soft-tissue deficiency, as seen in a burn or a complex palmar laceration with soft-tissue loss that has been allowed to heal by secondary intention, new, vascularized skin may be necessary to restore a gliding surface for the flexor tendon. Lack of active finger flexion suggests either flexor tendon adhesions or flexor tendon discontinuity (as discussed below for type 6). Exploration of the flexor sheath is necessary to discover the cause.

Type 4: Fingers that can be neither actively flexed nor actively extended are very uncommon, and these limitations are related to an incompetent flexor and extensor mechanism. There is full passive motion of these fingers. Passive flexion indicates no clinically important dorsal disease, and intact passive extension denotes the absence of a palmar flexion contracture. These fingers typically have intrasynovial flexor adhesions requiring tenolysis or they have flexor tendon discontinuity as well

as extensor dysfunction secondary to either lateral band subluxation palmar to the axis of rotation of the proximal interphalangeal joint (boutonniére deformity) or an extensor tendon repair that has healed in the lengthened position, or both. The extensor side is reconstructed first, as prolonged postoperative joint immobilization following extensor reconstruction is often required. Once maximum active extensor improvement has been achieved, flexor tenolysis or reconstruction is done as long as complete passive finger flexion is maintained.

Type 5: Fingers that cannot be extended passively are very common, and the limitation is caused by isolated palmar soft-tissue contracture. These fingers can, by definition, be fully flexed actively, but the presence of a flexion contracture prevents full digital extension. This situation is most commonly seen in patients with Dupuytren's contracture. It may also be seen in patients with volar soft-tissue defects that were allowed to heal by secondary intention. Patients often tolerate small degrees of deformity; however, when the contracture becomes severe, surgical release with or without soft-tissue reconstruction may be necessary.

Type 6: Fingers that have full active extension but lack active flexion have a deficient flexor mechanism. The dorsal joint capsules, collateral ligaments, and extensor tendons are continuous and of normal tension and compliance, but either intrasynovial adhesions of the flexor tendon or elongation or rupture of that tendon results in incomplete active finger flexion. Direct surgical exploration is the only definitive way to assess the cause of the lack of active flexion.

Exploration and restoration of ac-

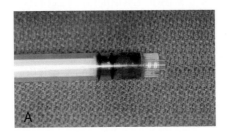
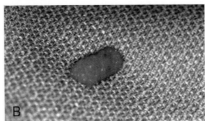

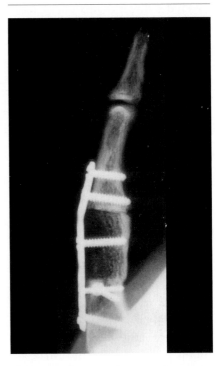

Figure 4 A compact cancellous graft is made with a small syringe packed with cancellous autogenous bone from the iliac crest graft **(A)**. This plug can replace a missing segment of bone **(B)**. (Reprinted with permission from Jesse B. Jupiter, MD.)

Figure 5 The cortical aspect of an autogenous bone graft should be placed opposite to the plate volarly, as this produces the strongest and therefore most stable fixation. (Reprinted with permission from Jesse B. Jupiter, MD.)

tive digital flexion may require one, two, or three surgical stages. All surgical protocols begin with a direct exploration of the flexor tendon, its pulley system, and its soft-tissue surroundings. The flexor tendon may be intact, intact but lengthened, or ruptured. In addition, the flexor sheath is assessed for the presence of restrictive intrasynovial adhesions. If the tendon is in continuity but has decreased intrasynovial excursion because of adhesions, a flexor tenolysis is performed and early postoperative mobilization rehabilitation is begun. If the flexor tendon is intact but elongated at the repair site and surrounded by restrictive adhesions, aggressive surgical lysis of adhesions is performed. A less vigorous rehabilitation protocol, a so-called frayed-tendon protocol, may be required to decrease the risk of subsequent tendon rupture. If the tendon is ruptured (or lengthened by >3 mm), the first decision to be made is whether a primary repair of the tendon is possible. If the proximal muscle-tendon unit is not adherent and has good excursion, and the proximal stump can be advanced without undue tension, repair may be performed. Usually, this is the case only in the first few weeks following laceration and repair, although in our experience repairs done as late as 3 months following injury are sometimes successful. If primary repair is not possible, either intrasy-

novial tendon grafting or placement of an inert silicone rod can be done. Primary tendon grafting can be performed if the A2 and A4 pulleys are intact; typically, a silicone rod is placed if a pulley must be reconstructed (or if the flexor tendon sheath bed is poor). If a silicone rod is placed, tendon-graft reconstruction is typically performed between 3 and 6 months later. Following rod placement and exchange, a third surgical procedure, flexor tenolysis, may be required depending on the patient's propensity toward scar formation and his or her adherence to the rigors of the rehabilitation protocol.

The treatment of a ruptured flexor digitorum profundus tendon with an intact flexor digitorum superficialis tendon is controversial; it is typically our preference to avoid grafting of a flexor digitorum profundus in the setting of an intact flexor digitorum superficialis tendon. We have found fingers with only an intact flexor digitorum superficialis to be highly functional and, if necessary, a distal interphalangeal stabilization procedure can be performed.

Bone Loss

Bone loss within the hand is defined as incomplete contact of the skeletal segment despite anatomic positioning of the main osseous fragments. The adverse sequelae of bone loss

include delayed union or nonunion, progressive deformity, and/or failure of internal fixation.

When analyzing this condition, one must consider several factors, including the bone involved, the location in the bone (intra-articular or extra-articular), whether the loss is terminal or intercalated within the bone, and the actual size of the defect. Coexistent problems may include loss of functional tissue, inadequate soft-tissue coverage, necrosis of adjacent bone segments, and active infection.[55-58]

Management of bone loss in the hand depends on both the functional deficit and the specific features of the reconstruction. Bone grafts or bone graft substitutes may function to fill a void, to provide structural support, or even to replace articular

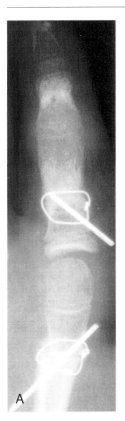
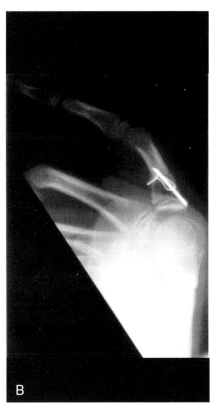
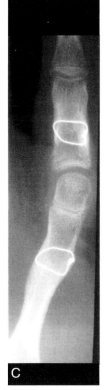
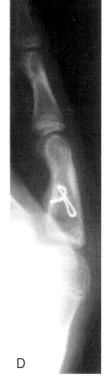

Figure 6 A and **B,** Initial anteroposterior and lateral radiographs made after a vascularized joint transfer from a toe to the thumb. **C** and **D,** Anteroposterior and lateral radiographs made 1 year later. (Reprinted with permission from Jesse B. Jupiter, MD.)

cartilage. Alternative techniques include skeletal shortening, arthroplasty, and distraction osteogenesis.

Bone grafts are classified by their type, the location of the donor site, and the intended function. Autogenous grafts include pure cancellous,[59] corticocancellous,[58,60] cortical strut,[61] osteochondral, and vascularized grafts either as isolated units or within composite transfers such as vascularized joints[62] or toe-to-hand transfers for the treatment of terminal loss.

Autogenous cancellous grafts offer the potential for both osteoinduction and osteoconduction, limited donor-site morbidity, ease of filling of the often three-dimensional aspects of an osseous defect, and rapidity of incorporation. The major disadvantage is a lack of structural support, which can be offset by either internal or external skeletal fixation.[63] A useful technique

is to create a compact cancellous graft for defect replacement. This is done by impacting cancellous bone into a small syringe with a diameter equivalent to that of the missing bone segment (Figure 4).

Corticocancellous bone grafts provide some element of structural support and are particularly useful when an osseous defect requires reconstruction. Restoration of skeletal length in phalangeal reconstruction is important to restore tendon balance and proper digital motion. Boulas and associates[64] described the use of interposition corticocancellous graft along with plate and screw fixation in the reconstruction of a traumatic proximal interphalangeal loss.

We recommended placement of the cortical aspect of the bone graft anteriorly to facilitate screw purchase as well as to enhance stability by having the stronger aspect of the

graft help to resist increased bending forces on the flexor side of the digit (Figure 5). Buchler and Aiken[65] described reconstruction of an area with partial articular loss with use of osteochondral grafts from the foot.

Vascularized bone transfers for the treatment of osseous defects in the tubular bones in the hand are either composite vascularized toe-joint transfers (Figure 6) or vascularized toe-to-hand transfers for the treatment of terminal osseous loss. These transfers also offer the potential for longitudinal growth in a child.

There are few indications for the use of allograft and bone graft substitutes to replace bone loss in the hand. Bone graft substitutes provide no structural support. Allograft bone replacement, while avoiding donor site morbidity, has several potential disadvantages, including resorption, infection, a potential immunogenic inflammatory response, and limited and slow revascularization. Perhaps the optimal application is to enhance the reconstruction of metacarpal lengthening by placing a corticocancellous allograft following distraction lengthening with external skeletal fixation.

Summary

The damage to a severely injured hand is varied and must be carefully assessed before surgical intervention is considered. The key aspect of a successful intervention is the identification of the anatomic abnormality; surgery or therapy can then be recommended on the basis of the pathological findings, the timing, and the previous interventions. The restoration of normal anatomy (bone) must precede efforts to restore function (soft tissue). Once the anatomy has been restored, consideration of the six types of stiff fingers will aid in surgical planning to allow the ideal clinical outcome.

References

1. Green DP, Butler TE: Fractures and dislocation in the hand, in Bucholz RW, Green DP, Heckman JD, Rockwood CA Jr (eds): *Rockwood and Green's Fractures in Adults*, ed 4. Philadelphia, PA, Lippincott-Raven, 1996, pp 607-744.

2. Jupiter JB, Axelrod TS, Belsky MR: Fractures and dislocations of the hand, in Browner BD, Jupiter JB, Levine AM, Trafton PG, (eds): *Skeletal Trauma: Fractures, Dislocations, Ligamentous Injuries*, ed 2. Philadelphia, PA, WB Saunders, 1998, pp 1225-1342.

3. Sanders RA, Frederick HA: Metacarpal and phalangeal osteotomy with miniplate fixation. *Orthop Rev* 1991;20:449-456.

4. Stern PJ: Fractures of the metacarpals and phalanges in Green DP, Hotchkiss RN, Pederson WC (eds): *Green's Operative Hand Surgery*, ed 3. New York, NY, Churchill Livingstone, 1993, pp 695-758.

5. Buchler U, Gupta A, Ruf S: Corrective osteotomy for post-traumatic malunion of the phalanges in the hand. *J Hand Surg [Br]* 1996;21:33-42.

6. Faierman E, Jupiter JB: Deformity and nonunion following fractures in Tubiana R, Gilbert A (eds): *Bone and Joint Disorders*. London, England, Martin Dunitz, 2002, pp 153-170.

7. Flatt AE: Closed and open fractures of the hand. Fundamentals of management. *Postgrad Med* 1966;39:17-26.

8. Reid DA: Corrective osteotomy in the hand. *Hand* 1974;6:50-57.

9. Green DP: Complications of phalangeal and metacarpal fractures. *Hand Clin* 1986;2:307-328.

10. Clinkscales GS Jr: Complications in the management of fractures in hand injuries. *South Med J* 1970;63:704-707.

11. Leonard MH: Blocking spur on proximal phalanx. *Hand* 1981;13:321.

12. Hunter JM, Cowen NJ: Fifth metacarpal fractures in a compensation clinic population: A report on one hundred and thirty-three cases. *J Bone Joint Surg Am* 1970;52:1159-1165.

13. Arafa M, Haines J, Noble J, Carden D: Immediate mobilization of fractures of the neck of the fifth metacarpal. *Injury* 1986;17:277-278.

14. Ford DJ, Ali MS, Steel WM: Fractures of the fifth metacarpal neck: Is reduction or immobilisation necessary? *J Hand Surg [Br]* 1989;14:165-167.

15. Royle SG: Rotational deformity following metacarpal fracture. *J Hand Surg [Br]* 1990;15:124-125.

16. Eichenholtz SN, Rizzon PC III: Fracture of the neck of the fifth metacarpal bone: Is over-treatment justified? *JAMA* 1961;178:425-426.

17. Barton NJ: Fractures of the shaft of the phalanges of the hand. *Hand* 1979;11:119-133.

18. Weeks PM, Wray RC: *Management of Acute Hand Injuries*. St Louis, MO, CV Mosby, 1973.

19. Smith RJ, Peimer CA: Injuries to the metacarpal bones and joints. *Adv Surg* 1977;11:341-374.

20. Manktelow RT, Mahoney JL: Step osteotomy: a precise rotation osteotomy to correct scissoring deformities of the fingers. *Plast Reconstr Surg* 1981;68:571-576.

21. Bouchon Y, Merle M, Foucher G, Michon J: [Malunions of the metacarpals and phalanges. Results of surgical treatment]. *Rev Chir Orthop Reparatrice Appar Mot* 1982;68:549-555.

22. Seitz WH Jr, Froimson AI: Management of malunited fractures of the metacarpal and phalangeal shafts. *Hand Clin* 1988;4:529-536.

23. Lucas GL, Pfeiffer CM: Osteotomy of the metacarpals and phalanges stabilized by AO plates and screws. *Ann Chir Main* 1989;8:30-38.

24. Menon J: Correction of rotary malunion of the fingers by metacarpal rotational osteotomy. *Orthopedics*. 1990;13:197-200.

25. Pichora DR, Meyer R, Masear VR: Rotational step-cut osteotomy for treatment of metacarpal and phalangeal malunion. *J Hand Surg [Am]* 1991;16:551-555.

26. van der Lei B, de Jonge J, Robinson PH, Klasen HJ: Correction osteotomies of phalanges and metacarpals for rotational and angular malunion: A long-term follow-up and a review of the literature. *J Trauma* 1993;35:902-908.

27. Wilson JN, Rowland SA: Fracture-dislocation of the proximal interphalangeal joint of the finger. *J Bone Joint Surg Am* 1966;48:493-502.

28. McCue FC, Honner R, Johnson MC, Gieck JH: Athletic injuries of the proximal interphalangeal joint requiring surgical treatment. *J Bone Joint Surg Am* 1970;52:937-956.

29. Zemel NP, Stark HH, Ashworth CR, Boyes JH: Chronic fracture dislocation of the proximal interphalangeal joint: Treatment by osteotomy and bone graft. *J Hand Surg [Am]* 1981;6:447-455.

30. Light TR: Salvage of intraarticular malunions of the hand and wrist: The role of realignment osteotomy. *Clin Orthop Relat Res* 1987;214:130-135.

31. Duncan KH, Jupiter JB: Intraarticular osteotomy for malunion of metacarpal head fractures. *J Hand Surg [Am]* 1989;14:888-893.

32. Vasko JR: An operation for old unreduced Bennett's fracture. *J Bone Joint Surg.* 1947;29:753-756.

33. Wagner CJ: Transarticular fixation of fracture-dislocations of the first metacarpal-carpal joint. *West J Surg Obstet Gynecol* 1951;59:362-365.

34. Giachino AA: A surgical technique to treat a malunited symptomatic Bennett's fracture. *J Hand Surg [Am]* 1996;21:149-151.

35. Jebson PJ, Blair WF: Correction of malunited Bennett's fracture by

intra-articular osteotomy: A report of two cases. *J Hand Surg [Am]* 1997;22:441-444.

36. Butler B, Rankin EA: in Epps CH, (ed), *Complications in Orthopaedic Surgery*, ed 3. Philadelphia, PA, Lippincott Williams and Wilkins; 1995, pp 389-401.

37. Coonrad RW, Pohlman MH: Impacted fractures in the proximal portion of the proximal phalanx of the finger. *J Bone Joint Surg Am* 1969;51:1291-1296.

38. Lister G: Intraosseous wiring of the digital skeleton. *J Hand Surg [Am]* 1978;3:427-435.

39. Segmuller G: *Surgical Stabilization of the Skeleton of the Hand*, Baltimore, MD, Williams and Wilkins, 1977.

40. Froimson AI: Osteotomy for digital deformity. *J Hand Surg [Am]* 1981;6:585-589.

41. Weckesser EC: Rotational osteotomy of the metacarpal for overlapping fingers. *J Bone Joint Surg Am* 1965;47:751-756.

42. Pieron AP: Correction of rotational malunion of a phalanx by metacarpal osteotomy. *J Bone Joint Surg Br* 1972;54:516-519.

43. Botelheiro JC: Overlapping of fingers due to malunion of a phalanx corrected by a metacarpal rotational osteotomy: Report of two cases. *J Hand Surg [Br]* 1985;10:389-390.

44. Gross MS, Gelberman RH: Metacarpal rotational osteotomy. *J Hand Surg [Am]* 1985;10:105-108.

45. Borgeskov S: Conservative therapy of phalangeal and metacarpal fractures. *Ugeskr Laeger* 1967;129:349-353.

46. Jupiter JB, Koniuch MP, Smith RJ: The management of delayed union and nonunion of the metacarpals and phalanges. *J Hand Surg [Am]*

1985;10:457-466.

47. Ireland ML, Taleisnik J: Nonunion of metacarpal extraarticular fractures in children: Report of two cases and review of the literature. *J Pediatr Orthop* 1986;6:352-355.

48. Goudot B, Voche PH, Bour C, Merle M: [Osteosynthesis using a L-shaped miniplate of metaphyseal and metaphyseal-epiphyseal fractures of metacarpals and phalanges]. *Rev Chir Orthop Reparatrice Appar Mot* 1991;77:130-134.

49. Schuind F, Cooney WP III, Burny F, An K: Small external fixation devices for the hand and wrist. *Clin Orthop Relat Res* 1993;293:77-82.

50. Wray RC Jr, Glunk R: Treatment of delayed union, nonunion, and malunion of the phalanges of the hand. *Ann Plast Surg* 1989;22:14-18.

51. Watson HK, Light TR, Johnson TR: Checkrein resection for flexion contracture of the middle joint. *J Hand Surg [Am]* 1979;4:67-71.

52. Curtis RM: Capsulectomy of the interphalangeal joints of the fingers. *J Bone Joint Surg Am* 1954;36:1219-1232.

53. Schneider LH: Tenolysis and capsulectomy after hand fractures. *Clin Orthop Relat Res* 1996;327:72-78.

54. Young VL, Wray RC Jr, Weeks PM: The surgical management of stiff joints in the hand. *Plast Reconstr Surg* 1978;62:835-841.

55. Freeland AE, Jabaley ME, Burkhalter WE, Chaves AM: Delayed primary bone grafting in the hand and wrist after traumatic bone loss. *J Hand Surg [Am]* 1984;9A:22-28.

56. Calkins MS, Burkhalter W, Reyes F: Traumatic segmental bone defects in the upper extremity. Treatment with exposed

grafts of corticocancellous bone. *J Bone Joint Surg Am* 1987;69:19-27.

57. Freeland AE, Jabaley ME: Stabilization of fractures in the hand and wrist with traumatic soft tissue and bone loss. *Hand Clin* 1988;4:425-436.

58. Segmuller G: Severe fractures including those with loss of bone, in Barton NJ (ed): *Fractures of the Hand and Wrist*. Edinburgh, Scotland, Churchill Livingstone, 1988, pp 173-190.

59. Jupiter JB, Ring DC (eds): *AO Manual of Fracture Management: Hand and Wrist*. New York, NY, Thieme, 2005, pp 125-130.

60. Freeland AE: External fixation for skeletal stabilization of severe open fractures of the hand. *Clin Orthop Relat Res* 1987;214:93-100.

61. Littler JW: Metacarpal reconstruction. *J Bone Joint Surg.* 1947;29:723-737.

62. Tsai TM, Jupiter JB, Kutz JE, Klenert HE: Vascularized autogenous whole joint transfer in the hand: A clinical study. *J Hand Surg [Am]* 1982;7:335-342.

63. Stahl S, Lerner A, Kaufman T: Immediate autografting in bones with open fractures with bone loss of the hand: A preliminary report. Case reports. *Scand J Plast Reconstr Surg Hand Surg* 1999;33:117-122.

64. Boulas HJ, Herren A, Buchler U: Osteochondral metatarsophalangeal autografts for traumatic articular metacarpophalangeal defects: A preliminary report. *J Hand Surg [Am]* 1993;18:1086-1092.

65. Buchler U, Aiken MA: Arthrodesis of the proximal interphalangeal joint by solid bone grafting and plate fixation in extensive injuries to the dorsal aspect of the finger. *J Hand Surg [Am]* 1988;13:589-594.

Dupuytren's Disease: Anatomy, Pathology, Presentation, and Treatment

Ghazi M. Rayan, MD

Abstract

The disorder called Dupuytren's disease has been recognized for approximately 400 years. Its presentation, although seemingly rather constant, is actually extremely variable, depending on which structures are involved. A thorough knowledge of palmar fascial anatomy is essential to the understanding of Dupuytren's disease.

Instr Course Lect 2007;56:101-111.

There have been recent advances in understanding the pathophysiology of Dupuytren's disease, and these have added to the knowledge about this disorder but have not yet changed its treatment. There are two distinct clinical entities, classic Dupuytren's disease and atypical, so-called non-Dupuytren's palmar fascial disease.[1,2] These two types differ in presentation, etiology, treatment, and prognosis. Authors of future epidemiologic and outcome studies should not confuse these two clinical entities. Surgical treatment is the conventional and most widely used method of managing Dupuytren's disease.

The earliest published reference to the disorder that was later to be called Dupuytren's disease was by Felix Platter, who in 1614 described a case, attributing the deformity to a flexor tendon contracture.[3] In 1777 Henry Cline recognized that the disorder involved the palmar fascia, in 1822 Sir Astley Cooper advocated closed fasciotomy as a treatment of the condition, and in 1831 Guillaume Dupuytren gave a detailed anatomic and pathologic description of the disease and demonstrated a surgical case in Paris that earned him the disease eponym.[4] By 1900 there were at least 256 publications related to Dupuytren's disease and at least 8 books on the subject.[2,5-11]

Age, gender, geography, and ethnicity influence the disease prevalence, which has been reported to be as low as 2% and as high as 42%.[12-14] Men are more likely to have the disease than women (9:1 ratio), and the overall incidence increases with age, with the frequency in women catching up to that in men later in life.[15] The disease is common in Scandinavia, Great Britain, Ireland, Australia, and North America. It is uncommon in southern Europe and South America and rare in Africa and China.[16,17]

Dupuytren's disease is associated with diabetes.[18-20] Burge and associates[21] and other authors[22,23] reported a higher risk of Dupuytren's disease in alcoholics, smokers, people with hypercholesterol, and patients infected with human immunodeficiency virus. There is controversy regarding a relationship between Dupuytren's disease and seizure disorders.[24,25] The etiology of Dupuytren's disease remains controversial as well, but inflammation, trauma, neoplasia, and genetics have been implicated as factors.[26-31] The evidence is strongest for at least a genetic predisposition. There is a clearly increased incidence in relatives of patients with Dupuytren's disease, and there has been at least one report of identical twins with the disease.[13,32] There seems to be an autosomal dominant transmission with variable penetrance.

Anatomy

The radial, ulnar, and central aponeuroses, palmodigital fascia, and digital fascia are all part of the palmar fascial complex[33] (Figure 1). These structures are involved to varying degrees in Dupuytren's disease. Each structure can be subdivided. The radial aponeurosis has four components: the thenar fascia (an extension of the central apo-

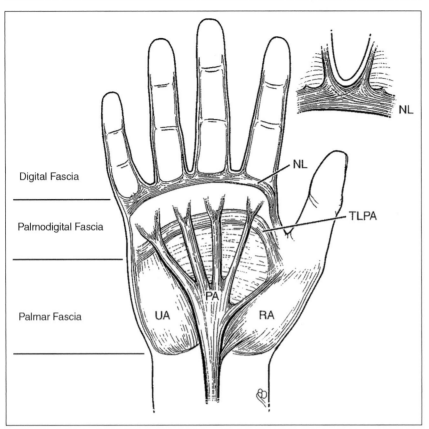

Figure 1 Palmar fascial complex with its five components: the radial aponeurosis (RA), ulnar aponeurosis (UA), central aponeurosis, palmodigital fascia, and digital fascia. NL = natatory ligament, PA = palmar aponeurosis, and TLPA = transverse ligament of the palmar aponeurosis. (Reprinted with permission from Rayan GM: Palmar fascial complex anatomy and pathology in Dupuytren's disease. *Hand Clin* 1999;15:75.)

neurosis), the thumb pretendinous band (small or absent), the distal commissural ligament, and the proximal commissural ligament.[34] The ulnar aponeurosis consists of the hypothenar muscle fascia (an extension of the central aponeurosis), the pretendinous band to the small finger (always present and very substantial), and the abductor digiti minimi confluence, which is enveloped by the fibers of the sagittal band.[35,36] The central aponeurosis is the core of Dupuytren disease activity. It is a triangular fascial layer with its apex proximal. Its fibers are oriented longitudinally, transversely, and vertically. The longitudinal fi-

bers fan out as pretendinous bands in the three central digits, and each bifurcates distally. Each bifurcation has three layers.[37] A superficial layer inserts into the dermis, a middle layer continues to the digit as the spiral band, and a deep layer passes almost vertically and dorsally. The transverse fibers make up the natatory ligament located in the distal part of the palm and the transverse ligament of the palmar aponeurosis. The transverse ligament of the palmar aponeurosis is proximal and parallel to the natatory ligament and deep to the pretendinous bands. Its distal, radial extent is the proximal commissural ligament. The trans-

verse ligament of the palmar aponeurosis gives origin to the septa of Legueu and Juvara, which protect the neurovascular structures and provide an additional proximal pulley to the flexor tendons.

The vertical fibers of the central aponeurosis are the minute vertical bands of Grapow and the septa of Legueu and Juvara. The vertical bands are numerous, small, strong, and scattered along the palmar fascial complex and are most abundant in the central aponeurosis.[38] The vertical septa of Legueu and Juvara are deep to the palmar fascia and form fibro-osseous compartments.[33,39,40] There are eight septa, one radial and one ulnar for each finger.[41] They form seven compartments of two types: four flexor septal canals that contain the flexor tendons and three web space canals that contain the common digital nerves and arteries and the lumbrical muscles (Figure 2). These septa are inserted in a soft-tissue confluence that consists of five structures: the A1 pulley, the palmar plate, the sagittal band, the interpalmar plate ligament, and the septa of Legueu and Juvara (Figure 3). The fascial structures in the palmodigital region are complex. The middle layer of the bifurcated pretendinous band spirals on its axis nearly 90°, and the peripheral fibers run vertically adjacent to the metacarpophalangeal joint capsule.[40] They continue distally deep to the neurovascular bundle and natatory ligaments and emerge distal to the natatory ligaments to continue as the lateral digital sheet. This spiral band therefore is the connection between the palmar and digital fascial structures. The proximal fibers of the natatory ligaments run in a transverse plane, but the distal fibers form a "u" and continue longitudinally along both sides of the digit, forming the lateral digital sheet. The lateral digital sheet therefore has deep and superficial contributions from the spiral band and the natatory ligament. The neurovascular bundle in the digit is surrounded by four fascial structures: the Grayson ligament (palmar), the Cleland ligament (dorsal), the Gosset lateral digital sheet laterally, and the Thomine retrovascular fascia medially and dorsally.[42]

Pathophysiology

The myofibroblast is the offending cell in Dupuytren's disease. It was described originally by Gabbiani and Majno[43] and further studied by Tomasek and associates.[44] The myofibroblast has morphologic characteristics of both a fibroblast and a smooth muscle cell, and it can actively contract.[45] The myofibroblast of Dupuytren's disease expresses α-smooth muscle actin that plays a role in contraction.[46] The Dupuytren myofibroblast synthesizes fibronectin, an extracellular glycoprotein, which connects myofibroblastic cells together and connects myofibroblastic cells to the extracellular stromal matrix with an integrin.[47,48] Myofibroblast contractility can be influenced by prostaglandins, which are found in nodules and active stages of the disease.[49-51] Fibroblast growth factor (FGF), transforming growth factor-α (TGF-α), epidermal growth factor, interleukin-1 (IL-1), and platelet-derived growth factor (PDGF) have been found to be expressed more in Dupuytren's disease.[52]

In Dupuytren's disease, normal fascial bands become diseased cords.[53] Dupuytren nodules and cords are pathognomonic of Dupuytren's disease.[54] A nodule usually appears first, but sometimes a cord develops without a nodule. Typically, the cords pro-

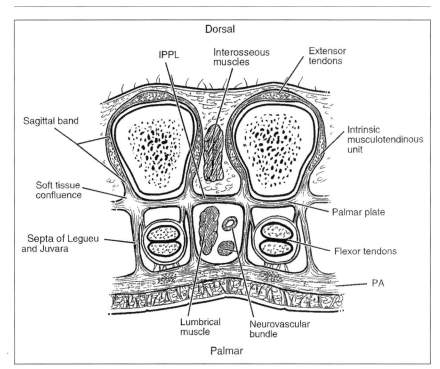

Figure 2   Interpalmar plate ligament (IPPL) and septa of Legueu and Juvara. PA = palmar aponeurosis. (Reprinted with permission from Rayan GM: Palmar fascial complex anatomy and pathology in Dupuytren's disease. *Hand Clin* 1999;15:79.)

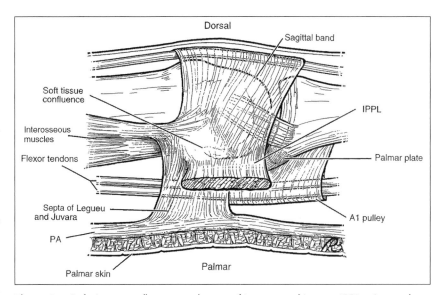

Figure 3   Soft-tissue confluence and septa of Legueu and Juvara. IPPL = interpalmar plate ligament; PA = palmar aponeurosis. (Reprinted with permission from Rayan GM: Palmar fascial complex anatomy and pathology in Dupuytren's disease. *Hand Clin* 1999;15:80.)

gressively shorten, leading to joint and soft-tissue contracture. The cords involve the palmar, palmodigital, or dig-ital regions. Shortened cords cause joint deformity, and long-standing flexion deformity leads to contracture of the capsuloligamentous tissue and flexion contractures of the metacarpophalangeal and proximal interphalangeal joints.

Grapow vertical bands become microcords leading to skin thickening, which is one of the earliest manifestations of Dupuytren's disease. Skin pits develop from the first layer of the split pretendinous band and are usually distal to the distal palmar crease.

The pretendinous cord develops from the pretendinous band and is the cord most frequently seen in Dupuytren's disease. It is responsible for flexion deformity of the metacarpophalangeal joint and often extends distally to continue with digital cords. Occasionally, the pretendinous cord bifurcates distally, with each branch extending into a different digit and forming a commissural "Y" cord. The vertical cord is less common and is connected to the pretendinous cord.[55] The vertical cord is short, thick, diseased tissue departing from the pretendinous cord and extending deeply in between the neurovascular bundle and the flexor tendon fibrous sheath. This cord is the diseased septa of Legueu and Juvara. Extensive palmar fascial disease is encountered in severe conditions and affects a large area of the palm, leading to diffuse thickening of many components of the palmar fascial complex including the transverse ligament of the palmar aponeurosis.

The spiral cord has four origins: the pretendinous band, the spiral band, the lateral digital sheet, and the Grayson ligament.[56] This cord is encountered most often in the small finger, but it may affect the ring finger. In the palm it is located superficial to the neurovascular bundle, just distal to the metacarpophalangeal joint; it passes deep to the neurovascular bundle; and in the digit it runs lateral to the neurovascular bundle as it involves the lateral digital sheet. Distally in the digit it is again superficial to the neurovascular bundle as it involves the Grayson ligament. Initially, the cord spirals around the neurovascular bundle, but as it contracts the cord straightens and the neurovascular bundle spirals around the cord. The distorted anatomy of the neurovascular bundle, which displaces medially and centrally, renders it at risk of injury during surgery.[57,58] The natatory cord develops from the natatory ligament, converting the u-shaped web-space fibers into a v shape and producing a contracture of the second, third, and fourth web spaces. The cord extends along the dorsal-lateral aspect of the adjacent digits and can be best detected by passively abducting the digits and at the same time flexing one digit and extending the other at the metacarpophalangeal joints. This maneuver allows the natatory cord to become more prominent.

The most frequently encountered digital cords are the central, spiral, and lateral cords. They are responsible for flexion deformity of the proximal interphalangeal joints. The central cord is an extension of the pretendinous cord in the palm. It courses in the midline and attaches into the flexor tendon sheath near the proximal interphalangeal joint or the periosteum of the middle phalanx on one side of the digit. The central cord usually does not displace the neurovascular bundle. The lateral cord originates from the lateral digital sheet and attaches to the skin or to the flexor tendon sheath near the Grayson ligament. The lateral cord leads to contracture of the proximal inter-phalangeal joint but can cause a flexion contracture of the distal interphalangeal joint. This cord can displace the digital neurovascular bundle toward the midline by its volume. The abductor digiti minimi cord is also known as the isolated digital cord. It originates from the abductor digiti minimi tendon, but it may also arise from the nearby muscle fascia or base of the proximal phalanx. It courses superficial to the neurovascular bundle and infrequently entraps and displaces it toward the midline. It frequently inserts on the ulnar side of the base of the middle phalanx, but it may attach on the radial side or have an additional insertion in the base of the distal phalanx, causing a contracture of the distal interphalangeal joint. The retrovascular cord is a poorly defined structure but is thought to develop from the retrovascular band of Thomine and is located deep to the neurovascular bundle.[58] It is different from the checkrein ligament. The retrovascular diseased tissue does not cause contracture of the proximal interphalangeal joint, but if the tissue is not removed, the proximal interphalangeal joint contracture may not be completely corrected.

The distal commissural cord is the diseased distal commissural ligament, which is the radial extension of the natatory ligament, whereas the proximal commissural cord originates from the proximal commissural ligament, which is the radial extension of the transverse ligament of the palmar aponeurosis. Both of these cords cause contracture of the first web space. The thumb pretendinous cord originates from the thumb pretendinous band and causes flexion deformity of the thumb metacarpophalangeal joint,[59] which is uncommon.

Diagnosis and Classification

In its early stages, Dupuytren's disease can be difficult to diagnose.[60-62] Skin changes are the earliest manifestation. Changes on the dorsum of the hand consist of either Garrod nodes, which are rare, or knuckle pads, which are more common. Garrod nodes are firm nodules at the proximal interphalangeal joints.[63,64] Knuckle pads are fibrosing lesions over the proximal interphalangeal joints. They are prevalent in patients with bilateral disease and in those with ectopic disease, such as in the feet and genitals.[63] Knuckle pads include loss of wrinkles, thickening, tethering, or hyperkeratosis. They are found in just fewer than half of patients with Dupuytren's disease, and the index finger is the most common digit involved.[65,66]

The changes in the palm begin with the formation of microcords from the Grapow fibers, which connect the dermis to the palmar fascia. This produces a pseudocallus or thickening of the skin and underlying subcutaneous tissue. These vertical bands are probably the first anatomic structures to become affected by Dupuytren's disease. The deep subcutaneous fat becomes fibrotic near the distal palmar crease.[67] As a result, the skin becomes tethered and adherent to the underlying fascial structures and loses its normal mobility. Skin thickening is often associated with surface rippling and dimpling. A skin pit is rarely confused or associated with other conditions and therefore it is a reliable sign of early Dupuytren's disease. Skin pits are caused by deep full-thickness skin retraction into the subcutaneous tissue. The diseased superficial fibers of the split pretendinous band form a dermal cord that pulls the dermal side of the skin inward. The apex of the cone-shaped skin pit is often buried deep within the subcutaneous space and cannot be seen by the examiner.

A Dupuytren nodule is a firm soft-tissue mass that is fixed to both the skin and the deep fascia. The nodule seems to originate in the superficial components of the palmar or digital fascia. It is usually well defined, localized, and raised above the surface, but it can be only a diffuse thickening of the deeper fascia. Nodules occur in the palm or digits. Palmar nodules are adjacent to the distal palmar crease, often in line with the ring and small fingers and sometimes proximal to the base of the thumb and small finger. Digital nodules are usually near the proximal interphalangeal joint or at the base of the digit. Nodules are often painless, but they can enlarge and become troublesome, causing pain when they are associated with stenosing tenosynovitis as a result of direct pressure on the flexor tendons and A1 pulley or from a vertical cord. Nodules have an abundance of myofibroblasts and a rich vascular supply.

Nodules tend to regress spontaneously and are replaced by a cord, but a cord can develop and mature without nodule regression. The normal bands discussed previously are the precursors of pathologic cords.[54] Early cords can adhere to the skin and blend with the nodule, making it difficult to ascertain where a nodule ends and a cord begins. The cord later becomes prominent and acquires the appearance and consistency of a tendon. Cords are located in the palm, the palmodigital area, or the digits. A mature cord has only sparse myofibroblasts but abundant collagen.

The disease has early, intermediate, and late phases. Skin changes with loss of normal architecture and formation of skin pits is the early phase. Nodules and cords form during the intermediate phase, and contractures mark the late phase. The late phase tends to go through four stages of contracture, with contracture of the metacarpophalangeal joint of the ring finger in stage I; contractures of the metacarpophalangeal and proximal interphalangeal joints of the ring finger and the metacarpophalangeal joint of the small finger in stage II; contractures of the metacarpophalangeal and proximal interphalangeal joints of the ring finger, the metacarpophalangeal and proximal interphalangeal joints of the small finger, and the metacarpophalangeal joint of the long finger in stage III; and stage III contractures as well as distal interphalangeal joint hyperextension of the ring or small finger in stage IV. This progression is not immutable. In many instances, palmar fascial disease or contracture remains confined to the palm and does not progress enough to cause digital flexion deformity. Palmar involvement usually precedes extension of the disease into the digits; however, the disease may also begin and remain in the digits. The ring finger is the most commonly involved digit, followed in order of frequency by the small, long, and index fingers and lastly by the thumb. The anatomy of the neurovascular bundle can be distorted as the spiral cord contracts. A palpable interdigital soft-tissue mass is an indication that the neurovascular bundle is involved, but it is not a reliable indicator.[57,68]

Dupuytren's disease may affect locations other than the hand, and patients with Dupuytren's disease should be examined for ectopic sites of involvement. Ectopic disease can be either regional in the upper extremity or distant in other parts of the body. Garrod nodes or knuckle pads occur on the dorsum of the hand and are almost always limited to the fingers. Three reports have noted disease extension into the wrist area.[69-71]

Dupuytren contractures have been reported in more proximal locations in the upper extremity.[72,73] Distant ectopic disease occurs occasionally, and patients with knuckle pads are more likely to have distant involvement.[66] The most common distant ectopic disease is fibromatosis restricted to the plantar fascia. This is usually asymptomatic and rarely causes flexion contracture of the toes.[74,75] Wheeler and Meals[76] reported on a patient with Dupuytren's disease who had bilateral palmar contracture, bilateral plantar nodules, and nodular fasciitis of the popliteal space.

There is a clinical condition that is similar to Dupuytren's disease but should not be confused with it. It is termed non-Dupuytren's disease.[1,2] Classic Dupuytren's disease occurs mostly in Caucasians, whereas non-Dupuytren's disease occurs mostly in a diverse ethnic group. Non-Dupuytren's disease is unilateral, usually involving a single digit, and it is not infrequently associated with trauma, including surgery. Patients with this disease rarely need surgical treatment, and the condition can spontaneously improve. Confusing these two conditions can produce contrasting epidemiologic data.

In addition to non-Dupuytren's disease, there are other soft-tissue changes that can mimic early Dupuytren's disease, and certain pathologic processes can be mistaken for established Dupuytren's disease. Epithelioid sarcoma has masqueraded as Dupuytren's disease.[77,78] Also, skin changes and nodules in Du-

puytren's disease should be distinguished from occupational thickening, hyperkeratosis, and callus formation that are caused by chronic friction and pressure on a working person's hand.[61] McGrouther[62] described changes in the edematous hand that cause bulging of the subcutaneous adipose tissue between fibrous bands with exaggeration of normal anchorage of the fascia to the skin, giving the appearance of early Dupuytren's disease. Large Dupuytren nodules should be differentiated from palmar soft-tissue subcutaneous lesions such as localized pigmented villonodular synovitis (soft-tissue giant-cell tumor), palmar ganglions, and inclusion cysts. Stenosing tenosynovitis without triggering can be associated with thickening and adherence of the skin to the underlying flexor tendon sheath. Prominence of flexor tendons due to attenuation of annular pulleys, as is found in rheumatoid arthritis, can be confused with pretendinous cords.[79] Digital joint flexion deformity such as that seen following ulnar nerve lesions and posttraumatic contracture also should be differentiated from long-standing Dupuytren's disease. The presence of other manifestations in the typical disease can reinforce its diagnosis. Accurate diagnosis and differentiation between the types of palmar fascial contracture are necessary to gain insight into the disease prognosis and to achieve a satisfactory treatment outcome.

Treatment

Observation is indicated for a patient who has static Dupuytren's disease with minimal contracture and without compromise of function. Recent basic science research has shown the potential of certain local agents in the treatment of Du-

puytren's disease. These include the calcium channel blockers nifedipine and verapamil[45] for early stages of the disease and collagenase[80] for advanced stages. Enzymatic fasciotomy with trypsin and hyaluronidase followed by forced extension of the digit has been reported.[81] Steroid injection into nodules has been used to suppress the disease.[82] Intralesional injections of gamma-interferon[83] decrease the symptoms and the size of the lesions in both Dupuytren's disease and hypertrophic scars, probably by decreasing expression of α-smooth muscle actin and production of collagen. There is no consensus regarding local injection for the treatment of Dupuytren's disease.

Surgery is the most widely used treatment of advanced Dupuytren's disease. Flexion contracture of the metacarpophalangeal joint of >30° and flexion contracture of the proximal interphalangeal joint of 15° interfere with function and, in the presence of a well-developed cord, are indications for surgical treatment. Treatment of metacarpophalangeal joint contractures is more successful than that of proximal interphalangeal joint contractures.

Percutaneous fasciotomy was first used by Astley Cooper and has been advocated for palmar cords in older patients.[84,85] In severe cases, this technique may be useful as a preliminary procedure.[86] There is a risk to the flexor tendons and the nerves, and reflex sympathetic dystrophy has been reported after percutaneous releases.[87] The technique of percutaneous release uses a stab wound adjacent to the cord and a number-11 blade to cut the cord while the digit is extended.

Fasciectomy is associated with a lower recurrence rate than is fasciotomy (15% compared with 43%).

Partial, regional, or limited fasciectomy remains the most conventional and widely used technique among hand surgeons today.[88,89] Partial fasciectomy is the excision of the diseased tissue only and was first described by Goyrand in 1834. Freehafer and Strong[88] recommended that treatment with use of multiple small longitudinal incisions.

In segmental aponeurectomy, multiple small incisions are created in the palm and digits, and segments of diseased tissue are excised without removal of all tissue. Russ[89] and Moermans[90] first described this minimally invasive technique, and the results are comparable with those of other methods of treatment, with a recurrence rate of 21%. The procedure is done through a series of c-shaped incisions, and 1-cm segments of diseased tissue are excised.

McIndoe and Beare[91] performed a total fasciectomy through a transverse palmar incision and digital z-plasties without excising the skin, which they reported on in 1958. Zachariae[92] compared this procedure with a limited fasciectomy and found nearly equal functional results, but other authors reported a higher incidence of complications with total fasciectomy.

Dermofasciectomy involves simultaneous excision of skin and diseased tissue.[10,93] The recurrence rate after this procedure is lower than that after other surgical techniques. When it was combined with skin grafting, there were no recurrences beneath the graft even when the method was used to treat recurrent disease.[93-95] A midterm review revealed recurrent nodule formation limited to graft insets in 10% of patients, without recurrence of cords. There were few other complica-

tions, but an increase in disease extension was found between 3 and 13 years after dermofasciectomy.[94,96] This technique is best suited for recurrent and severe primary disease, when the skin is adherent to the underlying Dupuytren's disease tissue, but it is not indicated for all recurrent and severe cases. Roush and Stern[97] reported the total range of motion after surgical treatment of recurrent Dupuytren's disease to be better after fasciectomy and flap coverage than after skin-grafting or arthrodesis. An attempt should always be made to dissect the skin from Dupuytren's disease tissue, but skin that cannot be saved should be excised and skin graft should be used if necessary.

Severe flexion deformity of the proximal interphalangeal joint can result in a residual contracture after excision of the offending digital cord. This contracture may be caused by attenuation of the central slip of the extensor tendon, which is placed at risk by a prolonged contracture of the proximal interphalangeal joint, especially when the deformity exceeds 60°. If the proximal interphalangeal joint remains contracted after a digital fasciectomy, extension splinting for several weeks can help to restore the tone of the central.[95,96,98-100] Surgical release of a proximal interphalangeal joint contracture after fasciectomy is indicated if the residual deformity is >40°.

Preoperative and postoperative skeletal traction with an external fixation device has been used to improve correction of severe contractures of the proximal interphalangeal joint. In severe cases, a continuous elongation technique before fasciectomy has been shown to decrease the deformity, facilitate surgery, minimize the need for am-

putation, and alter the collagen orientation and even the metabolism of the fascia.[101,102] Although this technique is an additional option for treating difficult cases, it is associated with a high rate of complications such as infection, pin loosening, recurrence, and even amputation.

Salvage procedures may be necessary for severe digital deformities (for example, a flexion contracture of the proximal interphalangeal joint in excess of 70°) and especially for recurrent cases with an exuberant amount of scarring. Dorsal wedge osteotomy of the proximal phalanx is a method to prevent amputation.[103] Another option is arthrodesis of the proximal interphalangeal joint combined with resection of a portion of the proximal phalanx to shorten the digit, allowing extension without tension on the neurovascular structures. Arthroplasty of the proximal interphalangeal joint with a silicone implant can correct some of the deformity and retain motion but is associated with the risk of further flexion deformity of the joint. Amputation at the proximal interphalangeal joint or through the proximal phalanx may be necessary when nerve and vascular damage results in loss of sensory function and cold intolerance.

Primary closure should be used whenever possible. McGrouther[62] illustrated about 60 diagrams in the literature of surgical incisions used for the treatment of Dupuytren's disease. However, the most commonly used are the Bruner zigzag incision and the midline longitudinal incision that is closed with multiple z-plasties.

When primary closure is not possible, the wounds can be left open. Dupuytren was the first to leave wounds open after making a transverse palmar incision. McCash[104] used the same method with minor modifications. The palmar incision is left open to heal by secondary intention. Reports of satisfactory results of this method, with less pain, better motion, and low complication rates, continue to appear in the literature.[105-108]

A full-thickness skin graft from the wrist, the ulnar side of the hand, or the antecubital area is most useful for recurrent or severe cases when primary closure is not possible. A distally based dorsal hand flap, rotation flaps from the side of the fourth and fifth digits, and a cross-finger flap from an adjacent digit can be used. A butterfly flap is useful for coverage after excision of a natatory cord from a digital web space to minimize web space contracture formation. Simple and four-flap z-plasties can be used for the first web space.

Complications of surgery for Dupuytren's disease are either technique-related, such as neurovascular injury, hematoma, and infection, or related to patient physiology, such as stiffness and reflex symptomatic dystrophy. Boyer and Gelberman[109] classified complications temporally as intraoperative, early postoperative, and late postoperative. The risk of digital nerve injury is associated with severe contractures of the metacarpophalangeal and proximal interphalangeal joints, with altered nerve anatomy by a spiral cord, and, especially in recurrent cases, with exuberant amounts of scar tissue. Preventive measures include isolation of the neurovascular bundle by careful dissection, with use of loop magnification and on the basis of knowledge of the pathologic anatomy. The dissection is performed in a proximal-to-distal direction, sometimes in combination with a distal-to-proximal approach,

before removal of the diseased cord. If the nerve is transected, a primary repair should be done.

A vascular injury can be an arterial laceration, arterial spasm, intimal hemorrhage, or vessel rupture resulting from vigorous correction of a severe digital joint contracture. Arterial laceration that results in vascular compromise requires immediate repair or placement of an interposition vein graft. Arterial spasm and intimal hemorrhage are treated first by repositioning the digit in flexion, then irrigating with warm saline solution, applying topical lidocaine, and even administering intravenous heparin. If all else fails, vascular reconstruction should be done.

Separating diseased tissue from adherent skin is difficult, especially in recurrent cases. To reduce the risk of buttonholing the skin, the use of a number-15C scalpel and the back of the knife as a dissector allows separation of diseased tissue from normal skin. In addition, using an operating room light to transilluminate from the epidermal side of the skin allows visualization of the thickness of the flap and can alert the surgeon when the dissection is becoming too superficial.

Hematoma is prevented by tourniquet deflation and then achievement of adequate hemostasis before wound closure. Deflating the tourniquet and assessing the skin vascularity before closure to ensure adequate circulation is the best way to prevent skin necrosis. Closure under tension should be avoided, and skin grafting or use of the open palm method should be considered if a primary closure is too tight. If skin necrosis develops, excision of necrotic tissue and skin grafting or flap coverage are performed.

Reflex sympathetic dystrophy, also referred to as a flare reaction

and complex regional pain syndrome, may occur after surgery. The patient has swelling, hyperemia, dysesthesias, and pain out of proportion to that expected. Direct trauma to the nerves and excessive dissection are thought to be predisposing factors. The simultaneous performance of a carpal tunnel release with the surgery for Dupuytren's disease is a predisposing factor, especially in women. An atraumatic surgical technique and gentle handling of nerves and other tissues during surgery should minimize the development of this complication. If a specific cause cannot be identified, the treatment is therapy for pain control. In recalcitrant cases, a series of stellate sympathetic ganglion blocks can be helpful.

Inclusion cysts can occur near the scar as a result of entrapment of dermal tissue in the subcutaneous space and can be prevented by careful attention to skin approximation during wound closure. Hypertrophic scar formation is lessened by careful attention to the placement of the skin incisions.

The recurrence rate ranges between 2% and 60%, with an average of 33%.[104-108,110] This may represent true recurrence (disease at the surgical site) or disease extension (disease outside of the area of the prior surgery). Recurrence is more common in patients with proximal interphalangeal joint involvement, a diseased small finger, and more than one digit affected as well as in those who present a longer time after surgery or after a secondary fasciectomy.

Summary

Dupuytren's disease is a genetic disorder that occurs throughout life, with an increasing frequency with age. A proliferation of myofibroblasts leads to abnormal collagen formation and a varying degree of contracture in the palm and fingers. There are two distinct clinical entities, classic Dupuytren's disease and, atypical, non-Dupuytren's palmar fascial disease. These two types differ in presentation, etiology, treatment, and prognosis. Nonsurgical treatment has yet to be of significant benefit; surgery is indicated for patients whose function is limited by the disease. A metacarpophalangeal joint flexion contracture of greater than 30° or a proximal interphalangeal joint flexion contracture of greater than 15° are conditions considered significant enough to warrant surgery. Partial fasciectomy is probably the most appropriate treatment initially, whereas more radical surgical procedures are indicated for symptomatic recurrent disease. An understanding of the pathophysiology and anatomy of the disease helps in managing these patients. Recurrence is common and complications from surgery are not infrequent.

References

1. Rayan G, Moore J: Non-Dupuytren's disease of the palmar fascia. *J Hand Surg [Br]* 2005;30:551-556.

2. Rayan GM: Clinical presentation and types of Dupuytren's disease. *Hand Clin* 1999;15:87-96.

3. Elliot D: The early history of Dupuytren's disease. *Hand Clin* 1999;15:1-19.

4. Dupuytren G: De la retraction des doigts par suite d'une affection de l'aponevrose palmaire – description de la maladie – operation Chirugicale qui convient dens de cas. *J Univ Hebd Med Chir Prat Inst Med* 1831;5:349-365.

5. Stack HG: *The Palmar Fascia.* Edinburgh, Scotland, Churchill Livingstone, 1973.

6. Hueston JT, Tubiana R (eds): *Dupuytren's Disease,* ed 2. New York, NY, Churchill Livingstone, 1985.

7. McFarlane RM, McGrouther DA, Flint MH (eds): *Dupuytren's Disease: Biology and*

Treatment. New York, NY, Churchill Livingstone, 1990.

8. Berger A, Delbruck A, Brenner P, Hinzmann R (eds): *Dupuytren's Disease: Pathobiochemistry and Clinical Management.* New York, NY, Springer, 1994.

9. Hueston JT, Seyfer AE: Some medicolegal aspects of Dupuytren's contracture. *Hand Clin* 1991;7:617-632.

10. Tubiana R, Leclercq C, Hurst LC, Badalamente MA, Mackin EJ (eds): *Dupuytren's Disease.* London, England, Martin Dunitz, 2000.

11. Brenner P, Rayan GM: *Dupuytren's Disease: A Concept of Surgical Treatment.* Vienna, Austria, Springer, 2003.

12. Ross DC: Epidemiology of Dupuytren's disease. *Hand Clin* 1999;15:53-62.

13. Ling RSM: The genetic factor in Dupuytren's disease. *J Bone Joint Surg Br* 1963;45:709-718.

14. Mikkelsen O: Epidemiology in a Norwegian population, in McFarlane RM, Mc-Grouther DA, Flint MH (eds): *Dupuytren's Disease: Biology and Treatment.* New York, NY, Churchill Livingstone, 1990, pp 199-200.

15. Early PF: Population studies in Dupuytren's contracture. *J Bone Joint Surg Br* 1962;44:602-613.

16. Hueston JT: Dupuytren's diathesis, in Hueston JT (ed): *Dupuytren's Contracture.* Edinburgh, Scotland, Livingstone, 1963, pp 51-63.

17. McFarlane R: On the origin and spread of Dupuytren's disease. *J Hand Surg [Am]* 2002;27:385-390.

18. McFarlane R, Ross D: Dupuytren's disease, in Weinzweig J (ed): *Plastic Surgery Secrets.* Philadelphia, PA, Hanley and Belfus, 1998, pp 554-559.

19. Arkkila PE, Kantola IM, Viikari JS: Dupuytren's disease: Association with chronic diabetic complications. *J Rheumatol* 1997;24:153-159.

20. Chammas M, Bousquet P, Renard E, Poirier JL, Jaffiol C, Allieu Y: Dupuytren's disease, carpal tunnel syndrome, trigger finger and diabetes mellitus. *J Hand Surg [Am]* 1995;20:109-114.

21. Burge P, Hoy G, Regan P, Milne R: Smoking, alcohol and the risk of Dupuytren's contracture. *J Bone Joint Surg Br* 1997;79:206-210.

22. Noble J, Arafa M, Royle SG, McGeorge G, Crank S: The association between alcohol, hepatic pathology and

Dupuytren's disease. *J Hand Surg [Br]* 1992;17:71-74.

23. An HS, Southworth SR, Jackson WT, Russ B: Cigarette smoking and Dupuytren's contracture of the hand. *J Hand Surg [Am]* 1988;13:872-874.

24. Critchley EM, Vakil SD, Hayward HW, Owen VM: Dupuytren's disease in epilepsy: Result of prolonged administration of anticonvulsants. *J Neurol Neurosurg Psychiatry* 1976;39:498-503.

25. Arafa M, Noble J, Royle SG, Trail IA, Allen J: Dupuytren's and epilepsy revisited. *J Hand Surg [Br]* 1992;17:221-224.

26. Chansky HA, Trumble TE, Conrad EU III, Wolff JF, Murray LW, Raskind WH: Evidence for a polyclonal etiology of palmar fibromatosis. *J Hand Surg [Am]* 1999;24:339-344.

27. Zachariae L: Dupuytren's contracture: the aetiological role of trauma. *Scand J Plast Reconstr Surg* 1971;5:116-119.

28. Meagher S: Manual work and industrial injury: A personal commentary, in McFarlane RM, McGrouther DA, Flint MH (eds): *Dupuytren's Disease: Biology and Treatment.* New York, NY, Churchill Livingstone, 1990, pp 261-263.

29. Hueston JT, Seyfer AE: Some medicolegal aspects of Dupuytren's contracture. *Hand Clin* 1991;7:617-634.

30. McFarlane R, Botz J, Cheung H: Epidemiology of surgical patients, in McFarlane RM, McGrouther DA, Flint MH (eds): *Dupuytren's Disease: Biology and Treatment.* New York, NY, Churchill Livingstone, 1990, pp 201-213.

31. Liss GM, Stock SR: Can Dupuytren's contracture be work related?: Review of the evidence. *Am J Ind Med* 1996;29:521-532.

32. Couch H: Identical Dupuytren's contracture in identical twins. *Can Med Assoc J* 1938;39:225-226.

33. Rayan GM: Palmar fascial complex anatomy and pathology in Dupuytren's disease. *Hand Clin* 1999;15:73-86.

34. Tubiana R, Simmons BP, DeFrenne HA: Location of Dupuytren's disease on the radial aspect of the hand. *Clin Orthop Relat Res* 1982;168:222-229.

35. White S: Anatomy of the palmar fascia on the ulnar border of the hand. *J Hand Surg [Br]* 1984;9:50-56.

36. Rayan GM, Murray D, Chung KW, Rohrer M: The extensor retinacular system at the metacarpophalangeal joint:

Anatomical and histological study. *J Hand Surg [Br]* 1997;22:585-590.

37. McGrouther DA: The microanatomy of Dupuytren's contracture. *Hand* 1982;14:215-236.

38. Grapow M: Die anatomie und physiologische bedeutung der palmaraponourose. Archiv fur Anatomie Und Physiologie Leipzig. *Anatomicsche Abtheilung.* 1887;143:2-3.

39. Legueu F, Juvara E: Des aponévroses de la paume de la main. *Bull Soc Anat Paris* 1892;6:383.

40. Gosset J: Dupuytren's disease and the anatomy of the palmodigital aponeurosis, in Hueston JT, Tubiana R (eds): *Dupuytren's Disease*, ed 2. New York, NY, Churchill Livingstone, 1985, pp 75-81.

41. Bilderback KK, Rayan GM: The septa of Legueu and Juvara: An anatomic study. *J Hand Surg [Am]* 2004;29:494-499.

42. Thomine JM: The development and anatomy of the digital fascia, in Hueston JT, Tubiana R (eds): *Dupuytren's Disease*, ed 2. New York, NY, Churchill Livingstone, 1985, pp 3-12.

43. Gabbiani G, Majno G: Dupuytren's contracture: Fibroblast contraction? An ultrastructural study. *Am J Pathol* 1972;66:131-146.

44. Tomasek JJ, Gabbiani G, Hinz B, Chaponnier C, Brown RA: Myofibroblasts and mechano-regulation of connective tissue remodelling. *Nat Rev Mol Cell Biol* 2002;3:349-363.

45. Rayan GM, Parizi M, Tomasek JJ: Pharmacologic regulation of Dupuytren's fibroblast contraction in vitro. *J Hand Surg [Am]* 1996;21:1065-1070.

46. Tomasek J, Rayan GM: Correlation of alpha-smooth muscle actin expression and contraction in Dupuytren's disease fibroblasts. *J Hand Surg [Am]* 1995;20:450-455.

47. Tomasek JJ, Haaksma CJ: Fibronectin filaments and actin microfilaments are organized into a fibronexus in Dupuytren's diseased tissue. *Anat Rec* 1991;230:175-182.

48. Halliday NL, Rayan GM, Zardi L, Tomasek JJ: Distribution of ED-A and ED-B containing fibronectin isoforms in Dupuytren's disease. *J Hand Surg [Am]* 1994;19:428-434.

49. Hurst LC, Badalamente MA, Makowski J: The pathobiology of Dupuytren's contracture: Effects of prostaglandins on myofibroblasts. *J Hand Surg [Am]* 1986;11:18-23.

50. Chiu HF, McFarlane RM: Pathogenesis of Dupuytren's contracture: A correlative clinical-pathological study. *J Hand Surg [Am]* 1978;3:1-10.

51. Magro G, Fraggetta F, Colombatti A, Lanzafame S: Myofibroblasts and extracellular matrix glycoproteins in palmar fibromatosis. *Gen Diagn Pathol* 1997;142:185-190.

52. Badalamente MA, Hurst LC: The biochemistry of Dupuytren's disease. *Hand Clin* 1999;15:35-42.

53. Luck JV: Dupuytren's contracture: A new concept of the pathogenesis correlated with surgical management. *J Bone Joint Surg Am* 1959;41:635-664.

54. McFarlane RM: Patterns of the diseased fascia in the fingers in Dupuytren's contracture: Displacement of the neurovascular bundle. *Plast Reconstr Surg* 1974;54:31-44.

55. Bilderback KK, Rayan GM: Dupuytren's cord involving the septa of Legueu and Juvara: A case report. *J Hand Surg [Am]* 2002;27:344-346.

56. McFarlane R: The finger, in McFarlane RM, McGrouther DA, Flint MH (eds): *Dupuytren's Disease: Biology and Treatment.* New York, NY, Churchill Livingstone, 1990, pp 155-167.

57. Umlas ME, Bischoff RJ, Gelberman RH: Predictors of neurovascular displacement in hands with Dupuytren's contracture. *J Hand Surg [Br]* 1994;19:664-666.

58. McFarlane R: The anatomy of Dupuytren's disease, in Hueston JT, Tubiana R (eds): *Dupuytren's Disease*, ed 2. New York, NY, Churchill Livingstone, 1985, pp 54-71.

59. Rayan GM: Dupuytren's disease. American Academy of Orthopaedic Surgeons (AAOS) Orthopaedic Knowledge Online. http://www5.aaos.org/oko

60. Hueston JT: *Dupuytren's Contracture.* Edinburgh, Scotland, Livingstone, 1963.

61. McFarlane RM: Dupuytren's disease: Relation to work and injury. *J Hand Surg [Am]* 1991;16:775-779.

62. McGrouther D: The extensor mechanism and knuckle changes: An overview of operative treatment, in McFarlane RM, McGrouther DA, Flint MH (eds): *Dupuytren's Disease: Biology and Treatment.* New York, NY, Churchill Livingstone, 1990, pp 295-310.

63. Garrod AE: On an unusual form of nodule upon the joints of the fingers. *St. Bartholomew's Hosp Rep* 1893;29:157-161.

64. Hueston JT: Dorsal Dupuytren's disease. *J Hand Surg [Am]* 1982;7:384-387.

65. Skoog T: Dupuytren's contracture with special reference to etiology and improved surgical treatment, its occurrence in epileptics. *Acta Chir Scand* 1948;96(Suppl 139):1.

66. Caroli A, Zanasi S, Marcuzzi A, Guerra D, Cristiani G, Ronchetti IP: Epidemiological and structural findings supporting the fibromatous origin of dorsal knuckle pads. *J Hand Surg [Br]* 1991;16:258-262.

67. Flint M: The genesis of the palmar lesion, in McFarlane RM, McGrouther DA, Flint MH (eds): *Dupuytren's Disease: Biology and Treatment.* New York, NY, Churchill Livingstone, 1990, pp 282-70.

68. Short WH, Watson HK: Prediction of the spiral nerve in Dupuytren's contracture. *J Hand Surg [Am]* 1982;7:84-86.

69. Boyes JH, Jones FE: Dupuytren's disease involving the volar aspect of the wrist. *Plast Reconstr Surg* 1968;41:204-207.

70. Simons AW, Srivastava S, Nancarrow JD: Dupuytren's disease affecting the wrist. *J Hand Surg [Br]* 1996;21:367-368.

71. Sinha A: Dupuytren's disease may extend beyond the wrist crease in continuity. *J Bone Joint Surg Br* 1997;79:211-212.

72. Okano M: Dupuytren's contracture (palmar fibromatosis) extending over the arm. *Acta Derm Venereol* 1992;72:381-382.

73. Bunnell S: *Surgery of the Hand.* Philadelphia, PA, JB Lippincott, 1944, p 613.

74. Classen DA, Hurst LN: Plantar fibromatosis and bilateral flexion contractures: A review of the literature. *Ann Plast Surg* 1992;28:475-478.

75. Donato RR, Morrison WA: Dupuytren's disease in feet causing flexion contracture in the toes. *J Hand Surg [Br]* 1996;21:364-366.

76. Wheeler ES, Meals RA: Dupuytren's diathesis: A broad spectrum disease. *Plast Reconstr Surg* 1981;68:781-783.

77. Erdmann MW, Quaba AA, Sommerlad BC: Epithelioid sarcoma masquerading as Dupuytren's disease. *Br J Plast Surg* 1995;48:39-42.

78. Yacoe ME, Bergman AG, Ladd AL, Hellman BH: Dupuytren's contracture: MR imaging findings and correlation between MR signal intensity and cellularity of lesions. *AJR Am J Roentgenol* 1993;160:813-817.

79. Elliot D, Khan J: Palmar bands in

rheumatoid arthritis and other chronic conditions of the upper limb. *J Hand Surg [Br]* 1996;21:369-374.

80. Badalamente MA, Hurst LC: Enzyme injection as nonsurgical treatment of Dupuytren's disease. *J Hand Surg [Am]* 2000;25:629-636.

81. McCarthy DM: The long-term results of enzymic fasciotomy. *J Hand Surg [Br]* 1992;17:356.

82. Ketchum LD, Donahue TK: The injection of nodules of Dupuytren's disease with triamcinolone acetonide. *J Hand Surg [Am]* 2000;25:1157-1162.

83. Pittet B, Rubbia-Brandt L, Desmouliere A, et al: Effect of gamma-interferon on the clinical and biologic evolution of hypertrophic scars and Dupuytren's disease: An open pilot study. *Plast Reconstr Surg* 1994;93:1224-1235.

84. Colville J: Dupuytren's contracture—the role of fasciotomy. *Hand* 1983;15:162-166.

85. Rowley DI, Couch M, Chesney RB, Norris SH: Assessment of percutaneous fasciotomy in the management of Dupuytren's contracture. *J Hand Surg [Br]* 1984;9:163-164.

86. Bryan AS, Ghorbal MS: The long-term results of closed palmar fasciotomy in the management of Dupuytren's contracture. *J Hand Surg [Br]* 1988;13:254-256.

87. Leclercq C, Hurst L, Badalamente M: Nonsurgical treatment, in Tubiana R, Leclercq C, Hurst LC, Badalamente MA, Mackin EJ (eds): *Dupuytren's Disease.* London, England, Martin Dunitz, 2000, pp 121-131.

88. Freehafer AA, Strong JM: The treatment of Dupuytren's contracture by partial fasciectomy. *J Bone Joint Surg Am* 1963;45:1207-1216.

89. Russ R: The surgical aspects of Dupuytren's contraction. *Am J Med Sci* 1908;135:856.

90. Moermans JP: Segmental aponeurectomy in Dupuytren's disease. *J Hand Surg [Br]* 1991;16:243-254.

91. McIndoe A, Beare R: The surgical management of Dupuytren's contracture. *Am J Surg* 1958;95:197-203.

92. Zachariae L: Extensive versus limited fasciectomy for Dupuytren's contracture. *Scand J Plast Reconstr Surg* 1967;1:150-153.

93. Heuston JT: The control of recurrent Dupuytren's contracture by skin replacement. *Br J Plast Surg* 1969;22:152-156.

94. Searle AE, Logan AM: A mid-term review of the results of dermofasciectomy for Dupuytren's disease. *Ann Chir Main Memb Super* 1992;11:375-380.

95. Ketchum LD, Hixson FD: Dermofasciectomy and full-thickness grafts in the treatment of Dupuytren's contracture. *J Hand Surg [Am]* 1987;12:659-664.

96. Kelly C, Varian J: Dermofasciectomy: A long term review. *Ann Chir Main Memb Super* 1992;11:381-382.

97. Roush TF, Stern PJ: Results following surgery for recurrent Dupuytren's disease. *J Hand Surg [Am]* 2000;25:291-296.

98. Smith P, Breed C: Central slip attenuation in Dupuytren's contracture: A cause of persistent flexion of the proximal interphalangeal joint. *J Hand Surg [Am]* 1994;19:840-843.

99. Weinzweig N, Culver JE, Fleegler EJ: Severe contractures of the proximal interphalangeal joint in Dupuytren's disease: Combined fasciectomy with capsuloligamentous release versus fasciectomy alone. *Plast Reconstr Surg* 1996;97:560-566.

100. Rives K, Gelberman R, Smith B, Carney K: Severe contractures of the proximal interphalangeal joint in Dupuytren's disease: Results of a prospective trial of

operative correction and dynamic extension splinting. *J Hand Surg [Am]* 1992;17:1153-1159.

101. Messina A, Messina J: The continuous elongation treatment by the TEC device for severe Dupuytren's contracture of the fingers. *Plast Reconstr Surg* 1993;92:84-90.

102. Bailey AJ, Tarlton JF, Van der Stappen J, Sims TJ, Messina A: The continuous elongation technique for severe Dupuytren's disease. A biochemical mechanism. *J Hand Surg [Br]* 1994;19:522-527.

103. Moberg E: Three useful ways to avoid amputation in advanced Dupuytren's contracture. *Orthop Clin North Am* 1973;4:1001-1005.

104. McCash CR: The open palm technique in Dupuytren's contracture. *Br J Plast Surg* 1964;17:271-280.

105. Gelberman RH, Panagis JS, Hergenroeder PT, Zakaib GS: Wound complications in the surgical management of Dupuytren's contracture: A comparison of operative incisions. *Hand* 1982;14:248-254.

106. Zachariae L: Operation for Dupuytren's contracture by the method of McCash. *Acta Orthop Scand* 1970;41:433-438.

107. Lubahn JD: Open-palm technique and soft-tissue coverage in Dupuytren's disease. *Hand Clin* 1999;15:127-136.

108. Schneider LH, Hankin FM, Eisenberg T: Surgery of Dupuytren's disease: A review of the open palm method. *J Hand Surg [Am]* 1986;11:23-27.

109. Boyer MI, Gelberman RH: Complications of the operative treatment of Dupuytren's disease. *Hand Clin* 1999;15:161-166.

110. Foucher G, Cornil C, Lenoble E: Open palm technique for Dupuytren's disease: A five-year follow-up. *Ann Chir Main Memb Super* 1992;11:362-366.

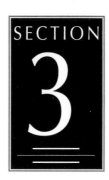

SECTION 3

Adult Reconstruction: Pain Management in Joint Arthroplasty

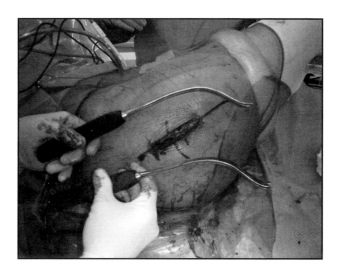

Patient-Controlled Analgesia for Total Joint Arthroplasty

Charles H. Crawford III, MD
Arthur L. Malkani, MD

Abstract

Pain control following total joint arthroplasty is critical for optimizing patient outcome. Both the real and perceived success of joint arthroplasty surgery depends on the patient's level of pain in the postoperative period. Patients who experience less pain will be more satisfied with their surgery and will be able to more fully participate in postoperative mobilization and rehabilitation. Optimal pain control must be balanced against the adverse effects of narcotics, including alteration of sensorium (especially in older patients) as well as respiratory depression. Modern strategies to control postoperative pain involve a multimodal approach that includes the use of intravenous patient-controlled analgesia.
Instr Course Lect 2007;56:115-119.

Although pain control is a major concern for every patient undergoing orthopaedic surgery, pain is often undertreated.[1] Inadequate treatment of pain may occur because of the surgeon's unfamiliarity with advances and options in pain management and from misconceptions concerning complications that can result from pain control measures. Pain management strategies range from spinal and epidural anesthesia, regional anesthetic blocks of peripheral nerves, oral and parenteral opioid administration, and the use of nonnarcotic pain modulators such as nonsteroidal anti-inflammatory drugs (NSAIDs). Patient-controlled analgesia (PCA) has become a preferred postoperative modality for many surgeons and patients. Knowl-edge of the concerns regarding PCA can help surgeons to optimize patient satisfaction and outcome while minimizing the complications associated with narcotic use.

Acute Pain and Its Sequelae

Pain is the body's response to local tissue damage; pain modulators are released including prostaglandins, histamine, serotonin, bradykinin, and substance P. Pain signals are transmitted along peripheral nerve fibers to the spinal cord tracts and the brain. Physical responses to pain occur at both the subconscious reflexive level and at the conscious level.

The importance of adequate pain control is well documented.[1-3] Acute pain can lead to multiple adverse consequences in the postoperative period including sympathetic activation, immobility, and neuroendocrine stress responses. These physiologic changes can lead to clinically significant complications including myocardial ischemia, thromboembolism, and pneumonia. Additionally, uncontrolled acute pain can lead to physical and psychological changes, which can contribute to chronic pain states.

Pain Control Options

There is great variation in individual tolerance and response to pain. Physical differences in neuronal and chemical pain modulators may play a role, as well as differences in psychological responses to pain.

In the postoperative period, delays and inconsistencies can occur in the interrelationship between the patient who experiences the pain, the doctor who prescribes the pain medicine, the nurse who assesses the patient and delivers the prescription, and the effective onset of pain relief provided by the medication. This delay in pain treatment can lead to increased pain and anxiety for the patient and to unnecessary demands on the physician and nurs-

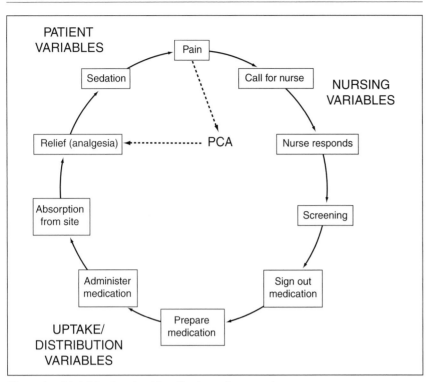

Figure 1   Variables involved in effective pain control.

Table 1
Examples of PCA Doses and Intervals With Commonly Used Opioids

Drug	Dose	Delay Interval
Morphine	1 to 3 mg/pulse	6 to 10 minutes
Hydromorphone	0.1 to 0.5 mg/pulse	6 to 10 minutes
Meperidine	10 mg/pulse	6 to 10 minutes

ing staff. Advances in PCA have reduced some of the inconsistencies and delays in the pain relief process (Figure 1). The actual time needed for the pain relief process, as well as the anxiety of the patient who was previously not in direct control of pain amelioration, can be decreased by the use of PCA devices.[4]

Historical Background

Traditional intramuscular injections of morphine have several drawbacks, including variable and erratic absorption and delay in time of onset. Intravenous routes of morphine introduction allow for more immediate and consistent blood concentrations. The use of PCA was popularized in the late 1970s to better treat the pain of hospitalized patients while avoiding the adverse effects of narcotic overdosage. Advances in technology have allowed the development of microprocessors and pumps that store and regulate delivery of a drug in response to the push of a button. PCA is now commonly used in most hospitals in the United States. Optimal protocols are actively being investigated and refined.

Original studies of intravenous on-demand opioid administration involved a bedside nurse who would administer small doses of opioid at the patient's request. Although pain relief was improved with these smaller total doses of opioid, the obvious demands on the nursing staff precluded widespread application of this protocol. Researchers developed and tested a variety of machines that allowed patients to safely self-administer opioids via their intravenous line. These PCA devices were triggered to administer a preset amount of opioid when the patient pushed a button on the end of a cord attached to the machine. A delay or lockout interval prevented the patient from administering more opioid before a set time had elapsed to allow the previous dose to take its maximal effect.[4-8]

Effectiveness and Choices

Many studies have reported safe and effective use of PCA devices with high patient satisfaction.[4,9-12] Morphine is the most commonly used and recommended first choice for intravenous opioid therapy. Morphine is typically administered in 1- to 3-mg increments every 6 to 10 minutes. Hydromorphone is a good alternative to morphine and is typically administered in 0.1- to 0.5-mg increments, because its potency is approximately five times that of morphine. Meperidine is another choice for analgesia; however, its use is often avoided because of the risk of seizures from buildup of its metabolite, normeperidine. Fentanyl also can be used but it is associated with a short duration of action. All of these analgesics can be used with bolus doses and basal rates. Basal rates should be used with great caution to avoid respiratory depression, especially in older patients. Commonly prescribed protocols are shown in Table 1.

Even with PCA, complete pain

relief is unrealistic. The goal of treatment is to effectively reduce pain while minimizing the side effects associated with narcotic use. For some patients, PCA may not provide better pain control than nurse-administered bolus doses as needed. Adjustments to dosage based on individual patient needs should be addressed.[11,12] Patient factors, such as physical and mental disabilities, may prevent successful use of a PCA device. PCA pumps can be expensive and the medical staff must be familiar with their proper operation.

One of the newer choices for PCA is the fentanyl hydrochloride patient-controlled transdermal system that uses a low intensity direct current to transfer fentanyl on demand across the skin into the systemic circulation. Clinical studies have shown that the system is safe, effective, and well tolerated by patients.[13] Fentanyl is also available as a 25- to 75-μg continuous-release patch that can be applied to the skin every 3 days.

Regional Versus Systemic PCA

In 1998, Singelyn and associates[14] performed a prospective study to compare the effects of pain control of PCA with morphine, continuous epidural analgesia, and continuous three-in-one block (of the lumbar plexus) in 45 patients undergoing knee rehabilitation after unilateral total knee arthroplasty. The authors concluded that local-regional analgesia (epidural or three-in-one block) provided better pain relief and faster rehabilitation than intravenous PCA with morphine. Because fewer side effects were found with the three-in-one block compared with the epidural analgesia, three-in-one block was recom-

mended as the pain control method of choice.

In a 1999 study by Singelyn and Gouverneur,[15] intravenous PCA with morphine, patient-controlled epidural analgesia, and continuous three-in-one block were compared for efficacy in pain control in 1,300 patients after unilateral total hip arthroplasty. The authors found similar pain relief in all three groups with a lower incidence of side effects in the group using the three-in-one block method. In 2000 and 2001, Singelyn and associates[16,17] published additional studies showing that PCA devices for the regional block catheters limit the amount of local anesthetic used, while maintaining pain control and patient satisfaction.

Despite these studies that support the use of regional anesthetic blocks after total knee and hip arthroplasty, these techniques may not be appropriate or available to every patient. The administration of regional analgesia requires specific tools and technical skills that are not available at all institutions. The invasive nature of the technique is not tolerated by all patients and can be associated with complications including difficulties with postoperative thromboembolism prophylaxis.

A new product for epidural analgesia uses a gradually releasing foam technology to provide a one-time depot of morphine into the epidural space, eliminating the need for epidural catheters that may interfere with patient mobilization and anticoagulation therapy.[18]

Adverse Events

Common adverse effects of opioid analgesia include respiratory depression, nausea, sedation, pruritus, and urinary retention. Nausea is the most common adverse event lead-

Table 2
Risk Factors for Respiratory Depression With PCA Use
Advanced age (older than 70 years)
Hypovolemia
Large incremental doses (> 1 mg morphine per dose)
Use of continuous infusion mode (basal rate)
Use of additional central nervous system depressants (benzodiazepines, antihistamines)
Comorbidities (pulmonary, cardiac, renal, hepatic)

ing to patient dissatisfaction with PCA.[2] Because respiratory depression is the most serious and life-threatening adverse event, it is the most widely studied.

The risk of respiratory depression increases with advanced age (older than 70 years), hypovolemia, large incremental doses (> 1 mg morphine), the use of a continuous infusion mode, the use of additional central nervous system depressants, and patient comorbidities including pulmonary, cardiac, and renal disease[4,9,19] (Table 2). Despite these findings, PCA can successfully be used in an elderly patient who is cognitively intact and who is provided with appropriate precautions and individualized therapies. A typical dose would be 1 mg of morphine every 6 to 10 minutes; continuous basal rates are not recommended.[11,20]

Management of adverse effects includes using antiemetic medications, changing the opioid, adjusting the interval dose, and discontinuing PCA therapy. The use of acetaminophen as an adjunct to morphine after major surgery has been studied extensively. In a recent meta-analysis, Remy and associates[21] showed that acetaminophen had a morphine-sparing effect but did not

Table 3
Multimodal Approach to Pain Control With PCA for Joint Arthroplasty Patients

Total Knee Arthroplasty	Total Hip Arthroplasty

Femoral nerve and sciatic nerve block
  Preoperative
  ± indwelling catheter
  Bupivacaine
	Lumbar plexus block
	  Preoperative
	  Bupivacaine

Intra-articular injection Intraoperative after closure Bupivacaine	PCA pump
PCA pump	Ketorolac: intramuscular/intravenous
Ketorolac: intramuscular/intravenous	Oral narcotics
Oral narcotics	

reduce the incidence of morphine-related adverse effects.

Multimodal Approach

The use of multiple complementary methods for treating pain is the standard practice in many centers. Effective multimodal pain control can facilitate rapid rehabilitation and discharge after total joint arthroplasty. Some centers have acute pain service teams that specialize in developing and implementing pain control protocols.[22] At the authors' hospital, a typical patient undergoing total hip arthroplasty is treated with a preoperative lumbar plexus block, supplemented in the postoperative period with analgesia using an intravenous morphine PCA pump, an oral narcotic or acetaminophen tablet, and an intramuscular/intravenous NSAID.

A typical patient undergoing total knee arthroplasty would receive all or some of the multimodal options for postoperative relief including a preoperative sciatic and femoral nerve block, an intraoperative intra-articular injection of a local anesthetic, analgesia administered with a postoperative intravenous morphine PCA pump, and administration of an oral narcotic/acetaminophen tablet

and an intramuscular/intravenous NSAIDs.

Femoral nerve blocks are supplemented with an indwelling catheter that is removed after 48 hours. The intravenous morphine PCA pump is programmed to deliver 1-mg doses every 6 minutes on demand with no continuous basal rate. An oral combination of hydrocodone 7.5 mg/acetaminophen 500 mg in tablet form is allowed every 4 to 6 hours as needed for pain. Ketorolac (15 mg intravenous injections) are given every 8 hours for the first 24 hours after surgery, if needed (Table 3). PCA pumps are typically discontinued on postoperative day one or two with nerve and urinary catheters to facilitate physical therapy and eventual discharge.

Summary

Optimal anesthetic and analgesic protocols are dependent on the patient, the surgeon, and institutional characteristics. Knowledge of the issues and techniques for pain control will help the surgeon and anesthesiologist to develop optimal pain control protocols for patients undergoing total joint arthroplasty. Without adequate pain control, patients will be less satisfied with the hospital ex-

perience, postoperative rehabilitation may be compromised, and postoperative complications may increase.

Strategies for developing and choosing protocols include the preoperative identification of patients who are at risk for complications, minimizing soft-tissue trauma during surgery, using effective regional and local anesthetics, using NSAIDs and other pain modulating nonnarcotic medications, and tailoring oral and parenteral narcotics to the individual needs of a patient. The use of PCA devices can assist in optimizing systemic concentrations of narcotics, as well as regional doses of local anesthetics. PCA devices provide patients with a sense of control over their pain, and decrease the need for care from the nursing staff. Proper monitoring and assessment of patients using a PCA device is essential to optimize efficacy and minimize adverse events. To minimize respiratory depression, adjustments to the level of PCA should be made based on an assessment of the changing condition of the patient. A multimodal approach that includes the use of regional blocks and NSAIDs also can reduce the need for postoperative narcotics and the inherent side effects associated with their use. Effective collaboration among the orthopaedist, the anesthesiologist, and the hospital staff to reduce postoperative pain after total joint arthroplasty can lead to improved patient satisfaction with recovery and overall outcome.

References

1. Joint Commission on Accreditation of Healthcare Organizations: *Pain Sandards for 2001.* Oakbrook Terrace, Illinois, JCAHO, 2000.

2. Sinatra RS, Torres J, Bustos AM: Pain management after major orthopaedic surgery: Current strategies and new concepts. *J Am Acad Orthop Surg*

2002;10:117-129.

3. Bourne MH: Analgesics for orthopedic postoperative pain. *Am J Orthop* 2004;33:128-135.

4. White PF: Use of patient-controlled analgesia for management of acute pain. *JAMA* 1988;259:243-247.

5. Sechzer PH: Objective measurement of pain. *Anesthesiology* 1968;29:209-210.

6. Forrest WH, Smethurst PW, Kientz ME: Self-administration of intravenous analgesics. *Anesthesiology* 1970;33:363.

7. Sechzer PH: Studies in pain with the analgesic-demand system. *Anesth Analg* 1971;50:1-10.

8. Graves DA, Foster TS, Batenhorst RL, Bennett RL, Baumann TJ: Patient-controlled analgesia. *Ann Intern Med* 1983;99:360-366.

9. Tamsen A, Hartvig P, Fagerlund C: Patient-controlled analgesic therapy: Clinical experience. *Acta Anaesthesiol Scand Suppl* 1982;74:157-160.

10. Colwell CW Jr: The use of the pain pump and patient-controlled analgesia in joint reconstruction. *Am J Orthop* 2004;33(suppl 5):10-12.

11. Macintyre PE: Safety and efficacy of patient-controlled analgesia. *Br J Anaesth* 2001;87:36-46.

12. Macintyre PE: Intravenous patient-controlled analgesia: One size does not fit all. *Anesthesiol Clin North America* 2005;23:109-123.

13. Sinatra R: The fentanyl HCl patient-controlled transdermal system (PCTS): An alternative to intravenous patient-controlled analgesia in the postoperative setting. *Clin Pharmacokinet* 2005;44(suppl 1):1-6.

14. Singelyn FJ, Deyaert M, Joris D, Pendeville E, Gouverneur JM: Effects of intravenous patient-controlled analgesia with morphine, continuous epidural analgesia, and continuous three-in-one block on postoperative pain and knee rehabilitation after unilateral total knee arthroplasty. *Anesth Analg* 1998;87:88-92.

15. Singelyn FJ, Gouverneur JM: Postoperative analgesia after total hip arthroplasty: I.V. PCA with morphine, patient-controlled epidural analgesia, or continuous "3-in-1" block?: A prospective evaluation by our acute pain service in more than 1,300 patients. *J Clin Anesth* 1999;11:550-554.

16. Singelyn FJ, Gouverneur JM: Extended "three-in-one" block after total knee arthroplasty: Continuous versus patient-controlled techniques. *Anesth Analg* 2000;91:176-180.

17. Singelyn FJ, Vanderelst PE, Gouverneur JM: Extended femoral nerve sheath block after total hip arthroplasty: Continuous versus patient-controlled techniques. *Anesth Analg* 2001;92:455-459.

18. Viscusi ER: Emerging techniques for postoperative analgesia in orthopedic surgery. *Am J Orthop* 2004;33(suppl 5):13-16.

19. Hagle ME, Lehr VT, Brubakken K, Shippee A: Respiratory depression in adult patients with intravenous patient-controlled analgesia. *Orthop Nurs* 2004;23:18-27.

20. Lavand'Homme P, DeKock M: Practical guidelines on the postoperative use of patient-controlled analgesia in the elderly. *Drugs Aging* 1998;13:9-16.

21. Remy C, Marret E, Bonnet F: Effects of acetaminophen on morphine side-effects and consumption after major surgery: Meta-analysis of randomized controlled trials. *Br J Anaesth* 2005;94:505-513.

22. Riegler FX: Update on perioperative pain management. *Clin Orthop Relat Res* 1994;305:283-292.

The Role of Minimally Invasive Hip Surgery in Reducing Pain

Fabio R. Orozco, MD
Alvin Ong, MD
Richard H. Rothman, MD

Abstract

The purported benefits of minimally invasive total hip arthroplasty (THA) compared with conventional approaches has stirred controversy in the orthopaedic community. Some studies performed by the pioneers of the minimally invasive techniques showed improvement in immediate patient outcomes. Less blood loss, shorter hospital stays, lessened immediate postoperative pain, and faster return to normal activities are potential benefits of any type of minimally invasive surgery. Most studies of minimally invasive THA have involved changes in the intraoperative and postoperative protocols that could independently affect patient outcome. Appropriate prospective studies that compare conventional and minimally invasive THA and the effects of different rehabilitation protocols on patient outcome are needed. The results of different approaches for minimally invasive THA also require study. A review of reported short-term outcomes and complications of small-incision THA performed using several modifications of existing surgical approaches and the possible effect on postoperative pain provide needed information on this controversial topic.

Instr Course Lect 2007;56:121-124.

Total hip arthroplasty (THA) is one of the most successful orthopaedic procedures performed in the United States; its overall success is documented by extensive research.[1,2] Patients undergoing THA can expect significant improvement in their quality of life and function, substantial pain relief, and an anticipated longevity of the prosthesis of more than 15 years.

Over the past few decades, THA has substantially evolved because of improvements in prosthetic designs, materials, surgical techniques, and re-habilitation protocols. Recently, less invasive procedures based on laparoscopic and arthroscopic principles have been developed for joint arthroplasty. These surgical techniques allow THA to be performed through a smaller incision with the potential for less tissue damage and less perioperative morbidity (Figures 1 and 2).

Classic Principles of Joint Arthroplasty

Current principles of joint arthroplasty include good visualization of the surgical field, gentle and atraumatic handling of the tissues, avoidance of damage to the nerves, absolute hemostasis, and skilled and expeditious execution of the chosen surgical technique. With the introduction of minimally invasive surgery, additional principles include improved cosmesis and a decrease in pain and length of hospitalization.

Advantages and Disadvantages of Minimally Invasive THA

Proponents of minimally invasive surgery believe that these new surgical techniques result in a decrease in immediate postoperative pain, soft-tissue trauma, and blood loss, along with a shortened period of hospitalization, and improved cosmesis.[3-5] Potential disadvantages of minimally invasive surgery include the increased difficulty of performing surgery in a restricted visual field, poor visualization, an increase in surgical time, and a significant increase in the time needed for the surgeon to acquire the required surgical skills, along with the attendant risks involved until an adequate level of skill is achieved.[6-8]

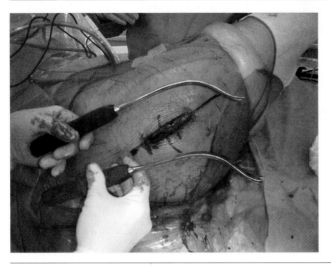
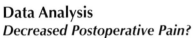

Figure 1 Intraoperative photograph shows that a small incision may require special acetabular and femoral instrumentation.

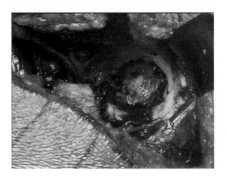

Figure 2 Intraoperative photograph shows adequate exposure of the acetabulum through a minimally invasive lateral approach.

Data Analysis

Decreased Postoperative Pain?

In a matched-pair analysis comparing regular incision THA with mini-incision THA through the anterolateral approach,[9] postoperative pain and requirements for narcotic medication were evaluated. Sixty patients in the control group underwent THA using a conventional technique and 60 patients underwent THA using a small-incision exposure. No detectable difference was found between the two groups in blood loss, narcotic requirements, and postoperative pain. Other studies have found similar results with no detectable differences in pain scores or analgesic use.[10,11]

Decreased Soft-Tissue Trauma?

It could be assumed that a smaller incision would lessen soft-tissue trauma; however, results do not support this assumption. Mardones and associates[12] performed minimally invasive THA on 20 cadaveric hips and found significant soft-tissue damage, particularly to the abductor mechanism.

A Safer Approach?

The literature shows conflicting results involving safety and the complication rate after minimally invasive THA. Several studies have shown no statistically significant difference in the complication rate when comparing THA using standard and small incisions.[4,7,10,11] In contrast, Woolson and associates[8] found a significantly higher risk of wound complications, a higher percentage of malpositioning of the acetabular component, and a poor fit and fill of cementless femoral components in patients treated with small-incision THA. Fehring and Mason[13] reported three catastrophic complications in patients treated with minimally invasive THA. In one patient, a segmental defect in the dome of the acetabulum was created. In another patient, multiple dislocations occurred after surgery because of a malpositioned cup; the patient later required revision surgery. In a third patient, an intraoperative fracture of the greater trochanter led to a severe Trendelenburg lurch caused by nonunion of the fracture. Bal and associates[14] reported on early complications in patients treated with two-incision minimally invasive THA and found a 10% revision rate. Repeat surgery was required because of femoral fractures, dislocations, wound complications, and subsidence and loosening of the femoral implant. The femoral cutaneus nerve was injured in 25% of patients.

Better Cosmesis?

Because it is intuitive to believe that a small incision will result in a more cosmetically appealing scar, improved cosmesis is one of the proposed benefits of minimally invasive THA; however, no scientific proof exists to support this belief. Mow and associates[15] studied the cosmetic appearances of healed incisions in 34 patients who underwent primary THA. Twenty patients were treated using minimally invasive THA and 14 were treated with standard-length incisions. The appearance of the scar was evaluated at an average of 2 years postoperatively. The appearance of each scar was graded independently by two plastic surgeons using a standardized rating system. Results showed that more mini scars (6 of 20) were rated poor compared with standard-length scars (1 of 14), and that more patients treated with standard-incision THA had scars that were rated good. More patients treated with mini-incision techniques (2 of 20) had wound-healing complications.

None of the 14 patients treated with standard-incision THA had wound-healing complications. All patients believed that their hip scar was acceptable in appearance, but 30 of 31 patients rated the relief of pain and the longevity of the hip prosthesis as higher in priority than scar cosmesis. The authors concluded that cosmesis of mini-incision THA scars may be inferior to standard-incision scars because of damage to skin and soft tissues produced by the high retractor pressures needed for exposure using a skin incision of limited length.

Comparative Studies

Few comparative studies are available that evaluate the outcomes of minimally invasive THA compared with standard-incision THA.[8,10] A study by Woolson and associates[8] evaluated 135 consecutive primary THAs (50 with a mini incision [≤ 10 cm] and 85 with a standard-length incision). Because of the patient selection process, those treated using the mini-incision technique had a significantly lower average body mass index and a lower average score on the American Society of Anesthesiologists rating, indicating that the patients treated with mini-incision techniques were thinner and healthier than the patients treated with standard-incision techniques. No significant differences in blood loss, transfusion requirements, postoperative pain, length of the hospital stay, and the patient's condition after discharge were found in the two groups. The group treated with the mini-incision technique had a significantly higher risk of wound complications, a higher percentage of acetabular component malpositioning, and poor fit and fill of femoral cementless components. In this particular study, the surgeons had no special prior training in minimally

invasive surgery nor did they use any special instrumentation.

Chimento and associates[10] performed a prospective randomized clinical trial to compare THA using a standard approach with THA using a minimally invasive approach. Sixty patients with a body mass index lower than 30 were randomly assigned to receive incisions of 8 cm or 15 cm. Patients in the group treated with the smaller incision had significantly less intraoperative blood loss ($P < 0.003$) and less total blood loss. Fewer patients treated with the minimally invasive surgery limped at 6-week follow-up. Surgical time, transfusion requirements, narcotic usage, length of hospital stay, achievement of rehabilitation milestones, cane usage, and complications were similar in both groups. Most importantly, there was no difference between the groups at 1- and 2-year follow-up.

A prospective study by DiGioia and associates[16] compared minimally invasive THA and standard-incision THA. The authors concluded that patients treated with the minimally invasive approach had significantly less limping and faster improvement in stair-climbing ability at 3-month follow-up. This accelerated improvement diminished with longer follow-up; at 1-year follow-up both groups had equal improvement.

Wenz and associates[17] compared the short-term outcome of patients treated with THA using a direct lateral approach with patients treated with minimally invasive THA. Patients in the minimally invasive group had decreased transfusion requirements, achieved significantly earlier ambulation, needed less transfer assistance, and had a more favorable disposition at the time of hospital discharge.

Pain Management
In theory, less surgical dissection should result in less postoperative pain; however, there is no proof of this outcome in the literature. Minimizing soft-tissue damage with or without the use of minimally invasive techniques has the potential to reduce postoperative pain. A decrease in pain should have a positive effect on the patient's participation in the rehabilitation process. By reducing analgesic need, the known adverse effects of these medications should also be decreased. Only one prospective randomized study provides a scientific evaluation of postoperative pain as a major outcome measure after minimally invasive and standard-incision THA. A randomized prospective study by Ogonda and associates[11] evaluated 219 THAs. No significant differences in pain scores and analgesic usage in the early postoperative period occurred in patients treated with minimally invasive THA compared with those treated with standard-incision THA.

A multidisciplinary approach to pain management after THA is required and involves the patient, the patient's family, the anesthesiologist, nurses, physical therapists, and the orthopaedic surgeon. Because patient expectations are of great importance, patient education should emphasize realistic goals and provide information on the expected postoperative course. The patient should also participate in a preoperative physical therapy session in which the postoperative regimen is explained.

Summary
Although the goals of minimally invasive surgery are to decrease soft-tissue trauma, reduce blood loss, shorten the length of the hospital stay, decrease postoperative pain, ac-

celerate rehabilitation, produce better cosmesis, and improve overall patient outcomes, the early studies on minimally invasive THA have not validated the achievement of these goals.

Classic surgical principles consisting of good visualization, gentle and atraumatic handling of the tissues, avoidance of nerve injuries, absolute hemostasis, and skilled and expeditious execution of the chosen surgical technique should be used. Shortening the length of the surgical incision is appropriate if classic surgical principles are not violated, risk of injury and complications are not increased, and the patient's long-term outcome is not compromised.

References

1. NIH Consensus Development Website. *Total Hip Replacement: NIH Consensus Statement, 1994*. Available at: http://consensus.nih.gov/1994/1994Hipreplacement098html.htm. Accessed June 1, 2006.

2. Sakalkale DP, Eng K, Hozack WJ, Rothman RH: Minimum 10-year results of a tapered cementless hip replacement. *Clin Orthop Relat Res* 1999;362:138-144.

3. Berger RA: Mini-incision total hip replacement using an anterolateral approach: Technique and results. *Orthop Clin North Am* 2004;35:143-151.

4. Sculco TP, Jordan LC, Walter WL: Minimally invasive total hip arthroplasty: The Hospital for Special Surgery experience. *Orthop Clin North Am* 2004;35:137-142.

5. Wright JM, Crockett HC, Delgado S, Lyman S, Madsen M, Sculco TP: Mini-incision for total hip arthroplasty: A prospective, controlled investigation with 5-year follow-up evaluation. *J Arthroplasty* 2004;19:538-545.

6. Goldstein WM, Branson JJ, Berland KA, Gordon AC: Minimal-incision total hip arthroplasty. *J Bone Joint Surg Am* 2003;85(suppl 4):33-38.

7. Howell JR, Masri BA, Duncan CP: Minimally invasive versus standard incision anterolateral hip replacement: A comparative study. *Orthop Clin North Am* 2004;35:153-162.

8. Woolson ST, Mow CS, Syquia JF, Lannin JV, Schurman DJ: Comparison of primary total hip replacements performed with a standard incision or a mini-incision. *J Bone Joint Surg Am* 2004;86:1353-1358.

9. Ciminiello M, Parvizi J, Sharkey PF, Eslampour A, Rothman RH: Total hip arthroplasty: Is small incision better? *J Arthroplasty* 2006;21:484-488.

10. Chimento GF, Pavone V, Sharrock N, Kahn B, Cahill J, Sculco TP: Minimally invasive total hip arthroplasty: A prospective randomized study. *J Arthroplasty* 2005;20:139-144.

11. Ogonda L, Wilson R, Archbold P, et al: A minimal-incision technique in total hip arthroplasty does not improve early postoperative outcomes: A prospective, randomized, controlled trial. *J Bone Joint Surg Am* 2005;87:701-710.

12. Mardones R, Pagnano MW, Nemanich JP, Trousdale RT: Muscle damage after total hip arthroplasty done with the two-incision and mini-posterior techniques. *Clin Orthop Relat Res* 2005;441:63-67.

13. Fehring TK, Mason JB: Catastrophic complications of minimally invasive hip surgery: A series of three cases. *J Bone Joint Surg Am* 2005;87:711-714.

14. Bal BS, Haltom D, Aleto T, Barrett M: Early complications of primary total hip replacement performed with a two-incision minimally invasive technique. *J Bone Joint Surg Am* 2005;87:2432-2438.

15. Mow CS, Woolson ST, Ngarmukos SG, Park EH, Lorenz HP: Comparison of scars from total hip replacements done with a standard or a mini-incision. *Clin Orthop Relat Res* 2005;441:80-85.

16. DiGioia AM III, Plakseychuk AY, Levison TJ, Jaramaz B: Mini-incision technique for total hip arthroplasty with navigation. *J Arthroplasty* 2003;18:123-128.

17. Wenz JF, Gurkan I, Jibodh SR: Mini-incision total hip arthroplasty: A comparative assessment of perioperative outcomes. *Orthopedics* 2002;25:1031-1043.

The Use of Local Periarticular Injections in the Management of Postoperative Pain After Total Hip and Knee Replacement: A Multimodal Approach

Hari K. Parvataneni, MD

Amar S. Ranawat, MD

Chitranjan S. Ranawat, MD

Abstract

Theoretically, an appropriately designed and implemented multimodal pain protocol should reduce postoperative pain levels, need for narcotic medication, and adverse events while improving functional recovery including ambulation, discharge from hospital, range of motion, and return to work. A complete, perioperative multimodal pain protocol for total hip replacement and total knee replacement, including use of a novel periarticular injection, has been described and early clinical results are reported.

Instr Course Lect 2006;56:125-131.

Pain is expected after trauma to the musculoskeletal system. Similarly, surgical trauma to soft tissues and bone results in pain. Orthopaedic procedures have been reported to be among the most painful of surgical procedures.[1,2] One of the most significant patient concerns regarding total hip replacement (THR) or total knee replacement (TKR) is the anticipated pain directly related to surgical trauma during the postoperative recovery period. It has been reported that more than half of postoperative patients receive suboptimal pain control[3,4] and half of all patients undergoing THR or TKR will experience severe pain[5] in the early postoperative period.

Significance of Pain

Surgeons often underestimate the severity and significance of postoperative pain, and this often results in significant physical and emotional discomfort for patients and their families.[3,4] The significance of pain, however, extends far beyond the humanitarian and ethical aspects of inadequate pain control. Postoperative pain often adversely affects clinical outcome and can have a significant economic impact.

Rehabilitation after THR or TKR is directly linked to pain and comfort levels. Earlier mobilization, ambulation, and return of normal gait is associated with more optimal pain control.[6,7] Additionally, arthrofibrosis and diminished postoperative range of motion are closely related to postoperative pain and related joint splinting and immobilization.[8] Complications may also be related to the physiologic response to pain and prolonged periods of diminished mobility and include pulmonary and vascular complications such as pneumonia and deep venous thrombosis.[9,10] Inadequately treated acute pain may ultimately lead to chronic pain via sensitization of the nervous system.[11,12]

Postoperative pain has a significant economic impact and is a common cause of delayed discharge from the hospital or rehabilitation facility and early readmission.[13-15] Additionally, delay in the return of function or prolonged disability negatively impact a patient's ability to return to work. Patient perceptions of surgical success are closely

One or more of the authors or the departments with which they are affiliated have received something of value from a commercial or other party related directly or indirectly to the subject of this chapter.

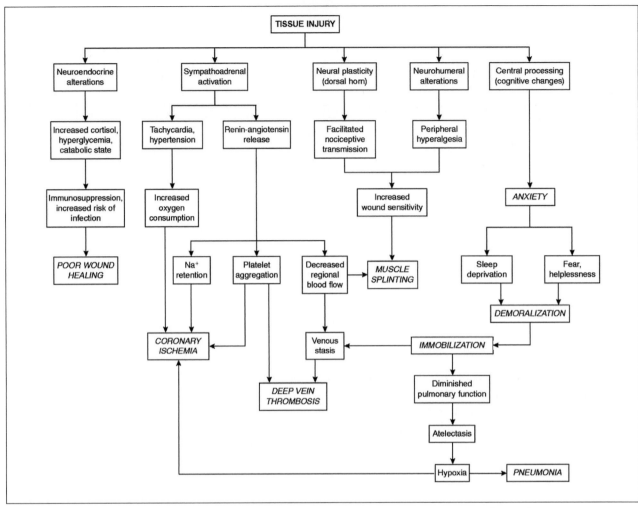

Figure 1   Cognitive and pathophysiologic responses associated with surgical trauma and their effect on key target organs. (Reproduced from Sinatra RS, Torres J, Bustos AM: Pain management after major orthopaedic surgery: Current strategies and new concepts. *J Am Acad Orthop Surg* 2002;10(2):117-129.)

matched to residual pain, functional limitations, and speed of recovery.[16,17]

Pathophysiology of Pain
Detailed descriptions of the pathways involved in pain generation, perception, and physiologic responses have been published by the American Academy of Orthopaedic Surgeons;[10,18,19] nonetheless, pain is still a poorly understood, complex phenomenon. Painful stimuli (thermal, chemical, or mechanical) result in a physio-

logic response that likely involves neural, cellular, and humoral components (Figure 1).

Besides the sensory aspects of pain, cognitive and emotional components are important factors that influence a patient's perception of pain.[20] Factors including age, gender, culture, education level, communication skills, prior pain experience, expectations, and preoperative education regarding pain all influence an individual's pain perception and experience in the postoperative period.

The Concept of a Multimodal Approach to Pain Control
To obtain more effective pain control, it seems logical that a pain protocol must act simultaneously on several of the pain pathways as well as both centrally and peripherally. A multimodal approach uses various techniques and pharmacologic agents, each operating through a different site or mechanism[21] (Figure 2). Synergism is obtained when the analgesic effects of the individual agents or modalities are potentiated and the resultant analgesic effect is greater.[22]

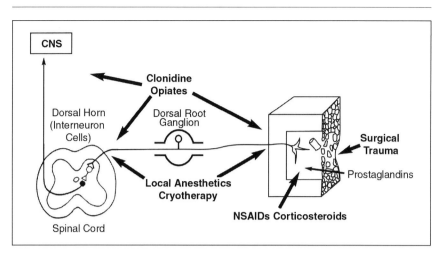

Figure 2 Schematic representation of the sites of action of analgesics along the pain pathway from the periphery to the central nervous system (CNS). NSAIDs = nonsteroidal anti-inflammatory drugs. (Reproduced with permission from Reuben SS, Sklar J: Pain management in patients who undergo outpatient arthroscopic surgery of the knee. *J Bone Joint Surg Am* 2000;82:1754-1766.)

Table 1
Components of a Multimodal Approach for THR or TKR

Preoperative patient education/clarification of expectations

Preemptive analgesia

Anesthesia technique

Surgical technique

Intraoperative agents (including use of a novel periarticular injection)

Postoperative analgesia

Table 2
Preoperative Pain Management Protocol for THR and TKR

Preemptive Analgesia/Medications (Admission Area)

1. Celecoxib 200/400 mg orally
2. Oxycodone SR 10/20 mg orally
3. Pantoprazole 40 mg orally
4. Warfarin 5 mg orally

SR = sustained release

Optimal pain control is the primary goal of this modality, but reduction of the dosages of individual medications decreases the risk of associated complications. This reduction of dosage and adverse effects is most beneficial with narcotics, particularly opioid narcotics.

The concept of multimodal pain control has received increasing interest in the recent literature.[10,21-23] There has been particular interest in total joint arthroplasty with various combinations of local, regional, and systemic modalities. Published results are promising in terms of improved perioperative pain control, reduced need for narcotic medications, and reduced associated adverse effects.[21,22]

Advanced Perioperative Multimodal Pain Protocol

The key aspects of the multimodal approach to pain control after THR or TKR are outlined in Table 1.

Preoperative Patient Education

As described previously, patient factors and background play an impor-

tant part in postoperative pain perception. As part of the authors' total joint replacement protocol, all patients are enrolled in a preoperative total joint replacement class and are given videos and handouts at the time of surgical consultation. Important aspects of the surgical procedure, postoperative course, and rehabilitation are reviewed in detail. Patient expectations are tempered toward realistic recovery goals, and typical timelines for recovery of function and for a pain-free joint are outlined. The overall goal is to reduce patient anxiety and misconceptions in the early postoperative period that can negatively affect a patient's perception of pain.

Preemptive Analgesia

Preemptive analgesia involves preoperative administration of various agents to reduce central sensitization and amplification of postoperative pain.[21] Prevention of pain is easier and more effective than control of established pain.[24] Ideally, preemptive analgesia should reduce both the neurogenic and inflammatory

responses to surgical trauma.[25] Preemptive analgesia must be combined with appropriate intraoperative and postoperative modalities for greater effectiveness. This concept can be expanded to include local or systemic administration of analgesic and anti-inflammatory agents before the physiologic neurogenic and inflammatory responses to surgery are complete during and after surgery.

The specific agents administered preoperatively are outlined in Table 2. These are administered approximately 2 hours before incision to achieve appropriate functional levels.

Controlled-release oxycodone has been shown to improve pain control and decrease the need for other narcotic agents and other analgesics, while improving functional recovery and reducing adverse effects.[26,27] The effects of controlled-release oxycodone are enhanced by

Table 3
Perioperative Pain Management Protocol for THR and TKR

Intraoperative Injection

1. 0.5% bupivacaine 200-400 mg
2. Morphine sulfate (0.8 cc) 8 mg
3. Epinephrine 1/1,000 (0.3 cc) 300 µg
4. Methylprednisolone acetate 40 mg
5. Cefuroxime (10 cc) 750 mg
6. Dilute with normal saline to a total volume of 60 cc

No steroids in diabetic/ immunocompromised patients/revisions

Vancomycin if allergic to penicillin

Clonidine transdermal patch applied in operating room (100 µg)

Table 4
Injection Sites for Intraoperative Periarticular Injection

THR

Prior to final reduction:

  Anterior capsule

  Iliopsoas tendon and insertion site

After final reduction (before irrigation and closure):

  Abductors

  Fascia lata

  Gluteus maximus and its insertion

  Posterior capsule and short external rotators

  Synovium

TKR

Prior to insertion of liner and reduction:

  Posterior capsule

  Posteromedial and posterolateral structures

After reduction:

  Extensor mechanism

  Synovium

  Capsule

  Pes anserinus, anteromedial capsule, and periosteum

  Iliotibial band

  Collateral ligaments and origins

preemptive administration (preoperatively as well as on a scheduled basis postoperatively).

Cyclooxygenase (COX)-2 selective inhibitors reduce pain and inflammation after tissue trauma while preserving the cytoprotective actions associated with the COX-1 enzyme. By administering this agent daily beginning preoperatively, continuous analgesic and anti-inflammatory effects are provided. Improved pain scores, improved joint range of motion, and reduced need for narcotics for breakthrough pain have been demonstrated with this group of agents.[28,29] Because of potential renal and cardiac toxicity, this agent is administered to patients with normal renal and cardiac function and only for a short course postoperatively.

Anesthesia Technique

All patients receive regional anesthesia (spinal, epidural, or combination) unless specific contraindications exist (numerous prior lumbar spinal procedures or coagulopathy). Administration is performed by anesthesiologists who are experienced in regional anesthetic techniques and familiar with the preferences of

the surgeon. All patients must achieve complete anesthesia before incision. Supplementation with general anesthesia or systemic analgesia is considered a failure of regional technique.

Surgical Technique

The technique of reduced tissue trauma surgery is used in all patients. Inappropriate stretching, tearing, and maceration of the soft tissues, including the skin, is minimized by sharp dissection, adequate exposure, and appropriate tissue releases. Incision length varies between 10 and 20 cm, depending on patient factors such as amount of fat, resistance of the soft tissues, level of deformity, prior surgical procedures, and amount of contracture. A deep

drain is used routinely for 24 hours to minimize hematoma formation.

For TKR, application of a standard thigh tourniquet is minimized. Direct mechanical trauma to the quadriceps and hamstring muscle compartments as well as ischemic injury to the entire distal extremity is therefore minimized. Additionally, the pressure applied during use is maintained at approximately 100 mm Hg above the systolic blood pressure. The tourniquet is used for a brief period only for the cementation of the final implants.

Intraoperative Periarticular Injection

The components of this novel combination of agents are detailed in Table 3. Meticulous injection is performed into the synovium, ligamentous attachments, deep fascia, capsule, muscle groups deep to the fascia, and into the arthrotomy sites. Direct free intra-articular injection is avoided. The sites of injection for THR and TKR are outlined in Table 4.

This intraoperative injection is considered to be the most important and effective component of this pain protocol. Direct analgesic effect is produced by long-acting local anesthetic as well as local opioid via different mechanisms. Additionally, epinephrine prolongs the action of the local agents by decreasing absorption by vasoconstriction via its α-adrenergic effects. It may also have an effect in decreasing postoperative bleeding and hematoma.

Morphine exerts its analgesic effects centrally, regionally, and locally by its effect on opioid receptors. Local administration allows sustained effect with a minimum of the typical opioid adverse effects (sedation, nausea, and respiratory depression), which occur through central opioid receptors. Local administration of morphine has demonstrated advantages in the reduction of postoperative pain in total joint arthroplasty.[30]

Clonidine exerts its effect via its α-2 adrenergic actions. It results in potentiation of the actions of local anesthetic agents and local opioids via synergistic effects.[31,32] Transdermal administration allows sustained action for several days while minimizing potential adverse effects, including bradycardia and hypotension.

Corticosteroid is a key component of this injection. Numerous studies have demonstrated potent local anti-inflammatory effects as well as reductions in the local stress responses to surgical trauma.[33,34] By potently suppressing these physiologic responses to surgery, pain is improved and functional recovery should be improved. Local injection of corticosteroids has been used extensively in musculoskeletal tissues and joints without impairment of wound healing. **(DVD 14.1)**

Postoperative Analgesia

The goals of the postoperative protocol include administration of a variety of agents that act via different mechanisms and exert local and systemic effects, use of agents with combined analgesic and anti-inflammatory properties, early conversion from parenteral to oral agents with prolonged effect, use of baseline analgesia to provide more uniform pain control, and minimization of narcotic use and associated adverse effects. The specific agents administered postoperatively are listed in Table 5.

COX-2 selective inhibitors and sustained-release oral narcotics are continued postoperatively on a scheduled basis to provide baseline analgesia and anti-inflammatory effects. Additionally, the need for

medications for breakthrough pain is reduced.

The use of parenteral narcotics is minimized by using ketorolac as the first-line parenteral as-needed medication. By its COX inhibition, ketorolac exerts both anti-inflammatory and analgesic effects. Parenterally, this effect is potent and has been shown to result in less opioid use with less opioid-related adverse effects while providing superior pain relief.[35,36] Parenteral opioids are prescribed for breakthrough pain if the ketorolac is ineffective.

Acetaminophen is also administered postoperatively on a scheduled basis. It has no anti-inflammatory effect, but provides baseline analgesic and antipyretic effects. The mechanism of action is unclear, but acetaminophen is thought to elevate the pain threshold, possibly by inhibition of the nitric oxide pathway via neurotransmitter receptors (including N-methyl-d-aspartate and substance P)[37] or via central inhibition of COX-3.[38]

Early Experience

Between October 1, 2003, and June 30, 2004, the authors performed 50 THRs (in 50 patients) and 52 TKRs (in 36 patients) using intraoperative periarticular injection combined with reduced tissue trauma surgery and the modified pain protocol described previously. Patients were assessed using postoperative pain scales and monitored for narcotic requirements. Additionally, patient assessment questionnaires were used to document recovery of functional milestones, such as unassisted walking, stair-climbing, straight leg raising, range of motion, and overall satisfaction.

For the group of patients who underwent TKR, narcotic pain requirements and the need for pro-

longed physical therapy were significantly reduced in comparison with historical control subjects. Overall patient satisfaction was greatly improved. Recovery was described as easy by 83% of patients undergoing unilateral procedures and by 64% of patients undergoing bilateral procedures. By 5 weeks after surgery, 77% of knees achieved 110° range of motion and no knees achieved less than 90° range of motion. By 5 weeks after surgery, all patients could climb stairs with assistance of the banister, and 20% of patients could climb and descend independently. Only 12% of patients required physical therapy beyond 2 months after surgery, and no patients required physical therapy beyond 6 months. There were no instances of delayed wound healing or wound infections, and no patients required manipulations or repeated surgery.

For the group of patients who

Table 5
Postoperative Pain Management Protocol for THR and TKR

Recovery Room

1. Ketorolac IV q 6 hr PRN (15 mg if > 65 yr, 30 mg if < 65 yr, hold if renal impairment)

2. If ketorolac is ineffective, morphine 2 to 4 mg IV q 15 min

Orthopaedic Floor

1. Ketorolac IM q 6 hr PRN (15 mg if > 65 yr, 30 mg if < 65 yr, hold if renal impairment)

2. If ketorolac is ineffective, morphine 2 to 4 mg IM q 2-4 hrs

3. Celecoxib 200 mg orally daily for 10 days

4. Oxycodone SR 10/20 mg orally q 12 hr for 24 hr

5. Oxycodone 5 mg orally q 6 hrs PRN

6. Acetaminophen 1,000 mg orally q 6 hr

7. Pantoprazole 40 mg orally daily

SR = sustained release, q = every, IV = intravenously, PRN = as needed, IM = intramuscularly

---

underwent THR, narcotic pain requirements and the need for prolonged physical therapy were also significantly reduced compared with historical control subjects. Recovery of functional milestones was achieved at an earlier period in 90% of patients. Overall patient satisfaction was greatly improved; 78% of patients described their recovery as easy. By 6 weeks postoperatively, 97% of patients had no or mild pain, 60% had no limp, and 66% were walking unlimited distances (1 to 2 miles) and without a cane. By 3 months postoperatively, 94% had no pain, 85% had no limp, and 98% were walking unlimited distances (1 to 2 miles) and without a cane. As with the TKR patients, there were no instances of delayed wound healing or wound infections, and no patients required repeat surgery.

Summary

Key components of the protocol described include the use of a variety of pharmacologic agents exerting effects via different mechanisms that result in superior pain control with reduction of adverse effects. Additionally, the use of these agents before the physiologic responses are at their peak results in a superior clinical response. Moreover, meticulous periarticular infiltration with the novel injection mixture described produces early, potent analgesic and anti-inflammatory effects. This injection forms the core of the advanced multimodal pain protocol described. By controlling acute pain in the critical early postoperative period after THR and TKR, the periarticular injection and modified pain protocol can promote faster recovery of function and improved patient satisfaction.

References

1. Chung F, Ritchie E, Su J: Postoperative pain in ambulatory surgery. *Anesth Analg* 1997;85:808-816.

2. Rawal N, Hylander J, Nydahl PA, Olofsson I, Gupta A: Survey of postoperative analgesia following ambulatory surgery. *Acta Anaesthesiol Scand* 1997;41:1017-1022.

3. Filos KS, Lehmann KA: Current concepts and practice in postoperative pain management: Need for a change? *Eur Surg Res* 1999;31:91-107.

4. Follin SL, Charland SL: Acute management: Operative or medical procedures and trauma. *Ann Pharmacother* 1997;31:1068-1076.

5. Bonica JJ: Postoperative pain, in Bonica JJ (ed): *The Management of Pain*. Malvern, PA, Lea & Febiger, 1990, pp 461-480.

6. Singelyn FJ, Deyaert M, Joris D, Pendeville E, Gouverneur JM: Effects of intravenous patient-controlled analgesia with morphine, continuous epidural analgesia, and continuous three-in-one block on postoperative pain and knee rehabilitation after unilateral total knee arthroplasty. *Anesth Analg* 1998;87:88-92.

7. Kroll MA, Otis JC, Sculco TP, et al: The relationship of stride characteristics to pain before and after total knee arthroplasty. *Clin Orthop Relat Res* 1989;239:191-195.

8. Ryu J, Saito S, Yamamoto K, Sano S: Factors influencing the postoperative range of motion in total knee arthroplasty. *Bull Hosp Jt Dis* 1993;53:35-40.

9. Craig DB: Postoperative recovery of pulmonary function. *Anesth Analg* 1981;60:46-52.

10. Sinatra RS, Torres J, Bustos AM: Pain management after major orthopaedic surgery: Current strategies and new concepts. *J Am Acad Orthop Surg* 2002;10:117-129.

11. Carr DB, Goudas LC: Acute pain. *Lancet* 1999;353:2051-2058.

12. Samad TA, Moore KA, Sapirstein A, et al: Interleukin-1-mediated induction of COX-2 in the CNS contributes to inflammatory pain hypersensitivity. *Nature* 2001;410:471-475.

13. Pavlin DJ, Chen C, Penaloza DA, Polissar NL, Buckly FP: Pain as a factor complicating recovery and discharge after ambulatory surgery. *Anesth Analg* 2002;95:627-634.

14. Pavlin DJ, Rapp SE, Polissar NL, Malmgren JA, Koerschgen M, Keyes H: Factors affecting discharge time in adult outpatients. *Anesth Analg* 1998;87:816-826.

15. Gold BS, Kitz DS, Lecky JH, Neuhaus JM: Unanticipated admission to the hospital following ambulatory surgery. *JAMA* 1989;262:3008-3010.

16. Bayley KB, London MR, Grunkemeier GL, Lansky DJ: Measuring the success of treatment in patient terms. *Med Care* 1995;33:AS226-AS235.

17. Dickstein R, Heffes Y, Shabtai EI, Markowitz E: Total knee arthroplasty in the elderly: Patients' self appraisal 6 and 12 months postoperatively. *Gerontology* 1998;44:204-210.

18. Phillips WJ, Currier BL: Analgesic pharmacology: I. Neurophysiology. *J Am Acad Orthop Surg* 2004;12:213-220.

19. Ekman EF, Koman LA: Acute pain following musculoskeletal injuries and orthopaedic surgery: Mechanisms and management. *Instr Course Lect* 2005;54:21-33.

20. Burns JW, Hodsman NB, McLintock TT, Gillies GW, Kenny GN, McArdle CS: The influence of patient characteristics on the requirements for postoperative analgesia: A reassessment using patient-controlled anesthesia. *Anaesthesia* 1989;44:2-6.

21. Skinner HB: Multimodal acute pain management. *Am J Orthop* 2004;33(Suppl 5):5-9.

22. Hartrick CT: Multimodal postoperative pain management. *Am J Health Syst Pharm* 2004;61:S4-10.

23. Viscusi ER: Emerging techniques for postoperative analgesia in orthopedic surgery. *Am J Orthop* 2004;33(Suppl 5):13-16.

24. Acute Pain Management Guideline Panel: Acute pain management in adults: Operative procedures. Quick reference guide for clinicians. *Medsurg Nurs* 1994;3:99-107.

25. Mallory TH, Lombardi AV Jr, Fada RA, Dodds KL, Adams JB: Pain management for joint arthroplasty: Preemptive analgesia. *J Arthroplasty* 2002;17(4 suppl 1):129-133.

26. Cheville A, Chen A, Oster G, McGarry L, Narcessian E: A randomized trial of controlled-release oxycodone during inpatient rehabilitation following unilateral total knee arthroplasty. *J Bone Joint Surg Am* 2001;83:572-576.

27. Reuben SS, Connelly NR, Maciolek H: Postoperative analgesia with controlled-release oxycodone for outpatient anterior cruciate ligament surgery. *Anesth Analg* 1999;88:1286-1291.

28. Buvanendran A, Kroin JS, Tuman KJ, et al: Effects of perioperative administration of a selective cyclooxygenase 2 inhibitor on pain management and recovery of function after knee replacement: A randomized controlled trial. *JAMA* 2003;290:2411-2418.

29. Camu F, Beecher T, Recker DP, Verburg KM: Valdecoxib, a COX-2-specific inhibitor, is an efficacious, opioid-sparing analgesic in patients undergoing hip arthroplasty. *Am J Ther* 2002;9:43-51.

30. Tanaka N, Sakahashi H, Sato F, Hirose K, Ishii S: The efficacy of intra-articular analgesia after total knee arthroplasty in patients with rheumatoid arthritis and in patients with osteoarthritis. *J Arthroplasty* 2001;16:306-311.

31. Joshi W, Reuben SS, Kilaru PR, Sklar J, Maciolek H: Postoperative analgesia for outpatient arthroscopic knee surgery with intraarticular clonidine and/or morphine. *Anesth Analg* 2000;90:1102-1106.

32. Paech MJ, Pavy TJ, Orlikowski CE, Lim W, Evans SF: Postoperative epidural infusion: A randomized double-blind dose-finding trial of clonidine in combination with bupivacaine and fentanyl. *Anesth Analg* 1997;84:1323-1328.

33. Holte K, Kehlet H: Perioperative single-dose glucocorticoid administration: Pathophysiologic effects and clinical implications. *J Am Coll Surg* 2002;195:694-712.

34. Mirzai H, Tekin I, Alincak H: Perioperative use of corticosteroid and bupivacaine combination in lumbar disc surgery: A randomized controlled trial. *Spine* 2002;27:343-346.

35. Alexander R, El Moalem HE, Gan TJ: Comparison of the morphine-sparing effects of diclofenac sodium and ketorolac tromethamine after major orthopedic surgery. *J Clin Anesth* 2002;14:187-192.

36. Barber FA, Gladu DE: Comparison of oral ketorolac and hydrocodone for pain relief after anterior cruciate ligament reconstruction. *Arthroscopy* 1998;14:605-612.

37. Bjorkman R, Hallman KM, Hedner J, et al: Acetaminophen blocks spinal hyperalgesia induced by NMDA and substance P. *Pain* 1994;57:259-264.

38. Chandrasekharan NV, Dai H, Roos KL, et al: COX-3, a cyclooxygenase-1 variant inhibited by acetaminophen and other analgesic/antipyretic drugs: Cloning, structure, and expression. *Proc Natl Acad Sci USA* 2002;99:13926-13931.

Nonsteroidal Anti-Inflammatory Drugs: Are They Safe After Joint Arthroplasty for Early Pain?

James J. Purtill, MD

Abstract

A significant proportion of patients will experience moderate to severe pain after hip or knee replacement surgery. Multimodal pain control regimens have been developed to address this issue. These regimens may include the use of nonsteroidal anti-inflammatory drugs (NSAIDs). Concern over excessive bleeding in the perioperative period, especially in joint arthroplasty patients receiving anticoagulation therapy, generally prohibits the use of nonspecific NSAIDs. Cyclooxygenase-2 inhibitors, a class of NSAIDs, are not believed to increase the risk of bleeding and may be useful in this population of patients. However, recent research shows increased cardiovascular and renal risks with cyclooxygenase-2 inhibitors and has limited their use for postoperative pain control in joint arthroplasty patients.

Instr Course Lect 2007;56:133-137.

As many as 80% of patients who undergo surgical procedures report moderate to severe postoperative pain. Because current postoperative pain management is suboptimal, new multimodal pain management strategies are being developed. Nonsteroidal anti-inflammatory drugs (NSAIDs) are often included in postoperative pain management protocols. A recently developed class of NSAIDs, cyclooxygenase-2 (COX-2) inhibitors, has shown particular promise for treating orthopaedic surgical patients.[1]

Aspirin, the best known NSAID, was developed in the 1890s and remains the most frequently used medication in the world. In the United States, 13 million people use aspirin and other NSAIDs on a daily basis. NSAIDs are commonly used for relief of musculoskeletal pain and inflammation and are also used for postoperative analgesia for patients having surgical procedures.[2] As an adjunct to standard narcotic pain medication protocols, NSAIDs improve patient comfort and enhance rehabilitation. NSAIDs, when used in postoperative pain management regimens, also reduce the need for narcotics, which may minimize the risk of potential complications associated with narcotic use alone. Excessive use of narcotics can result in respiratory depression, nausea, vomiting, and excessive sedation, all factors that may limit early rehabilitation.

Allergy, hypersensitivity to aspirin or other NSAIDs, peptic ulcer disease, and bleeding disorders are contraindications to the use of NSAIDs (Table 1). There is a relative contraindication to the use of these medications in elderly patients.[3] Because few studies have specifically examined patients older than 65 years, the profile of NSAID side effects is largely unknown in this patient population. This lack of data is of concern to orthopaedic surgeons because most patients who undergo joint arthroplasty are older than 65 years.

Significant potential side effects associated with the administration of NSAIDs include gastrointestinal disorders (such as ulceration, bleeding, perforation), renal failure, and cardiovascular side effects[4] (Table 1). These side effects may limit the use of NSAIDs for postoperative pain regimens. Concerns over the use of these medications in patients receiving anticoagulation therapy, as well as in elderly patients, may limit their usefulness in postoperative pain regimens for patients who undergo joint arthroplasty.

Pharmacology

Arachidonic acid is a polyunsaturated fatty acid that exists in the cell

Table 1
Contraindications and Adverse Effects Associated With NSAIDs

Contraindications

   Allergy

   Hypersensitivity to aspirin or other NSAIDs

   Peptic ulcer disease

   Bleeding disorders

Relative contraindications

   Elderly patients (> 65 years)

   Patients receiving anticoagulation therapy

Potential adverse effects

   Gastrointestinal disorders (ulceration, bleeding, and perforation)

   Renal failure

   Cardiovascular disorders

membrane and is modified by cyclooxygenases to form prostaglandins. Prostaglandins mediate inflammation and pain transmission throughout the body and have certain physiologic functions such as stimulating smooth muscle contraction, and repair functions such as mucosal maintenance in the stomach.[5] COX-1 and COX-2 are the two known cyclooxygenases.

NSAIDs are cyclooxygenase inhibitors. Traditional or nonspecific NSAIDs bind to both COX-1 and COX-2 and thereby block arachidonic acid from binding to the cyclooxygenases, which decrease or eliminate its subsequent transformation into various prostaglandins. NSAIDs exhibit different affinities for COX-1 and COX-2.[6] Aspirin, for example, irreversibly binds both COX-1 and COX-2. COX-2 inhibitors bind COX-2 preferentially and may leave COX-1 function unimpaired.

COX-1 and COX-2 Mediated Function and Inhibitors

COX-2 activity produces prostaglandins associated with pain and in-flammation in the body. COX-1 activity is believed to have a primarily constitutive function; prostaglandins formed by COX-1 activity regulate normal physiologic functions and biologic repair. Adverse stimuli, such as bacterial endotoxins, interleukins, physiologic stress, and proinflammatory cytokines induce COX-2 activity. COX-2 inhibitors block production of prostaglandins that mediate inflammation and the transmission of pain signals in the body.[7] COX-1 has a constitutive function in the stomach. Prostaglandins that are formed as a result of COX-1 activity in the stomach function in the repair of the mucosa. COX-2 is not believed to be involved in this process.

Because nonspecific NSAIDs bind both COX-1 and COX-2, the inhibition of COX-1 activity may interfere with mucosal maintenance in the stomach and may predispose patients to the development of peptic ulcers and bleeding elsewhere in the gastrointestinal tract. COX-2 specific inhibitors bind COX-2 tightly and may allow some of the beneficial effects of COX-1 activity in the gastrointestinal tract. Lower morbidity to the gastrointestinal tract is expected with the long-term use of COX-2 inhibitors compared with the use of nonspecific NSAIDs.

In the brain, COX-2 mediated prostaglandin synthesis moderates sleep and wake cycles. Prostaglandins, which are synthesized as a result of COX-2 activity in the central nervous system, may cause fever and aid in the transmission of pain signals in the central nervous system. COX-2 inhibitors reduce pain signal transmission in the central nervous system and function as antipyretics.[8]

In the kidney, COX-2 is induced as a result of decreased circulating blood volume, which in turn results in decreased renal blood flow. Decreasing renal blood flow occurs in conjunction with dehydration, with blood loss (such as in the postoperative period), and with renal disease. Prostaglandins in the kidney, which are formed as a result of COX-2 activity, increase sodium reabsorption as a compensatory function to combat decreased renal blood flow, resulting in water retention and increased intravascular volume. NSAIDS, especially COX-2 inhibitors, block this compensatory function and may contribute to renal failure.

NSAIDs and Postoperative Bleeding

Thromboxane A_2, which is produced in blood vessels as a result of damage to the vascular endothelium, stimulates platelet aggregation. Nonspecific NSAIDs are believed to reduce production of thromboxane A_2 in the vascular endothelium, thus causing decreased platelet aggregation and possible increased bleeding. This increased risk of bleeding is pertinent in patients undergoing surgical procedures and has traditionally limited the use of nonspecific NSAIDs in the perioperative period.[9,10] In a placebo-controlled study, the use of ibuprofen, a nonspecific NSAID, resulted in a 45% increase in perioperative blood loss following total hip arthroplasty.[11]

COX-2 inhibitors, unlike nonspecific NSAIDs, do not reduce thromboxane A_2 production. Therefore, patients using COX-2 specific inhibitors are believed to have no increased risk for bleeding. COX-2 specific inhibitors can be administered until the time of surgery as well as in the postoperative period with no significant increased risk of bleeding. Nonspecific NSAIDs with COX-1 inhibitor activity have been shown to increase bleeding and blood loss in the perioperative period. The use of nonspecific NSAIDs is usually stopped in the preoperative period; concern remains regarding their use in the postoperative period.[9,10]

NSAIDs and Postoperative Pain Management

NSAIDS, when used in combination with opiate pain medications in the postoperative period, improve overall analgesia and provide a so-called narcotic-sparing effect with the need for less intravenous or intramuscular narcotic medications for breakthrough pain. This narcotic-sparing effect has significant potential benefits for patients including increased respiratory function and decreased nausea, vomiting, and sedation.[12]

Nonspecific NSAIDs

A study of the use of nonspecific NSAIDs for postoperative analgesia after orthopaedic surgery by Hanna and associates[13] compared the use of ketoprofen with placebo and showed a 30% morphine-sparing effect for patients receiving ketoprofen. The patients using ketoprofen also reported better overall pain relief with less sedation. Although excessive bleeding is a concern with the use of nonspecific NSAIDs, no differences in wound bleeding were found in this study.

In another study, ketorolac (30 mg every 6 hours in 4 doses), another nonspecific NSAID, was compared with placebo (saline solution) for pain control in the 24-hour postoperative period following total knee arthroplasty. A 30% reduction in morphine use was noted. However, the group treated with ketorolac had 6% lower hemoglobin levels

in the postoperative period. Although lower hemoglobin levels in the ketorolac group was statistically significant, this finding had no clinical implications in this study.[14,15]

In another study, the bleeding propensity of patients using meloxicam, a COX-2 specific inhibitor, was compared with that of a group of patients treated with indomethacin, a nonspecific NSAID. The group receiving the nonspecific NSAID had a 17% greater blood loss than the group treated with the COX-2 specific inhibitor.[16]

COX-2 Specific Inhibitors

In a large meta-analysis comparing COX-2 inhibitors with nonspecific NSAIDs, both medications were found to be effective analgesics; however, COX-2 specific inhibitors showed improved gastrointestinal safety. Unimpaired platelet function was a significant added benefit of COX-2 inhibitors. Renal safety, however, was not improved with the use of COX-2 specific inhibitors compared with nonspecific NSAIDs.[4]

COX-2 inhibitors have been directly compared with opiates for efficacy in providing postoperative analgesia. In a study comparing a COX-2 inhibitor (rofecoxib) with acetaminophen with codeine, 22% fewer patients treated with rofecoxib required intravenous or intramuscular narcotic medications for breakthrough pain. The group receiving rofecoxib also showed lower rates of nausea (19% versus 40%) and less vomiting (7% versus 23%) than the group treated with acetaminophen with codeine.[17]

In patients who had total knee replacement, rofecoxib was compared with placebo for postoperative pain control. Significant opiate-sparing effect with less pain, nausea, and vomiting was confirmed for the

group treated with rofecoxib. Patients receiving rofecoxib also reported better sleep and improved function (including increased knee flexion and shorter time in physical therapy).[18]

Valdecoxib, another COX-2 specific inhibitor, showed a significant opiate-sparing effect for patients undergoing total knee replacement. Patients receiving valdecoxib reported lower maximum pain intensity and increased patient satisfaction compared with patients receiving a placebo.[19] Another study compared the efficacy of valdecoxib to placebo in patients who had hip replacement surgery. In the patients treated with valdecoxib for 48 hours postoperatively, a 40% morphine-sparing effect was reported. Patients in the valdecoxib group also reported lower levels of pain intensity and improved satisfaction. Valdecoxib was well tolerated with side effects equal to that of the placebo;[20] however, valdecoxib is no longer commercially available and has been withdrawn from the market.

In anther study of patients who had hip replacement surgery, paracoxib, a parenteral COX-2 inhibitor, had a significant opioid-sparing effect. Patients had lower pain scores and higher Global Evaluation rating scores compared with those treated with placebo.[21] Paracoxib was also compared with morphine and with ketorolac in another study. Paracoxib was found to be as effective as ketorolac and more effective than morphine for the control of acute pain after orthopaedic knee surgery;[22] however, paracoxib is not commercially available in the United States.

Complications With COX-2 Specific Inhibitors

Although COX-2 specific inhibitors offer improvements in postoperative analgesia and decreased risk of bleeding and gastrointestinal side effects compared with nonspecific NSAIDs, concerns remain regarding their safety in treating joint arthroplasty patients.

Osteointegration With Cementless Implants

COX-2 inhibitors may alter the process of osteointegration of cementless implants with the surrounding bone and interfere with long-term fixation. In a study, the COX-2 specific inhibitor celecoxib was compared with placebo in a 6-week trial of patients following cementless total hip arthroplasty. Periprosthetic bone mineral density and implant subsidence were measured; no difference was found in the celecoxib and placebo groups.[23]

Cardiovascular Risk

COX-2 inhibitors reduce prostaglandin I2 (prostacyclin) production in the vascular endothelium, where prostacyclin functions in the dilatation of the surrounding blood vessels. The decrease in prostacyclin caused by the use of COX-2 inhibitors is believed to result in vasoconstriction and subsequent hypertension. Prostacyclin in normal physiologic amounts also inhibits platelet aggregation. The use of a COX-2 inhibitor reduces prostacyclin and may increase the risk of platelet aggregation. In the coronary vessels, this hypertension and increased platelet aggregation may increase the risk of myocardial infarction.[24]

The theoretic increase in cardiovascular risk with the use of COX-2 inhibitors has been confirmed in two separate large clinical trials. The Vioxx and Gastrointestinal Outcomes Research Studies study showed increased cardiovascular risk in patients receiving rofecoxib (Vioxx, Merck, Whitehouse Station, NJ).[25] In a second clinical study, the Adenomatous Polyp Prevention on Vioxx study, a two times higher risk of myocardial infarction was shown in patients receiving rofecoxib.[26]

In contrast to rofecoxib, celecoxib has not been found to have the same cardiovascular risk profile.[26] In the Celecoxib Long-term Arthritis Safety Study, no increased cardiovascular risk was found in patients taking celecoxib.[27] However, in another large study analyzing celecoxib, a 2.5 to 3.4 times higher cardiovascular risk was found in patients taking celecoxib. The patients in this study were given supratherapeutic doses (400 or 800 mg per day) for an extended period of time; the increased cardiovascular risk appeared to be dose-related.[28]

Postoperative Pain Management Protocols

For approximately 2 years, rofecoxib was routinely administered at the dose of 50 mg per day for 5 days postoperatively in most patients undergoing hip or knee arthroplasty at the authors' institution. The use of rofecoxib was discontinued after the increased cardiovascular risk was defined and the drug was withdrawn from the commercial market. Celecoxib has been used since that time in selected patients following hip and knee arthroplasty. Before administering celecoxib, patients are screened for risk factors for coronary artery disease, hypertension, and renal disease. Celecoxib has an acute pain indication and therefore may be used postoperatively. It is administered at a dose of 400 mg on the first postoperative day and 200 mg twice a day for 5 days. Patients who were taking celecoxib preoperatively for arthritis pain are allowed to continue taking the medication until the day of surgery.

Summary

NSAIDs have a role in postoperative pain control in patients undergoing hip and knee replacement surgery. The significant advantages to the use of NSAIDs in conjunction with standard narcotic postoperative pain regimens include decreased narcotic use and improved pain control. Because lower narcotic requirements result in more alert patients, early rehabilitation efforts may be improved.

COX-2 inhibitors may have significant advantages over nonspecific NSAIDs, such as a lower risk of gastrointestinal toxicity. In addition, lack of platelet impairment (especially for patients on postoperative anticoagulation therapy) is an attractive characteristic of COX-2 inhibitors compared with nonspecific NSAIDs. COX-2 inhibitors do not impair platelets; therefore, with vasoconstriction (caused by decreased prostacyclin in the coronary vessels), there may be normal platelet aggregation in the vessels, which can result in decreased coronary blood flow and may lead to myocardial infarction.

Concerns with complications from COX-2 inhibitors such as renal impairment and increased cardiovascular risks have limited their use at the present time. As a recent editorial admonishes, "surgeons should avoid prescribing coxibs for patients with or at high risk for coronary artery disease."[29] Because a significant proportion of patients undergoing hip and knee replacement have inadequate pain control in the postoperative period, the need for better pain control and the benefits of the narcotic-sparing effect of COX-2 specific inhibitors must be balanced with their significant potential side effects.

References

1. Sinatra R: Role of COX-2-inhibitors in the evolution of acute pain management. *J Pain Symptom Manage* 2002;24(suppl 1):S18-S27.

2. Everts B, Wahrborg P, Hedner T: COX-2-specific inhibitors: The emergence of a new class of analgesic and anti-inflammatory drugs. *Clin Rheumatol* 2000;19:331-343.

3. Nuutinen LS, Laitinen JO, Salomaki TE: A risk-benefit appraisal of injectable NSAIDs in the management of postoperative pain. *Drug Saf* 1993;9:380-393.

4. Cicconetti A, Bartoli A, Ripari F, Ripari A: COX-2 selective inhibitors: A literature review of analgesic efficacy and safety in oral-maxillofacial surgery. *Oral Surg Oral Med Oral Pathol Oral Radiol Endod* 2004;97:139-146.

5. Cotran RS, Kumar V, Collins T, Robbins SL: *Robbins Pathologic Basis of Disease*, ed 6. Philadelphia, PA, WB Saunders Co, 1999.

6. Hawkey CJ: COX-2 inhibitors. *Lancet* 1999;353:307-314.

7. Urban MK: COX-2 specific inhibitors offer improved advantages over traditional NSAIDs. *Orthopedics* 2000;23(suppl 7):S761-S764.

8. Dubois RN, Abramson SB, Crofford L, et al: Cyclooxygenase in biology and disease. *FASEB J* 1998;12:1063-1073.

9. Reuben SS, Fingeroth R, Krushell R, Maciolek H: Evaluation of the safety and efficacy of the perioperative administration of rofecoxib for total knee arthroplasty. *J Arthroplasty* 2002;17:26-31.

10. Reuben SS, Ekman EF: The effect of cyclooxygenase-2 inhibition on analgesia and spinal fusion. *J Bone Joint Surg Am* 2005;87:536-542.

11. Slappendel R, Weber EW, Benraad B, Dirksen R, Bugter ML: Does ibuprofen increase perioperative blood loss during hip arthroplasty? *Eur J Anaesthesiol* 2002;19:829-831.

12. Moote C: Efficacy of nonsteroidal anti-inflammatory drugs in the management of postoperative pain. *Drugs* 1992;44:(suppl 5)14-29.

13. Hanna MH, Elliott KM, Stuart-Taylor ME, Roberts DR, Buggy D, Arthurs GJ: Comparative study of analgesic efficacy and morphine sparing effect of intramuscular dexketoprofen trometamol with ketoprofen or placebo after major orthopaedic surgery. *Br J Clin Pharmacol* 2003;55:126-133.

14. Fragen RJ, Stuhlberg SD, Wixson R, Glisson S, Librojo E: Effect of ketorolac tromethamine on bleeding and on requirements for analgesia after total knee arthroplasty. *J Bone Joint Surg Am* 1995;77:998-1002.

15. Milne JC, Russell JA, Woods GW, Dalton MD: Effect of ketorolac tromethamine (toradol) on ecchymosis following anterior cruciate ligament reconstruction. *Am J Knee Surg* 1995;8:24-27.

16. Weber EW, Slappendel R, Durieux ME, Dirksen R, van der Heide H, Spruit M: COX 2 selectivity of non-steroidal anti-inflammatory drugs and perioperative blood loss in hip surgery: A randomized comparison of indomethacin and meloxicam. *Eur J Anaesthesiol* 2003;20:963-966.

17. Korn S, Vassil TC, Kotey PN, Fricke JR: Comparison of rofecoxib and oxycodone plus acetaminophen in the treatment of acute pain: A randomized, double-blind, placebo-controlled study in patients with moderate to severe postoperative pain in the third molar extraction model. *Clin Ther* 2004;26:769-778.

18. Buvanendran A, Kroin JS, Tuman KJ, et al: Effects of perioperative administration of a selective cyclooxygenase 2 inhibitor on pain management and recovery of function after knee replacement: A randomized controlled trial. *JAMA* 2003;290:2411-2418.

19. Reynolds LW, Hoo RK, Brill RJ, North J, Recker DP, Verburg KM: The COX-2 specific inhibitor, valdecoxib, is and effective opioid-sparing analgesic in patients undergoing total knee arthroplasty. *J Pain Symptom Manage* 2003;25:133-141.

20. Camu F, Beecher T, Recker DP, Verburg KM: Valdecoxib, a COX-2 specific inhibitor is and efficacious, opioid-sparing analgesic in patients undergoing hip arthroplasty. *Am J Ther* 2002;9:43-51.

21. Malan TP, Marsh G, Hakki SI, Grossman E, Traylor L, Hubbard RC: Paracoxib sodium, a parenteral cyclooxygenase 2 selective inhibitor, improves morphine analgesia and is opioid-sparing following total hip arthroplasty. *Anesthesiology* 2003;98:950-956.

22. Rasmussen GL, Steckner K, Hogue C, Torri S, Hubbard RC: Intravenous paracoxib sodium for acute pain after orthopedic knee surgery. *Am J Orthop* 2002;31:336-343.

23. Lionberger DR, Noble PC: Celecoxib does not affect osteointegration of cementless total hip stems. *J Arthroplasty* 2005; 20(suppl 3):115-122.

24. Fitzgerald GA: Coxibs and cardiovascular disease. *N Engl J Med* 2004;351:1709-1711.

25. Bombardier C, Laine L, Reidin A, et al: Comparison of upper gastrointestinal toxicity of rofecoxib and naproxen in patients with rheumatoid arthritis: VIGOR Study Group. *N Engl J Med* 2000;343:1520-1528.

26. Levesque LE, Brophy JM, Zhang B: The risk for myocardial infarction with cyclooxygenase-2 inhibitors: A population study of elderly adults. *Ann Intern Med* 2005;142:481-489.

27. Silverstein FE, Faich G, Goldstein JL, et al: Gastrointestinal toxicity with celecoxib vs nonsteroidal anti-inflammatory drugs for osteoarthritis and rheumatoid arthritis: the CLASS study: A randomized controlled trial: Celecoxib Long-Term Arthritis Safety Study. *JAMA* 2000;284:1247-1255.

28. Topol EJ: Arthritis medicines and cardiovascular events: "House of coxibs". *JAMA* 2005;293:366-368.

29. Bhattacharyya T, Smith RM: Cardiovascular risks of coxibs: The orthopaedic perspective. *J Bone Joint Surg Am* 2005;87:245-246.

Developments in Spinal and Epidural Anesthesia and Nerve Blocks for Total Joint Arthroplasty: What Is New and Exciting in Pain Management

Eugene R. Viscusi, MD
Javad Parvizi, MD
T. David Tarity, BS

Abstract

The decision to use regional or general anesthesia for patients undergoing total joint arthroplasty continues to be controversial. Recent reviews of the literature support the growing trend for the use of regional anesthesia with a multifaceted approach, spanning nuances in block placement as well as pharmacologic agents and delivery systems. Innovative developments offer appealing options and encouraging results for the management of pain after major orthopaedic procedures. The ultimate decision, although varied, requires careful preoperative planning and protocols to ensure adequate pain control and patient satisfaction.

Instr Course Lect 2007;56:139-145.

Since the dawn of modern anesthesia techniques, there has been controversy regarding the benefits and shortcomings of regional versus general anesthesia. During the past decade, extensive literature confirming the benefits of regional anesthesia, particularly for patients undergoing total joint arthroplasty, have shifted the preferred modality toward regional anesthesia.[1] Regional anesthesia produces nearly ideal surgical conditions, including profound muscle relaxation, controlled reduction of blood pressure, and better control of postoperative pain.[2] Neuraxial techniques have also been shown to offer protection against deep venous thrombosis[3-5] and less consumption of opioids during the perioperative and postoperative rehabilitation periods.[6-8] The advent of vigorous anticoagulation protocols aimed at reducing the risk of thromboembolic events has placed some constraints on the use of regional anesthesia. The most feared complication resulting from the coadministration of anticoagulants and spinal or epidural anesthesia/analgesia is the development of a spinal hematoma that may lead to irreversible spinal cord ischemia and neurologic damage.[9]

Perioperative and postoperative pain, if mismanaged, may contribute to the surgical stress response leading to hypercoagulability, pulmonary or urinary problems, hyperdynamic circulation, increased oxygen consumption, and less than sufficient rehabilitation that contributes to poor outcomes.[10,11] This chapter highlights the current trends and emerging technologies in the field of regional anesthesia for pain management after total joint arthroplasty.

Spinal (Intrathecal) Analgesia

Spinal anesthesia, with the addition of spinal morphine, is a relatively simple anesthetic technique that provides excellent surgical conditions and extended postoperative analgesia.[12] Intrathecal morphine (typical dose, 0.2 to 0.5 mg) is combined with local anesthetic at the time of spinal injection. At the authors' institution, intrathecal morphine 0.2 mg is most commonly combined with isobaric bupivacaine 7.5 to 15 mg. Intrathecal morphine is reported to provide between 12 and 20 hours of pain relief. Most anesthesiologists believe smaller doses of morphine provide the best ratio of analgesia to adverse effects, although at least one recent study found that 0.5 mg of morphine produced better analgesia than 0.2 mg, with a similar profile of adverse effects.[13] Spinal anesthesia/analgesia is most commonly delivered through the placement of a small-bore 24- to 27-gauge spinal needle. The use of pencil-point needles, such as the Sprotte Pencil Point Spinal Needle (Pajunk GmbH, Geisingen, Germany), significantly reduces the incidence of postdural puncture headache (spinal headache). The coagulation profile of the patient must be normal before spinal injection to reduce the risk of epidural hematoma. Hematoma may result from traumatic needle/catheter placement, sustained anticoagulation with an indwelling epidural catheter, and with epidural catheter removal.[9] Dose intervals and coagulation monitoring must be coordinated with the anesthesiology/acute pain team to optimize safety. The American Society of Regional Anesthesia has published guidelines for neuraxial anesthesia and anticoagulation therapy.[14]

Typical opioid adverse effects such as nausea, vomiting, pruritus, respiratory depression, and hypotension have been reported with this combination.[10] All patients receiving opioids require monitoring for respiratory depression. Standard monitoring of patients who have received spinal or epidural opioids at the authors' institution includes hourly assessment of respiratory rate and sedation for 24

hours. Standing orders and protocols facilitate the management of these conditions. Strategies to reduce "breakthrough" pain typically use a multimodal approach, including both opioid and nonopioid analgesics (acetaminophen, cyclo-oxygenase-2 selective inhibitors, and nonselective anti-inflammatory drugs). Supplemental opioids such as intravenous patient-controlled analgesia can be safely coadministered with intrathecal morphine with proper patient surveillance. Appropriate monitoring and treatment of adverse effects allows this technique to be a useful tool for pain control, particularly for patients undergoing total hip arthroplasty.

Epidural Anesthesia and Analgesia

For patients undergoing total joint arthroplasty, some practitioners prefer epidural anesthesia. Similar to spinal anesthesia, epidural anesthesia offers reasonable muscle relaxation and controlled reduction in blood pressure, but it also provides extended duration of anesthesia delivered by means of an indwelling epidural catheter. Postoperatively, the catheter may be used for continuous analgesia. A recent meta-analysis concluded that continuous epidural analgesia provided better postoperative analgesia when compared with parenteral opioids regardless of agent, location of catheter placement, and type and time of pain assessment.[15] Typical infusions consist of local anesthetic (bupivacaine or ropivacaine) and/or opioid (morphine, fentanyl, or hydromorphone). Reports in the literature suggest significantly improved pain control with a mixture of local anesthetics and opioids after major orthopaedic surgery.[16-18] Epidural local anesthetic can contribute to postoperative hypotension and motor impairment. Hypotension is exacerbated by hypo-

volemia. Motor weakness is usually easily managed with adjustment of the rate of epidural infusion. Hypotension results from sympathetic chain blockade, which accompanies sensory and motor blockade.[18] Hypotension usually responds to appropriate fluid management. Epidural opioids may cause the typical opioid-related adverse effects. Standing orders for treatment of nausea, vomiting, and pruritus are generally effective. Epidural opioids, such as intrathecal morphine, can cause respiratory depression and hence require similar respiratory monitoring. Epidural catheters are not recommended for use with the most aggressive anticoagulation regimens because of the potential for epidural hematoma formation.

Continuous epidural analgesia via a catheter is a relatively burdensome technique, with a reported failure rate of approximately 30%.[19,20] Catheter, tubing, and epidural pumps often impede patient activity and may be cumbersome, especially during physical therapy. Catheter systems also require a considerable amount of maintenance by a knowledgeable and dedicated nursing staff. Furthermore, the possibility for programming and medication errors with epidural and intravenous patient-controlled analgesia pumps should not be discounted. The adequacy of analgesia and signs of epidural hematoma should be monitored at regular intervals. Although highly effective, epidural analgesia is labor intensive and generally requires an acute pain management team.

Combined Spinal-Epidural Anesthesia

Combined spinal-epidural anesthesia, most commonly administered via a needle through a needle approach, was first described in 1982[21] and has continued to gain popularity for use in patients undergoing orthopaedic surgery. After an epidural needle is introduced into the epidural space, a spinal needle is advanced though the epidural needle, and a standard spinal anesthetic is performed. The spinal needle is then removed, and an epidural catheter is advanced into the epidural space.

Other techniques of delivering combined spinal-epidural anesthesia include a two-needlestick approach in which an epidural catheter placement at L1-L2 is followed by placement of a subarachnoid needle at L3-L4[22] and the combined needle approach, which consists of joining a spinal needle along the length of an epidural needle with particular attention to ensure dural puncture separate from epidural catheter placement.[23,24]

A review of the various combined spinal-epidural anesthesia techniques by Cook[24] provides technical details as well as the causes of failure and failure rates associated with each method. Recent reports suggest a failure rate of the spinal component of the needle-through-needle approach to administering combined spinal-epidural anesthesia to be approximately 5%.[25,26] There has also been a reported failure rate of epidural analgesia for postoperative analgesia after combined spinal-epidural anesthesia ranging between 18% to 22% compared with a failure rate of 6% to 8% for epidurals alone.[24] The advantages of the combined spinal-epidural anesthesia technique include spinal anesthesia for surgery with the potential to use the epidural catheter if the surgery outlasts the spinal anesthetic. Moreover, the epidural catheter is available for postoperative analgesia. Despite the advantages of this technique, the

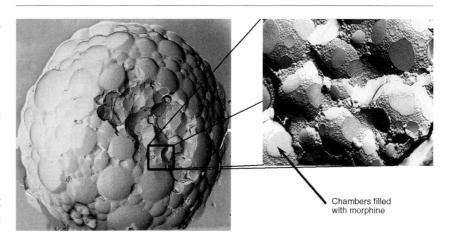

Figure 1   DepoDur scanning electron micrograph. Inset (*arrow*) shows chambers filled with morphine. (Courtesy of SkyePharma, London, England.)

epidural catheter cannot be tested at the time of placement, leading to a potentially nonfunctioning catheter and consequently a dissatisfied patient. All cautions related to epidural and spinal catheters apply to the combined spinal-epidural anesthesia technique; hence, this type of anesthesia should be administered by experienced clinicians.

Extended Release Epidural Morphine

The US Food and Drug Administration has recently approved a novel formulation of extended-release epidural morphine (EREM) known as DepoDur (SkyePharma, London, England) (Figure 1). This formulation consists of a lyposomal carrier (DepoFoam, SkyePharma) with preservative-free morphine. EREM is injected via a standard lumbar epidural injection for postoperative analgesia; however, an indwelling epidural catheter is not used with this preparation. EREM has been studied in patients undergoing hip and knee arthroplasty and demonstrated a 48-hour period of analgesia.[27] In a hip arthroplasty study, patients who received EREM showed a significant reduction in the need for supplemen-

tal analgesia (Figure 2). In the same study, patients who received EREM had significantly better pain intensity scores compared with intravenous patient-controlled analgesia alone. This technique offers the advantage of catheter-free and pump-free pain relief and is particularly appealing for patients receiving anticoagulation therapy.[28] The absence of an epidural catheter reduces the risk of epidural hematoma formation with anticoagulation. Adverse effects are similar to those of standard opioid therapy; careful monitoring by a knowledgeable staff is mandated. The absence of external paraphernalia should facilitate patient mobility and reduce the burden of care related to catheter maintenance. Furthermore, additional considerations of the decreased burden of use for the patient, nursing staff, and pain management team add to the appeal of this novel analgesic.

Single-Injection Peripheral Nerve Blocks and Continuous Peripheral Nerve Blocks

Peripheral neural blockade can be used as a sole anesthetic technique for patients undergoing total joint arthroplasty. In a comparison with intravenous patient-controlled anal-

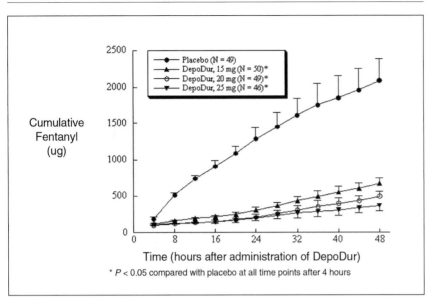

Figure 2   Graph showing cumulative fentanyl usage over 48 hours (mean, standard error) during hip arthroplasty. (Courtesy of SkyePharma.)

gesia using morphine after undergoing total knee arthroplasty, continuous lumbar plexus anesthesia (3-in-1 block) provided better pain relief and faster knee rehabilitation with fewer adverse events.[29] A prospective study by Singelyn and Gouverneur comparing a 3-in-1 block and patient-controlled analgesia with morphine after total hip arthroplasty found comparable pain relief with fewer technical problems and adverse effects with 3-in-1 block administration.[30] This approach completely eliminates central neuraxial manipulation and any potential for related problems such as epidural hematoma formation. Peripheral blocks are used more often as effective adjunctive analgesic techniques, particularly after total knee arthroplasty.[31] A recent study concluded that combining femoral nerve block with epidural analgesia after total knee arthroplasty significantly improved pain control compared with epidural anesthesia alone.[32] Furthermore, in a recent meta-analysis, Richman and associates[33] concluded that continuous peripheral nerve block analgesia significantly reduced opioid consumption and opioid-related adverse effects compared with opioid analgesia.

The blocks of interest for total joint arthroplasty involve the major plexi of the lower extremity: the lumbar plexus (L2, L3, and L4) and the lumbosacral plexus (L5, S1, S2, and S3). Blocks of the lumbar plexus will provide analgesia to the hip and anteromedial aspect of the knee. The lumbosacral plexus provides analgesia to the posterolateral aspect of the knee and the remainder of the leg below the knee. L2, L3, and L4 can be blocked posteriorly through the posterior lumbar plexus block or anteriorly by a femoral block. L5, S1, S2, and S3 can be blocked at the sciatic nerve posteriorly or in the popliteal fossa. The latter block is particularly useful for foot and ankle surgery and less commonly used for adult reconstruction.

Single-injection perineural local anesthetic blocks have the potential to provide extended analgesia after surgery. Depending on the specific local anesthetic used, analgesia may last 12 to 24 hours. In many circumstances, however, this duration of action fails to provide adequate analgesia as a sole strategy. Similar to epidural analgesia, single-injection blocks and continuous catheter blocks may provide less than complete analgesia, although continuous catheter systems have been demonstrated to markedly prolong the duration of pain relief compared with single-injection peripheral blocks.[6,34] Moreover, femoral nerve blocks have been found to provide incomplete anesthesia to the obturator nerve.[35] The short duration of single-injection perineural local anesthetic blocks can be overcome by catheter insertion and continuous infusion of perineural local anesthetic as well as parenteral opioids and nonopioid analgesics. Hence, additional analgesics should be available and ordered as part of a multimodal analgesia plan.

Standard inpatient infusion pumps may be used. Additionally, a variety of disposable electronic and mechanical pumps are available if the practitioner wishes to send the patient home with a continuous infusion of local anesthetic. These techniques provide localized analgesia, without the potential adverse effect of hypotension that may accompany epidural analgesia. Furthermore, an attractive quality of this approach is a localized motor block limited to one extremity.

The addition of a perineural catheter delivery system introduces some problems, although fewer problems occur than with an epidural catheter. With anticoagulation, perineural catheters may present some risk for bleeding and potential hematoma formation. Although not

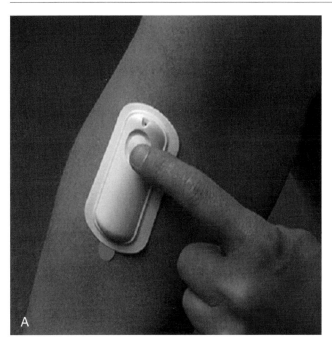

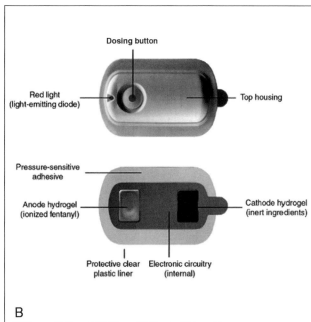

Figure 3   A, Photograph showing use of the patient-activated fentanyl iontophoretic transdermal system (Fentanyl Iontophoretic Transdermal System [IONSYS™], ALZA Corporation, Mountain View, CA). **B,** Illustration showing the components of the Fentanyl Iontophoretic Transdermal System (IONSYS™). (Courtesy of ALZA Corporation.)

as catastrophic as an epidural hematoma, several case reports have documented injury from psoas compartment hematomas.[36-38] As with any catheter delivery system, there is a slight chance of infection and other catheter-related problems. These problems include potential bleeding, increased systemic absorption of local anesthetic, and increased burden of care. Local anesthetic toxicity is rare, but potentially a risk. If patients are to be sent home with a catheter and infusion device, surveillance and follow-up is mandatory. In addition, patients should be instructed to avoid potential injury of the insensate limb. As with neuraxial techniques, there is a rare incidence of nerve injury associated with peripheral nerve blocks. Peripheral nerve blocks and particularly continuous blocks with indwelling catheters require particular skills from the anesthesia and acute pain team.

Intra-articular and Incisional Local Anesthetic Infusions

Wound infiltration of local anesthetic can provide short-term cutaneous analgesia. A catheter can be placed in the incision to provide an extended infusion of local anesthetic; however, catheter precautions apply with this technique. Intra-articular local anesthetic, with or without a catheter, has been reported to have mixed results after total joint replacement because of the complexity and severity of pain associated with these procedures.[39] After total knee arthroplasty, some studies advocate local anesthetic infusion with anesthetics, epinephrine, and morphine, which has been shown to result in increased flexion and reduced hospital stays.[40,41] These techniques are best reserved for procedures with less resulting pain or as a multimodal approach for pain management because the duration of this type of analgesia is short-lived.

Patient-Activated Transdermal Analgesia

Intravenous patient-controlled analgesia is used routinely as an adjunct to many of the techniques described. Although it is an effective method of delivering pain relief, problems frequently occur such as intravenous tube infiltration, pump malfunction, kinking of intravenous tubing, and interference with patient activity. Intravenous patient-controlled analgesia also has been implicated in medication errors that may lead to patient harm.[42] As a result, a novel iontophoretic patient-activated device has been developed to address some of these issues[43] (Figure 3). The device is the size of a credit card, uses no needle, and is patient activated. This device can be applied to the upper arm or the chest and is designed to manage moderate to severe pain requiring opioid analgesia. The system delivers a preprogrammed amount of fentanyl hydrochloride over 10 minutes for a total of 80 doses or for 24 hours.[44] In a double-blind, placebo-controlled trial, the iontophoretic fentanyl hydrochloride patient-administered transdermal analgesic system demonstrated superiority over placebo for acute postoperative pain management.[45] A recent study comparing this iontophoretic transdermal system (IONSYS, ALZA Corporation, Mountain View, CA) with standard morphine intravenous patient-controlled analgesia demonstrated therapeutic equivalence.[46] When approved, this system may be a useful adjuvant for total joint arthroplasty analgesia.

Summary

Regional anesthesia is an important part of the current approach to providing analgesia to patients who have undergone total joint arthroplasty. Multimodal analgesic regimens incorporate various agents and techniques, whose aim is to thwart pain at multiple sites of action. When considering the analgesic options, it is important to consider the implications of anticoagulation, ease of use, and burden of care. Less invasive delivery systems that provide continuous analgesia and are compatible with aggressive anticoagulation regimens may facilitate rehabilitation and ultimately improve patient outcomes. Moreover, emerging technologies may soon address currently unmet needs.

References

1. Borghi B, Laici C, Iuorio S, et al: Epidural vs general anaesthesia. [In Italian.] *Minerva Anestesiol* 2002;68:171-177.

2. Liu SS, Strodtbeck WM, Richman JM, Wu CL: A comparison of regional versus general anesthesia for ambulatory anesthesia: A meta-analysis of randomized controlled trials. *Anesth Analg* 2005;101:1634-1642.

3. Modig J: The role of lumbar epidural anaesthesia as antithrombotic prophylaxis in total hip replacement. *Acta Chir Scand* 1985;151:589-594.

4. Davis FM, Laurenson VG, Gillespie WJ, Wells JE, Foate J, Newman E: Deep vein thrombosis after total hip replacement: A comparison between spinal and general anaesthesia. *J Bone Joint Surg Br* 1989;71:181-185.

5. Sharrock NE, Cazan MG, Hargett MJ, Williams-Russo P, Wilson PD Jr: Changes in mortality after total hip and knee arthroplasty over a ten-year period. *Anesth Analg* 1995;80:242-248.

6. Indelli PF, Grant SA, Nielsen K, Vail TP: Regional anesthesia in hip surgery. *Clin Orthop Relat Res* 2005;441:250-255.

7. Vendittoli PA, Makinen P, Drolet P, et al: A multimodal analgesia protocol for total knee arthroplasty: A randomized, controlled study. *J Bone Joint Surg Am* 2006;88:282-289.

8. Watson MW, Mitra D, McLintock TC, Grant SA: Continuous versus single-injection lumbar plexus blocks: Comparison of the effects on morphine use and early recovery after total knee arthroplasty. *Reg Anesth Pain Med* 2005;30:541-547.

9. Horlocker TT, Wedel DJ, Benzon H, et al: Regional anesthesia in the anticoagulated patient: defining the risks (the second ASRA Consensus Conference on Neuraxial Anesthesia and Anticoagulation). *Reg Anesth Pain Med* 2003;28:172-197.

10. Lema MJ: Opioid effects and adverse effects. *Reg Anesth* 1996;21(Suppl):38-42.

11. Shoji H, Solomonow M, Yoshino S, D'Ambrosia R, Dabezies E: Factors affecting postoperative flexion in total knee arthroplasty. *Orthopedics* 1990;13:643-649.

12. Sinatra RS, Torres J, Bustos AM: Pain management after major orthopaedic surgery: Current strategies and new concepts. *J Am Acad Orthop Surg* 2002;10:117-129.

13. Bowrey S, Hamer J, Bowler I, Symonds C, Hall JE: A comparison of 0.2 and 0.5 mg intrathecal morphine for postoperative analgesia after total knee replacement. *Anaesthesia* 2005;60:449-452.

14. Horlocker TT, Wedel DJ, Benzon H, et al: Regional anesthesia and the anticoagulated patient: Defining the risks (The Second ASRA Consensus Conference on neuraxial anesthesia and anticoagulation). *Reg Anesth Pain Med* 2003;28:172-197.

15. Block BM, Liu SS, Rowlingson AJ, Cowan AR, Cowan JA Jr, Wu CL: Efficacy of postoperative epidural analgesia: A meta-analysis. *JAMA* 2003;290:2455-2463.

16. Kampe S, Weigand C, Kaufmann J, Klimek M, Konig DP, Lynch J: Postoperative analgesia with no motor block by continuous epidural infusion of ropivacaine 0.1% and sufentanil after total hip replacement. *Anesth Analg* 1999;89:395-398.

17. Kopacz DJ, Sharrock NE, Allen HW: A comparison of levobupivacaine 0.125%, fentanyl 4 microg/mL, or their combination for patient-controlled epidural analgesia after major orthopedic surgery. *Anesth Analg* 1999;89:1497-1503.

18. Wheatley RG, Schug SA, Watson D: Safety and efficacy of postoperative epidural analgesia. *Br J Anaesth* 2001;87:47-61.

19. Andersen G, Rasmussen H, Rosenstock C, et al: Postoperative pain control by epidural analgesia after transabdominal surgery: Efficacy and problems encountered in daily routine. *Acta Anaesthesiol Scand* 2000;44:296-301.

20. Ready LB: Acute pain: Lessons learned from 25,000 patients. *Reg Anesth Pain Med* 1999;24:499-505.

21. Coates MB: Combined subarachnoid and epidural techniques. *Anaesthesia* 1982;37:89-90.

22. Brownridge P: Central neural blockade and caesarian section: Part 1. Review and case series. *Anaesth Intensive Care* 1979;7:33-41.

23. Eldor J, Chaimsky G: Combined spinal-epidural needle (CSEN). *Can J Anaesth* 1988;35:537-539.

24. Cook TM: Combined spinal-epidural techniques. *Anaesthesia* 2000;55:42-64.

25. Herbstman CH, Jaffee JB, Tuman KJ, Newman LM: An in vivo evaluation of four spinal needles used for the combined spinal-epidural technique. *Anesth Analg* 1998;86:520-522.

26. Casati A, D'Ambrosio A, De NP, Fanelli G, Tagariello V, Tarantino F: A clinical comparison between needle-through-needle and double-segment techniques for combined spinal and epidural anesthesia. *Reg Anesth Pain Med* 1998;23:390-394.

27. Viscusi ER, Martin G, Hartrick CT, Singla N, Manvelian G: Forty-eight hours of postoperative pain relief after total hip arthroplasty with a novel, extended-release epidural morphine

formulation. *Anesthesiology* 2005;102:1014-1022.

28. Hartrick CT, Martin G, Kantor G, Koncelik J, Manvelian G: Evaluation of a single-dose, extended-release epidural morphine formulation for pain after knee arthroplasty. *J Bone Joint Surg Am* 2006;88:273-281.

29. Singelyn FJ, Deyaert M, Joris D, Pendeville E, Gouverneur JM: Effects of intravenous patient-controlled analgesia with morphine, continuous epidural analgesia, and continuous three-in-one block on postoperative pain and knee rehabilitation after unilateral total knee arthroplasty. *Anesth Analg* 1998;87:88-92.

30. Singelyn FJ, Gouverneur JM: Postoperative analgesia after total hip arthroplasty: IV PCA with morphine, patient-controlled epidural analgesia, or continuous "3-in-1" block? A prospective evaluation by our acute pain service in more than 1,300 patients. *J Clin Anesth* 1999;11:550-554.

31. Barrington MJ, Olive D, Low K, Scott DA, Brittain J, Choong P: Continuous femoral nerve blockade or epidural analgesia after total knee replacement: A prospective randomized controlled trial. *Anesth Analg* 2005;101:1824-1829.

32. YaDeau JT, Cahill JB, Zawadsky MW, et al: The effects of femoral nerve blockade in conjunction with epidural analgesia after total knee arthroplasty. *Anesth Analg* 2005;101:891-895.

33. Richman JM, Liu SS, Courpas G, et al: Does continuous peripheral nerve block provide superior pain control to opioids? A meta-analysis. *Anesth Analg* 2006;102:248-257.

34. Mollmann M: Continuous spinal anesthesia. [In German.] *Anaesthesist* 1997;46:616-621.

35. Macalou D, Trueck S, Meuret P, et al: Postoperative analgesia after total knee replacement: The effect of an obturator nerve block added to the femoral 3-in-1 nerve block. *Anesth Analg* 2004;99:251-254.

36. Hoek JA, Henny CP, Knipscheer HC, ten Cate H, Nurmohamed MT, ten Cate JW: The effect of different anaesthetic techniques on the incidence of thrombosis following total hip replacement. *Thromb Haemost* 1991;65:122-125.

37. Adam F, Jaziri S, Chauvin M: Psoas abscess complicating femoral nerve block catheter. *Anesthesiology* 2003;99:230-231.

38. Johr M: A complication of continuous blockade of the femoral nerve. [In German.] *Reg Anaesth* 1987;10:37-38.

39. Busch CA, Shore BJ, Bhandari R, et al: Efficacy of periarticular multimodal drug injection in total knee arthroplasty: A randomized trial. *J Bone Joint Surg Am* 2006;88:959-963.

40. Lombardi AV Jr, Berend KR, Mallory TH, Dodds KL, Adams JB: Soft tissue and intra-articular injection of bupivacaine, epinephrine, and morphine has a beneficial effect after total knee arthroplasty. *Clin Orthop Relat Res* 2004;428:125-130.

41. Rasmussen S, Kramhoft MU, Sperling KP, Pedersen JH: Increased flexion and reduced hospital stay with continuous intraarticular morphine and ropivacaine after primary total knee replacement: Open intervention study of efficacy and safety in 154 patients. *Acta Orthop Scand* 2004;75:606-609.

42. Vicente KJ, Kada-Bekhaled K, Hillel G, et al: Programming errors contribute to death from patient-controlled analgesia: Case report and estimate of probability. *Can J Anaesth* 2003;50:328-332.

43. Viscusi ER: Emerging techniques for postoperative analgesia in orthopedic surgery. *Am J Orthop* 2004;33(Suppl):13-16.

44. Sinatra R: The fentanyl HCl patient-controlled transdermal system (PCTS): an alternative to intravenous patient-controlled analgesia in the postoperative setting. *Clin Pharmacokinet* 2005;44(suppl 1):1-6.

45. Viscusi ER, Reynolds L, Tait S, Melson T, Atkinson LE: An iontophoretic fentanyl patient-activated analgesic delivery system for postoperative pain: A double-blind, placebo-controlled trial. *Anesth Analg* 2006;102:188-194.

46. Viscusi ER, Reynolds L, Chung F, Atkinson LE, Khanna S: Patient-controlled transdermal fentanyl hydrochloride vs intravenous morphine pump for postoperative pain: A randomized controlled trial. *JAMA* 2004;291:1333-1341.

SECTION

4

Adult Reconstruction: Hip

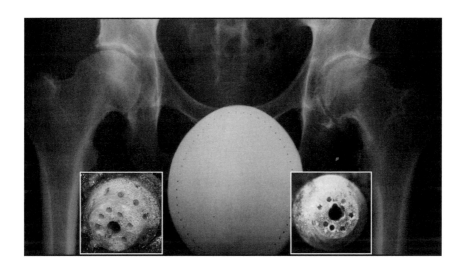

Metal-on-Metal Hip Resurfacing: What Have We Learned?

Harlan C. Amstutz, MD
Pat Campbell, PhD
Michel J. Le Duff, MA

Abstract

Surface hip arthroplasty has many attractive features for young, active patients, particularly because of the conservative nature of this treatment and its ability to preserve femoral bone. It is more anatomic and physiologic than stem-type hip replacements, and it represents a truly minimally osteoinvasive procedure, with no penetration into the femoral intramedullary canal. In addition, the construct has increased stability because of the near-normal diameter of the femoral component compared with most conventional hip replacement components. Although the short- to midterm clinical results for metal-on-metal hybrid hip resurfacing implants are definitely superior to those of earlier generations of resurfacing implants, the results of conventional total hip replacement using contemporary designs and bearing materials have also improved. As a result, it is imperative to assess what is known about the safety and efficacy of resurfacing to refine the indications and technique to improve the overall results and durability.

Instr Course Lect 2007;56:149-161.

The conservative nature of hip resurfacing makes it an attractive treatment option for young, active patients. Although the clinical results of metal-on-metal hybrid hip resurfacing implants are superior to those of earlier generations of resurfacing implants using polyethylene, to improve overall results and durability,

One or more of the authors or the departments with which they are affiliated have received something of value from a commercial or other party related directly or indirectly to the subject of this chapter.

the indications and technique for hip resurfacing should be refined.

Early Results

Between November 1996 and March 2003, 600 hips in 519 patients from a consecutive series of more than 950 hips were implanted with Conserve Plus resurfacing components (Wright Medical Technologies, Arlington, TN). The average age of the patients was 48.9 years, and 74% of the patients were male. The indications for treatment included osteoarthritis in 64% of patients, osteonecrosis in 8%, develop-

mental dysplasia of the hip in 12%, posttraumatic etiology in 8%, inflammatory etiology in 3%, Legg-Calvé-Perthes disease and slipped capital femoral epiphysis in 4%, and melorheostosis and pigmented villonodular synovitis in 1%. Previous surgeries had been performed in 7.3% of patients, including 12 core decompressions, 11 osteotomies, and 19 other procedures.

The average duration of follow-up was 5.6 years (range, 3.0 to 9.3 years). The University of California, Los Angeles (UCLA) hip scores showed improvement from preoperative to postoperative ratings in the following subcategories: pain, 3.5 versus 9.5; walking, 6.1 versus 9.6; function, 5.7 versus 9.5; and activity, 4.6 versus 7.5, respectively ($P < 0.0001$). The Medical Outcomes Study 12-Item Short Form Health Survey (SF-12) mental scores increased from 47.5 preoperatively to 52.8 postoperatively, and the SF-12 physical scores increased from 31.8 preoperatively to 50.6 postoperatively ($P < 0.0001$). The mean postoperative Harris hip score was 92.7. In the authors' initial publication on metal-on-metal hybrid hip resurfac-

Table 1
Femoral Neck Fracture Rates From Recent Studies

Study	Country	Type of Prosthesis	No. of Patients	No. of Fractures (%)
Chatterton et al[1] (2004)		BHR	71	1 (1.41%)
Cutts et al[2] (2004)		Corin	65	6 (9.23%)
DeSantis et al[3] (2005)		Conserve Plus	23	0 (0)
McMinn[4] (2003)	England	BHR	1209	4 (0.33%)
Pollard et al[5] (2003)	England	BHR	63	3 (4.76%)
Amstutz et al[6] (2004)	US	Conserve Plus	600	5 (0.83%)
Beaulé et al[7] (2004)	US	McMinn	42	1 (2.38%)
Chirodian et al[8] (2004)	England	Cormet-Hybrid	44	0 (0)
Bose (personal correspondence, 2005)	India	BHR	408	0 (0)
De Smet[9] (2005)	Belgium	BHR	252	1 (0.40%)
Hart and Scott[10] (2005)	England	1 McMinn and 3 BHR	4	0 (0)
Lilikakis et al[11] (2005)	England	Cormet (Cementless)	70	0 (0)
Little et al[12] (2005)	England	BHR	377	8 (2.12%)
Krikler and Nelson[13] (2005)		Not reported	345	5 (1.45%)
Shimmin and Back[14] (2005)	Australia	BHR	3497	50 (1.43%)
Sinha et al[15] (2006)	England	BHR	60	6 (10.00%)
Treacy et al[16] (2005)	England	BHR	144	1 (0.69%)
Grigoris et al[17] (2005)	US	Durom	200	0 (0)
Vendittoli et al[18] (2006)	Canada	Durom	96	0 (0)

BHR = Birmingham hip resurfacing

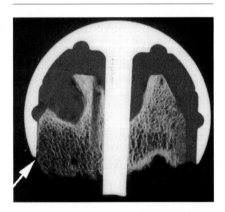

Figure 1 Cut section of a femoral head that was retrieved after revision for femoral neck fracture 5 months after resurfacing from a 57-year-old man with severe osteoarthritis and degenerative cystic changes secondary to developmental dysplasia of the hip. Note the excessive thickness of bone cement in the dome area, indicating incomplete seating of the component, and the uncovered reamed bone at the femoral-head neck junction (*arrow*).

ing, the results were satisfactory in patients with good bone quality. However, when failure occurred, femoral loosening and neck fracture were identified as the primary modes of failure. After the risk factors were identified, two options emerged to reduce the incidence of failure: (1) resurface only hips with good bone quality (having cystic defects less than 1 cm in size) and (2) improve the technique in patients presenting with significant risk factors for failure and assess the efficacy.[1,2]

Incidence and Prevention of Femoral Neck Fractures
The worldwide incidence of femoral neck fractures after hip resurfacing is approximately 1.25% (range, 0 to 10%) when combining all of the current reports in the literature[3-20]

(approximately 7,500 cases summarized in Table 1, with 3,500 of those being from the Australian Hip Registry). The apparent cause of femoral neck fractures is generally multifactorial. In the authors' series of patients who underwent hip resurfacing using the Conserve Plus implant, the incidence of femoral neck fractures is less than 0.6% of those whose hips were reconstructed with a 1-mm cement mantle. No such fractures have been reported in this series in the past 5 years (N = 500), which indicates that most femoral neck fractures may be preventable by using careful patient selection and optimal surgical technique.

Cut sections from implant failures in the authors' series showed that the implants were sometimes incompletely seated (Figure 1), which puts the femoral neck at risk in several ways. The surgeon may apply extra pressure or hammer blows to seat the proud component, leading to stress fractures if a patient has weak bone or component misalignment. In addition, reamed bone may remain uncovered and act as a stress riser, and the thick mantle may reduce bone cement penetration for fixation. Other risk factors include overaggressive removal of the large anterior osteophyte (which leaves uncovered reamed bone without a cortex), osteopenia, cystic degeneration, and overpressurization of acrylic into poor-quality bone.[1] Femoral neck notching and impingement were identified as additional risk factors after retrieval analysis of the implants from patients who experienced fractures in the 10-surgeon, multicenter, investigational device exemption (IDE) trial of the Conserve Plus.

In a study of retrieved femoral heads after failed hip resurfacing using Birmingham hip resurfacing (Smith & Nephew, Bromsgrove, England) and Cormet (Corin Medical, Cirencester, England) implants, Little and associates[14] reported a high incidence of osteonecrosis, which led to considerable investigation into the vascularity of the femoral head, review of surgical technique, and consideration of using approaches other than the posterior approach. Extensive penetration of cement into the femoral head has been observed in the authors' series. Although cement has been noted to nearly fill the femoral head in some retrievals, the relationship to femoral neck fractures has not been established. It is important for surgeons to recognize that the cement mantle thickness (clearance) between the cylindrically reamed part of the femoral head and the component varies in the different designs

Table 2
Resurfacing Systems and Target Cement Mantles

System	Manufacturer	Cement Mantle (mm)
Conserve Plus (US)	Wright Medical Technology, Arlington, TN	1
Conserve Plus (Europe)	Wright Medical Technology	0.5
BHR	Smith & Nephew, Memphis, TN	0
Cormet	Corin, Cirencester, England	0
Durom	Zimmer, Warsaw, IN	1
Articular Surface Replacement	DePuy, Warsaw, IN	< 1
ReCap Femoral Resurfacing	Biomet, Warsaw, IN	0.5
ICON Metal-on-Metal Hip Resurfacing	International Orthopaedics	0

from 0 to 1 mm (Table 2) and that different cementing strategies must be used for different recommended clearances. The viscosity of acrylic cement and the timing of application are important. For example, the lower the clearance, the lower viscosity of acrylic is required. Additionally, it is difficult to control cement penetration with low clearance, especially into the cylindrically reamed section. Excess cement must be extruded to avoid overpenetration of the cement and the component must be fully seated while minimizing the impaction force necessary. Designs with a 1-mm cement mantle are recommended because they permit the use of a doughier acrylic and the fingers can pressurize the cement into the cylindrically reamed portion of the head to ensure penetration of 1 to 2 mm. Additional pressurization of the acrylic into the dome and chamfered areas occurs as the component is seated, but the 1-mm clearance around the bone when using the Conserve Plus and Durom (Zimmer, Warsaw, IN) implants allows for extravasation of the excess cement and minimizes the risk of overpressurization.

Although the healing of stress

fractures under resurfacing components has been reported,[21,22] additional long-term analysis is required because bone undergoing repair following stress fracture is a site of weakness and histologic analysis from the authors' series has shown that fractures have occurred in these areas.

Incidence and Prevention of Loosening

In first- and second-generation hip resurfacing implants using metal-on-polyethylene bearings, component loosening was the primary failure mode whether the implants had a cemented or cementless interface on the acetabular or femoral side. Acetabular component loosening was greatly reduced with a cementless component, but there was an increase in femoral loosening and late neck fractures caused by polyethylene particle–induced osteolysis. In hip implants using metal-on-metal resurfacing, component loosening has been significantly reduced and acetabular component loosening is uncommon.

In the authors' series, acetabular component loosening has not been observed in any of the 950 Conserve Plus implants over a 10-year period.

The multicenter IDE study, which had 1,200 hip resurfacings not including those of the authors, reported a 0.5% incidence of acetabular component loosening that was likely the result of a lack of initial stability obtained at insertion and a failure to properly assess stability at that time. The incidence of acetabular component loosening for other types of hip resurfacing implants is less well described, but because the designs vary in the amount of hemispheric coverage (165° to 180°) and in the method of obtaining initial stability to compensate for variations in bead size and type of coating, it is important to be familiar with these variations to ensure enduring fixation.

With the Conserve Plus resurfacing system, the final reamed size should be 1 mm smaller than the final outside diameter of the acetabular component. The rigid metal ring gauge that is 1 mm under the outside diameter of the component should seat to the floor of the acetabulum in all planes. If the gauge does not reach the floor or is difficult to insert, this is probably because of a rim of bone posteriorly at the acetabular entrance that was created from the cutting teeth of the reamers being less than a full hemisphere. The ring gauge with the outside diameter of the component should not go to the floor to provide a press-fit of approximately 1 mm. The press-fit is essentially achieved in the anterior to posterior direction between the anterior and posterior columns of the acetabulum. It is recommended that the surgeon hold the socket firmly with the inserter attached, the angle finder indicating a 42° lateral opening when pointing straight up, and then have the technician or assistant impact the component until it is firmly seated. It is important to assess the fixation of the implant at this point by rocking the pelvis with the inserter still engaged in the socket. If the fixation is insufficient, the component should be removed, the acetabular cavity reamed more deeply, and the component reinserted.

Incidence and Prevention of Femoral Component Loosening

The incidence of femoral component loosening has been greatly reduced since the first generation of hip resurfacing implants that used polyethylene. In patients with good bone stock, particularly males younger than 55 years with osteoarthritis, the survivorship from four recent reports ranged from 98.5% to 99% at 3-year follow-up.[11,18,21,23] Femoral component loosening in the authors' series of patients with primary osteoarthritis and good bone quality has rarely occurred since this type of hip resurfacing was first performed in 1996. The incidence of femoral component loosening in the authors' series, especially when the patient has deficient bone stock in this hip, was 2% of patients, who subsequently required conversion to a total hip replacement. In most instances of femoral component loosening, the failure was associated with patients with risk factors such as large cystic degeneration in the hip and/or a small hip surface area.[2,8] Fifty percent of failures occurred in the first series of 110 patients; during the time these patients underwent hip resurfacing, the instrumentation and techniques were still being developed.

In a retrieval analysis that was done on failed prostheses from the authors' series and on prostheses with different designs that were submitted from around the world, femoral component loosening was noted to be associated with a variable quantity of cement present in the femoral component.[24] The total percentage of the femoral head sections occupied by cement (mantle, cement-filled fixation pegs or cysts, and penetration combined) ranged from 11% to 89%, and the percentage was significantly more in failures from loosening compared with all other modes of failure ($P = 0.001$). Cement-filled cysts were more prevalent in prostheses that failed because of femoral component loosening compared with nonfemoral component failures ($P < 0.025$).

In the first 600 hips in the authors' series, there were 18 revisions in 17 patients for definite femoral component loosening. After carefully studying retrievals and photographs of the femoral head before cementation, the major reason for failure was apparently inadequate fixation at the time of surgery secondary to poor bone preparation and/or a small area for fixation because of bone loss related to cystic defects (Figure 2). All but one loose femoral component occurred in the first 300 hips in the authors' series. Substantial femoral metaphyseal stem radiolucencies were noted in 13 hips during the same period, none of which required revision. As a result, changes in surgical technique were made to improve the quality of the bone preparation and fixation at the time of surgery.

The surgical technique changes are summarized in Table 3. A significant improvement was noted in the second 300 hips in the authors' series compared with the first 300 using time-dependent analysis and time to radiolucency as the end point ($P = 0.016$).[25] This improvement was attributable to the technical changes made during the implantation of the first 300 hips, including adding fixation holes in

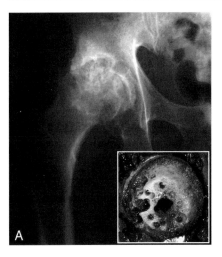
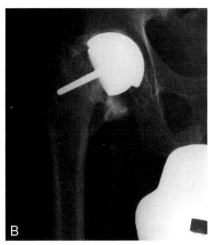
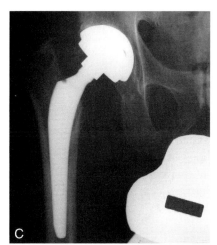

Figure 2 **A,** AP radiograph of the hip of a 66-year-old male long distance runner with end-stage osteoarthritis. Note the extensive cystic degeneration of the femoral head confirmed by the photograph (*inset*) of the femoral head after preparation. There is still cystic material present in the defects, and there are a limited number of drilled holes in the dome. The stem was not cemented as was the custom at that time. The patient required a small femoral component (46 mm) and his surface arthroplasty risk index was 5. **B,** AP radiograph obtained 65 months after resurfacing shows the femoral component has loosened and tipped into varus. Despite Brooker grade IV heterotopic ossification, the patient continued running long distances postoperatively. **C,** AP radiograph showing that the femoral component was replaced by a double-wedge, grit-blasted cementless femoral stem and a unipolar head articulating with the well-fixed acetabular component, which was left in place. Prophylactic radiation therapy was performed, and heterotopic ossification was removed during revision surgery. The patient subsequently switched his sporting activities to bicycling and is doing well 2 years after conversion to total hip replacement and 3 years after contralateral hip resurfacing.

Table 3
Technical Changes for the Two Generations of Femoral Fixation*

	First Generation	Second Generation
Suction	No suction (first 100 hips)	Dome suction
Drilled holes	A few dome holes (0 if good bone quality)	Increased number (chamfer added)
Stem cementation	Stem not cemented (only rarely in patients with bad bone quality)	Stem cemented in 152, regardless of cyst size
Target stem-shaft angle	Anatomic	140°
Removal of cystic debris	Incomplete (curette only)	Complete (high-speed burr)

*Based on the authors' experience with the Conserve Plus

the dome and chamfered areas and cleansing and drying using a suction tip in the dome hole. Positioning the femoral component in a more valgus position did not show any effect as an independent variable. No patients in the authors' series who have undergone implantation in the past 5 years have required revision or had signs of potential component loosening. However, because none of the components with cemented stems showed femoral radiolucencies or were revised for aseptic loosening and because to date no adverse consequences such as femoral neck narrowing or stress shielding have been observed, the authors recommend cementation in hips with cysts greater than 1 cm and in all hips with femoral component sizes smaller than 48 mm.

Although high-impact activities have not been associated with failure in the absence of risk factors, in the authors' study femoral component loosening occurred in six patients who participated in high-impact activities including a competitive tennis player, a fitness instructor, a marathon runner, a mountain biker (two hips), and an expert downhill skier. High-impact activities are defined as physical activities that use running or jumping as the primary mode of displacement or as any other activity mode that generates joint reaction forces greater than three times body weight. All of these patients received implants using first-generation surgical techniques and had hips with risk factors. With implantations using second-generation surgical techniques, the implant components have proved more durable in patients with risk factors who have continued to participate in high-impact activities. Nonetheless, patients with risk factors have been advised not to participate in high-impact activities or to minimize impact because it is unknown whether components implanted using second-generation surgical techniques will maintain the integrity of the hip joint over the long term. The rationale for advising patients to take these precautions is that the cystic areas of the femoral head are filled with cement, which has a different modulus of elasticity than the bone or metal resurfacing component, and it is likely that repetitive high impact may initiate or contribute to a component loosening process. Although long-term follow-up will provide more conclusive data, the incidence of femoral component loosening has been reduced from 5.7% of patients to 0.3% and the incidence of femoral radiolucencies has been reduced from 3.7% to 0.7%, which is a total reduction from 9.3% to 1% when comparing the first 300 hips implanted and the second 300 hips implanted in the authors' series. The minimum 3-year follow-up of the patients in the second group of 300 hips has already exceeded the average time to radiolucency (25.3 months ± 10.4 [1 standard deviation]). These findings suggest that significant improvement has been achieved, although the average follow-up for the second group of 300 hips was 55 months compared with 83 months for the first group of 300 hips in the authors' series.

Bone Conservation

First-generation metal-on-polyethylene surface arthroplasties were conservative on the femoral side but not

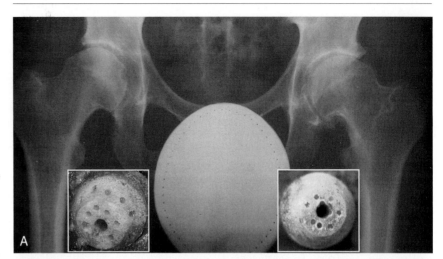

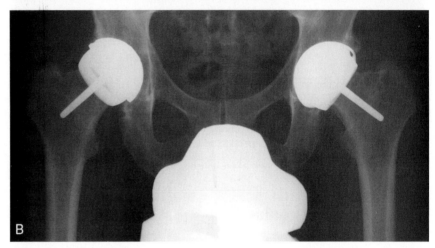

Figure 3   **A,** AP radiograph of a 47-year-old man with end-stage osteoarthritis of the left hip. The right hip shows early signs of osteoarthritis. The patient underwent bilateral procedures 6 years apart. Photographs (*insets*) show the femoral heads after preparation. Note the difference in the number and positioning of the drill holes, which illustrates an evolution of the authors' surgical technique between 1998 (left hip surgery) and 2004 (right hip surgery). **B,** AP radiograph obtained 8 years after undergoing left hip resurfacing (Conserve Plus) and 2 years after the right hip procedure. Note the difference in acetabular component thickness; the right side was reconstructed with the thin (3.5-mm) shell and for the left side the standard (5-mm) socket was used. The two femoral components are identical (48 mm), but the right socket has an outside diameter that is 3 mm smaller than that of the left.

on the acetabular side because the initial design had a cemented femoral component with approximately 4 to 5 mm of polyethylene and a cement layer.[26] Later versions with porous implants for the socket were also not conservative because a two-part socket (a 3- to 4-mm titanium shell and a 3- to 5-mm polyethylene liner) was necessary.[27] Although there was

a marked improvement in the fixation durability of the components, the main cause of failure was osteolysis associated with the large ball size and conventional polyethylene radiated in air.[28] Although the chamfered cylinder sockets with mesh blocked the particle access to the acetabulum, the intracapsular femoral neck and head remained vulnerable to osteoly-

Table 4
Acetabular Component Characteristics of Hip Resurfacing Systems

System	Coverage (°)	Shape	Surface	Shell Thickness (mm)
Conserve Plus	170	Truncated hemisphere	Sintered cobalt-chromium beads (50 to 150 mm) ± hydroxyapatite	3.5 or 5
BHR	160 ID, 180 OD	Hemisphere	Cobalt-chromium beads (0.9 to 1.3 mm) cast-in + hydroxyapatite	3 (rim), 6 (dome)
Cormet	180	Equatorial expansion	Titanium and plasma spray under vacuum and static load (Ti-VPS) + hydroxyapatite	3 and 4 (2 cups per head)
Durom	165	Truncated hemisphere	Ti-VPS	4
Articular Surface Replacement	168 to 170	Truncated hemisphere	Sintered cobalt-chromium beads (200 to 300 mm) + hydroxyapatite	5 to 6
ReCap	180	Hemisphere	Ti-VPS ± hydroxyapatite	3
ICON	180	Hemisphere	Cobalt-chromium beads (bead size not known) cast-in + hydroxyapatite	Not known

ID = inside diameter, OD = outside diameter

sis. The acetabulum of patients whose hips were resurfaced with hemispherical design, which used adjuvant screw fixation, may also have been vulnerable because the debris penetrated into the acetabulum through the screw holes.[29,30] In contrast, metal-on-metal resurfacing uses a thin, one-piece acetabular shell, which allows porous fixation without removing any more bone than conventional total hip arthroplasty. In the first 543 Conserve Plus implantations in the authors' series, a 5-mm shell was used routinely; and in patients with a low femoral head-neck ratio (< 1.2), such as those with osteoarthritis secondary to Legg-Calvé-Perthes disease or slipped capital femoral epiphysis, removal of more bone from the acetabulum was often necessary for hip resurfacing than for total hip replacement. However, with the introduction of the thin (3.5-mm) shells, 3 mm of bone is typically preserved either on the femoral head or acetabulum during hip resurfacing (Figure 3). It is also possible to implant the socket without reaming to the floor of the acetabulum (as is often done during total hip replacement), thus positioning the socket more anatomically. Other designs have shells of varying thickness, varying degrees of hemispheric coverage, and varying modes of fixation, but all of these designs appear to be more conservative and successful than first-generation designs (Table 4).

Femoral Bone Preservation
Compared with total hip replacement designs, the femoral head is preserved in hip resurfacing, and femoral stress shielding has been shown to cause complications to date. Bone preservation of the femoral neck using dual energy x-ray absorptiometry scanning has been demonstrated in a series of patients who underwent hemiresurfacing of the femoral head only to treat osteonecrosis.[31] At 6-year follow-up, there was no evidence of diminished bone mineral density, adverse stress shielding, or adverse remodeling in a series of six patients who underwent unilateral hemiresurfacing when compared with the normal hips of control subjects. These hemiresurfacing components, first implanted in 1981, did not have a short metaphyseal stem. However, similar amounts of bone preservation have been reported at 24-month follow-up in another study comparing 13 patients who underwent metal-on-metal resurfacing and 13 patients who underwent total hip replacement.[32] In this study, the bone mineral density of the proximal femur was maintained or increased with resurfacing, whereas a significant decrease was observed with total hip replacement.

Femoral Neck Narrowing
AP and lateral radiographic evidence of femoral neck narrowing (a loss of ≥ 10% of femoral neck diameter from original postoperative radiographs) has been observed in patients who have undergone various types of hip resurfacing over the past 30 years.[9] However, femoral neck narrowing is difficult to quantify in the AP plane because of the variable rotation observed in cross-table lateral radiographs. The only reliable information available regarding femoral neck narrowing, therefore, is that obtained in mediolateral radiographs. The reported incidence of femoral neck narrowing varies with prosthetic type.

In the authors' series, no known failures associated with femoral neck narrowing have occurred to date. The incidence of femoral neck narrowing in the first 600 Conserve Plus implantations in the authors' series (as observed on mediolateral radiographs) was 2.8 % (17 of 600), 7 of which occurred in the first 70 hips implanted. Although the etiology and significance of femoral neck narrowing are unknown, possible causes include stress shielding (because of a reduction of femoral head diameter in hips that have been resurfaced with thick shells) or external pressure because of synovitis. With the introduction of the thin socket shell, the reamed femoral bone diameter and component size, on average, are 2 mm larger than they were with the 5-mm shells, thereby adding area for fixation; the impact on femoral neck narrowing of this adjustment, however, is as yet unknown.

At an average 8.7-year follow-up (range, 7 to 10 years), the incidence of femoral neck narrowing in the authors' series of hip resurfacings performed using McMinn (Corin, Cirencester, England) components was 20%.[9] A complete loss of the anterior cortex of the femoral neck has been observed with the McMinn prostheses, which may be related to the size of the stem or external soft-tissue pressure.

At an average 28.5-month follow-up (range, 24.0 to 37.8 months), Lilikakis and associates[13] reported a 27% incidence of femoral neck narrowing of 10% or greater in a series of patients who underwent hip resurfacing with the Cormet hydroxyapatite-coated prosthesis. The coating of the stem may be related to this higher incidence. In an earlier experimental study conducted by Hedley and associates,[33] it was re-ported that a porous-coated stem in a canine model quickly became ingrown with resulting stress shielding peripherally, which may account for the greater incidence of femoral neck narrowing in this implant compared with other designs.

Wear and Metallurgy

The tribology of metal-on-metal resurfaced joints is now well understood. Every device today is made from a cobalt-chromium-molybdenum alloy. All of the current devices have a carbon level greater than 0.2%. To minimize wear in these components, precise machining and final finishing are critical. The design features, which are important to reduce wear, include (in descending order of importance) radial clearance, sphericity, and surface finish. Although there has been one report of pin and disk test results that suggest increased wear occurs with heat-treated and solution-annealed cobalt-chromium,[34] multiple simulator studies have been conducted under conditions comparable to those in the body that report the wear rates of as-cast, heat-treated, solution-annealed, and forged-wear cobalt-chromium are approximately the same.[35,36] New data suggest that wear can be reduced by as much as 50% by forging the femoral component (which makes it harder) and using it against the softer as-cast, heat-treated, and solution-annealed socket (A-CLASS Advanced Metal-on-Metal Bearing, Wright Medical, Arlington, TN), but this has not yet been verified in vivo. Other new technologies suggest there may be ways of reducing wear by using ceramic coating or hardening the component materials.[37]

The authors' retrieval analysis shows that one of the major improvements brought about by metal-on-metal bearings is a reduction in wear.[24] The wear rate of these failed components was generally low (often not measurable using a coordinate measuring machine), with the exception of poorly functioning implants, particularly those in which acetabular malpositioning resulted in steep cup angles (> 55° of abduction) in some retrievals.[38] These failed components commonly had metallosis of the tissues and a wear stripe pattern on the femoral component. Acetabular osteolysis occurred in two patients, which may be a unique complication of metal-on-metal resurfacing.

Hip Resurfacing and Vascularity

Although much is known about the vascularity of the hip, much is unknown about vascularity in association with hip resurfacing. One study reported a high incidence of femoral neck fractures in patients who underwent hip resurfacing and suggested avascularity as a possible cause.[14] In the authors' experience, rich vascularity of the femoral head has been observed after preparation of the arthritic bone into the chamfered cylinder shape, suggesting hypervascularity. This hyperemia associated with osteoarthritis has been verified in positron emission tomography studies conducted by Forrest and associates[39] In addition, Freeman[40] has observed that femoral osteophytes associated with the osteoarthritic disease progression appear to occlude the branches from the medial circumflex artery, which normally enter the femoral head at the head-neck junction.

Extensive histologic analyses of failed resurfaced femoral heads conducted in the authors' laboratory have demonstrated areas of bone in which new bone formation occurs around dead bone, particularly around the cement interfaces in short-term retrievals; however, necrosis of the entire femoral head rarely occurred.[10] These healing areas of necrotic bone may be the result of using the posterior surgical approach and technique, but a subsequent healing process generally occurs without adverse sequelae because of ample reserve to sustain overall general viability, presumably the result of a rich anastomosis. Several studies have been conducted to ascertain the amount of reduction in blood flow by oxygen/nitrogen saturations using a laser Doppler flowmeter, but the findings of these studies are inconclusive because of the limited areas of sampling.[41,42] Additional studies that sample a larger portion of the femoral head are needed to ascertain the accuracy of these results. Positron emission tomography appears be a useful tool in evaluating the entire femoral head as well as for assessing various surgical approaches.

Stability

Dislocation is rare after hip resurfacing because the femoral head is approximately the same size as a normal hip. Once the capsule is healed, the hip is stable. Stability, however, is highly dependent on component positioning. If there is excessive anteversion in the femoral neck and the cup is excessively anteverted, dislocation can occur anteriorly. Posterior dislocation may also occur because of impingement. Most experienced surgeons recommend a femoral component neck-shaft angle of approximately 140° and a socket orientation of approximately 42° that is open laterally, with a range of 40° to 50° being acceptable; a smaller lateral opening may result in impingement. Anterior impinge-

ment is assessed by internal rotation of the hip in 90° of flexion. It is desirable to have at least 40° of internal rotation. There should also be at least 40° of external rotation in extension. With the hip and knee extended, the hip should be pushed anteriorly to make sure it is stable and that there is no possibility of subluxation. Impingement of the lesser trochanter against the ischium has been observed by the authors in an unusual instance of developmental dysplasia of the hip after valgus femoral osteotomy in which the patient's femoral neck-shaft angle was increased and the offset was markedly reduced. In this patient, the impingement could have been prevented by removing the bony impingement caused by the lesser trochanter.

Toxicity of Wear Products

The wear rate of the metal-on-metal bearing is extremely low. Bearings will not wear through in a patient's lifetime, but particles from the bearing surface will form during activities of daily living and through a corrosion process. These particles are traceable as ions in the blood as well as in the urine because they are excreted by the kidneys. The levels of these ions are quite variable, and it is unknown at this time whether high ion levels result in any adverse consequences.[43] The authors have identified elevated ion levels in some patients who underwent metal-on-metal total hip replacement more than 30 years ago without any known adverse consequences. Although concerns exist that elevated ion levels may cause cancer, at the present time, there is no known cause and effect relationship between elevated ion levels and cancer. More than 300,000 metal-on-metal implantations have been done since

the reintroduction of metal-on-metal bearings in 1988. A smaller number of implantations were done in the late 1960s and early 1970s, with some of these patients having implants lasting 35 or more years. Currently, however, not enough patients with metal-on-metal implants have been studied over the long term to be absolutely certain that elevated ion levels pose no risk of cancer. If there is a risk, it is likely extremely low, and any adverse effect can be determined only with long-term follow-up (20 to 30 years) encompassing a large number of patients.

Brodner and associates[44] reported that patients who had undergone total hip replacement with metal-on-metal gliding contacts and subsequently experienced renal failure had increased ion concentrations. They also reported that dialysis was ineffective in reducing these high ion concentrations, but subsequent renal transplantation was successful in reducing the elevated ion levels. To address concerns regarding the advisability of implanting metal-on-metal prostheses in women of childbearing age because of speculation that increased ion levels may cause birth defects, Brodner and associates[45] conducted a study on three women with metal-on-metal total hip replacements and elevated ion levels and reported no increase in ion levels in the umbilical cord blood and no adverse consequences with the babies. The four women from the authors' series who have delivered five healthy babies provided additional data regarding the safety of metal-on-metal implants. Because sufficient data are not currently available to dismiss the question entirely, however, it is recommended that patients of childbearing age who undergo metal-on-metal implantation should be informed of the concerns and available data. At the present time, metal ion concentrations in the blood of more than 100 patients who have had metal-on-metal implants have been studied serially for more than 5 years at the authors' institution with no adverse effects noted.

Metal Hypersensitivity

Metal hypersensitivity caused by the implantation of metal-on-metal bearings is rare. Several case reports have been submitted to the authors' laboratory for review from Europe and Australia in which patients with pain and bone destruction associated with apparent hypersensitivity were successfully treated with implant revision using alternative bearings. Since 1993, no instances of metal hypersensitivity to metal-on-metal bearings have been identified that have resulted in any adverse consequences in a series of more than 1,000 devices implanted at the authors' institution. The methods of studying this rare complication are under investigation in collaboration with Rush-Presbyterian St. Luke's Medical Center in Chicago, IL, as well as by investigators in England and Germany. It has been suggested that the incidence of metal hypersensitivity to metal-on-metal bearings may be 1 in 10,000 patients and that the incidence may be even lower in the United States, but there are no definitive data to corroborate this information.[46] Although studies are currently underway, there is no known methodology for identifying someone who is likely to develop this rare, delayed type of hypersensitivity.

Surgical and Postoperative Morbidity

Sepsis

Immediate, deep postoperative sepsis (infection) has not been observed

in any of more than 950 hips that have been resurfaced using the Conserve Plus device in the authors' series. Six patients, however, were identified as having hematogenous sepsis from elsewhere in the body. All but two of these patients were successfully treated by débridement in combination with antibiotic treatment. In one patient with rheumatoid arthritis, the diagnosis and treatment of sepsis (*Streptococcus*) was delayed for 1 month, and the surface arthroplasty was successfully converted to a total hip replacement in a one-stage procedure because the septic tissue at the time of surgery appeared to track under the femoral component and thorough débridement was not thought to be possible. In the other patient, there was a diagnosis of *Actinomyces* from a culture, and débridement was attempted, but was not successful; the patient subsequently underwent revision total hip replacement in a two-stage procedure.

After hip resurfacing surgery, patients should use antibiotic prophylaxis for dental cleaning for 1 year as recommended by the American Dental Association and the American Academy of Orthopaedic Surgeons; antiobiotic prophylaxis is also recommended for patients undergoing subsequent root canal procedures or other procedures with greater risk for infection. Bacterial infections that occur anywhere in the body must be promptly treated because of possible hematogenous spread to the site of an implant.

Heterotopic Ossification

The incidence of heterotopic ossification in male patients who have had hip surgery without prophylaxis is greater than 40%, but it is uncommon in women. The amount of bone that forms in most hips is in-

consequential (Brooker grades I and II), with only the more severe amounts (Brooker grades III and IV) potentially limiting the range of motion. The cause of heterotopic ossification is unknown and is likely to be multifactorial, with muscle trauma and bone debris implicated as contributing factors. In the first 400 patients in the authors' series, the incidence of heterotopic ossification in male patients was 10% (Brooker grades III and IV) with relatively few patients (approximately 1%) with some reduction in the range of motion despite being treated with indomethacin prophylaxis (50 mg preoperatively and then 25 mg three times daily for 5 days).[6] In two patients (three hips), bone was removed in association with single-dose radiotherapy without recurrence of heterotopic ossification (Figure 2).

To reduce the incidence of heterotopic ossification, the surgical technique has been refined, additional irrigation is used (from 1,000 up to 3,000 mL), and the surrounding tissues are protected from bone debris by a plastic sheet while chamfering the femoral head. These improvements have resulted in a reduction of the incidence of heterotopic ossification to 2%, and no recent severe instance of heterotopic ossification causing a reduction of range of motion has been reported. Male patients who undergo bilateral surgery in addition to receiving indomethacin should also receive one dose of radiation therapy (700 rads) preoperatively to improve the effectiveness of prophylaxis in this patient population.

Nerve Palsy

A high incidence of femoral nerve palsy (> 1%) was identified early in the authors' series. This incidence was the result of placing the femoral head anterior to the acetabulum to prepare for socket implantation and use of an unsatisfactory anterior pelvic stabilizer that may have pressed on the femoral triangle. All instances of femoral nerve palsy recovered spontaneously. Nerve palsy has been essentially eliminated as a complication of hip resurfacing by displacing the femoral head more superiorly and making certain that pelvic stability is secured by a positioner that presses against the pubis but not against the femoral triangle. Using the posterior approach, sciatic and peroneal nerve complications have not occurred at the authors' institution. The use of electrocautery posteriorly is recommended to make certain that the sciatic nerve is not at risk; a pin should be placed inside the retained capsule to be used as a retractor. Sciatic and peroneal nerve complications have been more commonly identified with the posterolateral approach. It is important to avoid pinching the nerve between the trochanter and the ischium when the dislocated hip is positioned into extreme external rotation.

Thromboembolic Phenomena

All patients are at risk for blood clots after undergoing hip or knee surgery. Because of its demonstrated long-term safety and efficacy, a 10 mg loading dose of warfarin therapy is initiated on the night of surgery and is adjusted over a 3-week postoperative period to maintain an international normalized ratio between 1.85 and 2.5. Aspirin is recommended for 3 weeks after discontinuation of warfarin therapy. The results of this prophylactic protocol have been excellent at the au-

thors' institution, with only 5 instances of phlebitis reported in 950 patients who underwent hip resurfacing; no pulmonary embolus or death occurred in this group. One postoperative bleeding episode occurred that did not require evacuation and was resolved by withholding warfarin therapy for 2 days. It is important that warfarin therapy is carefully monitored to make sure the level of protection is safe and efficacious.

Learning Curve

The best way to reduce the steep learning curve for hip resurfacing is to learn from the experience of others. Surgeons who participated in the Conserve Plus multicenter trial and who observed the technique before initiation greatly benefited from the experience. Those who spent up to 1 week observing multiple procedures had the fewest complications when performing the procedure on their own. Therefore, observing and participating in surgery with a surgeon who is experienced in hip resurfacing may be one of the most important factors in learning the techniques of mobilizing the femoral head, facilitating accurate pin placement, guiding the instruments, and displacing the femur superiorly and anteriorly and to adequately visualize the socket. Acquiring a surgical technique that allows for correction of pin placement up to the final reaming is recommended. Optimal bone preparation and cementation are essential in preventing femoral neck fracture and loosening. Practice with cadaver specimens or even dry bones can facilitate learning the technique of bone preparation.

Templating is an absolute must in hip resurfacing. It is essential to ob-

tain an AP radiograph of the pelvis, a table-down lateral radiograph, and especially a true lateral radiograph to evaluate osteophytes, the femoral neck-shaft angle, and anteversion. A 140° neck-shaft angle is recommended in most patients. In patients with excessive valgus (> 155°), reducing the femoral neck-shaft angle by approximately 10° is recommended; in those with excessive varus (< 125°), increasing the femoral neck-shaft angle by approximately 10° is recommended. Adequate exposure is essential to obtain a circumferential view of the femoral head for accurate pin centering, to expose the acetabulum for reaming, and to implant the socket in the correct position. A photograph of the femoral head should be obtained before implantation so there is a visual record of the bone quality and preparation; it can also prove to be extremely useful in the analysis of failures.

Summary

Since the reintroduction of hip resurfacing with metal-on-metal bearings, much has been learned about implant, patient, and surgical factors that contribute to success and failure. Data culled from detailed and critical 10-year follow-up analyses of more than 950 patients who underwent hip resurfacing performed by a single surgeon using a single design implant coupled with a better understanding of failure modes through retrieval analysis has allowed risk factors to be determined and technique changes made to improve outcomes. It is essential that surgeons considering performing hip resurfacing with metal-on-metal bearings learn from experienced surgeons to avoid early technical errors.

References

1. Amstutz H, Campbell P, Le Duff M: Incidence and prevention of neck fractures after surface arthroplasty. *J Bone Joint Surg Am* 2004;86:1874-1877.

2. Beaulé P, Dorey F, Le Duff M, Gruen T, Amstutz H: Risk factors affecting early outcome of metal on metal surface arthroplasty of the hip in patients 40 years old and younger. *Clin Orthop Relat Res* 2004;418:87-93.

3. Chatterton M, Cranston C, Fordyce M: Patient satisfaction following hip resurfacing arthroplasty. *J Bone Joint Surg Br* 2004;86(suppl 3):293.

4. Cutts S, Datta A, Ayoub K, Lawrence T, Rahman H: Early failure modalities in hip resurfacing. *J Bone Joint Surg Br* 2004;86(suppl 3):279.

5. DeSantis V, Proietti L, Falcone G, Savatori S, Pola E, Conti C: Resurfacing total hip arthroplasty. European Federation of National Associations of Orthopaedics and Traumatology poster presentation, 2005, p 223. Abstract available at: http://www.portal2.efort.org/Portals/0/Content/PoP_Hip_Trauma_Knee.pdf. Accessed August 14, 2006.

6. McMinn DJ: Development of metal/metal hip resurfacing. *Hip Int* 2003;13(suppl 2):S41-S53. Available at: http://www.hip-int.com/index.asp?a=abstract&id=78D54E81-003D-4D38-8B49-50A49F7. Accessed August 14, 2006.

7. Pollard TC, Basu C, Ainsworth R, Lai W, Bannister GC: Is the Birmingham hip resurfacing worthwhile? *Hip Int* 2003;13:25-28.

8. Amstutz HC, Beaule P, Dorey F, Le Duff M, Campbell P, Gruen T: Metal-on-metal hybrid surface arthroplasty: Two to six year follow-up. *J Bone Joint Surg Am* 2004;86:28-39.

9. Beaulé P, Le Duff M, Campbell P, Dorey F, Park S, Amstutz H: Metal-on-metal surface arthroplasty with a cemented femoral component: A 7-10 year follow-up study. *J Arthroplasty* 2004;19:17-22.

10. Chirodian N, Saw T, Villar R: Results of hybrid total hip replacement and resurfacing: Is there a difference? *Hip Int* 2004;14:169-173.

11. De Smet K: Belgium experience with metal-on-metal surface arthroplasty. *Orthop Clin North Am* 2005;36:203-213.

12. Hart AJ, Scott G: Hip resurfacing following previous proximal femoral osteotomy. *Hip Int* 2005;15:119-122.

13. Lilikakis A, Vowler S, Villar R: Hydroxyapatite-coated femoral implant in metal-on-metal resurfacing hip arthroplasty: Minimum of two years follow-up. *Orthop Clin North Am* 2005;36:215-222.

14. Little C, Ruiz A, Harding I, et al: Osteonecrosis in retrieved femoral heads after failed resurfacing arthroplasty of the hip. *J Bone Joint Surg Br* 2005;87:320-323.

15. Krikler S, Nelson R: Mid-term results of a modern metal-on-metal hip resurfacing prosthesis. European Federation of National Associations of Orthopaedics and Traumatology oral presentation, 2005. Abstract available at: http://www.resurfacingofthehip.com/MyHip/hip_clinicalresults.htm. Accessed August 14, 2006.

16. Shimmin AJ, Back D: Femoral neck fractures following Birmingham hip resurfacing: A national review of 50 cases. *J Bone Joint Surg Br* 2005;87:463-464.

17. Sinha S, Murty AN, Wijeratne M, Singh S, Housden P: Periprosthetic fractures around resurfacing hip replacements. *J Bone Joint Surg Br* 2006;88(suppl 1):58.

18. Treacy R, McBryde C, Pynsent P: Birmingham hip resurfacing arthroplasty: A minimum follow-up of five years. *J Bone Joint Surg Br* 2005;87:167-170.

19. Grigoris P, Roberts P, Panousis K, Bosch H: The evolution of hip resurfacing arthroplasty. *Orthop Clin North Am* 2005;36:125-134.

20. Vendittoli PA, Lavigne M, Girard J, Roy AG: A randomised study comparing resection of acetabular bone at resurfacing and total hip replacement. *J Bone Joint Surg Br* 2006;88:997-1002.

21. Back DL, Dalziel R, Young D, Shimmin A: Early results of primary Birmingham hip resurfacings: An independent prospective study of the first 230 hips. *J Bone Joint Surg Br* 2005;87:324-329.

22. Cossey A, Back D, Shimmin A, Young D, Spriggins A: The nonoperative management of periprosthetic fractures associated with the Birmingham hip resurfacing procedure. *J Arthroplasty* 2005;20:358-361.

23. Daniel J, Pynsent PB, McMinn D: Metal-on-metal resurfacing of the hip in patients under the age of 55 years with osteoarthritis. *J Bone Joint Surg Br* 2004;86:177-188.

24. Campbell P, Beaulé P, Ebramzadeh E, et al: A study of implant failure in metal-on-metal surface arthroplasties. *Clin Orthop Relat Res*, in press.

25. Amstutz H, Le Duff M, Campbell P, Dorey F: The effects of technique changes on aseptic loosening of the femoral component in hip resurfacing: Results of 600 Conserve Plus with a 3-9 year follow-up. *J Arthroplasty*. in press.

26. Amstutz HC, Dorey F, O'Carroll PF: THARIES resurfacing arthroplasty: Evolution and long-term results. *Clin Orthop Relat Res* 1986;213:92-114.

27. Amstutz HC, Kabo M, Hermens K, O'Carroll PF, Dorey F, Kilgus D: Porous surface replacement of the hip with chamfer cylinder design. *Clin Orthop Relat Res* 1987;222:140-160.

28. Campbell P, Clarke I, Kossovsky N: Clinical significance of wear debris, in Amstutz HC (ed): *Hip Arthroplasty*. New York, NY, Churchill Livingstone, 1991, pp 555-570.

29. Nashed RS, Becker DA, Gustilo RB: Are cementless acetabular components the cause of excess wear and osteolysis in total hip arthroplasty? *Clin Orthop Relat Res* 1995;317:19-28.

30. Walter WL, Clabeaux J, Wright TM, Walsh W, Walter WK, Sculco TP: Mechanisms for pumping fluid through cementless acetabular components with holes. *J Arthroplasty* 2005;20:1042-1048.

31. Amstutz HC, Ebramzadeh E, Sarkany A, Le Duff M, Rude R: Preservation of bone mineral density of the proximal femur following hemisurface arthroplasty. *Orthopedics* 2004;27:1266-1271.

32. Kishida Y, Sugano N, Nishii T, Miki H, Yamaguchi K, Yoshikawa H: Preservation of the bone mineral density of the femur after surface replacement of the hip. *J Bone Joint Surg Br* 2004;86:185-189.

33. Hedley AK, Clarke IC, Kozinn SC, Coster I, Gruen T, Amstutz HC: Porous ingrowth fixation of the femoral component in a canine surface replacement of the hip. *Clin Orthop Relat Res* 1982;163:300-311.

34. Nevelos J, Shelton J, Fisher J: Metallurgical considerations in the wear of metal-on-metal hip bearings. *Hip Int* 2004;14:1-10.

35. Bowsher J, Nevelos J, Pickard J, Shelton J: Do heat treatments influence the wear of large diameter metal-on-metal hip joints? An in vitro study under normal and adverse gait conditions. *Trans Orthop Res Soc* 2003;28:1398.

36. Bowsher J, Shelton J: Influence of heat treatments on large diameter metal-metal hip joint wear, in *Symposium of The*

International Society for Technology and Arthroplasty, 2002. Available at: http://www.ista.to/symposium.shtml.

37. Fisher J, Hu X, Tipper J, et al: An in vitro study of the reduction in wear of metal-on-metal hip prostheses using surface-engineered femoral heads. *Proc Inst Mech Eng [H]* 2002;216:219-230.

38. Brodner W, Grubl A, Jankovsky R, Meisinger V, Lehr S, Gottsauner-Wolf F: Cup inclination and serum concentration of cobalt and chromium after metal-on-metal total hip arthroplasty. *J Arthroplasty* 2004;19:66-70.

39. Forrest N, Welch A, Murray AD, Schweiger L, Hutchison J, Ashcroft GP: Femoral head viability after Birmingham resurfacing hip arthroplasty: Assessment with use of [18F] fluoride positron emission tomography. *J Bone Joint Surg Am* 2006;88(suppl 3):84-89.

40. Freeman M: Some anatomical and mechanical considerations relevant to the surface replacement of the femoral head. *Clin Orthop Relat Res* 1978;134:19-24.

41. Beaulé P, Campbell P, Hoke R, Dorey F: Notching of the femoral neck during resurfacing arthroplasty of the hip: A vascular study. *J Bone Joint Surg Br* 2006;88:35-39.

42. Steffen RT, Smith SR, Urban JP, et al: The effect of hip resurfacing on oxygen concentration in the femoral head. *J Bone Joint Surg Br* 2005;87:1468-1474.

43. Tharani R, Dorey FJ, Schmalzried TP: The risk of cancer following total hip or knee arthroplasty. *J Bone Joint Surg Am* 2001;83-A:774-780.

44. Brodner W, Grohs J, Bitzan P, Meisinger V, Kovarik J, Kotz R: Serum cobalt and serum chromium level in two patients with chronic renal failure after total hip prosthesis implantation with metal-metal gliding contact. *Z Orthop Ihre Grenzgeb* 2000;138:425-429.

45. Brodner W, Grohs J, Bancher-Todesca D, et al: Does the placenta inhibit the passage of chromium and cobalt after metal-on-metal total hip arthroplasty? *J Arthroplasty* 2004;19:102-106.

46. Willert HG, Buchhorn GH, Fayyazi A, Lohmann CH: Histopathological changes around metal/metal joints indicate delayed type hypersensitivity: Preliminary results of 14 cases. *Osteologie* 2000;9:2-16.

Femoral Component Sizing and Positioning in Hip Resurfacing Arthroplasty

Paul E. Beaulé, MD, FRCSC
Philippe Poitras, BASc

Abstract

Hip resurfacing arthroplasty is now being done on a regular basis with excellent short-term results. Although the technologic improvements are important in achieving improved clinical results, surgical technique and implant positioning are also critical. To minimize the risk of impingement and preserve acetabular bone stock during hip resurfacing arthroplasty, it is important for orthopaedic surgeons to be familiar with the current principles of femoral component sizing and positioning.

Instr Course Lect 2007;56:163-169.

Now that hip resurfacing arthroplasty has progressed beyond the evaluation stage, it is regularly being offered as an alternative to total hip replacement for young and active adult patients.[1,2] As with other types of conservative hip surgery,[3-5] patient selection has helped minimize complications[6] and the risk of failure.[7] There are currently two major applications of hip resurfacing: hemiresurfacing for the treatment of early stage osteonecrosis and metal-on-metal resurfacing for the treatment of advanced arthritis. The clinical results of hemiresurfacing

have been variable because of the unpredictability of the pain relief achieved, with several series reporting survivorship rates of 80% and 60% at 5 and 10 years, respectively, with failures primarily related to acetabular cartilage wear or persistent pain.[8] Although these results are inferior to those for standard total hip replacement, they are comparable if not superior to other femoral head–sparing procedures (such as free vascularized fibular graft and proximal femoral osteotomy) and result in less morbidity.[8,9] Consequently, hemiresurfacing should be viewed as a "time-buying" procedure for patients younger than 40 years with a large osteonecrotic lesion at the precollapse or postcollapse stage.

Metal-on-metal hip resurfacing is comparable to hemiresurfacing in terms of bone preservation on both

the acetabular and femoral side.[10] Four major clinical series have reported 4- to 5-year survivorship rates of 97% to 99%.[6,7,11,12] All but one of these series[6] prospectively applied some form of patient selection that included but was not limited to a diagnosis of osteoarthritis, absence of osteopenia, and absence of large femoral head cysts. The two main modes of failure have been femoral component loosening and fracture of the femoral neck.[13,14] Based on a retrieval analysis of modern metal-on-metal hip resurfacings, Campbell and associates[13] noted that cement penetration within the femoral head varied tremendously, in some instances occupying 89% of the femoral head and associated with osteonecrotic lesions. As with the introduction of any new technology, surgical technique in respect to implant positioning also impacts survivorship and clinical function. Implant positioning is especially relevant to hip resurfacing because, as with unicompartmental knee arthroplasty,[15] it has unique technical aspects and is being reintroduced after a long absence from the surgical training curriculum. This chapter focuses on implant positioning and

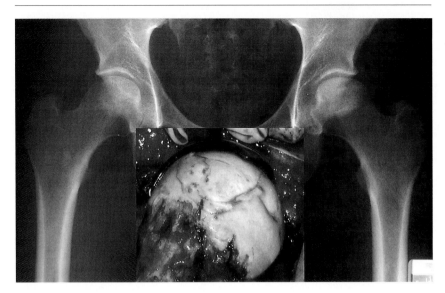

Figure 1   Radiograph and intraoperative photograph (inset) of the left hip of a 28-year-old man with Ficat stage III osteonecrosis. The inset photograph shows femoral head collapse and a spherometer being used to determine femoral head diameter.

sizing for hemiresurfacing in patients who are in the early stages of osteonecrosis and metal-on-metal hip resurfacing in patients with advanced arthritis.

Hemiresurfacing Arthroplasty

Proper component sizing and acetabular cartilage quality, which is related to the duration of symptoms, are probably the two most important factors affecting the clinical outcome of hemiresurfacing arthroplasty.[8] One of the most difficult challenges is accurate assessment of the acetabular cartilage and its ultimate durability against the femoral component. Beaulé and associates[16] reviewed a series of 37 hips with a mean follow-up of 6.5 years (range, 2 to 18 years). They found that patients with a longer duration of preoperative symptoms had more severe acetabular cartilage damage, and hips that had been converted to total hip replacement had a longer duration of symptoms before hemiresurfacing arthroplasty than the hips that were still functioning

(17 versus 12 months, respectively). The survivorship in this series was 79% at 5-year follow-up, 62% at 10-year follow-up, and 45% at 15-year follow-up. To minimize the stresses on the acetabular cartilage, the femoral component must be properly fitted and sized to minimize joint reaction forces (Figure 1). Langlais and associates[17] reviewed the results of 86 adjusted cup arthroplasties of different designs by radiographically studying the tolerance of the acetabulum when bearing weight with the cup. They reported that 85% of the patients had good to excellent results at mean follow-up of 6.5 years and stressed the importance of intraoperative precision fitting to the healthiest region of the acetabular cartilage whether it is peripheral or central. Thus, proper sizing of the femoral component in hemiresurfacing is primarily dictated by the inner diameter of the acetabulum, with most manufacturers offering components in 2-mm increments. However, because of the variable morphology of the hip joint, impre-

cision when matching the femoral component and acetabular cavity will always be present,[18] and a metal surface will articulate against articular cartilage as well as an articulating metal surface. Although one study showed that the use of ceramic or titanium femoral components did not result in a difference in clinical outcome of hemiresurfacing,[19] ceramic or titanium femoral components may nonetheless represent a future option because some series of hemiresurfacing arthroplasty have reported less satisfactory clinical outcomes using a cobalt-chromium femoral component.[20]

Another aspect of the surgical technique is the placement of the femoral component in the frontal plane.[21] In a classic article by Johnston and Larson[21] on the biomechanics of cup arthroplasty, medialization of the cup and lateral and distal transfer of the greater trochanter reduced the joint pressures by 57%. Although in hemiresurfacing the component is fixed and the acetabulum is not reamed, a vertical placement that is valgus of the cup arthroplasty increased abductor force by 20%, leading to an increase in joint reaction forces.[21] Interestingly, biomechanical analysis of the femoral component placement in metal-on-metal hip resurfacing led to similar findings.[22] Beaulé and associates[22] reported that going from a 130° to 140° femoral stem-shaft angle increased the joint reaction force by 18% (1.7 × body weight to 2.0 × body weight). Thus, if the main limitation of hemiresurfacing is acetabular cartilage wear and hip pain, surgeons should aim for a neutral alignment in the axis of the femoral neck to minimize joint reaction forces. In addition, if a patient is between implant sizes, choosing the smaller im-

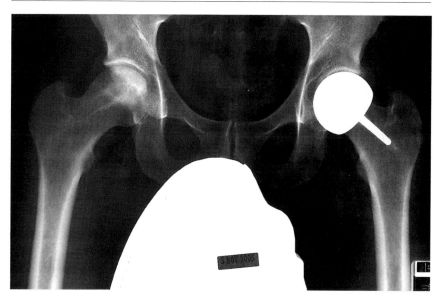

Figure 2 Radiograph showing a super-finished Conserve Plus (Wright Medical Technology, Arlington, TN) femoral component implanted during hemiresurfacing.

Table 1
Surface Arthroplasty Risk Index

Femoral head cyst > 1 cm	2 points
Weight < 82 kg	2 points
Previous hip surgery	1 point
UCLA Activity Score > 6	1 point.

plant is recommended so that at the time of conversion from hemiresurfacing to metal-on-metal hip resurfacing arthroplasty, acetabular bone stock is preserved (Figure 2).

Metal-on-Metal Hip Resurfacing Arthroplasty

As with the introduction of cementless designs in total hip replacements,[23] metal-on-metal bearings are not the only answer to the success of surface arthroplasty of the hip.[24] When reviewing the short-term results of patients 40 years old and younger who had metal-on-metal surface arthroplasty, Beaulé and associates[25] identified several independent factors that played a role in their premature failures. A surface arthroplasty risk index (SARI) was developed based on a 6-point scoring system (Table 1). A SARI score greater than 3 represented a fourfold increased risk in early failure or adverse radiologic changes and a survivorship of 89% at 4-year follow-up.[6] The SARI score also proved to be relevant in assessing the outcomes of the all-cemented McMinn resurfacing implant (Corin, Circentester, England) at a mean follow-up of 8.7 years.[26] Hip implants that had failed or had evidence of radiographic failure on the femoral side had a significantly higher SARI score than the remaining hip implants (3.9 versus 1.9), with an overall survivorship at 7-year follow-up for the femoral and acetabular components of 93% and 80%, respectively.[26]

Even with proper patient selection, hip resurfacing arthroplasty presents some challenging technical aspects in terms of implant positioning and sizing.[1] Structural abnormalities associated with certain diagnoses may pose some challenges in the positioning and fixation of the components. One such example is a patient with dysplasia in whom the presence of an acetabular deficiency combined with the inability to insert screws through the acetabular component may make initial implant stability unpredictable. Because this deformity in combination with a significant limb-length discrepancy or valgus femoral neck could compromise the functional results after hip resurfacing arthroplasty, a stem-type total hip replacement may provide a superior functional outcome.[27] In addition, because of the conservative nature of this treatment and the goal to closely reproduce the normal anatomy of the proximal femur, positioning of the implant components may have a greater impact on implant survivorship and patient function than a standard hip replacement[1] and will be influenced by the underlying pathology/ deformity that led to the degenerative changes.[22]

In the coronal plane, varus placement should be avoided; a relative valgus of 5° to 10° should be the goal, minimizing the tensile stresses at the superior bone-prosthesis junction.[22,28] For example, placement of the femoral component at 130° compared with 140° would increase the tensile stresses by 31%. As far as the sagittal/axial plane, restoring and/or maintaining femoral head-neck offset is quite different than when implanting stem-type total hip components. Although it has long been recognized that after total hip replacement impingement can limit range of motion[29] and in extreme instances result in hip instability,[30] the risk after surface arthroplasty may be greater because the femoral head-neck unit is preserved. Beaulé and associates (Chicago, IL, unpublished data presented at the Orthopaedic Research Society an-

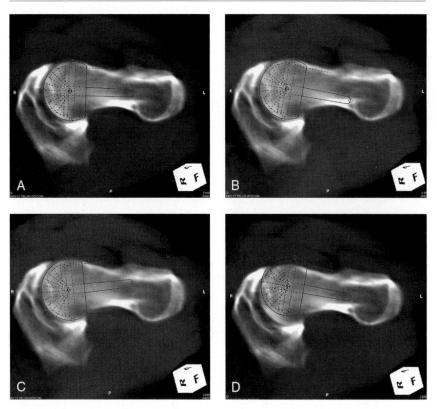

Figure 3 **A,** CT radial image of the femoral head-neck junction with a template of the resurfacing femoral component placed along the axis of the femoral neck without correction of offset anteriorly. CT radial image of the femoral head-neck junction with a template of the resurfacing femoral component shows that placement with increased anteversion does not change the anterior offset **(B)** and placement with increased retroversion does not change the anterior offset **(C)**. **D,** CT radial image of the femoral head-neck junction with a template of the resurfacing femoral component shows how anterior translation of the femoral component restores femoral head-neck offset.

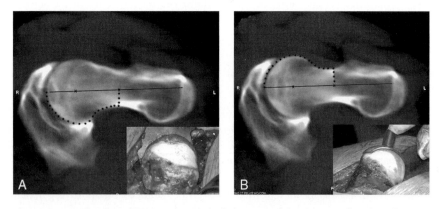

Figure 4 **A,** The dotted line on this CT radial image of the posterior head-neck junction demonstrates optimal offset. Intraoperative photograph (*inset*) of an arthritic femoral head. **B,** The dotted line on this CT radial image of the posterior head-neck junction demonstrates optimal anterior offset, which should be equal to the posterior offset. Intraoperative photograph (*inset*) showing spherometer gauges being used to restore head sphericity and anterior offset.

nual meeting, 2006) reported that 56% of hips treated by hip resurfacing have an abnormal offset ratio presurgically, with the two main diagnostic groups presenting with deficient femoral head-neck offset being patients with osteonecrosis and patients with osteoarthritis, both of which have been associated with femoroacetabular impingement in the prearthritic state.[31,32] This is particularly true in patients in whom the arthritis is secondary to femoroacetabular impingement.[32] This common cause of hip arthritis is believed to be secondary to a lack of femoral head-neck offset in the anterolateral area of the femoral head-neck junction (Figure 3, *A*).[33-35] If this pathology is not recognized at the time of hip resurfacing, patients could still experience impingement between the rim of the acetabulum or with the acetabular component itself[36] and/or have a restricted range of motion. Because of the lack of modularity on the femoral side, other means must be used to optimize femoral head-neck offset with hip resurfacing. One technique would be to modify the version of the femoral component, which is analogous to changing femoral component version in a regular total hip replacement. However, as illustrated in Figure 3, *B* and *C*, this has no impact on femoral head-neck offset. Anterior translation of the femoral component (Figure 3, *D*) certainly achieves proper anterior offset but at the expense of the posterior offset and an uneven cement mantle. For both techniques of version change and anterior translation of the femoral component, placement of the guidewire within the femoral neck is the key. More specifically, to increase the anteversion of the femoral component, the guidewire will be placed from anterior to posterior in relation to the femoral neck and vice versa for retroversion. In terms of anterior translation the guidewire is translated anteriorly with a relative anterior entry point in the femoral head. With the guidewire in place, reaming of the femoral head is initiated, being mindful that an excessive change in version can lead to notching of the anterior or posterior femoral neck, depending on the direction of the version change. Removal of prominent anterior neck osteophytes to restore femoral head sphericity is recommended[37] (Figure 4) because it not only optimizes the femoral head-neck offset, but also facilitates placement of the guidewire within the axis of the femoral neck (Figure 5). In addition, because the femoral head overlaps the neck cortex and projects most prominently posteriorly,[38] if the neck axis is not properly identified, there will be a tendency to place the femoral component more posteriorly on the neck, further adding to the deficient anterior offset. Although removal of the femoral head-neck osteophytes can significantly weaken the femoral neck if done too aggressively,[39] if these structures are left intact, the enlarged arthritic femoral head will require a larger femoral component. This technique will have the inevitable effect of implanting a larger acetabular component than would have been implanted in a standard total hip replacement[40] (Figure 6). **(DVD 18.1)**

However, impingement after total hip arthroplasty is multifactorial

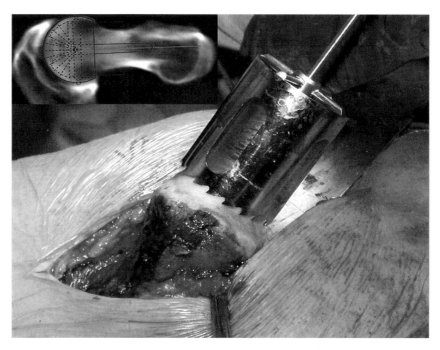

Figure 5   Intraoperative photograph showing the cylindrical reamer of the planned femoral component size being used for guidewire insertion once the axis is well defined using CT radial image templating (*inset*).

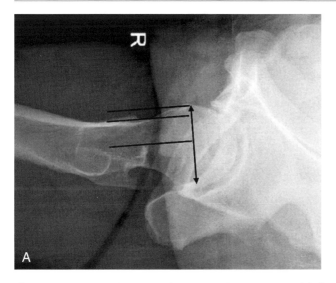
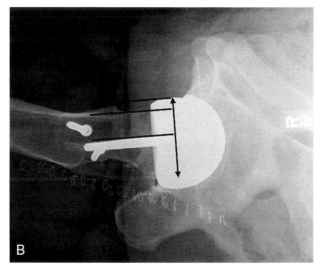

Figure 6   Preoperative **(A)** and postoperative **(B)** cross-table lateral radiographs demonstrating restoration of femoral head-neck offset after Conserve Plus (Wright Medical Technology) metal-on-metal hip resurfacing has been performed (device not FDA approved). The offset ratio was corrected from 0.09 to 0.14.

and includes factors such as soft-tissue and acetabular component orientation.[41,42] D'Lima and associates[41] demonstrated that there is a complex interaction between abduction of the acetabular component, anteversion of the acetabular component, and anteversion of the femoral component when determining the maximum prosthetic range of motion. Although no adverse events have been reported, a deficient offset ratio is analogous to an insufficient femoral head-neck ratio in standard total hip replacements, which, in the context of the McKee-Farrar prosthesis, contributed to its poor performance relative to the Ring prosthesis.[43]

Summary

Because the femoral head-neck junction is preserved with hip resurfacing, surgeons cannot rely on prosthetic femoral design to optimize patient clinical outcome. With hemiresurfacing arthroplasty, precise fitting of the femoral prosthesis and avoiding excessive valgus positioning will minimize the stresses within the acetabular cavity. Because the main limitation of this implant is predictable pain relief, careful patient counseling is recommended. For metal-on-metal hip resurfacing, restoring the anterior femoral head-neck offset by removing prominent osteophytes will minimize the risk of impingement and optimize femoral component sizing, which will in turn preserve acetabular bone stock. Finally, it is recommended that surgeons who will perform hip resurfacing visit centers with large experience.

References

1. Beaulé PE, Antoniades J: Patient selection and surgical technique for surface arthroplasty of the hip. *Orthop Clin North Am* 2005;36:177-185.

2. Grigoris P, Roberts P, Panousis K, Bosch H: The evolution of hip resurfacing arthroplasty. *Orthop Clin North Am* 2005;36:125-134.

3. Trousdale RT, Ekkernkamp A, Ganz R, Wallrichs SL: Periacetabular and intertrochanteric osteotomy for the treatment of osteoarthrosis in dysplastic hips. *J Bone Joint Surg Am* 1995;77:73-85.

4. Siebenrock KA, Scholl E, Lottenbach M, Ganz R: Bernese periacetabular osteotomy. *Clin Orthop Relat Res* 1999;363:9-20.

5. Beck M, Leunig M, Parvizi J, Boutier V, Wyss D, Ganz R: Anterior femoroacetabular impingement: Part II. Midterm results of surgical treatment. *Clin Orthop Relat Res* 2004;418:67-73.

6. Amstutz HC, Beaulé PE, Dorey FJ, Campbell PA, Le Duff MJ, Gruen TA: Metal-on-metal hybrid surface arthroplasty: Two to six year follow-up. *J Bone Joint Surg Am* 2004;86-A:28-39.

7. Daniel J, Pynsent PB, McMinn DJW: Metal-on-metal resurfacing of the hip in patients under the age of 55 years with osteoarthritis. *J Bone Joint Surg Br* 2004;86:177-184.

8. Beaulé PE, Amstutz HC: Treatment of Ficat stage III and IV osteonecrosis of the hip. *J Am Acad Orthop Surg* 2004;12:96-105.

9. Lieberman JR, Berry DJ, Mont MA, et al: Osteonecrosis of the hip: Management in the 21st century. *Instr Course Lect* 2003;52:337-355.

10. Beaulé PE: Surface arthroplasty of the hip: A review and current indications. *Semin Arthroplasty* 2005;16:70-76.

11. Back DL, Dalziel R, Young D, Shimmin A: Early results of primary Birmingham hip resurfacings: An independent prospective study of the first 230 hips. *J Bone Joint Surg Br* 2005;87:324-329.

12. Treacy R, Pynsent P: Birmingham hip resurfacing arthroplasty: A minimum follow-up of five years. *J Bone Joint Surg Br* 2005;87:167-170.

13. Campbell PA, Beaulé PE, Ebramzadeh E, et al: The John Charnley Award: A study of implant failure in metal-on-metal surface arthroplasties. *Clin Orthop Relat Res* 2006; in press.

14. Little CP, Ruiz AL, Harding IJ, et al: Osteonecrosis in retrieved femoral heads after failed resurfacing arthroplasty of the hip. *J Bone Joint Surg Br* 2005;87:320-323.

15. Lindstrand A, Stenstrom A, Ryd L, Toksvig-Larsen S: The introduction period of unicompartmental knee arthroplasty is critical: A clinical, clinical multicentered, and radiostereometric study of 251 Duracon unicompartmental knee arthroplasties. *J Arthroplasty* 2000;15:608-616.

16. Beaulé PE, Schmalzried TP, Campbell PA, Dorey F, Amstutz HC: Duration of symptoms and outcome of hemiresurfacing for hip osteonecrosis. *Clin Orthop Relat Res* 2001;385:104-117.

17. Langlais F, Barthas J, Postel M: Les cupules ajustees pour necrose idiopathique: Bilan radiologique. *Rev Chir Orthop Reparatrice Appar Mot* 1979;65(suppl 3):151-155.

18. Clarke IC, Amstutz HC: Human hip joint geometry and hemiarthroplasty selection, in *The Hip Proceedings*. St. Louis, MO, Mosby, 1975, pp 63-89.

19. Amstutz HC, Grigoris P, Safran MR, Grecula MJ, Campbell PA, Schmalzried TP: Precision-fit surface hemiarthroplasty for femoral head osteonecrosis: Long-term results. *J Bone Joint Surg Br* 1994;76:423-427.

20. Squire M, Fehring TK, Odum S, Griffin WL, Bohannon MJ: Failure of femoral surface replacement for femoral head avascular necrosis. *J Arthroplasty* 2005;20:108-114.

21. Johnston R, Larson CB: Biomechanics of cup arthroplasty. *Clin Orthop Relat Res* 1969;66:56-69.

22. Beaulé PE, Lee J, LeDuff M, Dorey FJ, Amstutz HC, Ebramzadeh E: Orientation of femoral component in surface arthroplasty of the hip: A biomechanical and clinical analysis. *J Bone Joint Surg Am* 2004;86-A:2015-2021.

23. Jones LC, Hungerford DS: Cement disease. *Clin Orthop Relat Res* 1987;225:192-206.

24. Beaulé PE, Amstutz HC: Surface arthroplasty of the hip revisited: Current indications and surgical technique, in Sinha RJ (ed): *Hip Replacement: Current Trends and Controversies*. New York, NY, Marcel Dekker, 2002, pp 261-297.

25. Beaulé PE, Dorey FJ, LeDuff MJ, Gruen T, Amstutz HC: Risk factors affecting outcome of metal on metal surface arthroplasty of the hip. *Clin Orthop Relat Res* 2004;418:87-93.

26. Beaulé PE, LeDuff M, Campbell P, Dorey FJ, Park SH, Amstutz HC: Metal-on-metal surface arthroplasty with a cemented femoral component: A 7-10

year follow-up study. *J Arthroplasty* 2004;19:17-22.

27. Silva M, Lee KH, Heisel C, dela Rosa M, Schmalzreid TP: The biomechanical results of total hip resurfing arthroplasty. *J Bone Joint Surg Am* 2004;86:40-41.

28. Freeman MAR: Some anatomical and mechanical considerations relevant to the surface replacement of the femoral head. *Clin Orthop Relat Res* 1978;134:19-24.

29. Amstutz HC, Markolf KL: Design features in total hip replacement, in Harris WH (ed): *The Hip Society: Proceedings of the Second Open Scientific Meeting.* St. Louis, MO, 1974, pp 111-124.

30. Bartz RL, Noble PC, Kadakia NR, Tullos HS: The effect of femoral component head size on posterior dislocation of the artificial hip joint. *J Bone Joint Surg Am* 2000;82:1300-1307.

31. Kloen P, Leunig M, Ganz R: Early lesions of the labrum and acetabular cartilage in osteonecrosis of the femoral head. *J Bone Joint Surg Br* 2002;84:66-69.

32. Ganz R, Parvizi J, Leunig M, Siebenrock KA: Femoroacetabular impingement: A cause for osteoarthritis of the hip. *Clin Orthop Relat Res* 2003;417:112-120.

33. Ito K: Minka-II MA, Leunig S, Werlen S, Ganz R. Femoroacetabular impingement and the cam-effect. *J Bone Joint Surg Br* 2001;83:171-176.

34. Eijer H, Leunig M, Mahomed N, Ganz R: Cross-table lateral radiographs for screening of anterior femoral head-neck offset in patients with femoro-acetabular impingement. *Hip International* 2001;11:37-41.

35. Beaulé PE, Zaragoza EJ, Motamedic K, Copelan N, Dorey J: Three-dimensional computed tomography of the hip in the assessment of femoroacetabular impingement. *J Orthop Res* 2005;23:1286-1292.

36. Wiadrowski TP, McGee M, Cornish BL, Howie DW: Peripheral wear of Wagner resurfacing hip arthroplasty acetabular components. *J Arthroplasty* 1991;6:103-107.

37. Beaulé PE: A soft-tissue sparing approach to surface arthroplasty of the hip. *Oper Tech Orthop* 2004;14:16-18.

38. Harty M: Surface replacement arthroplasty of the hip: Anatomic considerations. *Orthop Clin North Am* 1982;13:667-679.

39. Mardones RM, Gonzalez C, Chen Q, Zobitz M, Kaufman KR, Trousdale RT: Surgical treatment of femoroacetabular impingement: Evaluation of the effect of the size of the resection. *J Bone Joint Surg Am* 2005;87:273-279.

40. Loughead JM, Starks I, Chesney D, Matthews JNS, McCaskie AW, Holland JP: Removal of acetabular bone in resurfacing arthroplasty of the hip. *J Bone Joint Surg Br* 2006;88:31-34.

41. D'Lima DD, Urquhart AG, Buehler KO, Walker RH, Colwell CWJ: The effect of the orientation of the acetabular and femoral components on the range of motion of the hip at different head-neck ratios. *J Bone Joint Surg Am* 2000;82:315-321.

42. Scifert CF, Brown TD, Pedersen DR, Callaghan JJ: A finite element analysis of factors influencing total hip dislocation. *Clin Orthop Relat Res* 1998;355:152-162.

43. Ring PA: Total replacement of the hip joint: A review of a thousand operations. *J Bone Joint Surg Br* 1974;56:44-58.

Hip Resurfacing: Indications, Results, and Conclusions

Caroline Hing, BSc, MSc, MD, FRCS(Tr&Orth)
Diane Back, MBBS, FRCS Ed(Tr&Orth)
Andrew Shimmin, FAOrthA, FRACS, Dip Anat

Abstract

Hip resurfacing using metal-on-metal bearings has increased in popularity as a viable treatment option for young, active patients with osteoarthritis. Theoretic advantages of this procedure include preservation of bone stock, reduction in osteolysis, and a reduced risk of dislocation when compared with conventional hip arthroplasty with smaller diameter metal-on-polyethylene bearings. Concerns associated with the use of metal-on-metal bearings during hip resurfacing include the production of metal ions with unknown carcinogenic and immunologic effects. The long-term survival of the modern metal-on-metal hip resurfacing implant is also unknown. Hip resurfacing accounts for 7.5% of all hip replacements in Australia and has a 2.2% revision rate, with femoral fracture being the most common reason for revision. The cumulative survival rate at the authors' institution is 99.14% at 3-year follow-up.

Instr Course Lect 2007;56:171-178.

Hip resurfacing arthroplasty has continued to increase in popularity over the past decade as a treatment option for young, active patients with osteoarthritis.[1-3] Metal-on-metal bearings of cobalt-chromium alloy may reduce the risk of particulate-related osteolysis when compared with metal-on-polyethylene bearings but may increase potential risks because of the systemic and local effects of metal ions.[4-7] Various designs of hip resurfacing implants have evolved over the years since their original inception in the 1960s. The Birmingham hip resurfacing implant (BHR, Smith & Nephew, Bir-

mingham, England) in its present format has been in use since 1997, with an overall survival rate of 98% at 5-year follow-up reported by the center of its inception.[2,3] Radiostereophotogrammetric analysis to study the stability of resurfacing arthroplasty in the short term has also shown low values for cup migration and vertical and mediolateral migration of the implant head at 2-year follow-up. These results compared favorably with those for cemented components in conventional total hip replacements, confirming the favorable clinical and radiologic results of this implant in short-term use.[8]

Demographics of Hip Resurfacing in Australia

Metal-on-metal hip resurfacing has been performed in Australia since April 1999.[9] From September 1999 to December 2004, a total of 5,379 hip resurfacings were performed, accounting for 7.5% of all hip replacements. When compared with conventional total hip replacements, 2.2% of the hip resurfacings were revised as opposed to 1.9% of total hip replacements. Of the hip resurfacings, 86% used the BHR implant with a revision rate of 2%, and 14% used either the Cormet 2000 implant (Corin Medical, Cirencester, England), or the ASR (DePuy, Warsaw, IN) or Durom (Zimmer, Warsaw, IN) or Conserve Plus (Wright Medical Technology, Inc, Arlington, TN), with a revision rate of 3.6%.[9] The most common reason for revision was fracture of the femoral neck, with 59.3% of all resurfacing revisions performed for this reason; 84% of these fractures occurred within the first 6 months.[9]

When considering the 118 hip resurfacings that were revised, women had twice the risk of revision compared with men. Men older than 65 years had a higher percentage of revision compared with men younger than 65 years. For women, those 55 to 64 years of age had the highest risk of revision. Primary diagnosis also had an effect on the revision rate. Patients with osteoarthritis had the lowest number of early revisions (2%) compared with those with rheumatoid arthritis (8%), osteonecrosis (3.4%), and developmental dysplasia (3.2%).[9]

Conclusions from the Australian hip registry have confirmed that careful patient selection is important to ensure the longevity of a hip resurfacing implant, with the lowest number of revisions occurring in males younger than 65 years and in those with a primary diagnosis of osteoarthritis.

Indications for Hip Resurfacing

The ideal candidate for hip resurfacing is a man younger than 65 years with a primary diagnosis of osteoarthritis, good bone quality, and normal proximal femoral geometry.[3,9,10] Hip resurfacing cannot correct large limb-length inequality or change horizontal femoral offset.[10,11] Hence, patients with large limb-length inequality or significantly reduced horizontal offset are still best treated with conventional or extended offset stemmed implants.

Absolute contraindications to hip resurfacing include elderly and postmenopausal patients with osteoporosis, impaired renal function, and known metal hypersensitivity. Relative contraindications include inflammatory arthropathy, abnormal proximal femoral geometry, large femoral head geodes, and large areas of osteonecrosis.[1,10]

The proposed advantages of hip resurfacing as opposed to hip re-

placement are a lower dislocation rate, restoration of physiologic biomechanics, preservation of bone stock, and a return to a more active lifestyle.[1-3,11] Restoration of a normal femoral head size with preservation of hip biomechanics has contributed to a lower dislocation rate when compared with hip arthroplasty using a smaller femoral head.[1-3] A more physiologic pattern of femoral head loading following hip resurfacing is believed to produce compressive forces rather than hoop stresses, which may improve bone mineral density.[3] Favorable survivorship with a return to high-demand activities after hip resurfacing may be advantageous in younger patients who are actively employed in full-time positions.[1,3]

Early Results of Resurfacing at the Melbourne Orthopaedic Group

Between April 1999 and June 2001, 230 consecutive primary hip replacements using the BHR implant were performed by three surgeons at the Melbourne Orthopaedic Group. This series represented the first hip resurfacing performed using the BHR implant at this institution. All patients were available for follow-up. Patients were considered for the BHR implant rather than total hip replacement if they were active men younger than 75 years or active women younger than 60 years. Patients outside these age groups were considered on a case-by-case basis.[1] A clinical and radiologic review by an independent observer was performed at a mean follow-up of 3 years. Patients were assessed preoperatively using the Harris hip score,[12] the Medical Outcomes Study 12-Item Short Form Health Survey (SF-12),[13] and Charnley

grades.[14] Postoperatively, Oxford hip scores were also obtained.[15]

During radiologic review, radiolucent lines were recorded around the components in the zones described by Amstutz and associates[16] and DeLee and Charnley.[17] In addition, the preoperative femoral neck-shaft angle (A) was subtracted from the angle between the stem and the shaft (S) to determine varus or valgus implant positioning. If angle S was greater than angle A by more than 5°, the implant was considered to be valgus; if angle S was less than angle A by more than 5°, the implant was considered to be varus. The abduction angle of the acetabular component (C) was recorded, and the position of the stem relative to the femoral neck on the lateral radiograph was assessed[1] (Figure 1). The presence of heterotopic ossification was recorded using the classification of Brooker and associates.[18]

Demographics

Overall, 230 patients were included in the study (150 men and 80 women); 116 right hips and 114 left hips underwent resurfacing, and 17 patients underwent bilateral procedures. The mean age of patients at the time of surgery was 52 years (range, 18 to 82 years) (Figure 2). The mean patient height was 172.18 cm (standard deviation, 9.95 cm), the mean patient weight was 80.62 kg (standard deviation, 15.62 kg), and the mean body mass index was 27.02 kg/m^2 (standard deviation, 4.23 kg/m^2). The preoperative diagnoses are shown in Figure 3.

Results

At 3-year follow-up, one patient had died and one had undergone a revision to a total hip replacement because of a loose acetabular component. All surviving patients (228

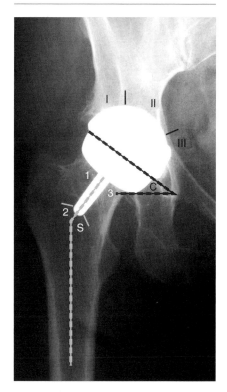

Figure 1 Postoperative radiographic measurements of implant position showing the zones of Amstutz (1, 2, and 3), the zones of DeLee and Charnley (I, II, and III), the stem shaft angle (S), and the cup angle (C).

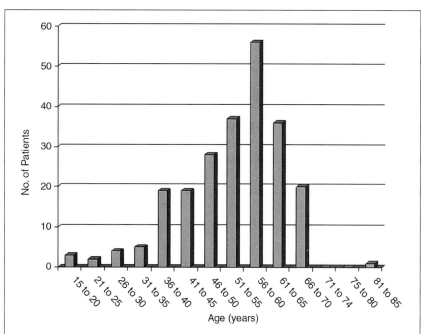

Figure 2   Graph showing age distribution of patients at the time of surgery.

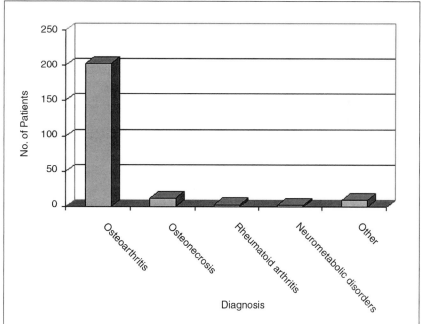

Figure 3   Graph showing preoperative diagnoses before hip resurfacing.

hips) returned questionnaires, and 204 hips were available for clinical and radiologic review. The remaining 24 hips had been reviewed at a minimum 2-year follow-up. The cumulative survival rate was 99.14% at 3 years. The range of movement improved in all patients from a mean flexion of 92° (range, 25° to 130°) preoperatively to 110° (range, 80° to 130°) postoperatively. The mean postoperative Oxford hip score was 13.5 (range, 12 to 28). The Harris hip scores and SF-12 scores are summarized in Table 1.

Complications
Medical and surgical complications are summarized in Table 2 . Patients also described clicking and squeaking. Fifty-three patients (22.9%) de-

scribed painless clicking that was believed to be caused by the psoas tendon impinging on the anterior surface of the acetabular component. Nine patients (3.9%) described painless squeaking at ex-

treme flexion that was believed to be caused by a disruption in the fluid film between the bearing surfaces. One implant was revised to a total hip replacement 18 months after the original surgery because of

Table 1
Preoperative and 3-Year Harris Hip and SF-12 Scores After Hip Resurfacing

Charnley Category	No. of Arthroplasties	Harris Hip Score (range)	SF-12 Score (physical component)	SF-12 Score (mental component)
A				
Preoperative	162	63.9 (8 to 93)	31.1	58.6
3-year	162	97.7 (60 to 100)	54.1	56.9
B				
Preoperative	53	56.2 (18 to 82)	30.3	60.5
3-year	52	99.4 (90 to 100)	54.1	57.7
C				
Preoperative	15	64.8 (30 to 98)	31.5	52.2
3-year	14	85.5 (30 to 100)	48.2	55.9

Table 2
Number of Surgical and Medical Complications After Hip Resurfacing

Surgical Complications (No.)	Medical Complications (No.)
Superficial wound infection (11)	Hypotension (14)
Notched neck (5)	Deep venous thrombosis (11)
Acetabular introducer wire breakage (4)	Urinary tract infection (9)
Sciatic nerve palsy (2)	Sinus tachycardia (5)
Femoral nerve palsy (2)	Pressure sores (4)
Retained guidewires (2)	Pulmonary embolus (2)
Fracture, healed (1)	
Component mismatch (1)	
Common peroneal nerve palsy (1)	
Profunda femoris artery pseudoaneurysm (1)	
Femoral artery damage (1)	
Rectus femoris intramuscular hematoma (1)	

loosening of the BHR acetabular component.

Radiologic Results at 3-Year Follow-Up

No radiolucent lines were noted around either component. The mean abduction angle of the acetabular component was 45.8° (range, 37° to 65°). In eight patients, the initial postoperative radiographs showed that the acetabular component was inadequately seated; however, by 2-year follow-up, there was bony ingrowth in all instances. The femoral implant position was valgus in most patients (2.9°), with poor seating noted in 7 patients, and an anterior position noted in 115 patients. Six patients had notching of the femoral neck on the immediate postoperative radiographs, with one patient developing a femoral neck fracture 6 weeks after surgery that united with marked femoral neck narrowing after a 6-week period of not bearing weight. Four other patients presented with pain and a possible stress fracture of the femoral neck within 1 year of surgery. All pain resolved after a period of not bearing weight.

Heterotopic ossification was noted in 59.56% of patients (Brooker grade I in 38.26%, grade II in 13.48%, and grade III in 7.83%). This relatively high percentage of patients with heterotopic ossification may have been caused by several factors: the patient age group (young males often have hypertropic osteoarthritis); no routine use of prophylactic indomethacin in this high-risk group; and the surgical approach with the extensile exposure used in this procedure had a learning curve that could have resulted in more soft-tissue stripping. Three patients underwent excision of heterotopic ossification for pain and a reduced range of motion. Clinical review at 3-year follow-up showed no difference in outcome scores compared with those of patients who had undergone resurfacing but had not undergone additional surgery.

Results

This consecutive series of patients who underwent hip replacement using BHR implants had a cumulative survival rate of 99.14% at 3-year follow-up, which compares favorably with the results of resurfacings at other centers.[2,3,9,16] Radiologic review showed no evidence of osteolysis of either component at 3-year follow-up, although one acetabular component was revised at 18 months for loosening. Most of the femoral components were valgus, but the significance of femoral component position on survival is unknown at this stage. In this series, one femoral neck fracture occurred, which united with a period of not bearing weight, and six patients had evidence of notching that was treated with a period of protected weight bearing; none of these patients progressed to displaced femoral neck fracture. This series had a lower rate of femoral neck fracture than that reported in Australia (1.46%), possibly because patients with femoral neck notching and pain were identified early and treated with a period of protected weight bearing.[10,19] Further follow-up to determine the long-term outcomes of this cohort is ongoing.

Complications Associated With Hip Resurfacing Arthroplasty

Complications specific to hip resurfacing include femoral neck fracture, osteonecrosis, increased metal ion levels, and metal hypersensitivity.[1-4,10] Complications associated with hip arthroplasty that also apply to hip resurfacing include dislocation, heterotopic ossification, thromboembolic disease, nerve palsies, and vascular damage.

Careful patient selection is important in reducing the risk of complications, as is meticulous surgical technique and restoration of hip biomechanics.[10] Recent short-term reviews of hip resurfacing outcomes and hip registries have addressed some of the issues contributing to complications.[1,2,9]

Femoral Neck Fracture

In Australia, the most common reason for revision of a hip resurfacing has been a femoral neck fracture[9] (Figure 4). A recent survey of surgeons who had experienced a femoral neck fracture in their practice showed an overall fracture rate of 1.46% associated with the BHR implant.[19] The Australian national fracture rate for men undergoing resurfacing was 0.98% and for women was 1.91%. The absolute risk of femoral neck fracture is 0.0191 in women and 0.0098 in men. There is

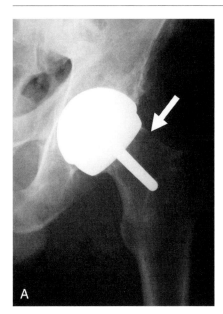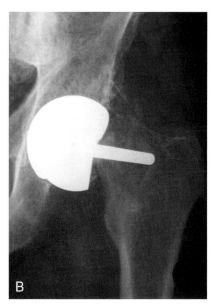

Figure 4   Radiographs showing a femoral neck stress fracture (*arrow*) (**A**) and propagation that occurred 6 weeks from hip resurfacing (**B**).

a statistically significant difference ($P < 0.001$) between men and women, with the relative risk for women versus men being 1.9496.[19] The mean time to fracture is 15 weeks from the time of initial surgery, with no significant difference between men and women.

Femoral neck notching and varus positioning have been implicated in increasing the risk of femoral neck fracture.[19-21] Finite element analysis using CT scans to reconstruct proximal femoral geometry and including the effect of muscle forces and hip loading in the boundary conditions has shown a change in bone mineral density up to 9 months from implantation. Bone resorption in this model was minimized by a valgus position of the femoral component, which may be the ideal alignment to prevent femoral neck fracture in the early postoperative period.[22] A cumulative effect of implant position and femoral neck bone density are likely to be important in the early postoperative period

for determining which patients are at risk of femoral neck fracture.

The effect of gender, age, and weight on the risk of femoral neck fracture and implant failure remains controversial. Obesity, which may contribute to poor surgical exposure, and osteoporosis in postmenopausal women may have osteoporosis, which may contribute to an increased risk of femoral neck fracture.[9,19] However, Beaulé and associates[23] have shown that weight less than 82 kg was significantly associated with a smaller femoral component size and a smaller fixation area and may result in adverse radiographic changes.

Femoral neck fracture has been shown to occur most commonly in the early postoperative period (mean time to fracture, 15 weeks); these fractures may be preceded by pain and limp that are not typically expected at that stage in the rehabilitation course.[19] Nondisplaced femoral neck fractures that are detected early may be successfully treated with a period of no weight bearing, which results in no compromise to clinical or radiologic outcomes.[24,25]

Osteonecrosis

Osteonecrosis as a result of femoral head resurfacing has been reported in the literature and may play a role in femoral neck fracture.[2,26] The true incidence of osteonecrosis with hip resurfacing is unknown because histologic studies have concentrated on failed retrieved resurfaced femoral heads.[26] Hip resurfacing has been shown to affect the oxygen concentration in the femoral head with an extended posterior approach, causing a mean 60% decrease in oxygen concentration; component insertion results in an additional 20% decrease.[27] Oxygen concentration does not improve significantly with wound closure, which raises concerns about the viability of the femoral head and neck after resurfacing. It can be postulated that osteonecrosis may be a cause of some femoral neck fractures if the interoperative reduction in oxygenation is permanent.[27]

Dual-energy x-ray absorptiometry (DEXA) can be used to measure changes in bone density around implants.[28] Most bone density changes occur within the first year after surgery. DEXA studies at 1 and 2 years postoperatively have shown that proximal femoral bone density is preserved, but the effect of implant position and notching on these measurements is unknown.[28] The findings from DEXA studies appear to concur with the finding of Freeman[21] that the vascular supply in the arthritic femoral head is mainly intraosseous, but do not concur with the findings of Steffen and associates[27] that femoral head oxygenation is reduced during surgery.[3]

Metal Ion Levels

Metal-on-metal bearing surfaces produce metal wear debris and corrode to produce metallic ions. The level of wear is dependent on metallurgy, implant design, and activity levels.[29] Theoretic risks of increased metal ion levels include local toxicity, osteolysis, and malignant change; however, the biologic long-term effects are unknown.[6,29,30] Various methods exist to measure serum chromium and serum cobalt, but the clinical relevance of raised metallic ions is uncertain.[10,29]

The BHR implant is made from a cobalt-chromium-molybdenum alloy, with a 4% carbide content that has been machine cast. A recent prospective longitudinal study of BHR implants found a peak in serum cobalt levels at 6 months postoperatively and a peak in serum chromium levels at 9 months postoperatively.[29] At 2-year follow-up, the mean serum ion levels were still higher than preoperative levels. No deterioration was found in renal function during the study period, and there was no radiographic evidence of lucency of either the femoral or acetabular components. Similar studies have also reported elevated cobalt and chromium levels with other bearing surface combinations, but it is difficult to compare these results because of differences in study designs and sampling. The local and systemic effects of elevated cobalt and chromium levels are still unknown.[7,29,31]

The mutagenic potential of metal ions is unknown because epidemiologic studies with these implants are of short duration. At present, orthopaedic implants are not classified based on carcinogenicity.[30] A recent in vitro study has demonstrated DNA damage in human cultured fibroblasts from synovial fluid of failed cobalt-chromium alloy prostheses, but this finding does not imply that DNA damage causes malignancy in humans.[6] Additional epidemiologic studies are needed to ascertain the malignant potential of metal ions in the context of hip resurfacing.

Dermal hypersensitivity to metal affects 10% to 15% of the population, with nickel being the most common sensitizer and cobalt-chromium being the second most common sensitizer.[32] Recent studies on metal hypersensitivity have shown a higher incidence in patients who have undergone arthroplasty than in the general population, but the relationship to osteolysis is unknown.[33] Patients with metal hypersensitivity may present with pain or an effusion. At a cellular level, free metal ions bind to native proteins to form allergens that activate a delayed cell-mediated immune response. Sensitized T-lymphocytes are activated and release cytokines with resultant macrophage activation. The histologic appearances of tissue samples from these patients are characterized by aseptic lymphocytic vasculitis associated lesions.[33] At present, no commercial hematologic tests are available for metal hypersensitivity, and the relevance of dermal hypersensitivity to metal in implant failure is yet to be defined.

Dislocation

Resurfacing the femoral head with a large femoral component and restoring the normal hip biomechanics may contribute to the low published dislocation rates of 0.75% at a mean of 3-year follow-up compared with conventional arthroplasty, which has a reported dislocation rate of up to 10%.[1,2,11,34] Smaller diameter metal-on-metal bearings have also been shown to exhibit suction

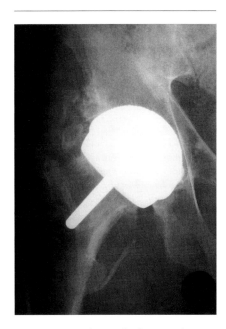

Figure 5   Radiograph showing heterotopic ossification (Brooker grade III) that occurred after hip resurfacing.

fit, which may contribute to stability. However, larger diameter metal-on-metal bearings have a greater diametric clearance and suction fit is less likely in the context of resurfacing.[35]

Heterotopic Ossification

Formation of heterotopic bone after hip resurfacing has been reported in 28% to 60% of patients[1,2,16] (Figure 5). Predisposition to formation of heterotopic bone is associated with male gender, bilateral simultaneous hip resurfacing, previous heterotopic bone formation, and extensive soft-tissue stripping.[36] Although the effect on clinical outcome scores is minimal, heterotopic ossification may reduce range of motion.[1,2,16] Indomethacin prophylaxis has been shown to reduce the risk of heterotopic bone formation.[33] Indications for the use of indomethacin vary from selective in high-risk patients to routine in all patients.[16,36]

Other Complications

Neurovascular injuries and thromboembolic disease have also been reported as complications of hip resurfacing, but these complications occur at rates comparable to those for conventional hip arthroplasty.[1,2,16]

Learning Curve

Implantation of the BHR using a posterior approach has an associated learning curve. A prospective study of two orthopaedic surgeons in the same unit, using the same approach and standard instrumentation, showed a significant improvement ($P < 0.001$) in surgical time and implant position, but no difference in clinical outcome when comparing the first to the second cohort of 50 patients who underwent implantation.[37] Because a significant learning curve is associated with hip resurfacing, this factor should be considered on initial introduction of this implant into clinical practice.

Summary

Hip resurfacing appears to provide a viable treatment option in the short term for young patients with degenerative arthritis. Careful patient selection is needed, with the best results obtained in young men with good bone stock. There is a learning curve associated with the procedure, and although short-term results are favorable, the long-term clinical and radiographic outcomes are still unknown. Concerns with hip resurfacing include the risk of femoral neck fracture in the early postoperative period, which is associated with varus implantation and intraoperative femoral neck notching. In addition, hip resurfacing is not ideal if the patient requires increased limb length or horizontal offset. The long-term effects of increased se-

rum metal ion levels is unknown. Serum cobalt levels appear to peak at 6 months postoperatively, whereas serum chromium levels appear to peak at 9 months postoperatively. Metal sensitivity has been implicated as a cause of groin pain in patients who have undergone hip resurfacing, but the relationship to osteolysis and whether it causes implant failure is unknown. Long-term independent studies of survivorship and complications are needed to determine ideal patient selection and reduce the risk of complications.

References

1. Back DL, Dalziel R, Young D, Shimmin A: Early results of primary Birmingham hip resurfacings. *J Bone Joint Surg Br* 2005;87:324-329.

2. Treacy RC, McBryde CW, Pynsent PB: Birmingham hip resurfacing arthroplasty. *J Bone Joint Surg Br* 2005;87:167-170.

3. Daniel J, Pynsent PB, McMinn DJ: Metal-on-metal resurfacing of the hip in patients under the age of 55 years with osteoarthritis. *J Bone Joint Surg Br* 2004;86:177-184.

4. MacDonald SJ: Metal-on-metal total hip arthroplasty: The concerns. *Clin Orthop Relat Res* 2004;429:86-93.

5. Dumbleton JH, Manley MT: Metal-on-metal total hip replacement: What does the literature say? *J Arthroplasty* 2005;20:174-188.

6. Davies AP, Sood A, Lewis AC, Newson R, Learmonth ID, Case CP: Metal-specific differences in levels of DNA damage caused by synovial fluid recovered at revision arthroplasty. *J Bone Joint Surg Br* 2005;87:1439-1444.

7. Jacobs JJ, Skipor AK, Doorn PF, et al: Cobalt and chromium concentrations in patients with metal on metal hip replacements. *Clin Orthop Relat Res* 1996;329(suppl):S256-263.

8. Itayem R, Arndt A, Nistor L, McMinn D, Lundberg A: Stability of the Birmingham hip resurfacing arthroplasty at two years. *J Bone Joint Surg Br* 2005;87:158-162.

9. Australian Orthopaedic Association: *National Joint Replacement Registry Annual*

Report. 2005, pp 29-63. Available at: www.dmac.adelaide.edu.au/aoanjrr/documents/corrigenda_2005.pdf. Accessed August 3, 2006.

10. Shimmin AJ, Bare J, Back DL: Complications associated with hip resurfacing arthroplasty. *Orthop Clin North Am* 2005;36-A:187-193.

11. Silva M, Haeng Lee K, Heisel C, Dela Rosa M, Schmalzried TP: The biomechanical results of total hip resurfacing arthroplasty. *J Bone Joint Surg Am* 2004;86-A:40-46.

12. Harris WH: Traumatic arthritis of the hip after dislocation and acetabular fractures: Treatment by mold arthroplasty: An end result study using a new method of result evaluation. *J Bone Joint Surg Am* 1969;51:737-755.

13. Dawson J, Fitzpatrick R, Murray D, Carr A: Comparison of measures to assess outcomes in total hip replacements. *Qual Health Care* 1996;5:81-88.

14. Charnley J: The long-term results of low-friction arthroplasty of the hip performed as a primary intervention. *J Bone Joint Surg Br* 1972;54:61-76.

15. Dawson J, Fitzpatrick R, Carr A, Murray D: Questionnaire on the perceptions of patients about total hip replacement. *J Bone Joint Surg Br* 1996;78:185-190.

16. Amstutz HC, Beaulé PE, Dorey FJ, Le Duff MJ, Campbell PA, Gruen TA: Metal-on-metal hybrid surface arthroplasty: Two to six-year follow-up study. *J Bone Joint Surg Am* 2004;86-A:28-39.

17. DeLee JG, Charnley J: Radiological demarcation of cemented sockets in total hip replacement. *Clin Orthop Relat Res* 1976;121:20-32.

18. Brooker AF, Bowerman J, Robinson RA, Riley LH Jr: Ectopic ossification following total hip replacement: Incidence and a method of classification. *J Bone Joint Surg Am* 1973;55:1629-1632.

19. Shimmin AJ, Back DL: Femoral neck fractures associated with hip resurfacing: A national review of 50 cases. *J Bone Joint Surg Br* 2005;87:463-464.

20. Freeman MA, Cameron HU, Brown GC: Cemented double-cup arthroplasty of the hip: A 5 year experience with the ICLH prosthesis. *Clin Orthop Relat Res* 1978;134:45-52.

21. Freeman MA: Some anatomical and mechanical considerations relevant to the surface replacement of the femoral head. *Clin Orthop Relat Res* 1978;134:19-24.

22. Kohan L, Gillies M: Effect of femoral component alignment on femoral neck remodelling after hip resurfacing: A finite element analysis. *Proceedings of the 65th Annual Scientific Meeting.* Australian Orthopaedic Academy, 2005, p 69.

23. Beaulé PE, Dorey FJ, LeDuff ML, Gruen T, Amstutz HC: Risk factors affecting outcome of metal-on-metal surface arthroplasty of the hip. *Clin Orthop Relat Res* 2004;418:87-93.

24. Cumming D, Fordyce M: The non-operative management of a peri-prosthetic subcapital fracture after metal-on-metal Birmingham hip resurfacing: A case report. *J Bone Joint Surg Br* 2003;85:1055-1056.

25. Cossey AJ, Back DL, Shimmin A, Young D, Spriggins AJ: The non-operative management of peri-prosthetic fractures associated with the Birmingham hip resurfacing procedure. *J Arthroplasty* 2005;20:358-361.

26. Little CP, Ruiz AL, Harding IJ, et al: Osteonecrosis in retrieved femoral heads after failed resurfacing arthroplasty of the hip. *J Bone Joint Surg Br* 2005;87:320-330.

27. Steffen RT, Smith SR, Urban JP, et al: The effect of hip resurfacing on oxygen concentration in the femoral head. *J Bone Joint Surg Br* 2005;87:1468-1474.

28. Kishida Y, Sugano N, Nishii T, Miki H, Yamaguchi K, Yoshikawa H: Preservation of the bone mineral density of the femur

after surface replacement of the hip. *J Bone Joint Surg Br* 2004;86:185-189.

29. Back DL, Young DA, Shimmin AJ: How do serum cobalt and chromium levels change after metal-on-metal hip resurfacing? *Clin Orthop Relat Res* 2005;438:177-181.

30. McGregor D, Baan RA, Portensky C, Rice JM, Wilbourne JD: Evaluation of the carcinogenic risks to humans associated with surgical implants and other foreign bodies: A report of an IARC Monographs Programme Meeting. *Eur J Cancer* 2000;36:307-313.

31. Jacobs JJ, Skipor AK, Patterson LM, et al: Metal release in patients who have had a primary total hip arthroplasty: A prospective controlled longitudinal study. *J Bone Joint Surg Am* 1998;80:1447-1458.

32. Hallab N, Merritt K, Jacobs JJ: Metal sensitivity in patients with orthopaedic implants. *J Bone Joint Surg Am* 2001;83-A:428-436.

33. Willert HG, Buchhorn GH, Fayyazi A, et al: Metal-on-metal bearings and hypersensitivity in patients with artificial hip joints. *J Bone Joint Surg Am* 2005;87:28-36.

34. Kelley SS, Lachiewicz PF, Hickman JM, Paterno SM: Relationship of femoral head and acetabular size to the prevalence of dislocation. *Clin Orthop Relat Res* 1998;355:163-170.

35. Clarke MT, Lee PT, Arora A, Villar RN: Levels of metal ions after small- and large-diameter metal-on-metal hip arthroplasty. *J Bone Joint Surg Br* 2003;85:913-917.

36. Back DL, Dalziel R, Young D, Shimmin A: The incidence of heterotopic bone formation following hip resurfacing. *J Bone Joint Surg Br* 2005;87(suppl I):44.

37. Back DL, Shimmin AJ: Learning curve associated with hip resurfacing arthroplasty. *J Bone Joint Surg Br* 2005;87(suppl I):45.

The Pathogenesis of Osteonecrosis

Lynne C. Jones, PhD
David S. Hungerford, MD

Abstract

Although numerous studies concerning the pathogenesis of osteonecrosis have been published, the pathophysiologic mechanisms that may be involved continue to be debated. In the early 1980s, the concept of accumulative cell stress was advanced, which is a theory that proposes that bone cells are exposed to multiple insults or stresses, the effects of which accumulate to the point that the cells cannot sustain themselves and die. Technologic advances have led scientists to a better understanding of cell and molecular biology, and recent studies of osteonecrosis and its risk factors have indicated that this concept should be revisited. It now appears that using the term "necrosis" may be incorrect and that apoptosis may play a significant role. Research on osteoporosis, fracture healing, bone graft incorporation, hematology, and genetics may lend insight into the etiology and pathogenesis of osteonecrosis. Several studies on osteoporosis have focused on the effect of exogenous glucocorticoids on the behavior of osteocytes, osteoblasts, osteocytes, and their precursors. Recent findings on osteonecrosis and bone biology are placed into the context of what has been previously reported.

Instr Course Lect 2007;56:179-196.

Osteonecrosis, a musculoskeletal disease characterized by death of osteocytes and the loss of associated hematopoietic elements, usually occurs as focal lesions in weight-bearing joints. Although osteonecrosis can occur in any diarthrodial joint, it most frequently involves the epiphysis of the convex side of the hip, knee, shoulder, and ankle—in that order. Osteonecrosis can involve the diaphysis or metaphysis of any bone, but in these locations it seldom becomes clinically significant. Progression of the epiphyseal lesions is dependent on the size and location and may proceed to collapse of the subchondral bone and destruction of the overlying cartilage. It is uncommon for the entire weight-bearing surface to be involved. Osteonecrosis occurs in individuals of either gender at any age, although it is detected mostly frequently in patients between 30 and 59 years of age.

This disease has been referred to by several different names: osteonecrosis, avascular necrosis, ischemic necrosis of bone, ischemic necrosis of the femoral head, aseptic necrosis, and nontraumatic necrosis. Recently, the term "osteonecrosis" has been more widely accepted by the scientific community because it does not connote a specific pathogenic mechanism.

Several different classification systems that have been used to separate the development of osteonecrosis into several stages include those described by the Association Research Circulation Osseous Committee on Terminology and Classification,[1] Marcus and associates,[2] Steinberg and associates,[3] Ficat and Arlet,[4] and Ohzono and associates.[5] These systems are based on radiographic or MRI features of the disease as noted for the hip, although they can also be adapted to other joints. Regardless of the system, the earliest stage is characterized by hip pain in patients with radiographs and MRI scans within normal limits. Osteonecrosis is suspected because the painful hip has been noted in a patient who has either one or more risk factors or osteonecrosis has been diagnosed in the contralateral hip. The next stage of the disease, called stage I by all systems, is characterized by normal radiographs but an abnormal MRI or bone scan. At this stage, a decrease in signal intensity on T1-weighted MRI scans can be observed. The next stage, called stage II in all systems, is distinguished by radiographic changes in the subchondral bone that may include evidence of osteosclerosis, cyst formation, or osteopenia. In patients with stage II osteonecrosis, there is no evidence of subchondral fracture and the articular surface is intact. The next stage, called stage III in all systems, is distinguished by radiographic evidence of a crescent sign indicating subchondral collapse. It is at this point that the various staging systems diverge, depending on whether the staging system distinguishes the amount of head depression (flattened contour). After subchondral collapse, joint narrowing with or without acetabular involvement occurs. In end-stage osteonecrosis, advanced degenerative changes are associated with both the femoral head and acetabulum, and the integrity of the joint is destroyed.

Natural History

The inconsistency of the natural history of the disease has impacted the ability of clinicians to adequately evaluate current and future treatment regimens for osteonecrosis. As osteonecrosis may be asymptomatic in its early stages, the onset is difficult to establish. Some of what is known about the natural history of osteonecrosis is derived from the study of the biologic response to traumatic osteonecrosis (displaced fractures, radiation, and caisson disease). With respect to atraumatic osteonecrosis, studies have focused on characterizing the contralateral asymptomatic side in patients with confirmed osteonecrosis.[6-9] However, these studies assume that both sides have followed similar tracks, when in fact the contralateral side may be exposed to different external stimuli such as abnormal weight bearing/kinematics and internal stimuli such as increased exposure to inflammatory mediators.

Patients frequently ask whether osteonecrosis can spread or recur. Spreading implies an infectious process; there is no evidence at this time that this is a significant etiology for osteonecrosis. However, one infrequent manifestation of osteonecrosis, multifocal osteonecrosis, occurs when lesions are detected in three or more separate anatomic sites.[10] Although multifocal osteonecrosis may give the impression that the disease is spreading, the lesions develop at different rates in the affected joints for unknown reasons. In 1979, Inoue and Ono[11] evaluated the histopathology of 40 femoral heads (29 femoral heads and 11 biopsies) and concluded that there was evidence that repeated episodes of infarction can occur. However, in a histologic study of osteonecrotic femoral heads, Yamamoto and associates[12] found evidence of extension of osteonecrosis in only 2 of 606 consecutive patients (0.3%). Using MRI scans, Kim and associates[13] reported on three instances of multifocal osteonecrosis (unknown denominator) showing evidence of two low-signal intensity bands on T1-weighted MRI scans. In one patient, a thickening of the second band was described after 6 months. All of the evidence of recurrent osteonecrosis has been based on relatively few case reports, indicating the rarity of this manifestation of the disease. In addition, Yamamoto and associates[12] cautioned that care should be taken in how tissue is classified as recurrence and suggested that it should not include focal necrosis that results from collapse at the junction between the lesion and the juxtaposed viable bone. The incidence of recurrence needs to be evaluated further using serial MRI scans over an extended period.

Osteonecrosis appears on MRI scans and/or radiographs, in most patients, within 2 years of a probable inciting event (for example, high doses of steroids). It is unknown what the time lag is between its pathologic appearance and the appearance of radiographic evidence of osteonecrosis. With regard to osteonecrosis of a "definite" etiology, Calandruccio and Anderson[14] observed that of the patients with displaced fractures who develop osteonecrosis, 80% have radiographic evidence of osteonecrosis within 2 years of the fracture. Fink and associates[15] identified femoral head osteonecrosis in 6 hips of 4 patients (out of 43 patients) within 3 months of undergoing renal transplantation. For steroid-associated osteonecrosis, Koo and associates[16] detected the onset of osteonecrosis, using serial MRI, at 1 to 16 months after the initiation of corticosteroid therapy, with most patients diagnosed within 1 year. Using serial MRI (at 1, 3, 6, and 12 months), Oinuma and associates[17] reported that 32 of 72 patients with systemic lupus erythematosus were diagnosed with osteonecrosis within 39.6 and 100.2 days of the initiation of corticosteroid treatment. The time it takes for subchondral and subsequent femoral head collapse to occur once osteonecrosis is diagnosed is less predictable because most patients undergo some form of treatment, ranging from protected weight bearing to total joint arthroplasty. Estimates of time to femoral head collapse have ranged up to 5 years, depending on the size (volume and amount of surface involvement) and location of the lesion.[8,9,16,18-20] In patients with sickle cell disease, Hernigou and associates[18] reported that 87% of the patients (all stages without collapse) experienced femoral head collapse within 5 years of diagnosis. For patients diagnosed with Steinberg stage I disease, 14 of

32 patients experienced flattening of the femoral head by 3 years after diagnosis, whereas 8 experienced femoral head collapse after 5 years (mean, 42 months). As would be anticipated, more advanced stages had shorter times to femoral head collapse: the average was 30 months for patients with stage II osteonecrosis and within 6 months for those with stage III. In patients who had osteonecrosis associated with corticosteroid therapy, Koo and associates[19] observed that 79% of the nonoperated femoral heads collapsed within 18 months after diagnosis. Ito and associates[8] observed that in those patients who had osteonecrosis associated with corticosteroid therapy, most experienced clinical failure (Harris hip score ≤ 70) by 2 years (56.7%) and 5 years (61.1%) after diagnosis, with subchondral collapse leading to a flattened or markedly deformed femoral head. There does appear to be a subset of patients who do not go on to experience subchondral collapse. Ito and associates also reported that 37.2% of the patients with osteonecrosis that they studied had not experienced clinical failure at 10 years after diagnosis.

Etiology

A large number of diseases and risk factors are known to be associated with osteonecrosis[12-27] (Table 1). Etiologic associations that have been identified can be separated into direct, strong, or probable/possible risk factors. A direct etiology indicates that the cause-and-effect relationship is firmly established. A strong association signifies that there is a considerable body of evidence linking these risk factors to osteonecrosis. A probable/possible etiology presumes that although there is a high prevalence of patients with osteonecrosis in the referenced

Table 1
Potential Risk Factors for Osteonecrosis[21-27]

Direct Association	
Trauma (including fractures, burns, frostbite, dislocations, vascular trauma, Kienböck disease)	Gaucher's disease
	Major arterial disease
	Sickle cell disease and thalassemias
Caisson disease	Postirradiation

Strong Association	
Alcohol consumption	Corticosteroid therapy

Possible/Probable Association*	
Cigarette smoking	Iatrogenic
Connective tissue disease/rheumatologic	Hemodialysis
Ankylosing spondylitis	Organ transplantation
Ehlers-Danlos syndrome	Laser surgery
Polymyalgia rheumatica	Highly active antiretroviral therapy
Polymyositis	Infectious (osteomyelitis, HIV,
Raynaud's disease	meningococcemia)
Rheumatoid arthritis	Metabolic/endocrinologic
Sjögren syndrome	Chronic renal failure
Septic lupus erythematosus	Cushing disease
Diet (obesity, starvation)	Diabetes
Gastrointestinal	Fabray's disease
Inflammatory bowel disease	Gout and hyperuricemia
Pancreatitis	Hypercholesterolemia
Hematologic and vascular	Hyperparathyroidism
Arteriosclerosis	Lipodystrophies (hyperlipidemia)
Disseminated intravascular coagulation	Minor trauma
Giant cell arteritis	Neurodamage
Hemophilia	Neoplastic
Hypofibrinolysis	Orthopaedic
Idiopathic thrombocytopenia	Congenital hip dislocation / hip
Leukemia	dysplasia
Polycythemia	Hereditary dysostosis
Postvenous thrombosis	Legg-Calvé-Perthes disease
Thrombophilia	Osteoporosis/osteomalacia
Thrombophlebitis	Slipped capital femoral epiphysis
Vasculitis	Pregnancy

*There are reports of an association between these diseases and osteonecrosis. However, it may be the treatment (such as with corticosteroids) or another associated comorbidity that actually is the primary risk factor.

group, the cause-and-effect relationship is more difficult to confirm in individual patients. However, a significant number of these comorbidities are associated with either corticosteroid therapy or hematologic abnormalities.

One of the difficulties with establishing an etiology of osteonecrosis is that many individuals with a specific risk factor do not develop osteonecrosis. For example, in several published series, a large percentage

of patients with osteonecrosis consume excess alcohol, but only a small percentage of people consuming excess alcohol develop osteonecrosis.[28] A significant percentage of patients with osteonecrosis have also been reported to have a history of corticosteroid therapy; however, most patients receiving corticosteroids do not develop osteonecrosis.[29] The same is true for all of the probable/possible risk factors. In the past, clinical research has focused on qualifying risk factors. For example, the dose and duration of corticosteroid therapy influences whether an individual is at risk. Basic science research has also focused on the consequences of specific risk factors (such as corticosteroid administration) on bony tissue. However, based on the results of both basic science and clinical research, it is likely that osteonecrosis is a multifactorial disease.[30,31] It may be that there is an accumulation of risk factors that ultimately crosses the threshold to initiate the onset of osteonecrosis. Another possibility is that a person may be genetically predisposed to the development of osteonecrosis that is triggered by one or more secondary factors. Epidemiologic studies are needed to evaluate the interrelationships of multiple factors and the pathogenesis of osteonecrosis.

During the late 1980s and early 1990s, several reports concerning the incidence of osteonecrosis in patients with human immunodeficiency virus (HIV) were published.[32-35] Since then, most studies have indicated that the incidence of osteonecrosis in this patient population is quite small, ranging from 0.12% to 4.4%.[36-41] Risk factors that have been implicated in this patient population include those associated with patients who do not have HIV, including alcoholism, and corticosteroid therapy as well as disease-specific risk factors (highly active retroviral therapy, other protease inhibitors, and the disease itself).[42,43] Whether antiviral therapy contributes to the development of osteonecrosis has been widely debated.[36,38,39,41,44-48] Valencia and associates[41] reported that the mean time from initiation of highly active retroviral therapy to the diagnosis of osteonecrosis was 12 months

(range, 2 to 24 months), suggesting an association similar to that found for patients receiving corticosteroid therapy. However, several investigators have cast doubt as to whether antiviral therapy is really a risk factor for osteonecrosis.[36,42,44,47] There are several significant antiretroviral adverse effects associated with highly active retroviral therapy for patients with acquired immunodeficiency syndrome, including lactic acidosis, hepatic steatosis, hyperlactatemia, hepatotoxicity, hyperglycemia, fat maldistribution, hyperlipidemia, bleeding disorders, osteoporosis, and skin rash.[46] Some of these adverse effects are risk factors for osteonecrosis. Ries and associates[49] screened 50 patients with HIV for risk factors known to be associated with osteonecrosis, including corticosteroid therapy, alcohol use, and specific disease associations (sickle cell disease, Gaucher's disease, or caisson disease). Although these authors concluded that the absence of these risk factors in four of seven patients suggests that HIV may be a risk factor, their screen (the number of risk factors examined) was quite limited, and other risk factors (including antiviral therapy) may be present.

Severe acute respiratory syndrome (SARS) was first reported in Asia in November 2002, and a global alert was issued by the World Health Organization in March 2003.[50,51] Beginning in the summer of 2004, reports of SARS and osteonecrosis were published.[52,53] The incidence of osteonecrosis in this patient population is generally believed to be related to corticosteroid therapy.[52,54-56] Hong and Du[52] found that the mean time to the diagnosis of osteonecrosis was 119 days after the onset of SARS or 116 days after the initiation of corticosteroid ther-

apy. Patients were treated with intravenous methylprednisolone (80 to 800 mg daily) for 3 to 20 days, which was followed by oral prednisolone therapy (the cumulative dose ranged from 640 to 20,000 mg). Joint pain was noted 12 to 120 days after the onset of SARS. These authors also found that there was a high incidence of multifocal osteonecrosis in this patient population. Li and associates[55] reported similar findings. In patients who developed osteonecrosis, osteonecrosis was detected within 6 months of initiation of corticosteroid therapy. The dosage of corticosteroid was noted to be higher for those who developed osteonecrosis than those who did not, and osteonecrosis was identified as multifocal in a large percentage of patients. Griffith and associates[54] reported that 134 of 254 patients with SARS developed joint pain, but osteonecrosis was not diagnosed in most of them. Patients unresponsive to antibiotic therapy received ribavirin (24 mg/kg/day) and hydrocortisone (10 mg/kg/day). Patients with progressive deterioration were given pulsed methylprednisolone intravenously (500 to 1,000 g/day). Although only 12 patients in this study had osteonecrosis of either the hip or knee, nonspecific subchondral or intramedullary bone marrow abnormalities (not clearly defined by the authors) were found in 77 patients. It is important to note that, in addition to receiving corticosteroid therapy, many patients also received antiviral therapy with ribavirin,[52,54] which may also be a risk factor for osteonecrosis.

As correlation is not a synonym for causation, it is important to determine whether different mechanisms are involved with each proposed etiology. Although the pathway that ends in osteonecrosis may have different initiating agents and mechanisms, the pathways may converge at some point. In attempting to identify a common link between the vastly different etiologic associations, it is important to identify unifying pathologies common to all etiologies. For osteonecrosis of the femoral head these unifying pathologies may include but are not limited to vascular disturbances, elevated intramedullary pressure, fat cell abnormalities, and coagulation disorders.

Pathogenesis

Pathogenesis is defined as mechanisms of disease production and progression. Several theories have been proposed concerning the pathogenesis of osteonecrosis. Schroer[50] argued that a theory on the pathogenesis of osteonecrosis must explain several pathologic findings that are consistently found regardless of the associated risk factors. Several outstanding articles have been published on this topic.[21-25,57-60]

The initial pathology of osteonecrosis is characterized by bone marrow changes eventually resulting in necrosis and loss of hematopoietic elements. Intramedullary edema and evidence of hemorrhage have been documented.[61-65] Lipocyte hypertrophy and hyperplasia have been noted, especially in instances of osteonecrosis associated with corticosteroid therapy or alcoholism.[66-68] The finding of thrombi in the microvasculature has been debated and may be either related to instances of osteonecrosis with specific etiologies or occur early in the presymptomatic stages.[21,69,70] As the osteonecrosis progresses, increasing numbers of dead osteocytes are found within the trabecular lacunae. It has been assumed that cell death is by necrosis,

but there is recent evidence that cell death may be a consequence of apoptosis.[71-75] The interface between the necrotic segment and the surrounding bone is characterized by increased biologic activity characteristic of bone repair. One of the pathognomonic features of osteonecrosis is the presence of creeping substitution—that is, new bone formation overlying necrotic trabeculae. The area surrounding the lesion is rich in newly formed blood vessels. In more advanced stages, a thin sclerotic margin surrounds the lesion. A crescent sign can be detected on radiographs, signifying a separation of the subchondral plate from the underlying supporting cancellous bone. The location of most necrotic lesions is primarily in the weight-bearing region of the convex-shaped articulation (the anterosuperior aspect of the femoral head). Physiologic features of this disease include increased intraosseous pressure, abnormal angiography, and abnormal venography. Any theory concerning the pathophysiology of osteonecrosis should explain not only the pathophysiologic features of the disease but also its natural history.

Theories relating to the pathogenesis of osteonecrosis can be grouped as cellular theories, extraosseous theories, and intraosseous theories. Examples of osteonecrosis developing as a consequence of direct cytotoxicity include radiation necrosis, chemotherapy-related necrosis, and thermal injuries. Although the direct cytotoxic effects of steroids and alcohol have been implicated, the evidence for this has not been convincing when studied at physiologic concentrations.[57] Possible extraosseous mechanisms may be either arterial or venous mechanisms. There is a clear relationship between

the interruption of the blood supply to bone and the development of traumatic osteonecrosis. However, the possible role of this mechanism in the development of atraumatic osteonecrosis is less clear. Intravascular vascular occlusion has been documented, although it is unknown as to whether it is a cause or effect. Likewise, although venous stasis has also been observed to occur in association with osteonecrosis, it has not been determined whether this is an inciting factor or a consequence of the disease.

Intraosseous mechanisms may be either extravascular or intravascular. Intraosseous intravascular mechanisms are involved in osteonecrosis related to sickle cell disease and, possibly, dysbaric exposure. The underlying cause is the embolization of the microvasculature by diseased cells (sickle cell disease) or gas bubbles (dysbaric exposure). Osteonecrosis related to these etiologies can be found not only in the femoral head and neck but also in the metaphyseal regions extending down into the diaphysis. An extension of this hypothesis proposes that fat emboli can disrupt the blood flow within bone.[69] Experiments have used injections of microspheres or oil droplets (lipiodol) to show that microvascular occlusion and bone necrosis can result from embolization of the vasculature.[76,77] Clinically, the presence of fat emboli within the diseased femoral head has been documented.[69] However, those who disagree with this theory point to the fact that hyperlipidemia exists in patients who do not develop osteonecrosis; in addition, the presence of fat emboli is not pathognomonic for this disease and can also be found in the femoral head outside of the necrotic lesions.[21,78]

There has been renewed interest

in the possibility of intravascular co-agulation as a key to understanding the pathogenesis of osteonecrosis. Jones[57,69] proposed that the final common pathway for the diverse etiologies of osteonecrosis was intra-vascular coagulation. A substantial number of factors that may activate intravascular coagulation have been identified,[26] including thrombo-philia (increased likelihood of blood clots) and hypofibrinolysis (de-creased ability to lyse blood clots). Several studies have shown that pa-tients with osteonecrosis have a higher incidence of abnormal levels of coagulation factors than control subjects.[79-82] Analyzing nine coagu-lation factors, Jones and associates[81] reported that 37 of 45 patients (82.2%) with osteonecrosis had at least one coagulation disorder com-pared with 30% of control subjects ($P < 0.0001$); 21 of 45 patients (46.7%) were identified with two or more abnormalities compared with 2.5% of control subjects ($P < 0.0001$). It may be that the presence of any coagulation factor abnormali-ty (not a specific coagulopathy) is the risk factor. Furthermore, be-cause of the sophistication of the co-agulation system (feedback mecha-nisms and redundancies), it may also be that the coagulation factor that is the primary risk factor has not yet been identified. These findings may be a consequence of inherited defects or they may be associated with specific comorbidities or treat-ments. It is possible that one or more coagulation abnormalities may act as a primary risk factor and that other secondary factors that may have an impact on blood circulation to bone (such as smoking, alcohol, or corticosteroids) trigger the onset of the disease.

Intraosseous extravascular mech-anisms may also be involved. It has been established that there is a direct relationship between blood flow and intraosseous pressure: increased pressure results in decreased flow. It has been proposed that bone, partic-ularly within convex articulations, acts as a Starling resister.[24,83] In this model of a rigid canister that con-tains a thin-walled tube, any in-crease in the pressure within the compartment results in the collapse of the thin-walled tube contained within the compartment. Adapting this model to osteonecrosis, the bone would be the rigid compart-ment, whereas veins and venules would be the thin-walled tubes. Clinical studies have demonstrated the presence of elevated in-traosseous pressures and increased hydraulic resistance in diseased fem-oral heads.[24,84,85] Downey and asso-ciates[84] also observed abnormally high hydraulic resistance in the in-tertrochanteric bone away from the osteonecrotic lesion and concluded that this supports the concept that venous impairment is part of the cause and not an effect of osteone-crosis. With osteonecrosis, the in-crease in pressure within the bony compartment may be a consequence of edema, lipocyte hypertrophy, or an increased number of lipocytes.

A recently published study ar-gued that the final common path-way leading to collapse of the femo-ral head is an uncoupling of the rates of osteoclastic bone resorption and osteoblastic bone regeneration.[86] Currently, however, it is not known whether this argument is true. Un-like osteoporosis and other bone metabolic diseases,[71,87-92] it is not known whether bone remodeling is affected during the pathogenesis of osteonecrosis. What is known is de-rived primarily from the evaluation of histologic specimens. Osteoblasts are present and new bone is formed on the surface of the dead trabeculae (creeping substitution). In fact, a sclerotic area forms at the periphery of the lesion. It is unclear whether the osteoclasts are affected. Al-though most descriptions of the pa-thology do not mention osteoclast activity, one report suggested there is an increased number of osteo-clasts.[93] The area of dead bone, or necrotic lesion, resembles an infarct. The lack of living tissue and mi-crovasculature are the reasons this disease was called avascular. How-ever, the response to the lesion is not avascular. The lesion is surrounded by a hyperemic area. Repair is often attempted but unsuccessful, perhaps because of the size of the lesion, the accumulation of unrepaired micro-fractures, and the change in biome-chanical properties. Perhaps some signal stops the repair or causes apop-tosis of cells to occur.

Osteonecrosis resembles diseases in other tissues in which the body's response to the stimulus (infarct) actually contributes to the disease, as with delayed hypersensitivity reac-tions or autoimmune diseases. One example of this is the body's re-sponse to tubercular lesions.[94] The body responds by attempting to wall off a site of persistent infection. The cells surrounding the lesion release inflammatory mediators and cyto-kines that cause activation of mac-rophages that release substances that ultimately cause tissue damage. A granuloma forms with liquefaction necrosis surrounded by fibrous tis-sue. In osteonecrosis, the area of dead bone is walled off from the healthy tissue by fibrosis and scle-rotic bone. This wall may then act as a barrier to revascularization, recon-stitution of the marrow elements, and the transport of the cytokines and other cellular mediators needed to adequately repair the bone. In fact, it is common to see areas of liquefaction necrosis in the late stages of osteonecrosis.[61] Perhaps more can be learned about the mechanisms involved by applying what is known about osteopetrosis and osteosclerosis to the study of osteonecrosis.

Different hypotheses concerning the pathogenesis of osteonecrosis have been debated for decades. There are many key questions that remain unanswered concerning the pathogenesis of atraumatic osteonecrosis. What cells are affected? How are they affected? How do they contribute to the disease process? Why is the attempt at repair unsuccessful? What causes the disease to occur in some people and not others with the same risk factors? With advances in technology, researchers are now able to better explore potential mechanisms at the molecular, protein, and cellular levels. Recent studies on osteonecrosis have used this technology to advance understanding of the potential mechanisms involved in this disease. Research has focused on the identification of the cellular modulators that may be involved in the promotion and inhibition of fracture healing[95-103] and bone graft incorporation.[104-108] Detecting the presence or absence of these same substances surrounding osteonecrotic lesions may help determine why the repair of these lesions is limited. Significant advances have been made in the understanding of the coagulation factors involved in hypofibrinolysis and thrombophilia. Serologic and genetic studies have provided evidence that the presence of genetic mutations in at least one of the alleles for these factors may be associated with the development of osteonecrosis.[79-82,109-112] Additional studies have identified other mutations in genes coding for collagen II,

a drug-transport protein, and an alcohol-metabolizing enzyme that may also influence which individuals may be at risk to develop osteonecrosis.[113-115]

Steroids and Alcohol

Two of the major risk factors for osteonecrosis are corticosteroid therapy and alcoholism. Although the incidence of osteonecrosis in each of these patient populations is not known, it is estimated that fewer than 5% of patients subjected to high doses of corticosteroids or alcohol develop osteonecrosis.[22,116-118] However, patients with these two risk factors comprise a significant proportion of those diagnosed with osteonecrosis. The prevalence of corticosteroid use ranges from 3% to 38%; the prevalence of alcohol use ranges up to 29%.[22,116] Both risk factors are associated with comorbidities (such as hyperlipidemia, pancreatitis, smoking, and coagulopathies) that may also contribute to the development of osteonecrosis. Because alcohol use is more ubiquitous and less well defined than corticosteroid use, it is more straightforward to evaluate the effects of corticosteroid therapy in basic science and clinical studies; therefore, more data are available about the effects of corticosteroids on the musculoskeletal system.

Osseous Vasculature

Corticosteroids may affect the cardiovascular system in several ways, including elevated blood pressure, increased atherosclerosis, vascular injury, and endothelial cell damage[119] In a study using rabbits treated with methylprednisolone acetate (4 mg/week for 8 weeks), Nishimura and associates[120] observed foam cells in the intima and vacuolization of the tunica media in

veins taken from the femoral head (4 of 30 rabbits), ear (2 of 30 rabbits), femoral vein (2 of 30 rabbits), and the inferior vena cava (1 of 30 rabbits). Using the same model, Ichiseki and associates[121] found evidence of oxidative stress (decreased glutathione and increased lipid peroxide) and increased vascular permeability (albumin leakage) in animals after corticosteroid administration. Hirano and associates[122] studied cadaveric femoral heads taken from patients who had no history of hip problems. Of the 37 patients from whom specimens were obtained, 13 had received corticosteroid therapy for various reasons. The authors found no difference in the degree of stenosis of the superior retinacular arteries when comparing the corticosteroid and noncorticosteroid groups, whereas the number of stenotic superior retinacular veins was significantly increased in the corticosteroid group ($P < 0.0001$). In the femoral heads of patients with aseptic osteonecrosis of the hip, Laroche and associates[123] detected atherosclerotic lesions (3 of 20 patients) and thromboses (4 of 20 patients) in intraosseous arterioles of the capillaries. Saito and associates[124] evaluated core biopsy samples obtained from 16 femoral heads in patients with asymptomatic osteonecrosis and found necrotic debris associated with old intramedullary hemorrhage as well as evidence of new hemorrhage. They attempted to evaluate the walls of the blood vessels and reported that there were a few vessels that had collapsed or had broken wall structures. In a later study of 24 core biopsy samples, Saito and associates[125] observed evidence of structural damage to the vascular wall of arterioles and necrotic debris of blood vessels, but reported no evidence of damage to veins or sinusoids. Nishimura and associates[120] provide an outstanding discussion on this topic.

Osteocytes

The location of osteocytes within the trabeculae of cancellous bone and within the haversian canals of cortical bone have inhibited researchers from studying their biology. Osteocytes are osteoblasts that have become embedded in the ossifying tissue. Osteocytes are believed to play roles in the regulation of the overall metabolism of bone and in the mechanotransduction within bone.[126-128] It has been suggested that the consequence of the loss of osteocytes may be a breakdown in the system that senses fatigue microfractures and the pathways signaling cells to initiate repair.[71,87,128] This could then lead to an accumulation of the microfractures and eventually lead to collapse of the osseous infrastructure.

One of the pathognomonic features of osteonecrosis is the presence of dead osteocytes and empty lacunae. Additionally, the lacunae may become enlarged as a consequence of periosteocytic osteolysis.[85] It has generally been assumed that osteocytes die via cell necrosis; however, Calder and associates[72] and Weinstein and associates[75] observed apoptosis of osteocytes in the femoral heads of patients with osteonecrosis after glucocorticoid treatment. Shibahara and associates[74] also reported increased osteocyte apoptosis in the femoral heads of an animal model of osteonecrosis. In mice treated with prednisolone, Weinstein and associates[92] found decreased bone density, bone formation, and turnover as well as impaired osteoblastogenesis and osteoclastogenesis associated with

an increased number of apoptotic cells in the metaphyseal cortical bone of the femur. Weinstein and associates[75,92] have suggested that osteocyte apoptosis may be the primary etiology of glucocorticoid-induced bone diseases such as osteonecrosis and osteoporosis. O'Brien and associates[129] studied the potential role of glucocorticoids on osteocyte apoptosis using a transgenic mouse model in which a gene for an enzyme that inactivates glucocorticoids was inserted. They found that glucocorticoids can act directly on osteocytes to stimulate apoptosis. However, it remains to be proven that glucocorticoids cause apoptosis directly. Indirect signals—whether autocrine, paracrine, or endocrine—may also be involved. If corticosteroid-induced apoptosis is the primary etiology, systemic but not focal osteonecrosis would be expected. However, as suggested by Zalavras and associates,[71] the predilection of osteonecrosis for specific sites may be because ischemia and apoptosis act together in corticosteroid-associated osteonecrosis and because ischemia and apoptosis are not mutually exclusive events.

Osteoclasts

Little is known about the potential role of osteoclasts in osteonecrosis. Theoretically, a decoupling of the remodeling process with excessive osteoclasis could lead to destabilization of the necrotic segment leading to subchondral collapse. Bullough[93] has reported that there is increased osteoclastic activity at the interface between living bone and the necrotic lesion. Weinstein and associates[92] found diminished bone turnover in the vertebrae of mice treated with prednisolone. In the bone marrow cultures taken from the animals re-

ceiving 2.1 mg/kg/day of prednisolone for 27 days, the authors reported a significant decrease in the number of osteoclastic cells formed in response to 1,25 dihydroxy vitamin D3. In the transgenic mouse described previously, O'Brien and associates[129] found that cancellous osteoclasts were not affected by the transgene for the enzyme that inactivates glucocorticoids. Hofbauer and associates[129] found that glucocorticoids may also act to increase the number of osteoclasts and activity indirectly by inhibiting osteoprotegerin production and stimulating production of the ligand for osteoprotegerin by osteoblastic cells. Studies investigating the effect of glucocorticoids on bone cells indicate that glucocorticoids do not induce osteoclast apoptosis.[87] The results of these studies indicate that osteoclasts respond to the necrotic infarct; however, because collapse of the necrotic segment frequently occurs within the lesion and not at its periphery, the role that osteoclasts play in the pathogenesis of osteonecrosis is more likely to be reactive than causative.

Osteoblasts

Corticosteroids directly and indirectly affect osteoblasts. Clinically, corticosteroid therapy is associated with reduced bone formation.[71,87,88] This could be affected through several different osteoblastic responses to glucocorticoids[72,87-92,129-139] (Table 2). Treatment with exogenous glucocorticoids results in a decrease in the overall number of osteoblasts, which can be realized through either a decrease in the number of progenitor cells that develop into osteoblasts or by an increase in cell death (apoptosis or necrosis). Glucocorticoid therapy can also affect the cellular activity of bone cells as well as

Table 2
Osteoblastic Responses to Corticosteroids[72,87-92,129-139]

Cell Type and Action

Osteocytes

  Increased apoptosis

  Increased activity

  Decreased number of cells

  Increased skeletal fragility?

Osteoblasts

  Increased differentiation (humans)

  DNA synthesis affected depending on type of glucocorticoid, dose, and length of exposure

  Increased expression of genes associated with mature osteoblasts

  Decreased stability of mRNA for *Cbfa-1*

  Increased *C-fos*

  Reduces the parathyroid hormone action on osteoblasts

  Increased bone morphogenetic protein generation and notch receptors

  Suppresses bone morphogenetic protein-2

  May reduce transforming growth factor-β activity

  May reduce insulin-like growth factor-1 activity

  Decreased osteocalcin

  Increased osteocalcin secretion

  Decreased collagen 1

  Increased collagenase

  Decreased alkaline phosphatase (mature osteoblasts)

  Increased alkaline phosphatase activity

  Decreased proliferation

  Increased proliferation

  Decreased generation

  Increased apoptosis

  Protects against apoptosis

  Reduction in bone formation

  Decreased matrix mineralization?

  Upregulation of receptor activator of necrosis factor-κB ligand expression on cell surface

  Decreased production of osteoprotegerin

  Upregulation of mitogen-activated protein kinase phosphatase-1

Osteoclasts

  Increased resorption

  Decreased resorption

  Increased survival

  Increased proliferation

  Decreased generation

  Increased formation

the response to various cellular modulators.

In vitro studies concerning the effect of dexamethasone on the commitment of mesenchymal stem cells toward the osteoblast lineage have yielded conflicting results. Dexamethasone is added to the media of cultured precursor cells to push cells toward the osteoblast lineage and to maintain the osteoblastic phenotype. Treatment with gluco-corticoids also results in the expression of osteoblast-specific genes and proteins associated with osteo-blasts.[88] Cui and associates[131] found, however, that dexamethasone treatment resulted in a suppression of osteoblast differentiation with decreased expression of α1 type I collagen mRNA and osteocalcin in cultured pluripotential mesenchymal cells (D1 cells) with a concomitant expansion of adipocytes (increased expression of *422(aP2)* gene). In a subsequent study, Li and associates[132] found that dexamethasone also caused an increased expression of *PPARγ2*, a gene associated with adipocyte differentiation, and a decreased expression of the gene for *Cbfa1/Runx2*, a transcription factor associated with osteoblast differentiation. If confirmed in vivo and in humans, the shunting of pluripotential stem cells to the lipocyte lineage also has implications concerning the role of an increased number of lipocytes in the pathogenesis of osteonecrosis.

Contradictory results have also been reported concerning whether glucocorticoid administration increases or decreases apoptosis in osteoblasts. Apoptosis of osteoblasts has been detected in tissue samples obtained from patients with osteoporosis and those with osteonecrosis.[72,75,92] Weinstein and associates[75] found apoptotic bone cells lining the cancellous bone near the site of the subchondral fracture in patients with glucocorticoid-associated osteonecrosis. Calder and associates[72] detected apoptosis in osteoblasts in the femoral head of patients with osteonecrosis. Both groups found little evidence of apoptosis in the group of patients with sickle cell disease and osteonecrosis. Gohel and associates[133] observed that the treatment of primary rat osteoblasts with 100 nM of corticosterone for 72 hours caused a dose-dependent increase in the percentage of apoptotic cells. Weinstein and associates[92] treated 7-month-old mice for 27 days with 2.1 mg/kg/day of prednisolone and found a significant increase in the percentage of apoptotic cells compared with controls (2.03% ± 0.34% versus 0.66% ± 0.07%, $P < 0.05$). O'Brien and associates[129] also showed that prednisolone (2.1 mg/kg/day) increased osteoblast apoptosis, which was not seen in mice that were transgenic for an enzyme that inactivates glucocorticoids. In contrast, Yang and associates[140] did not detect apoptosis in osteoblasts exposed to dexamethasone for 3 days. Pereira and associates[141] found that cortisol (1 μmol/L) prevented apoptosis in osteoblasts grown under mineralizing conditions. Others have found that dexamethasone may protect against apoptosis, depending on the apoptotic model studied.[71,142,143]

Several factors may contribute to the conflicting results of the in vitro and in vivo studies on the effects of corticosteroids on osteoblasts. Differences between the types of cells used and the culturing conditions can significantly impact the results of these studies.[71,87] The cells have included both transformed and primary cultures as well as cells during different stages of differentiation and confluence. With respect to culturing conditions, there are differences in serum concentrations and differentiation-promoting agents, including the concentration of dexamethasone that is added, which highlights one of the limitations of using cell culture to model the in vivo environment. Furthermore, Cooper[87] questioned the relevance of evaluating osteoblasts in isolation when they are actually a part of a complex bone remodeling unit.

Behavior of Mesenchymal Stem Cells in Osteonecrosis

The behavior of human multipotential mesenchymal stem cells and the presence of apoptosis of bone cells have also been studied in cells obtained from patients with osteonecrosis.

Lee and associates[144] examined the differentiation potential of mesenchymal stem cells harvested from the proximal femurs of patients with osteonecrotic hips. The cells were able to proliferate and were homogeneously positive for β1-integrin. These mesenchymal stem cells could be directed toward chondrocytic or osteocytic differentiation depending on culture conditions. When cultured with transforming growth factor-β3, the cells expressed mRNA for aggrecan and collagen type II and produced collagen type II and sulfated proteoglycans, which are characteristic of chondrocytes. When cultured with dexamethasone, β-glycerophosphate, and L-ascorbic acid-2-phosphate, the cells showed increased expression of alkaline phosphatase activity and mineral deposition, which is characteristic of osteoblasts. These findings confirm that even though the cells were retrieved from patients who were diagnosed with osteonecrosis, marrow stromal cells retain their multipotential nature.

In a comparison of cells from patients with different etiologies, Hernigou and Beaujean[145] found that stromal cell activity (indicated by fibroblastic colony-forming units) and hematopoietic stem cell activity (indicated by granulocyte-macrophage progenitor cells) were more depressed for the alcohol-associated and steroid-associated groups when compared with the control group. Cells derived from idiopathic patients had slightly higher responses than those derived from the other patients with osteonecrosis, but these responses were still lower than those derived from the control group. The abnormal activity levels were found even though the biopsy samples were obtained from the iliac crest. In another study, Hernigou and associates[146] found that the steroid-associated osteonecrosis group had a significantly lower number of fibroblast colony-forming units (1.88 ± 4.02 per 10^6 bone marrow cells) compared with the sickle cell-osteonecrosis group (30.09 ± 33.1 per 10^6 bone marrow cells; $P = 0.000001$) or the control group (33.5 ± 21.7 per 10^6 bone marrow cells; $P = 0.000007$). They suggested that a decrease in the stem cell pool may result in the number of pluripotential mesenchymal cells being insufficient to meet the needs of bone remodeling or repair.

Gangji and associates[147] compared the replicative capacity of bone cells retrieved from biopsy samples obtained during core decompression and from the iliac crest of patients with osteonecrosis and compared them with bone cells obtained from patients with osteoarthritis. The proliferation rate of cells retrieved from the intertrochanteric region of the osteonecrotic femur was significantly slower than that of the cells retrieved from the osteoarthritic femoral heads ($P = 0.031$). In contrast, the cells taken from the iliac crest of patients with osteonecrosis had faster proliferation rates than the femoral cells and behaved similarly to cells taken from the femurs and from the iliac crest of the patients with osteoarthritis. There were no statistical differences in alkaline phosphatase activity or in collagen synthesis between patients with osteonecrosis and those with osteoarthritis, although both the basal level and 1,25 dihydroxyvitamin D_3 stimulated level of the patients with osteonecrosis were lower than those of the patients with osteoarthritis; moreover, collagen synthesis was slightly higher in patients with osteonecrosis. The authors suggested that their findings concerning proliferation rates and biochemistries may have an impact on the onset of osteonecrosis itself or in the bone repair that occurs following the insult. They did not find a change in the osteoblast phenotype.

Alcohol-Associated Osteonecrosis
The effect of alcohol on mesenchymal stem cells has been studied in cells retrieved from humans and in a rabbit model. Suh and associates[148] found a significant increase in the doubling time and a significant decrease in the osteogenic differentiation ability (as determined by alkaline phosphatase activity) in mesenchymal stem cells from patients with alcohol-associated osteonecrosis compared with the doubling time and osteogenic differentiation ability in cells from patients with femoral neck fractures. There was no significant difference between the groups with respect to adipogenic differentiation ability (as determined by assay of Oil Red O staining). Wang and associates[149] studied the effect of alcohol administered daily to New Zealand white rabbits for up to 6 months. Alcohol treatment resulted in elevations of serum lipid peroxides, triglycerides, and cholesterol level and a reduction in superoxide dismutase. Within the femoral head, fat cell hypertrophy and proliferation, diminished hematopoiesis, and an increased percentage of empty lacunae were noted. Using electron microscopy, low-density lipid droplets were ob-

served in the subchondral osteocytes. In mouse bone marrow stromal cell cultures, they found decreasing levels of alkaline phosphatase activity and osteocalcin release with increasing levels of ethanol. Using cell morphology and the appearance of cytoplasmic lipid droplets within the cell to assess adipocyte differentiation, they reported increasing numbers of adipocytes with increasing ethanol concentration. Both of these studies are limited by the methodology chosen to determine adipogenesis; further study using cell or genetic markers is warranted.

There are conflicting reports as to whether bone cell apoptosis occurs in alcohol-associated osteonecrosis. Weinstein and associates[75] reported that apoptotic bone cells were rare in the femoral heads of this patient population. In contrast, Calder and associates[72] noted apoptosis in the bone cells within the femoral head of the patients with alcohol-associated osteonecrosis that they evaluated. Both of these studies were limited by the number of patients with alcohol-associated osteonecrosis patients that were included (only three patients in each study). Further study of this patient subset as well as patients with other established or unknown (idiopathic) etiologies is required.

Cell Modulators
As demonstrated histologically, there is an attempt to repair the osteonecrotic lesions by creeping substitution. Although there are some reports of healing, or at least a reduction of the size of the lesion, these reports are relatively rare,[150-152] and most lesions do not heal. It is unclear what contributes to this inhibition or cessation of repair. Several different mechanisms

may be involved, but a better understanding of bone cell physiology and the modulation of cell activity in the healthy cell compared with the pathologic cell is needed. Little is known about what modulators are present in the zone surrounding the necrotic lesion and how they are regulated. It may be possible to glean some insight into this process from the results of experience with nonvascularized bone graft.

Enneking and Campanacci[104] described the pathology of retrieved human allografts. Characterizing the cancellous-cancellous junctions (a region most similar to the environment of the interface surrounding the osteonecrotic lesion), they noted fibrovascular repair that invaded the marrow spaces of the allograft. There was evidence of creeping substitution, and seams of reparative bone on the surfaces of the trabeculae of the allograft produced thickened trabeculae that were radiodense. The repair penetrated into the allograft approximately 2 to 4 mm. Farther into the graft, the original architecture was preserved, and the marrow spaces were filled with dense hypovascular fibrous tissue. Deeper yet, there were acellular remnants of fatty marrow. What is striking about this is the similarity of this description to pathologic descriptions of osteonecrotic lesions. Enneking and Campanacci suggested that the repair of the graft may be limited by host reparative fibrovascular tissue that appeared to block additional penetration of the allograft.[104] With respect to osteonecrosis, Schroer[21] also suggested that a thick scar of fibrous tissue could isolate the necrotic lesion from viable tissue, thereby preventing the penetration of revascularization of the damaged tissue. This type of response is found frequently in biologic responses to infectious agents and foreign bodies. It is plausible that the body's response to the necrotic segment may actually contribute to the pathology associated with osteonecrosis.

It is also possible that the body has a limited capacity to traverse an open space or a certain thickness of dead bone. Animal studies have proven that there is a critical distance that bone can bridge.[153] Studies of bone graft have shown that the innermost regions of structural grafts remain unrepaired after extensive periods of time.[104,154] This limitation may reflect hindrance to a decreasing oxygen supply at the outer limits of revascularization.

A limited capacity to repair an osteonecrotic lesion may reflect abnormal cell regulation. Studies of fracture healing and bone graft incorporation have identified several cytokines, enzymes, and other proteins that can influence bone repair and remodeling.[155] Khan and associates[106] have reported that tumor necrosis factor, fibroblast growth factor, platelet-derived growth factor, insulin-like growth factor, transforming growth factor-β, and bone morphogenetic proteins-2, -4, and -7 influence graft incorporation and bone healing. Matrix metalloproteinases also play a role. Henle and associates[99] suggest that delays in bone healing or even nonunion may be related to the concentrations of matrix metalloproteinases or their behavior over time. They also propose that an altered balance of the matrix metalloproteinase/tissue inhibitor of metalloproteinase system in favor of proteolytic activity may be involved in the pathophysiologic processes leading to fracture nonunion. It would be of interest to know whether the mechanism(s) involved in nonunions associated

with fracture healing are also involved in the biologic response to osteonecrotic lesions.

Smith[156] speculates whether angiogenesis is inhibited in osteonecrosis and states that glucocorticoids and interferons used to treat some of the comorbidities associated with osteonecrosis are inhibitors of angiogenesis. Neovascularization encourages the healing process in bone healing and graft incorporation. Vascular endothelial growth factor (VEGF) plays a primary role in stimulating angiogenesis in these instances[107,150,155,157,158] and has been shown to stimulate osteogenesis.[159,160] Hypoxia results in increased VEGF mRNA expression and, consequently, VEGF production.[161] Hypoxia activates the transcription factor hypoxia-inducible factor-1α and consequently increases VEGF expression in fracture repair.[158] VEGF has been detected in the proliferative zone above the necrotic hypertrophic zone in an animal model of Legg-Calvé-Perthes disease.[162] In adult patients with osteonecrosis, VEGF was primarily detected in the edematous area but was also noted in the marrow fibrosis area.[163] Of note was that VEGF was not detected in the transition zone between the necrotic segment and the edematous zone. The factors that may contribute to the lack of VEGF in the transitional zone remain to be defined.

Some of the necrotic cysts have been described as having an appearance of saponified fat,[93] which reflects the rupture of adipocytes.[61] There have been several hypotheses as to the role of the marrow fat cells in the pathogenesis of osteonecrosis that focus primarily on a potential role in venous congestion caused by increasing lipocyte number and size. Additionally, the necrosis of the fat

cells may release substances that inhibit bone formation, angiogenesis, or the distribution of factors that promote these activities. Further study is needed.

The changing biomechanical environment surrounding the osteonecrotic lesion may also influence the repair process. The intraosseous biomechanics are altered by the accumulation of unrepaired microfractures, the fibrovascular scar, and the presence of sclerosis. The effect of these variables on the biologic response is unknown for osteonecrosis, but it is known to have a significant impact in other bone pathologies.

Repair may also be hindered through a loss of the effectors of osteogenesis. As previously discussed, mesenchymal stem cells may be shunted to the adipocyte lineage, thereby decreasing the pool of osteoblasts needed.[131,132] An increase in osteoblast apoptosis with no effect on osteoclast viability may also unbalance the remodeling unit; however, the presence of a sclerotic rim suggests that osteoblasts are able to form bone in response to the lesion.

Genetics

It has been frequently suggested that osteonecrosis is a multifactorial disease and that certain individuals are more at risk or may be predisposed. Following this hypothesis, some patients may have a genetic predisposition to develop osteonecrosis after they are exposed to agents that serve as a secondary trigger. If this is true, it would explain why most patients exposed to known risk factors, such as corticosteroids and alcohol, do not develop osteonecrosis. Recently, researchers have explored several gene candidates that may play a role in the pathogenesis of osteonecrosis.

As discussed previously, patients with abnormal levels of coagulation factors associated with either thrombophilia or hypofibrinolysis may be at risk for osteonecrosis.[79-82] Abnormal levels of coagulation factors can be related to the other comorbidities associated with osteonecrosis (systemic lupus erythematosus) or treatments of osteonecrosis (corticosteroid therapy). Some of these coagulation alterations may also be the result of autosomal dominant disorders. Several investigators have shown a possible relationship between osteonecrosis and gene mutations for factor V Leiden,[164-166] the plasminogen activator inhibitor-1,[110,167,168] and methylenetetrahydrofolate reductase,[168,169] and prothrombin-genetic mutations associated with thrombophilia and hypofibrinolysis.[164-166]

In a recent report by Liu and associates,[170] a rare form of the disease—familial osteonecrosis—was identified in three families with 32 living members in whom osteonecrosis was diagnosed. They reported that all patients with familial osteonecrosis carried COL2A1 gene mutations. Patients with the sporadic form (nonfamilial) did not have these mutations. The role that a mutation in a gene for type II collagen may have in the development of osteonecrosis is yet to be defined.

Asano and associates[171] suggested that a mutation in a gene for the drug-transport protein, P-glycoprotein, may be associated with the development of osteonecrosis. In a study of 136 patients who underwent kidney transplantation (30 with osteonecrosis, 106 without osteonecrosis), they evaluated single-nucleotide polymorphisms in the multidrug-resistance gene 1 (ABCB1, MDR1). Patients with the ABCB1 3435TT genotype showed a significantly lower incidence of osteonecrosis. The incidence of osteonecrosis was higher in patients following the large-dose protocol. There was also evidence that the pump activity of P-glycoprotein is increased in 3435TT and, therefore, may result in increases in intracellular steroid concentrations in specific tissues.

In a study of alcoholic patients with hip osteonecrosis, Chao and associates[114] proposed that genetic polymorphisms in an alcohol-metabolizing enzyme may influence whether a patient develops osteonecrosis. Polymorphisms of several alcohol-metabolizing enzymes were evaluated in alcoholics with hip osteonecrosis, pancreatitis, cirrhosis of the liver, and combinations thereof. With respect to liver alcohol dehydrogenase, the alleles ADH2*1 and ADH2*2 were evaluated. The frequency of the allele ADH2*1 was significantly lower for the osteonecrosis group compared with the frequency of the alcoholic-cirrhosis group but not that of the alcoholic-pancreatitis group. These findings suggest that specific subpopulations of alcoholics may be more at risk to develop osteonecrosis than others.

The findings of these genetic studies may not only lead to a better understanding of the pathogenesis of osteonecrosis, but may also allow clinicians to screen for patients at risk. If this can be achieved, it may allow the initiation of measures that can delay disease progression and may have significant implications in pharmacologic treatment.

Summary

There are several potential risk factors that have been indicated for osteonecrosis. It is plausible that these risk factors work through different pathophysiologic mechanisms that converge to lead to the clinical entity known as osteonecrosis. Because a large percentage of patients with osteonecrosis have either received corticosteroid therapy or consume excessive amounts of alcohol, most of the research has focused on identifying the mechanisms that may be involved with these factors. For these potential etiologies, theories have ranged from direct effects on bone cells (toxicity and apoptosis) to indirect effects such as venous congestion resulting from disturbances in the intraosseous extravascular compartment. Both corticosteroids and alcohol have been shown to have specific effects on bone cells and their precursors. Whether these effects play a role in the initiation of the osteonecrotic lesion or the response to the lesion remains to be determined. Recent findings have identified mutations in the genes encoding for proteins within the cellular machinery associated with corticosteroid transport or alcohol metabolism. Further study is needed to determine whether these ultimately affect osteocyte health in vivo. Findings from future studies may have implications for both the understanding of osteonecrosis as well as the ability of clinicians to predict who may be at risk.

References

1. ARCO (Association Research Circulation Osseous): Committee on Terminology and Classification. ARCO News 1992;4:41-46.

2. Marcus ND, Enneking WF, Massam RA: The silent hip in idiopathic aseptic necrosis: Treatment by bone grafting. J Bone Joint Surg Am 1973;55:1351-1366.

3. Steinberg ME, Hayden GD, Steinberg DR: A quantitative system for staging avascular necrosis. J Bone Joint Surg Br 1995;77:34-41.

4. Ficat P, Arlet J: Necrosis of the femoral head, in Hungerford DS (ed): Ischemia

and Necroses of Bone. Baltimore, MD, Williams & Wilkins, 1980, pp 53-74.

5. Ohzono K, Saito M, Sugano N, Takaoka K, Ono K: The fate of nontraumatic avascular necrosis of the femoral head: A radiologic classification to formulate prognosis. Clin Orthop Relat Res 1992;277:73-78.

6. Bradway JK, Morrey BF: The natural history of the silent hip in bilateral atraumatic osteonecrosis. J Arthroplasty 1993;8:383-387.

7. Jergesen HE, Khan AS: The natural history of untreated asymptomatic hips in patients who have non-traumatic osteonecrosis. J Bone Joint Surg Am 1997;79:359-363.

8. Ito H, Matsuno T, Omizu N, Aoki Y, Minami A: Mid-term prognosis of non-traumatic osteonecrosis of the femoral head. J Bone Joint Surg Br 2003;85:796-801.

9. Ohzono K, Saito M, Takaoka K, Ono K, Nishina T, Kadowaki T: Natural history of nontraumatic avascular necrosis of the femoral head. J Bone Joint Surg Br 1991;73:68-72.

10. LaPorte DM, Mont MA, Mohan V, Jones LC, Hungerford DS: Multifocal osteonecrosis. J Rheumatol 1998;25:1968-1974.

11. Inoue A, Ono K: A histological study of idiopathic avascular necrosis of the head of the femur. J Bone Joint Surg Br 1979;61:138-143.

12. Yamamoto T, DiCarlo EF, Bullough PG: The prevalence and clinicopathological appearance of extension of osteonecrosis in the femoral head. J Bone Joint Surg Br 1999;81:328-332.

13. Kim YM, Rhyu KH, Lee SH, Kim HJ: Can osteonecrosis of the femoral head be recurrent? Clin Orthop Relat Res 2003;406:123-128.

14. Calandruccio RA, Anderson WE III: Post-fracture avascular necrosis of the femora head: Correlation of experimental and clinical studies. Clin Orthop Relat Res 1980;152:49-84.

15. Fink B, Degenhardt S, Paselk C, Schneider T, Modder U, Ruther W: Early detection of avascular necrosis of the femoral head following renal transplantation. Arch Orthop Trauma Surg 1997;116:151-156.

16. Koo KH, Kim R, Kim YS, et al: Risk period for developing osteonecrosis of the femoral head in patients on steroid treatment. Clin Rheumatol 2002;21:299-303.

17. Oinuma K, Harada Y, Nawata Y, et al: Osteonecrosis in patients with systemic lupus erythematosus develops very early after starting high dose corticosteroid treatment. Ann Rheum Dis 2001;60:1145-1148.

18. Hernigou P, Bachir D, Galacteros F: The natural history of symptomatic osteonecrosis in adults with sickle-cell disease. J Bone Joint Surg Am 2003;85:500-504.

19. Koo K-H, Kim R, Ko G-H: Preventing collapse in early osteonecrosis of the femoral head: A randomized clinical trial of core decompression. J Bone Joint Surg Br 1995;77:870-874.

20. Stulberg BN, Davis AW, Bauer TW: Osteonecrosis of the femoral head: A prospective randomized treatment protocol. Clin Orthop Relat Res 1991;268:140-151.

21. Schroer WC: Current concepts on the pathogenesis of osteonecrosis of the femoral head. Orthop Rev 1994;23:487-497.

22. Assouline-Dayan Y, Chang C, Greenspan A, Shoenfeld Y, Gershwin ME: Pathogenesis and natural history of osteonecrosis. Semin Arthritis Rheum 2002;32:94-124.

23. Chang CC, Greenspan A, Gershwin ME: Osteonecrosis: Current perspectives on pathogenesis and treatment. Semin Arthritis Rheum 1993;23:47-69.

24. Hungerford DS: Pathogenetic considerations in ischemic necrosis of bone. Can J Surg 1981;24:583-587.

25. Lavernia CJ, Sierra RJ, Grieco FR: Osteonecrosis of the femoral head. J Am Acad Orthop Surg 1999;7:250-261.

26. Jones JP Jr: Risk factors potentially activating intravascular coagulation and causing nontraumatic osteonecrosis, in: Urbaniak JR, Jones Jr JP (eds): Osteonecrosis: Etiology, Diagnosis and Treatment. Rosemont, IL, American Academy of Orthopaedic Surgeons, 1997, pp 89-96.

27. Ficat RP, Arlet J: Bone necroses with probable etiologic relationships, in Hungerford DS (ed): Ischemia and Necroses of Bone. Baltimore, MD, Williams & Wilkins, 1977, pp 131-161.

28. Orlic D, Jovanovic S, Anticevic D, Zecevic J: Frequency of idiopathic aseptic necrosis in medially treated alcoholics. Int Orthop 1990;14:383-386.

29. Zizic TM, Marcoux C, Hungerford DS, Dangereau JV, Stevens MB: Corticosteroid therapy associated with ischemic necrosis of bone in systemic lupus erythematosus. Am J Med 1985;79:596-604.

30. Jones JP: Epidemiological risk factors for nontraumatic osteonecrosis. Orthopaede 2000;29:370-379.

31. Kenzora JE, Glimcher MJ: Accumulative cell stress: The multifactorial etiology of idiopathic osteonecrosis. Orthop Clin North Am 1985;16:669-679.

32. Gerster JC, Camus JP, Chave JP, Koeger AC, Rappoport G: Multiple site avascular necrosis in HIV infected patients. J Rheumatol 1991;18:300-302.

33. Goorney BP, Lacey H, Thurairajasingam S, Brown JD: Avascular necrosis of the hip in a man with HIV infection. Genitourin Med 1990;66:451-452.

34. Schwartz O, Pindborg JJ, Svenningsen A: Tooth exfoliation and necrosis of the alveolar bone following trigeminal herpes zoster in HIV-infected patient. Tandlaegebladet 1989;93:623-627.

35. Tschakaloff A, Schahn E, Wagner W: Acute necrotizing bone destruction of the maxillary and mandibular midline area in HIV infection cases. Dtsch Z Mund Kiefer Gesichtschir 1989;13:249-251.

36. Calza L, Manfredi R, Mastroianni A, Chiodo F: Osteonecrosis and highly active antiretroviral therapy during HIV infection: Report of a series and literature review. AIDS Patient Care STDS 2001;15:385-389.

37. Gutierrez F, Padilla S, Ortega E, et al: Avascular necrosis of the bone in HIV-infected patients: Incidence and associated factors. AIDS 2002;16:481-483.

38. Keruly JC, Chaisson RE, Moore RD: Increasing incidence of avascular necrosis of the hip in HIV-infected patients. J Acquir Immune Defic Syndr 2001;28:101-102.

39. Miller KD, Masur H, Jones EC, et al: High prevalence of osteonecrosis of the femoral head in HIV-infected adults. Ann Intern Med 2002;137:17-25.

40. Roudiere L, Viard JP: Osteonecrosis of the hip, lipodystrophy and antiretroviral treatment. AIDS 2000;14:2056.

41. Valencia ME, Barreiro P, Soriano V, Blanco F, Moreno V, Lahoz JG: Avascular necrosis in HIV-infected patients receiving antiretroviral treatment: Study of seven cases. HIV Clin Trials 2003;4:132-136.

42. Allison GT, Bostrum MP, Glesby MJ: Osteonecrosis in HIV disease: Epidemiology, etiologies, and clinical management. AIDS 2003;17:1-9.

43. Blacksin MF, Kloser PC, Simon J: Avascular necrosis of bone in human immunodeficiency virus infected patients. *Clin Imaging* 1999;23:314-318.

44. Glesby MJ, Hoover DR, Vaamonde CM: Osteonecrosis in patients infected with human immunodeficiency virus: A case-control study. *J Infect Dis* 2001;184:519-523.

45. Monier P, McKown K, Bronze MS: Osteonecrosis complicating highly active antiretroviral therapy in patients infected with human immunodeficiency virus. *Clin Infect Dis* 2000;31:1488-1492.

46. Montessori V, Press N, Harris M, Akagi L, Montaner JSG: Adverse effects of antiretroviral therapy for HIV infection. *CMAJ* 2004;170:229-238.

47. Scribner AN, Troia-Cancio PV, Cox BA, et al: Osteonecrosis in HIV: A case-control study. *J Acquir Immune Defic Syndr* 2000;25:19-25.

48. Sighinolfi L, Carradori S, Ghinelli F: Avascular necrosis of the femoral head: A side effect of highly active antiretroviral therapy (HAART) in HIV patients? *Infection* 2000;28:254-255.

49. Ries MD, Barcohana B, Davidson A, Jergesen HE, Paiement GD: Association between human immunodeficiency virus and osteonecrosis of the femoral head. *J Arthroplasty* 2002;17:135-139.

50. Centers for Disease Control and Prevention: Outbreak of severe acute respiratory syndrome: Worldwide, 2003. *MMWR Morb Mortal Wkly Rep* 2003;289:1775-1776.

51. Booth CM, Matukas LM, Tomlinson GA, et al: Clinical features and short-term outcomes of 144 patients with SARS in the greater Toronto area. *JAMA* 2003;289:2801-2809.

52. Hong N, Du XK: Avascular necrosis of bone in severe acute respiratory syndrome. *Clin Radiol* 2004;59:602-608.

53. Li YM, Wang SX, Gao HS, et al: Factors of avascular necrosis of femoral head and osteoporosis in SARS patients' convalescence *Zhonghua Yi Xue Za Zhi* 2004;84:1348-1353.

54. Griffith JF, Antonio GE, Kumta SM, et al: Osteonecrosis of hip and knee in patients with severe acute respiratory syndrome treated with steroids. *Radiology* 2005;235:168-175.

55. Li ZR, Sun W, Qu H, et al: Clinical research of correlation between osteonecrosis and steroid. *Zhonghua Wai Ke Za Zhi* 2005;43:1048-1053.

56. Shen J, Liang BL, Zeng QS, et al: Report on the investigation of lower extremity osteonecrosis with magnetic resonance imaging in recovered severe acute respiratory syndrome in Guangzhou. *Zhonghua Yi Xue Za Zhi* 2004;84:1814-1817.

57. Jones JP Jr: Etiology and pathogenesis of osteonecrosis. *Semin Arthroplasty* 1991;2:160-168.

58. Lieberman JR, Berry DJ, Mont MA, et al: Osteonecrosis of the hip: Management in the 21st century. *Instr Course Lect* 2003;52:337-355.

59. Meyers MH: Osteonecrosis of the femoral head: Pathogenesis and long-term results of treatment. *Clin Orthop Relat Res* 1988;231:51-61.

60. Mont MA, Jones LC, Sotereanos DG, Amstutz HC, Hungerford DS: Understanding and treating osteonecrosis of the femoral head. *Instr Course Lect* 2000;49:169-185.

61. Bauer TW, McCarthy JJ, Stulberg BN: Osteonecrosis of the femoral head: Histological diagnosis and findings after core biopsy, in Urbaniak JR, Jones Jr JP (eds): *Osteonecrosis: Etiology, Diagnosis and Treatment.* Rosemont, IL, American Academy of Orthopaedic Surgeons, 1997, pp 73-79.

62. Koo KH, Ahn IO, Kim R, et al: Bone marrow edema and associated pain in early stage osteonecrosis of the femoral head: prospective study with serial MR images. *Radiology* 1999;213:715-722.

63. Korompilias AV, Gilkeson GS, Seaber AV, Urbaniak JR: Hemorrhage and thrombus formation in early experimental osteonecrosis. *Clin Orthop Relat Res* 2001;386:11-18.

64. Kubo T, Yamamoto T, Inoue S, et al: Histological findings of bone marrow edema pattern on MRI in osteonecrosis of the femoral head. *J Orthop Sci* 2000;5:520-523.

65. Saito S, Inoue A, Ono K: Intramedullary haemorrhage as a possible cause of avascular necrosis of the femoral head: The histology of 16 femoral heads at the silent stage. *J Bone Joint Surg Br* 1987;69:346-351.

66. Jaffe WL, Epstein M, Heyman N, Mankin HJ: The effect of cortisone on femoral and humeral heads in rabbits. *Clin Orthop Relat Res* 1972;82:221-228.

67. Solomon L: Idiopathic necrosis of the femoral head: pathogenesis and treatment. *Can J Surg* 1981;24:573-578.

68. Wang GJ, Sweet DE, Reger SI, Thompson RC: Fat-cell changes as a mechanism of avascular necrosis of the femoral head in cortisone-treated rabbits. *J Bone Joint Surg Am* 1977;59:729-735.

69. Jones JP Jr: Fat embolism, intravascular coagulation, and osteonecrosis. *Clin Orthop Relat Res* 1993;292:294-308.

70. Starklint H, Lausten GS, Arnoldi CC: Microvascular obstruction in avascular necrosis: Immunohistochemistry of 14 femoral heads. *Acta Orthop Scand* 1995;66:9-12.

71. Zalavras C, Shah S, Birnbaum MJ, Frenkel B: Role of apoptosis in glucocorticoid-induced osteoporosis and osteonecrosis. *Crit Rev Eukaryot Gene Expr* 2003;13:221-235.

72. Calder JDF, Buttery L, Revell PA, Pearse M, Polak JM: Apoptosis: A significant cause of bone cell death in osteonecrosis of the femoral head. *J Bone Joint Surg Br* 2004;86:1209-1213.

73. Sato M, Sugano N, Ohzono K, et al: Apoptosis and expression of stress protein (ORP150, H01) during development of ischemic necrosis in the rat. *J Bone Joint Surg Br* 2001;83:751-759.

74. Shibahara M, Nishida K, Asahara H, et al: Increased osteocyte apoptosis during the development of femoral head osteonecrosis in spontaneously hypertensive rats. *Acta Med Okayama* 2000;54:67-74.

75. Weinstein RS, Nicholas RW, Manolagas SC: Apoptosis of osteocytes in glucocorticoid-induced osteonecrosis of the hip. *J Clin Endocrinol Metab* 2000;85:2907-2912.

76. Jones JP Jr, Sakovich L: Fat embolism of bone: A roentgenographic and histological investigation, with use of intra-arterial lipiodol in rabbits. *J Bone Joint Surg Am* 1966;48:149-164.

77. Gregg PJ, Walder DN: Regional distribution of circulating microspheres in the femur of the rabbit. *J Bone Joint Surg* 1980;62:222-226.

78. Kenzora JE: Ischemic necrosis of femoral head: Part I. Accumulative cell stress: A hypothesis for the etiology of idiopathic osteonecrosis. *Instr Course Lect* 1983;32:242-252.

79. Glueck CJ, Freiberg R, Glueck HI, et al: Hypofibrinolysis: A common, major cause of osteonecrosis. *Am J Hematol* 1994;45:156-166.

80. Glueck CJ, Freiberg R, Tracy T, Stroop D, Wang P: Thrombophilia and

hypofibrinolysis: Pathophysiologies of osteonecrosis. *Clin Orthop Relat Res* 1997;334:43-56.

81. Jones LC, Mont MA, Le TB, et al: Procoagulants and osteonecrosis. *J Rheumatol* 2003;30:783-791.

82. Korompilias AV, Ortel TL, Urbaniak JR: Coagulation abnormalities in patients with hip osteonecrosis. *Orthop Clin North Am* 2004;35:265-271.

83. Wilkes CH, Visscher MB: Some physiological aspects of bone marrow pressure. *J Bone Joint Surg Am* 1975;57:49-57.

84. Downey DJ, Simkin PA, Lanzer WL, Matsen FA II: Hydraulic resistance: A measure of vascular outflow obstruction in osteonecrosis. *J Orthop Res* 1988;6:272-278.

85. Ficat RP, Arlet J: The syndrome of bone ischemia, in Hungerford DS (ed): *Ischemia and Necroses of Bone*. Baltimore, MD, Williams & Wilkins; 1977, pp 75-102.

86. Lai KA, Shen WJ, Yang CY, Shao CJ, Hsu JT, Lin RM: The use of alendronate to prevent early collapse of the femoral head in patients with nontraumatic osteonecrosis: A randomized clinical study. *J Bone Joint Surg Am* 2005;87:2155-2159.

87. Cooper MS: Sensitivity of bone to glucocorticoids. *Clin Sci* 2004;107:111-123.

88. Cooper MS, Hewison M, Stewart PM: Glucocorticoid activity, inactivity and the osteoblast. *J Endocrinol* 1999;163:159-164.

89. Engelbrecht Y, de Wet H, Horsch K, Langeveldt CR, Hough FS, Hulley PA: Glucocorticoids induce rapid up-regulation of mitogen-activated protein kinase phosphatase-1 and dephosphorylation of extracellular signal-regulated kinase and impair proliferation in human and mouse osteoblast cell lines. *Endocrinology* 2003;144:412-422.

90. Kasperk C, Schneider U, Sommer U, Niethard F, Ziegler R: Differential effects of glucocorticoids on human osteoblastic cell metabolism in vitro. *Calcif Tissue Int* 1995;57:120-126.

91. Walsh S, Jordan GR, Jefferiss C, Stewart K, Beresford JN: High concentrations of dexamethasone suppress the proliferation but not the differentiation or further maturation of human osteoblast precursors in vitro: Relevance to glucocorticoid-induced osteoporosis. *Rheumatology* 2001;40:74-83.

92. Weinstein RS, Jilka RL, Parfitt AM, Manolagas SC: Inhibition of osteoblastogenesis and promotion of apoptosis of osteoblasts and osteocytes by glucocorticoids: Potential mechanisms of their deleterious effects on bone. *J Clin Invest* 1998;102:274-282.

93. Bullough PG: The morbid anatomy of subchondral osteonecrosis, in Urbaniak JR, Jones Jr JP (eds): *Osteonecrosis: Etiology, Diagnosis and Treatment*. Rosemont, IL, American Academy of Orthopaedic Surgeons; 1997, pp 69-72.

94. Mims CA: *The Pathogenesis of Infectious Disease*. New York, NY, Academic Press, 1991.

95. Bouletreau PJ, Warren SM, Spector JA, et al: Hypoxia and VEGF up-regulate BMP-2 mRNA and protein expression in microvascular endothelial cells: Implications for fracture healing. *Plast Reconstr Surg* 2002;109:2384-2397.

96. Dimitriou R, Tsiridis E, Giannoudis PV: Current concepts of molecular aspects of bone healing. *Injury* 2005;36:1392-1404.

97. Diwan AD, Wang MX, Jang D, Zhu W, Murrell GA: Nitric oxide modulates fracture healing. *J Bone Miner Res* 2000;15:342-351.

98. Gerstenfeld LC, Cullinane DM, Barnes GL, Graves DT, Einhorn TA: Fracture healing as a post-natal developmental process: Molecular, spatial, and temporal aspects of its regulation. *J Cell Biochem* 2003;88:873-884.

99. Henle P, Zimmermann G, Weiss S: Matrix metalloproteinases and failed fracture healing. *Bone* 2005;37:791-798.

100. Lehmann W, Edgar CM, Wang K, et al: Tumor necrosis factor alpha (TNF-alpha) coordinately regulates the expression of specific matrix metalloproteinases (MMPs) and angiogenic factors during fracture healing. *Bone* 2005;36:300-310.

101. Li X, Quigg RJ, Zhou J, Ryaby JT, Wang H: Early signals for fracture healing. *J Cell Biochem* 2005;95:189-205.

102. Simon Am: MAnigrasso MB, O'Connor JP. Cyclo-oxygenase 2 function is essential for bone fracture healing. *J Bone Miner Res* 2002;17:963-976.

103. Zhang X, Schwarz EM, Young DA, Puzas JE, Rosier RN, O'Keefe RJ: Cyclooxygenase-2 regulates mesenchymal cell differentiation into the osteoblast lineage and is involved in bone repair. *J Clin Invest* 2002;109:1405-1415.

104. Enneking WF, Campanacci DA: Retrieved human allografts: A

clinicopathological study. *J Bone Joint Surg Am* 2001;83:971-986.

105. Goldberg VM: The biology of bone grafts. *Orthopedics* 2003;26:923-924.

106. Khan SN, Cammisa FP, Sandhu HS, Diwan AD, Girardi FP, Lane JM: The biology of bone grafting. *J Am Acad Orthop Surg* 2005;13:77-86.

107. Rabie ABM, Lu M: Basic fibroblast growth factor up-regulates the expression of vascular endothelial growth factor during healing of allogeneic bone graft. *Arch Oral Biol* 2004;49:1025-1033.

108. Virolainen P, Elima K, Metsaranta M, Aro HT, Vuorio E: Incorporation of cortical bone allografts and autografts in rats: expression patterns of mRNAs for the TGF-betas. *Acta Orthop Scand* 1998;69:537-544.

109. Ferrari P, Schroeder V, Anderson S, et al: Association of plasminogen activator inhibitor-1 genotype with avascular osteonecrosis in steroid-treated renal allograft recipients. *Transplantation* 2002;74:1147-1152.

110. Glueck CJ, Fontaine RN, Gruppo R, et al: The plasminogen activator inhibitor-1 gene, hypofibrinolysis, and osteonecrosis. *Clin Orthop Relat Res* 1999;366:133-146.

111. Zalavras C, Malizos KN, Dokou E, Vartholomatos G: The 677C→T mutation of the methylene-tetrahydrofolate reductase gene in the pathogenesis of osteonecrosis of the femoral head. *Haematologica* 2002;87:111-112.

112. Zalavras C, Vartholomatos G, Dokou E, Malizos KN: Genetic background of osteonecrosis: Associated with thrombophilic mutations? *Clin Orthop Relat Res* 2004;422:251-255.

113. Liu Y-F, Chen W-M, Lin Y-F, et al: Type II collagen gene variants and inherited osteonecrosis of the femoral head. *N Engl J Med* 2005;352:2294-2301.

114. Asano T, Takahashi KA, Fujioka M, et al: ABCB1 C3435T and G2677T/A polymorphism decreased the risk for steroid-induced osteonecrosis of the femoral head after kidney transplantation. *Pharmacogenetics* 2003;13:675-682.

115. Chao YC, Wang SJ, Chu HC, Chang WK, Hsieh TY: Investigation of alcohol metabolizing enzyme genes in Chinese alcoholics with avascular necrosis of hip joint, pancreatitis and cirrhosis of the liver. *Alcohol Alcohol* 2003;38:431-436.

116. Jacobs B: Epidemiology of traumatic and nontraumatic osteonecrosis. *Clin Orthop Relat Res* 1978;130:51-67.

117. Wing PC, Nance P, Connell DG, Gagnon F: Risk of avascular necrosis following short term megadose methylprednisolone treatment. *Spinal Cord* 1998;36:633-636.

118. Wong GK, Poon WS, Chiu KH: Steroid-induced avascular necrosis of the hip in neurosurgical patients: Epidemiological study. *ANZ J Surg* 2005;75:409-410.

119. Maxwell SRJ, Moots RJ, Kendall MJ: Corticosteroids: Do they damage the cardiovascular system? *Postgrad Med J* 1994;70:863-870.

120. Nishimura T, Matsumoto T, Nishino M, Tomita K: Histopathologic study of veins in steroid treated rabbits. *Clin Orthop Relat Res* 1997;334:37-42.

121. Ichiseki T, Matsumoto T, Nishino M, Kaneuji A, Katsuda S: Oxidative stress and vascular permeability in steroid-induced osteonecrosis model. *J Orthop Sci* 2004;9:509-515.

122. Hirano K, Tsutsui H, Sugioka Y, Sueishi K: Histopathologic alterations of retinacular vessels and osteonecrosis. *Clin Orthop Relat Res* 1997;342:192-204.

123. Laroche M, Ludot R, Thiechart M, Viguier G, Dromer C, Maziéres B. Histological appearance of the intra-osseous vessels of the femoral head in aseptic osteonecrosis of the hip, with or without antiphospholipid antibodies. *Clin Rheumatol* 1997;16:367-371.

124. Saito S, Inoue A, Ono K: Intramedullary haemorrhage as a possible cause of avascular necrosis of the femoral head: The histology of 16 femoral heads at the silent stage. *J Bone Joint Surg Br* 1987;69:346-351.

125. Saito S, Ohzono K, Ono K: Early arteriopathy and postulated pathogenesis of osteonecrosis of the femoral head: The intracapital arterioles. *Clin Orthop Relat Res* 1992;277:98-110.

126. Bonewald LF: Osteocytes: A proposed multifunctional bone cell. *J Musculoskelet Neuronal Interact* 2002;2:239-241.

127. Cullinane DM: The role of osteocytes in bone regulation: Mineral homeostasis versus mechanoreception. *J Musculoskelet Neuronal Interact* 2002;2:242-244.

128. Noble BS, Stevens H, Loveridge N, Reeve J: Identification of apoptotic changes in osteocytes in normal and pathological human bone. *Bone* 1997;20:273-282.

129. O'Brien CA, Jia D, Plotkin LI, et al: Glucocorticoids act directly on osteoblasts and osteocytes to induce apoptosis and reduce bone formation and strength. *Endocrinology* 2004;145:1835-1841.

130. Hofbauer LC, Gori F, Riggs BL, et al: Stimulation of osteoprotegerin ligand and inhibition of osteoprotegerin production by glucocorticoids in human osteoblastic lineage cells: Potential paracrine mechanisms of glucocorticoid-induced osteoporosis. *Endocrinology* 1999;140:4382-4389.

131. Cui Q, Wang G-J, Balian G: Steroid-induced adipogenesis in a pluripotential celline from bone marrow. *J Bone Joint Surg Am* 1997;79:1054-1063.

132. Li X, Jin L, Cui Q, Wang G-J, Balian G: Steroid effects on osteogenesis through mesenchymal cell gene expression. *Osteoporos Int* 2005;16:101-108.

133. Gohel A, McCarthy M-B, Gronowicz G: Estrogen prevents glucocorticoid-induced apoptosis in osteoblasts in vivo and in vitro. *Endocrinology* 1999;140:5339-5347.

134. Gohel AR, Hand AR, Gronowicz GA: Immunogold localization of beta 1-integrin in bone: Effect of glucocorticoids and insulin-like growth factor I on integrins and osteocytes formation. *J Histochem Cytochem* 1995;43:1085-1096.

135. Gronowicz GA, Fall PM, Raisz LG: prostaglandin E2 stimulates preosteoblast replication: An autoradiographic study in cultured fetal rat calvariae. *Exp Cell Res* 1994;212:314-320.

136. Weinstein RS, Manolagas SC: Apoptosis and osteoporosis. *Am J Med* 2000;108:153-164.

137. Namkung-Matthäi: Seale JP, Brown K, Mason RS: Comparative effects of anti-inflammatory corticosteroids in human bone-derived osteoblast-like cells. *Eur Respir J* 1998;12:1327-1333.

138. Nakashima T, Sasaki H, Tsuboi M, et al: Inhibitory effect of glucocorticoid for osteoblast apoptosis induced by activated peripheral blood mononuclear cells. *Endocrinology* 1998;139:2032-2040.

139. Hirayama T, Sabokbar A, Athanasou NA: Effect of corticosteroids on human osteoclast formation and activity. *J Endocrinol* 2002;175:155-163.

140. Yang L, Tao T, Wang X, et al: Effects of dexamethasone on proliferation, differentiation and apoptosis of adult human osteoblasts in vitro. *Chin Med J (Engl)* 2003;116:1357-1360.

141. Pereira RM, Delany AM, Canalis E: Cortisol inhibits the differentiation and apoptosis of osteoblasts in culture. *Bone* 2001;28:484-490.

142. Chae HJ, Chae SW: Kang JS, et al: Dexamethasone suppresses tumor necrosis factor-alpha-induced apoptosis in osteoblasts: Possible role for ceramide. *Endocrinology* 2000;141:2904-2913.

143. Davies JH, Evans BA, Jenney ME, Gregory JW: In vitro effects of combination chemotherapy on osteoblasts: Implications for osteopenia in childhood malignancy. *Bone* 2002;31:319-326.

144. Lee H-S, Huang G-T, Chiang H, et al: Multipotential mesenchymal stem cells from femoral bone marrow near the site of osteonecrosis. *Stem Cells* 2003;21:190-199.

145. Hernigou P, Beaujean F: Abnormalities in the bone marrow of the iliac crest in patients who have osteonecrosis secondary to corticosteroid therapy or alcohol abuse. *J Bone Joint Surg Am* 1997;79:1047-1053.

146. Hernigou P, Beaujean F, Lambotte JC: Decrease in the mesenchymal stem-cell pool in the proximal femur in corticosteroid-induced osteonecrosis. *J Bone Joint Surg Br* 1999;81:349-355.

147. Gangji V, Hauzeur J-P, Schoutens A, Hinsenkamp M, Appelboom T, Egrise D: Abnormalities in the replicative capacity of osteoblastic cells in the proximal femur of patients with osteonecrosis of the femoral head. *J Rheumatol* 2003;30:348-351.

148. Suh KT, Kim SW, Roh HL, Youn MS, Jung JS: Decreased osteogenic differentiation of mesenchymal stem cells in alcohol-induced osteonecrosis. *Clin Orthop Relat Res* 2005;431:220-225.

149. Wang Y, Li Y, Mao K, Li J, Cui Q, Wang G-J: Alcohol-induced adipogenesis in bone and marrow: A possible mechanism for osteonecrosis. *Clin Orthop Relat Res* 2003;410:213-224.

150. Ito H, Matsuno T, Omizu N, Aoki Y, Minami A: Mid-term prognosis of non-traumatic osteonecrosis of the femoral head. *J Bone Joint Surg Br* 2003;85:796-801.

151. Kopecky KK, Braunstein EM, Brandt KD: Apparent avascular necrosis of the hip: Appearance and spontaneous resolution of MR findings in renal

allograft recipients. *Radiology* 1991;179:523-527.

152. Sakamoto M, Shimizu K, Iida S, Akita T, Moriya H, Nawata Y: Osteonecrosis of the femoral head: A prospective study with MRI. *J Bone Joint Surg Br* 1997;79:213-219.

153. Hollinger JO, Kleinschmidt JC: The critical size defect as an experimental model to test bone repair materials. *J Craniofac Surg* 1990;1:60-68.

154. Tomford WV, Mankin HJ: Massive bone allografts, in Urist MR, O'Connor BT, Burwell RG (eds): *Bone Grafts, Derivatives & Substitutes*. Boston, MA, Butterworth-Heinemann, 1994, pp 187-192.

155. Gray JC, Elves MW: Early osteogenesis in compact bone isografts: A quantitative study of contributions of the different graft cells. *Calcif Tissue Int* 1979;29:225-237.

156. Smith DWE: Is avascular necrosis of the femoral head the result of inhibition of angiogenesis? *Med Hypotheses* 1997;49:497-500.

157. Gamradt SC, Lieberman JR: Bone graft for revision hip arthroplasty: Biology and future applications. *Clin Orthop Relat Res* 2003;417:183-194.

158. Komatsu DE, Hadjiargyrou M: Activation of the transcription factor HIF-1 and its target genes, VEGF, HO-1, iNOS, during repair. *Bone* 2004;34:680-688.

159. Furumatsu T, Shen ZN, Kawai A, et al: Vascular endothelial growth factor principally acts as the main angiogenic factor in early stage of human osteoblastogenesis. *J Biochem (Tokyo)* 2003;133:633-639.

160. Gerber HP, Vu TH, Ryan AM, Kowalski J, Werb Z, Ferrara N: VEGF couples hypertrophic cartilage remodeling, ossification and angiogenesis during endochondral bone formation. *Nat Med* 1999;5:623-628.

161. Steinbrech DS, Mehrara BJ, Saadeh PB, et al: VEGF expression in an osteoblast-like cell line is regulated by a hypoxia response mechanism. *Am J Physiol Cell Physiol* 2000;278:C853-C860.

162. Kim HKW, Bian H, Randall T, Garces A, Gerstenfeld LC, Einhorn TA: Increased VEGF expression in the epiphyseal cartilage after ischemic necrosis of the capital femoral epiphysis. *J Bone Miner Res* 2004;19:2041-2048.

163. Radke S, Battman A, Jatzke S, Eulert J, Jakob F, Schutze N: Expression of the angiomatrix and angiogenic proteins CYRG1, CTGF, and VEGF in osteonecrosis of the femoral head. *J Orthop Res* 2006;24:945-952.

164. Bjorkman A, Svensson PJ, Hillarp A, Burtscher IM, Runow A, Benoni G: Factor V Leiden and prothrombin gene mutation: Risk factors for osteonecrosis of the femoral head in adults. *Clin Orthop Relat Res* 2004;425:168-172.

165. Bjorkman A, Burtscher IM, Svensson PJ, Hillarp A, Besjakov J, Benoni G: Factor V Leiden and the prothrombin 20210A gene mutation and osteonecrosis of the knee. *Arch Orthop Trauma Surg* 2005;125:51-55.

166. Zalavras CG, Vartholomatos G, Dokou E, Malizos KN: Genetic background of osteonecrosis: Associated with thrombophilic mutations? *Clin Orthop Relat Res* 2004;422:251-255.

167. Ferrari P, Schroeder V, Anderson S, et al: Association of plasminogen activator inhibitor-1 genotype with avascular osteonecrosis in steroid-treated renal allograft recipients. *Transplantation* 2002;74:1147-1152.

168. Glueck CJ, Freiberg RA, Fontaine RN, Tracy T, Wang P: Hypofibrinolysis, thrombophilia, osteonecrosis. *Clin Orthop Relat Res* 2001;386:19-33.

169. Zalavras CG, Malizos KN, Dokou E, Vartholomatos G: The 677C T mutation of the methylene-tetra-hydrofolate reductase gene in the pathogenesis of osteonecrosis of the femoral head. *Haematologica* 2002;87:111-112.

170. Liu YF, Chen WM, Lin YF, et al: Type II collagen gene variants and inherited osteonecrosis of the femoral head. *N Engl J Med* 2005;352:2294-2301.

171. Asano T, Takahashi KA, Fujioka M, et al: ABCB1 C3435T and G2677T/A polymorphism decreased the risk for steroid-induced osteonecrosis of the femoral head after kidney transplantation. *Pharmacogenetics* 2003;13:675-682.

New Treatment Approaches for Osteonecrosis of the Femoral Head: An Overview

Michael A. Mont, MD
Lynne C. Jones, PhD
Thorsten M. Seyler, MD
German A. Marulanda, MD
Khaled J. Saleh, MD, MSc, FRCSC, FACS
Ronald E. Delanois, MD

Abstract

Osteonecrosis of the femoral head is a debilitating disease that ultimately leads to hip joint destruction. Various efforts have been made in an attempt to enhance the healing of osseous defects in the femoral head before collapse occurs. Examples of noninvasive treatment modalities include pharmacologic measures, electrical stimulation, shock wave therapy, and electromagnetic field therapy. In addition, biologic alternatives will induce new bone formation. Many of these agents or techniques are still undergoing preclinical and clinical trials, and some are not approved by the Food and Drug Administration for the treatment of osteonecrosis of the femoral head. It is important to review new treatment opportunities that are currently available or on the horizon.

Instr Course Lect 2007;56:197-212.

Osteonecrosis of the femoral head is a devastating disease that often leads to total hip arthroplasty.[1-3] Despite the continuous advances in prosthetic design and surgical technique, total hip arthroplasty is still a less than optimal choice for young patients with this disease. Thus, for these patients a reasonable goal

would be to delay the need for arthroplasty and preserve the joint. The results of joint-preserving procedures vary and ways of enhancing their efficacy are being intensively studied.

Various alternatives using growth and differentiation factors, such as bone morphogenetic proteins (BMPs), have been used in efforts to preserve the femoral head. Noninvasive treatment modalities include pharmacologic measures, electromagnetic field therapy, electrical stimulation, and shock wave therapy. Short-term follow-up for many

of these methods has demonstrated promising results in delaying the need for total hip arthroplasty.

This chapter will describe the use of nonsurgical modalities, new surgical approaches and the use of biologic substrates to preserve the femoral head (Table 1). Nonsurgical treatments include pharmacologic measures,[4-12] hyperbaric oxygen treatment,[13,14] electrical stimulation with direct current,[15-21] pulsed electromagnetic field therapy,[2,20-28] and extracorporeal shock wave therapy.[29-39] Surgical modalities will include cementation of the femoral head,[40-45] arthrodiastasis,[46-50] and the use of tantalum.[51-54] (T Gruen, MD, MJ Christie, MD, AD Hanssen, MD and R Lewis, MD, A Unger, MD, Dallas, TX, unpublished data presented at the AAOS Annual Meeting, 2002). The biologic substrates described will include demineralized bone matrix,[55-61] BMPs,[62-82] various growth factors,[80,81,83-97] stem cell therapy,[98-104] and gene therapy.[108-115] These methods can be used alone or

Table 1
Overview and Indications for New Treatment Approaches for Osteonecrosis*

Treatment Modality	Treatment Type	Indication
Pharmacologic Treatment		
Naftidrofuryl	Nonsurgical	Precollapse
Statins	Nonsurgical	Precollapse
Stanozolol	Nonsurgical	Precollapse
Heparin	Nonsurgical	Precollapse
Coumadin	Nonsurgical	Precollapse
Enoxaparin	Nonsurgical	Precollapse
Iloprost	Nonsurgical	Precollapse
Bisphosphonates	Nonsurgical	Precollapse
Innovative Nonsurgical Approaches		
Pulsed electromagnetic fields	Nonsurgical	Precollapse
Electrical stimulation with current	Nonsurgical/ Surgical	Precollapse
Extracorporal shock wave therapy	Nonsurgical	Precollapse
Hyperbaric oxygen therapy	Nonsurgical	Precollapse
Innovative Surgical Approaches		
Cementation femoral head	Surgical	Precollapse/early collapse
Tantalum	Surgical	Precollapse/early collapse
Arthrodiastasis	Surgical	Precollapse/early collapse
Biologic Treatment Modalities		
Demineralized bone matrix	Surgical	Precollapse/early collapse
Bone morphogenetic proteins	Surgical	Precollapse/early collapse
Transforming growth factor-β	Surgical	Precollapse/early collapse
Fibroblast growth factor	Surgical	Precollapse/early collapse
Insulin-like growth factor	Surgical	Precollapse/early collapse
Platelet-derived growth factor	Surgical	Precollapse/early collapse
Vascular endothelial growth factor	Surgical	Precollapse/early collapse
Mesenchymal stem cells	Surgical	Precollapse/early collapse

*For most new treatment modalities, the results of both preclinical animal and clinical human studies are very promising. The data in the literature are insufficient and more long-term results are needed to confirm the efficacy of these new treatment approaches.

in combination in the future based on results from evidence-based medicine in efforts to determine their true efficacy.

Nonsurgical Treatment Modalities for Osteonecrosis
Pharmacologic Measures
Various pharmacologic agents have been used throughout the years in an attempt to treat and prevent osteonecrosis of the femoral head.[3] These agents all have possible efficacy in the early stages of the disease before femoral head collapse. Treating patients with pharmacologic agents after the appearance of a crescent sign (collapse of the femoral head) or biomechanical compromise would not appear to be appropriate. The rationale for using pharmacologic agents is that they help correct pathophysiologic features of the disease, as well as allow revascularization or new bone formation. Information on the use of these agents has for the most part been gained through anecdotal reports, although recently a few prospective studies have been done. The following section will describe the use of lipid-lowering agents, vasodilators, prostacyclin analogs, various types of anticoagulants, and the use of bisphosphonates. The rationale for the use of each of these agents will be discussed along with what has been reported in terms of efficacy for the treatment of early stages of osteonecrosis. The pathophysiology of this disease is discussed in chapter 20 (Jones/Pathophysiology of Osteonecrosis).

Vasodilators have been used in the treatment of this disease on the theory that certain patients will have associated hypertension and these agents can further enhance the vascularization of ischemic areas. Zizic and associates (unpublished data) have observed a reduction in intraosseous pressure intraoperatively when patients were treated with vasodilators while performing a core decompression. In addition, a study by Arlet and associates[4] on the use of naftidrofuryl showed a reduction in bone marrow pressure in six of nine patients, without alteration of systemic pressure. It appears that there might be a scientific basis for using vasodilators in some patients; however, future prospective randomized studies are needed to determine their true efficacy.

Many patients who have osteonecrosis in association with systemic lupus erythematosus or other associated diseases will have high lipid levels or hypercholesterolemia. Lipid-lowering agents would reduce lipid levels in the blood and can either prevent osteonecrosis or treat the disease in its early stages. In addition, alterations in lipid metabolism have been implicated in the pathophysiology of the disease and various lipid-lowering agents may aid in this mechanism. An animal study by Motomura and associates[5] showed that lipid-lowering agents in combination with anticoagulants lower the risk of corticosteroid-associated osteonecrosis. Pritchett[113] studied 284 patients who were taking high-dose corticosteroids. Prolonged corticosteroid use produces a hyperlipidemic state that places patients at risk for osteonecrosis. The study analyzed patients who were using various statin drugs at the time they were started on high-dose corticosteroids and assessed the development of osteonecrosis. After a mean of 7.5 years (minimum follow-up, 5 years), only three patients (1%) from the statin group developed osteonecrosis. This 1% incidence is much less than the 3% to 20% incidence usually reported for patients receiving high-dose corticosteroids. Statins might offer protection against this disease when corticosteroid treatment is necessary. Because many of these medications (vasodilators and statins) cause few side effects and adverse events, these agents have been used for the prophylactic treatment of patients who require corticosteroids for systemic lupus erythematosus.

As discussed in chapter 20, many patients with osteonecrosis have associated disorders of hypofibrinolysis or thrombophilia. Various agents have been used to reverse these coagulation abnormalities. Stanozolol is an anabolic agent that decreases the amount of lipoprotein A, which has been associated with enhanced coagulation leading to arteriosclerosis and sludging of blood vessels.[114] Glueck and associates[6] reported the use of this agent in five patients with precollapse osteonecrosis and found a cessation of disease progression in the short term.

Other anticoagulants such as heparin or warfarin sodium also have been used in early stages of the disease. Glueck and associates[7] used enoxaparin in the treatment of patients with early stage osteonecrosis with thrombophilic-hypofibrinolytic disorders. After 2-year follow-up, 31 of 35 hips (88%) did not require surgery and maintained a precollapse state of disease without radiographic progression.

The use of anticoagulants such as heparin/warfarin sodium in a select group of patients with coagulation abnormalities needs further study, but appears to be a promising method of possibly preventing osteonecrosis or its progression in its early stages.

Iloprost is a prostacyclin analog, an effective inhibitor of platelet aggregation that promotes vascularization. It may be promising for the treatment of osteonecrosis. It has been most commonly used in two studies for the treatment of bone marrow edema syndrome, another disorder of the femoral head in which collapse can occur. Aigner and associates[8] compared the use of iloprost to core decompression in 36 patients with bone marrow edema syndrome. Iloprost was used in 17 patients (18 hips, mean age 49 years); a control group of 19 patients (20 hips, mean age 41 years) were treated with core decompression. After a mean follow-up of 11 months, all patients were evaluated clinically, radiographically, and with MRI. Hips treated with iloprost showed equal or better results than hips treated with core decompression. In a recent study by Meizer and associates,[9] 104 patients (mean age 53 years) with bone marrow edema syndrome of different localizations and etiologies were treated with iloprost. Bone marrow edema of the femoral head was treated in 18 of 104 patients. This study showed that the use of iloprost can help diminish pain at rest and during activity. Of the 104 patients with bone marrow edema, only 64.5% showed improvement between baseline MRI and follow-up MRI. It seems reasonable to believe that iloprost may promote vasodilatation and inhibit platelet aggregation to prevent collapse in osteonecrosis; however, further studies are needed.

Bisphosphonates are a group of agents that decrease osteoclastic resorption of bone and promote bone formation. They have been used in animal models of the disease as well as in a few recent prospective randomized studies. Rat, canine, and porcine studies have revealed that collapse of the femoral head may be reduced when treated with bisphosphonates.[12] In a recent prospective study, Agarwala and associates[10,115] treated 60 patients (100 hips) with osteonecrosis of the femoral head with the bisphosphonate alendronate. Follow-up ranged from 3 months to 5 years. Reduction in pain and disability scores as well as an increase in standing and walking time was significant at last follow-up. MRI evaluation showed a decrease of bone marrow edema in most patients, whereas radiographically hips either maintained the same stage or progressed by one stage. In another recent study by Lai and associates,[11] 20 patients (29 hips, mean patient age 43 years) were treated with alendronate and compared with a control group of 20 patients (25 hips, mean patient age 42 years). All patients had osteonecrosis of the femoral head and a large lesion. During the follow-up period from 24 to 28 months, only 2 of 29 hips (7%) treated with alendronate collapsed, whereas 19 of 25 hips (76%) in the control group collapsed. Total hip arthroplasty was performed in only 1 hip (3%) in the alendronate group at 26 months after the beginning of the treatment, compared with 16 of 25 hips (64%) in the control group that needed total hip arthroplasty during the treatment period. Further evaluation of these patients is necessary to see if these early efficacious effects will be maintained over the long term.

Additional clinical studies are needed to analyze the true efficacy of various pharmacologic agents in the prevention and treatment of osteonecrosis.

Hyperbaric Oxygen Treatment

Hyperbaric oxygen has been used to treat osteonecrosis of the femoral head, providing a ready source of oxygenation to prevent further death of bone and to promote healing.[116] The concept of hyperbaric oxygen therapy in orthopaedics is relatively new and remains highly controversial.[2,117]

Peskin and associates[13] examined the effects of hyperbaric oxygen therapy combined with no weight bearing in the treatment of osteonecrosis of the femoral head in rats. The authors stratified the study population in three groups. Group one included 16 rats treated with the combination of hyperbaric oxygen therapy and no weight bearing, group two included 20 rats treated solely with no weight bearing, and group three consisted of 18 rats who received no treatment regimen. Preservation and new bone forma-

tion of the femoral head was observed in a larger proportion in the group treated with hyperbaric oxygenation compared with the other two groups. Reis and associates[14] studied the effects of hyperbaric oxygen therapy on 12 selected patients with early-stage osteonecrosis of the femoral head as confirmed on MRI sequences. All patients received six daily sessions of hyberbaric oxygen therapy for a total of 100 consecutive days. At the conclusion of the study, 83% of the patients' femoral heads demonstrated a return to a nonpathologic state on MRI. In a meta-analysis of 15 reports, hyperbaric oxygen therapy showed superior results (81% success rate) compared with the outcomes of core decompression, osteotomy, bone grafting, electrical stimulation, and pharmacologic treatment (66% success rate) for early stage osteonecrosis.

Levin and associates[116] evaluated hyperbaric oxygen treatment in a model of vascular deprivation-induced necrosis of the femoral head in rats exposed to hyperbaric oxygen and compared it with untreated rats. There was no difference in new bone formation between both groups on the 2nd, 7th, and 21st days. Strauss[118] reported a meta-analysis of approximately 100 articles on hyperbaric oxygen therapy for osteonecrosis of the femoral head. He concluded that there are no superior outcomes of hyperbaric oxygen therapy compared with surgical treatment modalities for osteonecrosis of the femoral head.

Despite the present evidence of successful treatment of early-stage osteonecrosis with hyperbaric oxygen therapy in the scientific literature, additional studies are needed to assess the feasibility of this treatment on a larger scale.

Electrical Stimulation With Current

Various types of electrical stimulation have been used to stimulate osteoblasts, with the expectation that this method will lead to the formation of new bone and prevent collapse of the femoral head. In the treatment of osteonecrosis of the femoral head, it was first used in the 1980s and early 1990s to supplement core decompression and bone grafting.[15-19] In a less invasive surgical approach, electrodes were implanted in the femoral head after retrograde drilling of a small hole in the diseased bone. This is done in the hopes of creating new bone growth in the diseased area of the femoral head.[15,19]

Brighton and associates[21] analyzed the relationship between charge, current density, and the amount of bone formed in the medullary canal of the intact rabbit tibia. The findings of this study indicated that the amount of bone formed is directly related to both current density and charge. Trancik and associates[16] reported on 8 patients (11 hips) with precollapse osteonecrosis who were treated with electrical stimulation and followed a mean time of 3.5 years. Reoperation was required for 5 of 11 hips (45%) after a mean of 13 months after electrical stimulation. Further deterioration was found in the remaining six hips. Histologic examination of the retrieved femoral heads demonstrated only minimal evidence of new bone formation. This study showed that the treatment of osteonecrosis of the femoral head with electrical stimulation was ineffective in preventing disease progression in hips with early-stage osteonecrosis. In a study by Steinberg and associates,[119] capacitive coupling as an adjunct treatment of osteonecrosis of the femoral head was evaluated. In a case-control study of 40 patients treated with core decompression and grafting, capacitive coupling was used as an adjunct therapy in 20 patients. The patients were followed for 2 to 4 years and the results indicated that the addition of capacitive coupling did not improve outcome compared with core decompression and bone grafting alone.

Several studies have shown that electrical stimulation, when used in conjunction with treatment options such as core decompression and bone grafting, is effective in improving function of the femoral head and relieving pain.[15,17-20] Steinberg and associates[17] examined 42 hips at a minimum follow-up of 1 year after electrical stimulation in conjunction with core decompression and bone grafting. Most of the hips showed improved function and pain relief, although no effects of electrical stimulation on new bone formation could be noted at 1-year follow-up.

The treatment of osteonecrosis with electrical stimulation seems to be most effective in early-stage osteonecrosis and may promote clinical improvement, especially pain relief. However, long-term outcome studies are needed to evaluate the efficacy of this treatment.

Pulsed Electromagnetic Field Therapy

Modern bone growth stimulators use pulsed electromagnetic fields that affect disorders of dense connective tissue such as bone and tendons.[20,22] Electromagnetic fields have been used for more than 20 years in microwaves, cellular phones, and for MRI. Animal studies have shown the efficacy of pulsed magnetic fields in improving osteoblast activity. Cane and associates[23] investigated the healing process of

transcortical holes in the metacarpal bones in horse femurs. The pulsed electromagnetic fields were applied to the skin over the bone for 30 days, and then the metacarpal bones were evaluated histologically. The formation of new bone and mineral apposition rate were significantly greater in treated defects than in the control femurs, suggesting that electromagnetic fields stimulate bone repair and improve the osteogenic phase of the healing process.

In a preliminary report by Eftekhar and associates,[24] 24 patients (28 hips) with osteonecrosis of the femoral head were treated with pulsed electromagnetic fields and followed for a mean of 8 months (range, 6 to 36 months). Pain relief and improvement in hip function was noted in 19 of 23 patients (83%), who had reported moderate to severe pain before treatment. However, pain worsened in six postcollapse femoral heads after pulsed electromagnetic fields were applied, and two femoral heads experience progression of early-stage osteonecrosis. In a study by Lluch and associates,[25] 21 patients (30 hips) underwent noninvasively external electrostimulation by means of an electromagnetic field generator. The outcome was evaluated using MRI at 3-month intervals. Based on the size of the lesion, the overall success rate was 73.3%. Bassett and associates[26] treated 95 patients (118 hips) with a mean age of 38 years and an average follow-up time of 5.3 years. Based on radiographic analysis, the overall findings showed that patients with early-stage osteonecrosis had no progression of the disease and even experienced an improvement in grading. However, 103 hips with late-stage osteonecrosis did not improve and conditions worsened in 18.4% (19 hips). Seber and associ-

ates[27] reported the results of two patients (three hips) with early stage osteonecrosis treated with pulsed electromagnetic fields only. Pulsed electromagnetic fields were applied to both patients for 10 hours daily over a mean treatment time of 6 months. At 12-year follow-up all hips showed clinical improvement with no radiologic deterioration.

The use of pulsed electromagnetic waves in the treatment of osteonecrosis remains controversial. Several studies suggest that application of pulsed electromagnetic fields may be an alternative treatment modality in patients with early stages of osteonecrosis.[2,24-28]

Extracorporeal Shock Wave Therapy

The use of noninvasive shock wave therapy has been recently introduced to orthopaedics.[29] The use of shock wave therapy demonstrated consistent excellent results for the treatment of kidney and urethral stones. Over the past few years efforts have been made to treat patients with tendinitis and necrotic bone alterations. The mechanism by which shock wave treatment leads to bone regeneration is still unknown. It is believed that shock waves stimulate bone healing by causing microfractures in the necrotic area, inducing osteoblast activity and consequently revitalizing the affected bone.[29-32] In recent animal studies, it was shown that shock waves also promote neovascularization through an increased expression of endothelial nitric oxide synthase, vessel endothelial growth factor, and proliferating cell nuclear antigen.[33,34]

Gerdesmeyer and associates[37] found that the applied pressure of extracorporeal shock waves is almost diminished in dense bone and, consequently, questioned the value of this treatment modality in osteonecrosis. In an in vitro setting, Hausdorf and associates[38] analyzed the effect of extracorporeal shock-wave therapy in pig femurs. They postulated that a precise localization of the necrotic lesion of the femoral head seems to be crucial concerning the outcome of shock wave treatment.

Ludwig and associates[35] reported on 22 patients with osteonecrosis of the femoral head treated with extracorporeal shock waves. The clinical outcome was evaluated based on MRI findings, Harris hip scores, and pain in the affected hip joint. Significant therapeutic success was noted in 14 of 22 patients (64%) at 1-year follow-up. Wang and associates[36] studied 48 patients (mean age 40 years) with osteonecrosis of the femoral head. They stratified the study population in two groups: 23 patients (29 hips) were treated with shock waves and 25 patients (28 hips) underwent core decompression with bone grafting. After a mean follow-up of 25 months, the results showed an improvement in 23 of the 29 hips (79%) in the shock wave group, whereas only 8 of the 28 hips (29%) in the surgical group improved.

In short, shock wave therapy might alter the course of early stage osteonecrosis and lead to short-term pain relief, but needs further evaluation. Most reports are from Europe, where shock wave therapy has been used for the treatment of early disease.[39]

New Surgical Treatment Approaches
Cementation of the Femoral Head
The principle of using cementation of the femoral head is that the bone cement (or material) added to the femoral head immediately hardens and provides a mechanical construct to prevent collapse. Hernigou and associates[40] were the first to replace dead bone in a femoral head with cement in patients with sickle cell disease. In 10 patients (16 hips), cement was injected to elevate the cartilage and restore the sphericity of the femoral head. At 5-year follow-up, 14 of the 16 hips (87.5%) were still improved, showing no radiographic progression.

In a recent study by Wood and associates,[42,43] 21 patients (22 hips) with a collapsed femoral head were treated by open reduction augmented by methylmethacrylate cementation. All patients experienced immediate pain relief and improvement in mobility postoperatively. At a mean follow-up of 1.7 years (range, 1 to 3 years), however, six patients underwent total hip arthroplasty. When results were stratified according to size of the lesion, patients with smaller lesions showed better results than patients with larger lesions of the femoral head.

Cementation of the femoral head has the added potential of preventing additional collapse and maintaining sphericity.[41,44,45] It helps with immediate postoperative pain relief and improvement in mobility, without compromising subsequent revision to total hip arthroplasty. Nevertheless, cementation halts the revascularization and remodeling processes and presently should only be recommended for early-stage osteonecrosis. More studies reporting long-term outcomes are anticipated.

Arthrodiastasis
Arthrodiastasis is a method in which the joint is kept distracted while healing of the lesion of the femoral head can proceed without high weight-bearing forces that may disrupt the joint. The method was first described in 1979 to treat various disorders such as osteoarthritis, chondrolysis, and osteonecrosis of the femoral head.

The main principle of arthrodiastasis is to relieve joint loading and to circumvent femoral head collapse. Thacker and associates[46] reported on hinged distraction of the adolescent arthritic hip. The joint distraction was used in the treatment of 11 patients (mean age 13.9 years). All patients presented with constant pain before treatment. After use of a mean fixator for 4.4 months (range, 3 to 7 months), eight patients (73%) reported complete pain relief and three patients (27%) had pain after exercise. Hip flexion improved from a mean of 60° (range, 25° to 75°) preoperatively to a mean of 95° (range, 80° to 110°) postoperatively. Improvement was also reported in joint space size, which increased from 2.6 mm (range, 2 to 3 mm) before fixation to 4.8 mm (range, 4 to 7 mm) after fixation. According to these findings, this treatment appears to be effective in eliminating pain, improving function, and preventing progressive degenerative changes of the hip.

Arthrodiastasis as a treatment option to preserve the femoral head has been extensively studied in Legg-Calvé-Perthes disease. Maxwell and associates[47] reported preliminary results of arthrodiastasis in 15 children with minimal epiphyseal collapse and compared the outcome with that of a historical conservatively treated control group (30 hips). The mean age at the time of surgery was 10.4 years (range, 8.0 to 12.7 years) and the mean length of follow-up was 38.4 months (range, 15.8 to 56.6 months). At final follow-up, 1 of 15 hips (6%) in the arthrodiastasis group had disease progression, whereas in the control group 19 of 30 hips (63.3%) had disease progression. Kocaoglu and associates,[48] Kucukkaya and associates,[49] and Guamiero and associates[120] have found similar promising results using this technique.

Mont and associates[50] first described the combination of a nonvascularized bone grafting technique with arthrodiastasis using recombinant human osteogenic protein-1 (rhOP-1), cancellous autograft, and autogenous bone marrow for the treatment of adult patients with osteonecrosis. Early follow-up results have been promising for improved healing of the unloaded joint, and this technique potentially allows salvage of hips with late stage osteonecrosis.

Arthrodiastasis may be an effective treatment option for eliminating pain, improving function, preserving the joint, and preventing disease progression. However, substantial data and prospective studies are lacking and further work needs to be done to evaluate this method.

Tantalum
Tantalum has been used in the treatment of osteonecrosis of the femoral head to provide mechanical support to prevent collapse. The chemical element tantalum was first purified in 1905. It is a very hard transition metal that possesses a high strength-to-weight ratio and high volume porosity with communicating pores that allow rapid bone ingrowth. Several clinical applications made of commercially pure porous tantalum,[51,52] such as joint prostheses (T Gruen, MD, MJ Christie, MD, AD Hanssen, MD and R Lewis, MD, A Unger, MD, Dallas TX, unpublished data presented at the AAOS Annual Meeting, 2002), special prostheses for reconstruction fol-

lowing tumor resection, and spine fusion devices, have been used since 1977.

For the treatment of osteonecrosis, porous tantalum rods have been developed. The rod is inserted into the femoral neck and head from a lateral position. It provides support for the femoral head and there is no further need for bone grafting and its associated morbidity. In a prospective Food and Drug Administration-regulated Investigational Device Exemption study,[54] 98 patients (113 hips) with noncollapse osteonecrosis of the femoral head were treated with porous tantalum rods. The mean age of the patients was 43 years (range, 20 to 69 years) and they were followed for 5 years after surgery. Radiographic evaluation was performed by independent radiologists. Of the 113 hips, 94 hips were diagnosed with precollapse of the femoral head and 19 hips showed collapse of the femoral head. At final follow-up, 91 implants had survived (survival rate 81%), whereas 22 implants required removal because of progression of the disease and/or associated pain. Of the hips with implant revision, 19 hips presented without femoral head collapse preoperatively and 3 hips showed crescent signs at radiographic analysis before treatment. The mean Harris hip score for all hips with noncollapsed osteonecrosis of the femoral head increased from 63 preoperatively to 83 at 4-year follow-up. None of the tantalum implants failed mechanically or showed any signs of loosening.

The porous tantalum implants show encouraging results with regard to short-term survival rates and may have great impact on the treatment of osteonecrosis in the future, but further study is needed.

Biologic Substrates for the Treatment of Osteonecrosis
Demineralized Bone Matrix
Demineralized bone matrix contains bone growth factors and can induce the formation of new bone,[121-124] which may release or heal dead bone and help prevent femoral head collapse.[125]

Urist[55] was the first to report on the osteoinductive capacity of demineralized bone matrix,[56] produced by acid extraction of human allogenetic bone. It can be used as an excellent alternative to autogenous bone grafting.[57,126-128] Demineralized bone matrix contains collagen (predominantly collagen type I) and noncollagenous osteoinductive proteins such as BMPs and various growth factors, but lacks the structural integrity necessary to support a weight-bearing joint.[58]

Oakes and associates[59] evaluated the osteoconductive and osteoinductive potential of two different human demineralized bone matrices in a rat femur model with a critical-sized defect. Ninety animals were divided into three groups; one group was treated with demineralized bone matrix and an acid carrier, one group was treated with the acid carrier alone, and one group with no implants served as the surgical control group. At 16-week follow-up, 8 of the 48 defects (17%) treated with demineralized bone matrix showed complete radiographic healing, whereas none of the defects treated with the carrier alone or surgery alone demonstrated complete healing.

Peterson and associates[60] analyzed the osteoinductivity of three commercially available demineralized bone matrices in rat spinal fusion models. Their study demonstrated excellent osteoinductive capacity of commercially available demineralized bone matrix in a spinal fusion compared with surgical spinal decortication alone. Similar results have been reported by Lee and associates,[61] who analyzed the efficacy of eight different commercially available demineralized bone matrices in a rat spinal fusion model.

In a clinical study, Mont and associates[80] analyzed the outcome of nonvascularized bone grafting for osteonecrosis of the hip. In 21 hips the necrotic segment was replaced with a combination of demineralized bone matrix and a mixture of processed allograft with BMPs. At a mean follow-up of 48 months (range, 36 to 55 months), 86% of the patients had a successful outcome as defined by Harris hip scores greater than 80 points and no additional surgical intervention. The authors concluded that this technique successfully delays the need for total hip arthroplasty.

Lieberman and associates[129] evaluated 15 patients (17 hips) with osteonecrosis of the femoral head. Fifteen hips had early-stage osteonecrosis. After core decompression, all patients underwent bone grafting with an allogenic, antigen-extracted, autolyzed fibula allograft and 50 mg of partially purified human cortical demineralized bone matrix introduced into the core decompression site. In this study, 12 patients (14 hips) had a successful outcome in terms of preserving the femoral head and delaying the need for a total hip arthroplasty.

Demineralized bone matrix is readily available and may be an excellent bone graft extender or even substitute in the treatment of precollapse stages of osteonecrosis of the femoral head.[57,130,131]

Bone Morphogenetic Proteins
BMPs, as contained in demineralized bone matrix, can be beneficial in the stimulation of angiogenesis and new bone formation for the treatment of osteonecrosis of the femoral head.[81,132,133] Growth factors may help in various aspects of the repair and bone formation process.

BMPs are growth factors expressed by the extracellular matrix of bone. In 1973, Reddi and Huggins[63] characterized those proteins involved in the bone formation cascade. To date, more than 15 different BMPs have been identified. BMPs have the ability to initiate new bone formation by recruiting mesenchymal stem cells and stimulating cell differentiation of stem cells into osteoprogenitor cells.[134,135] With recombinant gene technology, some of these BMPs have been manufactured for musculoskeletal applications.[64]

Numerous animal studies on the use of recombinant human BMPs have helped to establish their efficacy and a solid foundation for further clinical development[64,110,136-138] (JR Lieberman, MD, A Conduah, MD, MR Urist, MD, unpublished data).

Mont and associates[50] reported on the effect of rhOP-1 (BMP-7) in a canine femoral head defect model. The rhOP-1 was used in 34 dogs with implemented defects of the femoral head as an adjunct to strut autografting. Their study showed that defects in groups treated with grafting and rhOP-1 healed faster radiographically than did those in the group treated with grafting only. Defects in animals that were left untreated did not heal. Augmentation of bone grafting with rhOP-1 improved the outcome of osteonecrosis of the femoral head.

Cook and associates[62] used rhOP-1 (BMP-7) in the treatment of bilateral osteochondral defects of the knee in 65 dogs. Of the 130 defects, 76 were treated with OP-1 implants, whereas 54 defects served as the control group and were implanted with bovine bone-derived collagen. At 52 weeks follow-up, the mean total score for gross appearance of all defects treated with OP-1 was higher than the score for the control groups.

Simank and associates[65,139] treated a sheep model with partial necrosis of the femoral head with absorbable BMP-2 and growth differentiation factor-5 (GDF-5). Femoral defects were induced in 27 sheep by direct ethanol injection. BMP-2 and GDF-5 were applied in nine sheep each, whereas nine other sheep were implanted with carrier only and served as the control group. Three weeks after operation and application of the growth factor, bone formation was noticeably induced in defects treated with GDF-5, whereas sheep treated with BMP-2 showed only enhanced bone formation.

Clinically, BMPs and their applications have extensively been studied in fracture healing,[66-68,79] (SP Scully, MD, WS Riszk, MD, AV Seaber, MD, JR Urbaniak, MD, Orlando FL, unpublished data presented at the Orthopaedic Research Society Annual Meeting, 1995) spinal fusions,[69-76,140] total joint arthroplasty, and nonunions.[77,78] In patients with osteonecrosis, BMPs have been used as an adjunct to enhance outcome after core decompression,[141] osteotomies, and bone grafting.

In a prospective, controlled, randomized study by Govender and associates,[82] 450 patients with open tibial fractures were treated with BMP-2. Of the 450 patients, 149 patients (mean age 33 years) received an implant containing 1.50 mg/mL BMP-2, 151 patients (37) were implanted with 0.75 mg/mL BMP-2, and 150 patients received standard care as a control group. At 6-week follow-up, 83% of fractures treated with 1.50 mg/mL BMP-2 had healed, whereas 72% of fractures in the group treated with 0.75 mg/mL BMP-2 had healed. In the control group only 65% of treated fractures exhibited signs of healing. Results of this study showed enhancement of bone repair in fractures when treated with BMP-2, which may be advantageous as an adjunct to standard care. Riedel and Valentin-Opran[142] treated 82 patients with tibial fractures with BMP-2 implants and presented similar results.

In a multicenter, open-label, randomized pilot study by Chiron and associates (Rhodes, Greece, unpublished data presented at the Fifth Congress of the European Federation of National Associations of Orthopaedics and Traumatology, 2001), 24 patients with osteonecrosis of the femoral head were treated with recombinant human BMP-2. All patients received the protein mixed to an autologous blood clot mixture at the time of core decompression. In a control group of 19 patients, core decompression was followed by a conventional treatment algorithm. The incidence of progression of osteonecrosis was lower in the patients who received human BMP-2; however, eight patients who received the blood-BMP-2 mixture developed heterotopic ossifications, compared with four patients in the control group. Nonetheless, the results of this study are promising and further research on applied dosage and intervention stage will be necessary.

Mont and associates[64] used a nonvascularized bone-grafting technique with rhOP-1 (BMP-7) in 15 patients with osteonecrosis of the femoral head. All patients were pre-operatively and postoperatively evaluated clinically and with MRI or CT to assess new bone formation. Preliminary results at mean follow-up of 6 months (range, 3 to 12 months) were promising, with only one failure in 15 patients (93% success rate).

Several BMPs have indicated excellent healing capabilities in various musculoskeletal applications,[65] and when used as a supplement to several therapy modalities in osteonecrosis, results are promising.[81]

Other Growth Factors

Other growth factors such as transforming growth factor-β, fibroblast growth factor, insulin-like growth factor, platelet-derived growth factor, and vascular endothelial growth factor (VEGF) may serve as potential therapeutic substrates[83-86,143-147] to augment fracture repair,[84,87-92,148-151] nonunions, spinal fusions,[93] and osteonecrosis.[94] Based on the evidence of basic science and animal studies on the efficacy of these growth factors, it is difficult to make predications and recommendations regarding clinical indications. Some of the factors might have the potential to enhance bone formation[95] when used alone or when used in combination with other growth factors,[152] demineralized bone matrix, mesenchymal stem cells, or BMPs.[96,97] In comparison with BMPs, some of these growth factors have only limited osteoinductive capabilities, but it is believed that growth factors enhance bone formation by stimulating cell proliferation, differentiation, and extracellular matrix synthesis. Further study in the field of growth factor application is needed to draw conclusions regarding the efficacy of growth factors in the treatment of osteonecrosis.[2]

Stem Cell Therapy

The implantation of autologous bone marrow containing stem cells may benefit the clinical treatment of osteonecrosis of the femoral head,[98-103,143,153] because the osteogenetic precursors are capable of differentiating into bone, cartilage, muscle, tendon, and other connective tissue.[154] In various studies the potential for using autologous stem cell therapy to augment bone repair and regeneration has been evaluated.

Gangji and associates[99] evaluated 13 patients (18 hips) with precollapse osteonecrosis, Ficat stage I to II, who were treated with core decompression. Bone marrow was implanted in 10 hips at the site of core decompression, whereas 8 hips served as a control group. After a 2-year follow-up, patients in the bone marrow-graft group showed significant reduction in pain and in joint symptoms ($P = 0.021$). In the control group, five of the eight hips revealed radiographic deterioration, whereas only one hip showed disease progression ($P = 0.016$) in the group with implanted bone marrow.

Hernigou and Beaujean[101] obtained autologous bone marrow from the iliac crest of 116 patients (189 hips). All patients were treated with core decompression and bone grafting using the obtained bone marrow. The patients were followed for 5 to 10 years. The evaluations were based on changes in Harris hip score, radiographic progression of the disease, and the need for a total hip arthroplasty. Of 145 hips with early stage osteonecrosis, 9 (6%) underwent total hip arthroplasty. Among 44 hips with Ficat stage III or IV, 25 hips (57%) needed total hip arthroplasty performed after core decompression and bone grafting with autologous bone marrow.

Muschler and associates[104] evaluated the use of bone marrow-derived stem cells in spinal fusion in a canine model. In this study, 12 beagles (mean age, 13 months) were prepared with three fusion sites in the spine. All sites were separated by one mobile segment. Induction of fusion was evaluated for three compositions—demineralized cortical bone powder without additives, demineralized cortical bone powder with aspirated bone marrow, and enriched demineralized cortical bone powder with aspirated bone marrow. The enrichment resulted in an approximately fivefold increase in the number of stem cells. In 8 of the 12 sites (67%) treated with enriched demineralized cortical bone powder with aspirated bone marrow, fusion was achieved. In the group of sites treated with demineralized cortical bone powder with aspirated bone marrow, 6 of 12 sites (50%) showed successful fusion. The sites treated with demineralized cortical bone powder only revealed fusion in 2 of 12 attempts (17%). This study concludes that a higher number of progenitor cells at the graft site is effective in the enhancement of spinal fusion.

The transplantation of autologous bone marrow as a treatment of osteonecrosis of the femoral head was first proposed in 1990. Since then, techniques for bone marrow aspiration have continuously improved and have become a common treatment option as an adjunct to core decompression and bone grafting. Clinical studies show great improvement in femoral head preservation after stem cell implantation in early stages of osteonecrosis.

Gene Therapy

Gene therapy seeks to harvest and manipulate endogenous cells to express specific proteins with osteoinductive capacity. Gene therapy is a newer technique used in the treatment of osteonecrosis. Even though the implantation of autologous bone marrow containing stem cells into sites of core decompression greatly improves clinical results, this treatment modality has restrictions such as limited supply and high cost, and associated donor site morbidity.[105-108] To manipulate the expression of endogenous cells, the desired gene has to be integrated into the DNA of the target cells through a process called transduction, using viral or nonviral vectors in an ex vivo or in vivo approach.[109] The manipulated cells will transcript the altered DNA into mRNA, which is then translated by ribosomes into polypeptides. These polypeptides can be growth factors with osteoinductive capability such as BMPs, interleukins, and/or angiogenetic growth factor that will activate multipotent mesenchymal stem cells found in bone marrow, fat tissue, and muscles. Multipotent mesenchymal stem cells act as progenitors and are still capable of differentiation in mesodermal tissue such as bone. Because the gene of the desired protein has been embedded in the DNA of the target cell, the information will be passed on to new generations of this cell line, possibly providing a long therapeutic effect.

Lieberman and associates[110] created bone marrow cells expressing BMP-2 by ex vivo adenoviral gene transfer to treat 8-mm critical-sized full-thickness femoral defects in rats. BMP-2-producing bone marrow cells were implanted into 24 femoral defects, whereas recombinant human BMP-2 was used to treat the defects in 16 mice femora. Control groups consisted of 32 femora that were injected with placebo. Two months after treatment, radiographic analysis showed that 22 of the 24 defects (91.7%) in rat femora treated with BMP-2 expressing bone marrow cells had healed. Femora treated with rhBMP-2 exhibited 100% healing, whereas only 1 of 32 femora (3.1%) in the control group exhibited successful healing.

In a recent study, Peterson and associates[111] treated femoral defects in a nude rat model with human lipoaspirate containing mesenchymal stem cells. The cells were obtained from healthy donors, grown in culture, infected with a BMP-2-carrying adenovirus, and applied to a collagen-ceramic carrier. The study group consisted of 20 femurs with induced femoral defects. The femoral defects in 12 of the 20 femora were treated with obtained human lipoaspirate cells that were genetically altered to overexpress BMP-2, whereas the remaining 8 femora were implanted with rhBMP-2. The control groups consisted of 12 femora that were injected with either the carrier only, or uninfected human lipoaspirate cells. All animals were sacrificed after 8 weeks and then evaluated radiographically. Of 12 femora treated with genetically altered human lipoaspirate cells, 11 (91.7%) had healed. Femora treated with rhBMP-2 exhibited 100% healing, whereas none of the 12 femora in the control showed any sign of healing.

Katsube and associates[155] enhanced the outcome of vascularized bone grafting by transferring VEGF into the implanted blood vessels. They did so by using an adenoviral vector containing the VEGF gene or an identical virus as placebo to be transduced in endothelial cells in rabbit saphenous arteries. The artery was introduced into necrotic iliac crest bone in vivo and angiogenesis was evaluated by blood flow measurements as well as vessel density following microangiography. At 1 week postoperatively, the blood flow in the group treated with VEGF was measured 14.19 ± 3.22 mL/min/100 g tissue and was significantly higher than 7.75 ± 1.84 mL/min/100 g of tissue in the control group ($P = 0.028$). Microangiography revealed neoangiogenesis in both groups 1 week postoperatively; however, the mean vessel length in the VEGF-transduced group (111.0 ± 10.1 mm) was significantly greater than in the control group (73.1 ± 4.6 mm) ($P = 0.007$). In addition, blood vessel density was shown to be higher in the VEGF transduction ($12.6 \pm 1.0\%$) than in 1-week controls ($8.9 \pm 0.9\%$) ($P = 0.039$). These findings indicate that VEGF may be used to supplement vascularized bone grafting for improvement of blood flow to the femoral head.[146,156]

In another study, Yang and associates[157] assessed the implantation of a recombinant plasmid containing the VEGF gene ($hVEGF_{165}$) directly into the necrotic femoral head of a rabbit model. Three randomized groups containing 24 rabbits were created and osteonecrosis of the femoral head was induced through a freeing technique in all of the animals. Through a 2-mm channel drilled into the femoral neck from a lateral position, 200 μg of the $hVEGF_{165}$ plasmid mixed with collagen and saline was implanted in the first group of rabbits, whereas the second group was implanted with collagen only. The third group was left untreated. Specimens were obtained at 2, 4, 6, and 8 weeks and evaluated by histologic and histomorphometric analysis. The formation of new blood vessels 4 weeks postoperatively was significantly in-

creased in the study group (7.14 ± 1.25) compared with that of rabbits implanted with collagen only (4.84 ± 0.78) and the group that was left untreated (3.69 ± 0.65) ($P < 0.01$). Formation of new bone 6 weeks after operation was also noted to be significantly increased in the group treated with the $hVEGF_{165}$ plasmid (7.69 ± 0.37) compared with the two control groups—the group treated with collagen (5.64 ± 1.47) and the untreated group (4.26 ± 0.34) ($P < 0.01$). VEGF gene transduction shows the potential to accelerate healing of osteonecrosis, but needs further study and clinical evaluation.

The few studies analyzing gene therapy[110-113,155-157] and expression of certain osteoinductive and angiogenetic proteins demonstrated promising results. Gene therapy is a relatively new field in orthopaedics, but has the potential for future treatment modalities in nonunions and bone defects as well as in the treatment of osteonecrosis of the femoral head.

Summary

Limitations in the treatment of early stage osteonecrosis of the femoral head have prompted increasing interest in alternative therapies. Bone grafts and their alternatives are attractive sources for the treatment of early stage disease to prevent femoral head collapse. There are currently many growth factors and BMPs under investigation as adjunct therapies to enhance and/or accelerate bone repair. The results vary and depend on the appropriate carrier or delivery system. Nevertheless, most of the results of both preclinical animal and clinical human studies are very promising. Orthopaedic surgeons may not only use biologic substances such as growth factors, BMPs, and demineralized bone matrix for the treatment of fractures, spinal fusion, and nonunions but also to treat osteonecrosis of the femoral head.

Recent advances in noninvasive treatment modalities such as pharmacologic measures, magnetic field stimulation, and shock wave therapy for early disease demonstrated the same or even more effective results combined with less morbidity than invasive procedures such as core decompression or nonvascularized bone grafting. More long-term results are needed to confirm the efficacy of these novel treatment approaches.

The variety of potentially viable alternatives or adjunctive treatment options to invasive procedures for femoral head preservation is exciting. The application of bone graft substitutes and growth factors continues to be a rapidly growing field in orthopaedics. Further clinical studies on efficacy and safety of these emerging new materials are needed.

References

1. Lieberman JR, Berry DJ, Mont MA, et al: Osteonecrosis of the hip: Management in the 21st century. *Instr Course Lect* 2003;52:337-355.

2. Hofmann S, Mazieres B: [Osteonecrosis: natural course and conservative therapy]. *Orthopade* 2000;29:403-410.

3. Mont MA, Hungerford DS: Non-traumatic avascular necrosis of the femoral head. *J Bone Joint Surg Am* 1995;77:459-474.

4. Arlet J, Mazieres B, Thiechert M, Vallieres G: The effect of IV injection of naftidrofuryl (praxilene) in intramedullary pressure in patients with osteonecrosis of the femoral head, in Arlet J, Mazieres B (eds): *Bone Circulation and Bone Necrosis*. Berlin, Germany, Springer, 1990, pp 405-406.

5. Motomura G, Yamamoto T, Miyanishi K, Jingushi S, Iwamoto Y: Combined effects

of an anticoagulant and a lipid-lowering agent on the prevention of steroid-induced osteonecrosis in rabbits. *Arthritis Rheum* 2004;50:3387-3391.

6. Glueck CJ, Freiberg R, Glueck HI, Tracy T, Stroop D, Wang Y: Idiopathic osteonecrosis, hypofibrinolysis, high plasminogen activator inhibitor, high lipoprotein(a), and therapy with Stanozolol. *Am J Hematol* 1995;48:213-220.

7. Glueck CJ, Freiberg RA, Sieve L, Wang P: Enoxaparin prevents progression of stages I and II osteonecrosis of the hip. *Clin Orthop Relat Res* 2005;435:164-170.

8. Aigner N, Petje G, Schneider W, Krasny C, Grill F, Landsiedl F: Juvenile bone-marrow oedema of the acetabulum treated by iloprost. *J Bone Joint Surg Br* 2002;84:1050-1052.

9. Meizer R, Radda C, Stolz G, et al: MRI-controlled analysis of 104 patients with painful bone marrow edema in different joint localizations treated with the prostacyclin analogue iloprost. *Wien Klin Wochenschr* 2005;117:278-286.

10. Agarwala S, Jain D, Joshi VR, Sule A: Efficacy of alendronate, a bisphosphonate, in the treatment of AVN of the hip: A prospective open-label study. *Rheumatology (Oxford)* 2005;44:352-359.

11. Lai KA, Shen WJ, Yang CY, Shao CJ, Hsu JT, Lin RM: The use of alendronate to prevent early collapse of the femoral head in patients with nontraumatic osteonecrosis: A randomized clinical study. *J Bone Joint Surg Am* 2005;87:2155-2159.

12. Tagil M, Astrand J, Westman L, Aspenberg P: Alendronate prevents collapse in mechanically loaded osteochondral grafts: A bone chamber study in rats. *Acta Orthop Scand* 2004;75:756-761.

13. Peskin B, Shupak A, Levin D, et al: Effects of non-weight bearing and hyperbaric oxygen therapy in vascular deprivation-induced osteonecrosis of the rat femoral head. *Undersea Hyperb Med* 2001;28:187-194.

14. Reis ND, Schwartz O, Militianu D, et al: Hyperbaric oxygen therapy as a treatment for stage-I avascular necrosis of the femoral head. *J Bone Joint Surg Br* 2003;85:371-375.

15. Aaron RK, Steinberg ME: Electrical stimulation of osteonecrosis of the femoral head. *Semin Arthroplasty* 1991;2:214-221.

16. Trancik T, Lunceford E, Strum D: The effect of electrical stimulation on osteonecrosis of the femoral head. *Clin Orthop Relat Res* 1990;256:120-124.

17. Steinberg ME, Brighton CT, Hayken GD, Tooze SE, Steinberg DR: Electrical stimulation in the treatment of osteonecrosis of the femoral head: A 1-year follow-up. *Orthop Clin North Am* 1985;16:747-756.

18. Steinberg ME, Brighton CT, Hayken GD, Tooze SE, Steinberg DR: Early results in the treatment of avascular necrosis of the femoral head with electrical stimulation. *Orthop Clin North Am* 1984;15:163-175.

19. Steinberg ME, Brighton CT, Steinberg DR, Tooze SE, Hayken GD: Treatment of avascular necrosis of the femoral head by a combination of bone grafting, decompression, and electrical stimulation. *Clin Orthop Relat Res* 1984;186:137-153.

20. Walter TH: Bioelectrical osteogenesis: acceleration of fracture repair and bone growth: An alternative to bone grafting in nonunions. *Clin Podiatry* 1985;2:41-57.

21. Brighton CT, Friedenberg ZB, Black J, Esterhai JL Jr, Mitchell JE, Montique F Jr: Electrically induced osteogenesis: relationship between charge, current density, and the amount of bone formed: introduction of a new cathode concept. *Clin Orthop Relat Res* 1981;161:122-132.

22. Linovitz RJ, Pathria M, Bernhardt M, et al: Combined magnetic fields accelerate and increase spine fusion: A double-blind, randomized, placebo controlled study. *Spine* 2002;27:1383-1389.

23. Cane V, Botti P, Soana S: Pulsed magnetic fields improve osteoblast activity during the repair of an experimental osseous defect. *J Orthop Res* 1993;11:664-670.

24. Eftekhar NS, Schink-Ascani MM, Mitchell SN, Bassett CA: Osteonecrosis of the femoral head treated by pulsed electromagnetic fields (PEMFs): A preliminary report. *Hip* 1983;306-330.

25. Lluch BC, Garcia-Andrade DG, Munoz FL, Stern LL: [Usefulness of electromagnetic fields in the treatment of hip avascular necrosis: A prospective study of 30 cases]. *Rev Clin Esp* 1996;196:67-74.

26. Bassett CA, Schink-Ascani M, Lewis SM: Effects of pulsed electromagnetic fields on Steinberg ratings of femoral head osteonecrosis. *Clin Orthop Relat Res* 1989;246:172-185.

27. Seber S, Omeroglu H, Cetinkanat H, Kose N: [The efficacy of pulsed electromagnetic fields used alone in the treatment of femoral head osteonecrosis: A report of two cases]. *Acta Orthop Traumatol Turc* 2003;37:410-413.

28. Aaron RK, Lennox D, Bunce GE, Ebert T: The conservative treatment of osteonecrosis of the femoral head: A comparison of core decompression and pulsing electromagnetic fields. *Clin Orthop Relat Res* 1989;249:209-218.

29. Ogden JA, Alvarez RR: Extracorporeal shock wave therapy in orthopaedics. *Clin Orthop Relat Res* 2001;387:2-3.

30. Haupt G: [Shock waves in orthopedics]. *Urologe A* 1997;36:233-238.

31. Ogden JA, Toth-Kischkat A, Schultheiss R: Principles of shock wave therapy. *Clin Orthop Relat Res* 2001;387:8-17.

32. Schaden W, Fischer A, Sailler A: Extracorporeal shock wave therapy of nonunion or delayed osseous union. *Clin Orthop Relat Res* 2001;387:90-94.

33. Wang CJ, Huang HY, Pai CH: Shock wave-enhanced neovascularization at the tendon-bone junction: An experiment in dogs. *J Foot Ankle Surg* 2002;41:16-22.

34. Wang CJ, Wang FS, Yang KD, et al: Shock wave therapy induces neovascularization at the tendon-bone junction: A study in rabbits. *J Orthop Res* 2003;21:984-989.

35. Ludwig J, Lauber S, Lauber HJ, Dreisilker U, Raedel R, Hotzinger H: High-energy shock wave treatment of femoral head necrosis in adults. *Clin Orthop Relat Res* 2001;387:119-126.

36. Wang CJ, Wang FS, Huang CC, Yang KD, Weng LH, Huang HY: Treatment for osteonecrosis of the femoral head: comparison of extracorporeal shock waves with core decompression and bone-grafting. *J Bone Joint Surg Am* 2005;87:2380-2387.

37. Gerdesmeyer L, Hauschild M, Ueberle F: ESWT bei Hüftkopfnekrose - Fokusmessungen. 3. Drei-Länder-Treffen der Österreichischen, Schweizer und Deutschen Fachgesellschaften für Stoßwellentherapie am 21-22 March, 2003, München. Abstractband p 63.

38. Hausdorf J, Lutz A, Rohrig H, Maier M: [Extracorporeal shock wave therapy and femur head necrosis–pressure measurements in the femur head]. *Z Orthop Ihre Grenzgeb* 2004;142:122-126.

39. Lauber S: [High energy extracorporeal shockwave therapy in femur head necrosis]. *Z Orthop Ihre Grenzgeb* 2000;138:Oa3-Oa4.

40. Hernigou P, Bachir D, Galacteros F:

Avascular necrosis of the femoral head in sickle-cell disease: Treatment of collapse by the injection of acrylic cement. *J Bone Joint Surg Br* 1993;75:875-880.

41. Wood ML, Kelley SS: Cement supplementation as a treatment for osteonecrosis. *Curr Opin Orthop* 2003;14:23-29.

42. Wood ML, McDowell CM, Kelley SS: Cementation for femoral head osteonecrosis: A preliminary clinic study. *Clin Orthop Relat Res* 2003;412:94-102.

43. Wood ML, McDowell CM, Kerstetter TL, Kelley SS: Open reduction and cementation for femoral head fracture secondary to avascular necrosis: Preliminary report. *Iowa Orthop J* 2000;20:17-23.

44. Hernigou P: [Treatment of hip necrosis by sequestrectomy and replacement with bone cement]. *Acta Orthop Belg* 1999;65(suppl 1):89-94.

45. Bresler F, Roche O, Chary-Valckenaire I, Blum A, Mole D, Schmitt D: [Femoral head osteonecrosis: Original extra-articular cementoplasty technique. A series of 20 cases]. *Acta Orthop Belg* 1999;65(Suppl 1):95-96.

46. Thacker MM, Feldman DS, Madan SS, Straight JJ, Scher DM: Hinged distraction of the adolescent arthritic hip. *J Pediatr Orthop* 2005;25:178-182.

47. Maxwell SL, Lappin KJ, Kealey WD, Mc-Dowell BC, Cosgrove AP: Arthrodiastasis in Perthes' disease: Preliminary results. *J Bone Joint Surg Br* 2004;86:244-250.

48. Kocaoglu M, Kilicoglu OI, Goksan SB, Cakmak M: Ilizarov fixator for treatment of Legg-Calve-Perthes disease. *J Pediatr Orthop B* 1999;8:276-281.

49. Kucukkaya M, Kabukcuoglu Y, Ozturk I, Kuzgun U: Avascular necrosis of the femoral head in childhood: The results of treatment with articulated distraction method. *J Pediatr Orthop* 2000;20:722-728.

50. Mont MA, Jones LC, Elias JJ, et al: Strut-autografting with and without osteogenic protein-1: A preliminary study of a canine femoral head defect model. *J Bone Joint Surg Am* 2001;83:1013-1022.

51. Black J: Biological performance of tantalum. *Clin Mater* 1994;16:167-173.

52. Pudenz RH: The repair of cranial defects with tantalum: An experimental study. *JAMA* 1943;121:478-481.

53. Bobyn JD, Poggie RA, Krygier JJ, et al: Clinical validation of a structural porous tantalum biomaterial for adult reconstruction. *J Bone Joint Surg Am*

2004;86(sSuppl 2):123-129.

54. Tsao AK, Roberson JR, Christie MJ, et al: Biomechanical and clinical evaluations of a porous tantalum implant for the treatment of early-stage osteonecrosis. *J Bone Joint Surg Am* 2005;87(suppl 2):22-27.

55. Urist MR: Bone: Formation by autoinduction. *Science* 1965;150:893-899.

56. Edwards JT, Diegmann MH, Scarborough NL: Osteoinduction of human demineralized bone: Characterization in a rat model. *Clin Orthop Relat Res* 1998;357:219-228.

57. Chakkalakal DA, Strates BS, Garvin KL, et al: Demineralized bone matrix as a biological scaffold for bone repair. *Tissue Eng* 2001;7:161-177.

58. Russell JL, Block JE: Clinical utility of demineralized bone matrix for osseous defects, arthrodesis, and reconstruction: Impact of processing techniques and study methodology. *Orthopedics* 1999;22:524-531.

59. Oakes DA, Lee CC, Lieberman JR: An evaluation of human demineralized bone matrices in a rat femoral defect model. *Clin Orthop Relat Res* 2003;413:281-290.

60. Peterson B, Whang PG, Iglesias R, Wang JC, Lieberman JR: Osteoinductivity of commercially available demineralized bone matrix: Preparations in a spine fusion model. *J Bone Joint Surg Am* 2004;86:2243-2250.

61. Lee YP, Jo M, Luna M, Chien B, Lieberman JR, Wang JC: The efficacy of different commercially available demineralized bone matrix substances in an athymic rat model. *J Spinal Disord Tech* 2005;18:439-444.

62. Cook SD, Patron LP, Salkeld SL, Rueger DC: Repair of articular cartilage defects with osteogenic protein-1 (BMP-7) in dogs. *J Bone Joint Surg Am* 2003;85(suppl 3):116-123.

63. Reddi AH, Huggins CB: Influence of geometry of transplanted tooth and bone on transformation of fibroblasts. *Proc Soc Exp Biol Med* 1973;143:634-637.

64. Mont MA, Ragland PS, Biggins B, et al: Use of bone morphogenetic proteins for musculoskeletal applications: An overview. *J Bone Joint Surg Am* 2004;86(suppl 2):41-55.

65. Simank HG, Manggold J, Sebald W, et al: Bone morphogenetic protein-2 and growth and differentiation factor-5 enhance the healing of necrotic bone in a sheep model. *Growth Factors* 2001;19:247-257.

66. Bostrom MP, Camacho NP: Potential role of bone morphogenetic proteins in fracture healing. *Clin Orthop Relat Res* 1998;(355 suppl):S274-S282.

67. Bostrom MP: Expression of bone morphogenetic proteins in fracture healing. *Clin Orthop Relat Res* 1998;(355 suppl):S116-S123.

68. Reddi AH: Initiation of fracture repair by bone morphogenetic proteins. *Clin Orthop Relat Res* 1998;(355 suppl):S66-S72.

69. Carlisle E, Fischgrund JS: Bone morphogenetic proteins for spinal fusion. *Spine J* 2005;5(6 suppl):240S-249S.

70. Zlotolow DA, Vaccaro AR, Salamon ML, Albert TJ: The role of human bone morphogenetic proteins in spinal fusion. *J Am Acad Orthop Surg* 2000;8:3-9.

71. Muschik M, Schlenzka D, Ritsila V, Tennstedt C, Lewandrowski KU: Experimental anterior spine fusion using bovine bone morphogenetic protein: A study in rabbits. *J Orthop Sci* 2000;5:165-170.

72. Morone MA, Boden SD: Experimental posterolateral lumbar spinal fusion with a demineralized bone matrix gel. *Spine* 1998;23:159-167.

73. Boden SD: Biology of lumbar spine fusion and use of bone graft substitutes: Present, future, and next generation. *Tissue Eng* 2000;6:383-399.

74. Berven S, Tay BK, Kleinstueck FS, Bradford DS: Clinical applications of bone graft substitutes in spine surgery: Consideration of mineralized and demineralized preparations and growth factor supplementation. *Eur Spine J* 2001;10(suppl 2):S169-S177.

75. Islam AA, Rasubala L, Yoshikawa H, Shiratsuchi Y, Ohishi M: Healing of fractures in osteoporotic rat mandible shown by the expression of bone morphogenetic protein-2 and tumour necrosis factor-alpha. *Br J Oral Maxillofac Surg* 2005;43:383-391.

76. Kain MS, Einhorn TA: Recombinant human bone morphogenetic proteins in the treatment of fractures. *Foot Ankle Clin* 2005;10:639-650.

77. Johnson EE, Urist MR: Human bone morphogenetic protein allografting for reconstruction of femoral nonunion. *Clin Orthop Relat Res* 2000;371:61-74.

78. Dimitriou R, Dahabreh Z, Katsoulis E, Matthews SJ, Branfoot T, Giannoudis PV: Application of recombinant BMP-7 on persistent upper and lower limb non-unions. *Injury* 2005;36(suppl

4):S51-S59.

79. Mont MA, Einhorn TA, Sponseller PD, Hungerford DS: The trapdoor procedure using autogenous cortical and cancellous bone grafts for osteonecrosis of the femoral head. *J Bone Joint Surg Br* 1998;80:56-62.

80. Mont MA, Etienne G, Ragland PS: Outcome of nonvascularized bone grafting for osteonecrosis of the femoral head. *Clin Orthop Relat Res* 2003;417:84-92.

81. Mazieres B: Bone morphogenetic protein and bone necrosis: A perspective. *ARCO News* 1994;6:3-5.

82. Govender S, Csimma C, Genant HK, et al: Recombinant human bone morphogenetic protein-2 for treatment of open tibial fractures: A prospective, controlled, randomized study of four hundred and fifty patients. *J Bone Joint Surg Am* 2002;84:2123-2134.

83. Mont MA, Jones LC, Einhorn TA, Hungerford DS, Reddi AH: Osteonecrosis of the femoral head. Potential treatment with growth and differentiation factors. *Clin Orthop Relat Res* 1998;(355 suppl):S314-S335.

84. Trippel SB: Growth factors as therapeutic agents. *Instr Course Lect* 1997;46:473-476.

85. Hungerford MW, Mont MA: [Potential uses of cytokines and growth factors in treatment of osteonecrosis]. *Orthopade* 2000;29:442-448.

86. Linkhart TA, Mohan S, Baylink DJ: Growth factors for bone growth and repair: IGF, TGF beta and BMP. *Bone* 1996;19(1 suppl):1S-12S.

87. Rosier RN, O'Keefe RJ, Hicks DG: The potential role of transforming growth factor beta in fracture healing. *Clin Orthop Relat Res* 1998;(355 suppl):S294-S300.

88. Bolander ME: Regulation of fracture repair by growth factors. *Proc Soc Exp Biol Med* 1992;200:165-170.

89. Joyce ME, Jingushi S, Bolander ME: Transforming growth factor-beta in the regulation of fracture repair. *Orthop Clin North Am* 1990;21:199-209.

90. Bostrom MP, Asnis P: Transforming growth factor beta in fracture repair. *Clin Orthop Relat Res* 1998;(355 suppl):S124-S131.

91. Lind M, Schumacker B, Soballe K, Keller J, Melsen F, Bunger C: Transforming growth factor-beta enhances fracture healing in rabbit tibiae. *Acta Orthop Scand* 1993;64:553-556.

92. Radomsky ML, Thompson AY, Spiro RC, Poser JW: Potential role of fibroblast growth factor in enhancement of fracture healing. *Clin Orthop Relat Res* 1998;(355 suppl):S283-S293.

93. Lewandrowski KU, Ozuna RM, F.X. P, Hecht AC: Advances in the biology of spinal fusion: Growth factors and gene therapy. *Curr Opin Orthop* 2000;11:167-175.

94. Yang C, Yang SH, Du JY, Li J, Xu WH, Xiong YF: Basic fibroblast growth factor gene transfection to enhance the repair of avascular necrosis of the femoral head. *Chin Med Sci J* 2004;19:111-115.

95. Lind M: Growth factor stimulation of bone healing: Effects on osteoblasts, osteomies, and implants fixation. *Acta Orthop Scand Suppl* 1998;283:2-37.

96. Canalis E, McCarthy TL, Centrella M: Effects of platelet-derived growth factor on bone formation in vitro. *J Cell Physiol* 1989;140:530-537.

97. Geiger F, Bertram H, Berger I, et al: Vascular endothelial growth factor gene-activated matrix (VEGF(165)-GAM) enhances osteogenesis and angiogenesis in large segmental bone defects. *J Bone Miner Res* 2005;20:2028-2035.

98. Gangji V, Toungouz M, Hauzeur JP: Stem cell therapy for osteonecrosis of the femoral head. *Expert Opin Biol Ther* 2005;5:437-442.

99. Gangji V, Hauzeur JP, Matos C, De Maertelaer V, Toungouz M, Lambermont M: Treatment of osteonecrosis of the femoral head with implantation of autologous bone-marrow cells: A pilot study. *J Bone Joint Surg Am* 2004;86:1153-1160.

100. Gangji V, Hauzeur JP: Treatment of osteonecrosis of the femoral head with implantation of autologous bone-marrow cells: Surgical technique. *J Bone Joint Surg Am* 2005;87(suppl 1(Pt 1)):106-112.

101. Hernigou P, Beaujean F: Treatment of osteonecrosis with autologous bone marrow grafting. *Clin Orthop Relat Res* 2002;405:14-23.

102. Hernigou P, Poignard A, Manicom O, Mathieu G, Rouard H: The use of percutaneous autologous bone marrow transplantation in nonunion and avascular necrosis of bone. *J Bone Joint Surg Br* 2005;87:896-902.

103. Bruder SP, Jaiswal N, Ricalton NS, Mosca JD, Kraus KH, Kadiyala S: Mesenchymal stem cells in osteobiology and applied bone regeneration. *Clin Orthop Relat Res* 1998;(355

Suppl):S247-S256.

104. Muschler GF, Matsukura Y, Nitto H, et al: Selective retention of bone marrow-derived cells to enhance spinal fusion. *Clin Orthop Relat Res* 2005;432:242-251.

105. Goulet JA, Senunas LE, DeSilva GL, Greenfield ML: Autogenous iliac crest bone graft. Complications and functional assessment. *Clin Orthop Relat Res* 1997;339:76-81.

106. Musgrave DS, Bosch P, Ghivizzani S, Robbins PD, Evans CH, Huard J: Adenovirus-mediated direct gene therapy with bone morphogenetic protein-2 produces bone. *Bone* 1999;24:541-547.

107. Summers BN, Eisenstein SM: Donor site pain from the ilium: A complication of lumbar spine fusion. *J Bone Joint Surg Br* 1989;71:677-680.

108. Vail TP, Urbaniak JR: Donor-site morbidity with use of vascularized autogenous fibular grafts. *J Bone Joint Surg Am* 1996;78:204-211.

109. Oakes DA, Lieberman JR: Osteoinductive applications of regional gene therapy: ex vivo gene transfer. *Clin Orthop Relat Res* 2000;(379 suppl):S101-S112.

110. Lieberman JR, Daluiski A, Stevenson S, et al: The effect of regional gene therapy with bone morphogenetic protein-2-producing bone-marrow cells on the repair of segmental femoral defects in rats. *J Bone Joint Surg Am* 1999;81:905-917.

111. Peterson B, Zhang J, Iglesias R, et al: Healing of critically sized femoral defects, using genetically modified mesenchymal stem cells from human adipose tissue. *Tissue Eng* 2005;11:120-129.

112. Lieberman JR: Orthopaedic gene therapy. Fracture healing and other nongenetic problems of bone. *Clin Orthop Relat Res* 2000;(379 suppl):S156-S158.

113. Pritchett JW: Statin therapy decreases the risk of osteonecrosis in patients receiving steroids. *Clin Orthop Relat Res* 2001;386:173-178.

114. Soma MR, Meschia M, Bruschi F, et al: Hormonal agents used in lowering lipoprotein(a). *Chem Phys Lipids* 1994;67-68:345-350.

115. Agarwala S, Sule A, Pai BU, Joshi VR: Alendronate in the treatment of avascular necrosis of the hip. *Rheumatology (Oxford)* 2002;41:346-347.

116. Levin D, Norman D, Zinman C, et al: Treatment of experimental avascular necrosis of the femoral head with hyperbaric oxygen in rats: histological evaluation of the femoral heads during the early phase of the reparative process. *Exp Mol Pathol* 1999;67:99-108.

117. Kawashima M, Tamura H, Nagayoshi I, Takao K, Yoshida K, Yamaguchi T: Hyperbaric oxygen therapy in orthopedic conditions. *Undersea Hyperb Med* 2004;31:155-162.

118. Strauss M: A meta-analysis and economic appraisal of osteonecrosis of the femoral head treated with hyperbaric oxygen. *ARCO News* 1995;7:110.

119. Steinberg ME, Brighton CT, Bands RE, Hartman KM: Capacitive coupling as an adjunctive treatment for avascular necrosis. *Clin Orthop Relat Res* 1990;261:11-18.

120. Guamiero R, Luzo CAM, Montenegro NB, Godoy RM: Legg-Calve-Perthes disease: A comparative study between two types of treatment: Femoral varus osteotomy an arthrochondrodiastasis with external fixation. *EPOS* 2000; Milan.

121. Emerson RH Jr, Malinin TI, Cuellar AD, Head WC, Peters PC: Cortical strut allografts in the reconstruction of the femur in revision total hip arthroplasty: A basic science and clinical study. *Clin Orthop Relat Res* 1992;285:35-44.

122. Khouri RK, Koudsi B, Reddi H: Tissue transformation into bone in vivo: A potential practical application. *JAMA* 1991;266:1953-1955.

123. Sampath TK, Reddi AH: Homology of bone-inductive proteins from human, monkey, bovine, and rat extracellular matrix. *Proc Natl Acad Sci USA* 1983;80:6591-6595.

124. Wang JS: Basic fibroblast growth factor for stimulation of bone formation in osteoinductive or conductive implants. *Acta Orthop Scand Suppl* 1996;269:1-33.

125. Etienne G, Ragland PS, Mont MA: Use of cancellous bone chips and demineralized bone matrix in the treatment of acetabular osteolysis: Preliminary 2-year follow-up. *Orthopedics* 2004;27(1 suppl):s123-s126.

126. Einhorn TA, Lane JM, Burstein AH, Kopman CR, Vigorita VJ: The healing of segmental bone defects induced by demineralized bone matrix: A radiographic and biomechanical study. *J Bone Joint Surg Am* 1984;66:274-279.

127. Kelly CM, Wilkins RM, Gitelis S,

Hartjen C, Watson JT, Kim PT: The use of a surgical grade calcium sulfate as a bone graft substitute: Results of a multicenter trial. *Clin Orthop Relat Res* 2001;382:42-50.

128. Sammarco VJ, Chang L: Modern issues in bone graft substitutes and advances in bone tissue technology. *Foot Ankle Clin* 2002;7:19-41.

129. Lieberman JR, Conduah A, Urist MR: Treatment of osteonecrosis of the femoral head with core decompression and human bone morphogenetic protein. *Clin Orthop Relat Res* 2004;429:139-145.

130. Martin GJ Jr, Boden SD, Titus L, Scarborough NL: New formulations of demineralized bone matrix as a more effective graft alternative in experimental posterolateral lumbar spine arthrodesis. *Spine* 1999;24:637-645.

131. Gitelis S, Piasecki P, Turner T, Haggard W, Charters J, Urban R: Use of a calcium sulfate-based bone graft substitute for benign bone lesions. *Orthopedics* 2001;24:162-166.

132. Moser M, Patterson C: Bone morphogenetic proteins and vascular differentiation: BMPing up vasculogenesis. *Thromb Haemost* 2005;94:713-718.

133. Valentin-Opran A, Wozney J, Csimma C, Lilly L, Riedel GE: Clinical evaluation of recombinant human bone morphogenetic protein-2. *Clin Orthop Relat Res* 2002;395:110-120.

134. Rengachary SS: Bone morphogenetic proteins: Basic concepts. *Neurosurg Focus* 2002;13:e2.

135. Schultze-Mosgau S, Lehner B, Rodel F, et al: Expression of bone morphogenic protein 2/4, transforming growth factor-beta1, and bone matrix protein expression in healing area between vascular tibia grafts and irradiated bone-experimental model of osteonecrosis. *Int J Radiat Oncol Biol Phys* 2005;61:1189-1196.

136. Kawai M, Bessho K, Maruyama H, Miyazaki J, Yamamoto T: Human BMP-2 gene transfer using transcutane-ous in vivo electroporation induced both intramembranous and endochondral ossification. *Anat Rec A Discov Mol Cell Evol Biol* 2005;287:1264-1271.

137. Simank HG, Sergi C, Jung M, et al: Effects of local application of growth and differentiation factor-5 (GDF-5) in a full-thickness cartilage defect model. *Growth Factors* 2004;22:35-43.

138. Tabuchi M, Miyazawa K, Kimura M, et al: Enhancement of crude bone morphogenetic protein-induced new bone formation and normalization of endochondral ossification by bisphosphonate treatment in osteoprotegerin-deficient mice. *Calcif Tissue Int* 2005;77:239-249.

139. Simank HG, Herold F, Schneider M, Maedler U, Ries R, Sergi C: [Growth and differentiation factor 5 (GDF-5) composite improves the healing of necrosis of the femoral head in a sheep model: Analysis of an animal model]. *Orthopade* 2004;33:68-75.

140. Peterson B, Iglesias R, Zhang J, Wang JC, Lieberman JR: Genetically modified human derived bone marrow cells for posterolateral lumbar spine fusion in athymic rats: Beyond conventional autologous bone grafting. *Spine* 2005;30:283-289.

141. Schedel H, Schneller A, Vogl T, et al: [Dynamic magnetic resonance tomography (MRI): A follow-up study after femur core decompression and instillation of recombinant human bone morphogenetic protein-2 (rhBMP-2) in avascular femur head necrosis]. *Rontgenpraxis* 2000;53:16-24.

142. Riedel GE, Valentin-Opran A: Clinical evaluation of rhBMP-2/ACS in orthopedic trauma: A progress report. *Orthopedics* 1999;22:663-665.

143. Gamradt SC, Lieberman JR: Genetic modification of stem cells to enhance bone repair. *Ann Biomed Eng* 2004;32:136-147.

144. Lieberman JR, Daluiski A, Einhorn TA: The role of growth factors in the repair of bone: Biology and clinical applications. *J Bone Joint Surg Am* 2002;84:1032-1044.

145. Nakamae A, Sunagawa T, Ishida O, et al: Acceleration of surgical angiogenesis in necrotic bone with a single injection of fibroblast growth factor-2 (FGF-2). *J Orthop Res* 2004;22:509-513.

146. Suzuki O, Bishop AT, Sunagawa T, Katsube K, Friedrich PF: VEGF-promoted surgical angiogenesis in necrotic bone. *Microsurgery* 2004;24:85-91.

147. Trippel SB, Rosenfeld RG: Growth factor treatment of disorders of skeletal growth. *Instr Course Lect* 1997;46:477-482.

148. Nakamura T, Hara Y, Tagawa M, et al: Recombinant human basic fibroblast growth factor accelerates fracture healing by enhancing callus remodeling

in experimental dog tibial fracture. *J Bone Miner Res* 1998;13:942-949.

149. Nash TJ, Howlett CR, Martin C, Steele J, Johnson KA, Hicklin DJ: Effect of platelet-derived growth factor on tibial osteotomies in rabbits. *Bone* 1994;15: 203-208.

150. Thaller SR, Dart A, Tesluk H: The effects of insulin-like growth factor-1 on critical-size calvarial defects in Sprague-Dawley rats. *Ann Plast Surg* 1993;31:429-433.

151. Trippel SB: Potential role of insulinlike growth factors in fracture healing. *Clin Orthop Relat Res* 1998;(355 suppl):S301-S313.

152. Kasten P, Vogel J, Luginbuhl R, et al: Ectopic bone formation associated with mesenchymal stem cells in a resorbable calcium deficient hydroxyapatite carrier. *Biomaterials* 2005;26:5879-5889.

153. Connolly JF: Clinical use of marrow osteoprogenitor cells to stimulate osteogenesis. *Clin Orthop Relat Res* 1998;(355 suppl):S257-S266.

154. Fleming JE Jr, Cornell CN, Muschler GF: Bone cells and matrices in orthopedic tissue engineering. *Orthop Clin North Am* 2000;31:357-374.

155. Katsube K, Bishop AT, Simari RD, Yla-Herttuala S, Friedrich PF: Vascular endothelial growth factor (VEGF) gene transfer enhances surgical revascularization of necrotic bone. *J Orthop Res* 2005;23:469-474.

156. Yang C, Yang S, Du J, Li J, Xu W, Xiong Y: Experimental study of vascular endothelial growth factor gene therapy for avascular necrosis of the femoral head. *J Huazhong Univ Sci Technolog Med Sci* 2003;23:297-299.

157. Yang C, Yang S, Du J, Li J, Xu W, Xiong Y: Vascular endothelial growth factor gene transfection to enhance the repair of avascular necrosis of the femoral head of rabbit. *Chin Med J (Engl)* 2003;116:1544-1548.

Core Decompression and Nonvascularized Bone Grafting for the Treatment of Early Stage Osteonecrosis of the Femoral Head

Michael A. Mont, MD
German A. Marulanda, MD
Thorsten M. Seyler, MD
Johannes F. Plate, BS
Ronald E. Delanois, MD

Abstract

Osteonecrosis of the femoral head is a devastating disease with many patients ultimately requiring a total hip arthroplasty. When the disease is diagnosed in its early stages (before collapse of the femoral head), various procedures such as core decompression (with and without bone grafting), osteotomies, as well as nonvascularized and vascularized bone grafting can be used in an effort to preserve the joint. The efficacy of core decompression has been peer-reviewed in more than 40 studies. In general, this treatment is most successful for patients with early stage, small- and medium-sized lesions, before collapse of the femoral head. Various methods of nonvascularized bone grafting have been used. Results have varied; however, a 60% to 80% success rate has been achieved at 5- to 10-year follow-up. In the future, these procedures may be used with various other biologic adjunctive growth and differentiation factors, which may lead to higher rates of successful treatment.

Instr Course Lect 2007;56:213-220

One or more of the authors or the departments with which they are affiliated have received something of value from a commercial or other party related directly or indirectly to the subject of this chapter.

Osteonecrosis is a devastating disease that typically affects young patients 20 to 40 years of age.[1] When untreated, the disease may progress and cause collapse of the femoral head, making a total hip arthroplasty necessary.[2] A certain percentage of patients are diagnosed before collapse of the femoral head and are amenable to joint-preserving procedures.[3] Typical femoral head-sparing procedures include core decompression with and without bone grafting,[4] osteotomies,[5-7] nonvascularized bone grafting,[8] and vascularized bone grafting.[9] Many of these procedures have success rates of 60% to 80% at short-term and mid-term follow-up, and all have the possibility for use with various growth and differentiation factors that may enhance their efficacy. The rationale, results, technique, and indications for treatment using core decompression and nonvascularized bone grafting will be discussed in this chapter.

Core Decompression

Core decompression was first described by Hungerford[10] and Ficat and Arlet[11] for use as both a diagnostic and therapeutic alternative for osteonecrosis of the femoral head. An 8- to 10-mm cylindrical core of bone from the affected femoral head was removed and analyzed to allow histologic diagnosis and to provide symptomatic relief. With the advent of MRI, the diagnostic use of this technique became irrelevant. The therapeutic effectiveness of core decompression may be the result of a mechanical reduction of bone marrow pressure as well as a possible induction of neovascularization.

Variable reports of the effectiveness of core decompression have appeared in the literature. Mont and associates[12] analyzed 24 reports[13-35] that appeared in the literature in 1995 or earlier, which included 1,206 hips treated with core decompression. Since 1995, 23 additional peer-reviewed reports have been published that included 1,491 hips. The results of these 47 studies (involving 2,697 hips) are summarized in Table 1. Outcomes were best for patients with precollapse disease, with an overall success rate of about 70% at follow-ups ranging from 2 to 10 years.

Attempts have been made to analyze the reasons for the varying results reported in studies using core decompression. It is possible that studies reporting high success rates had a larger proportion of patients who had less severe osteonecrosis. Some centers may also achieve more favorable results because of an increased awareness of the importance of early diagnosis, and because of the experience of the surgeons. Fewer complications would be expected at centers where a large number of procedures are performed. Various studies have also emphasized that factors such as size and location of the lesion are important prognosticators of outcome.[36,37] Studies reporting lower success rates with core decompression may have included patients with more advanced disease or patients taking high doses of steroids.[38,39] Interpreting and analyzing the results for core decompression from numerous studies has been difficult because of the small number of patients in some studies, different stages of the disease in patients, differing underlying causes and associated risk factors (such as corticosteroids), the use of differ-

ent surgical techniques, varying follow-up periods, and dissimilar postoperative rehabilitation protocols. More prospective, randomized, double-blinded studies are still needed to determine the true effectiveness of this procedure.

Studies in the literature indicate that the effectiveness of core decompression is negatively affected by more advanced stages of osteonecrosis.[3,12,14,15,22,35,38] Core decompression is an accepted alternative treatment for patients with stage I and II disease. The presence of stage III disease (subchondral collapse, presence of crescent sign) or stage IV disease (osteoarthritis, articular collapse) is a current contraindication for the use of this technique. Smith and associates[35] studied 114 hips and reported an 81% success rate for core decompression in patients with Ficat and Arlet stage I osteonecrosis. In hips with the crescent sign (stage III) or definitive collapse of the femoral head (stage IV), the success rates were 20% and 0%, respectively. Because core decompression relieves pain, has low morbidity, and is minimally invasive, it should be considered as palliative treatment for patients with advanced disease who are not candidates for hip arthroplasty because of medical or personal reasons.

There is increasing interest in combining core decompression of the femoral head with other treatments such as bone grafting, electrical stimulation, extracorporeal shock wave therapy, and arthroscopy. Steinberg and associates[40] reported on the effectiveness of core decompression and bone grafting in 116 hips with osteonecrosis. Seventy-four hips were also treated with direct electrical stimulation performed through a coil inserted

directly into the femoral head. Hips treated with electrical stimulation showed less radiographic disease progression and achieved a better clinical score than hips treated with decompression and grafting alone.

Core decompression has also been studied using added demineralized or decalcified bone matrix (DBM). Aaron and associates[4] evaluated 118 hips with Ficat and Arlet stage II or III osteonecrosis. Ninety hips in 66 patients had a mean follow-up of 40 months (range, 24 to 59 months) after treatment with core decompression. Twenty-eight hips in 21 patients were treated with core decompression and human DBM and had a mean follow-up of 34 months (range, 24 to 52 months). Results showed no difference in survival of hips in patients with Ficat and Arlet stage II osteonecrosis who were treated with core decompression compared with those treated with core decompression and DBM. However, in hips with Ficat and Arlet stage III osteonecrosis, core decompression and DBM resulted in substantially more successful outcomes than core decompression alone. At 24-month follow-up, the success rate in hips treated with core decompression alone was 47%, whereas those treated with core decompression and DBM had a success rate of 88%.

The surgical technique used for core decompression is quite variable.[15] Some surgeons prefer one core tract, whereas other surgeons perform multiple drillings using fluoroscopic guidance. The patient is positioned on a standard surgical table and the leg is placed in an anterior-posterior or a frog-leg position. The lesion should be preoperatively identified with the use of standard radiographs or MRI for radiographically occult lesions. The

Table 1
Results of Core Decompression

Authors	Year	Number of Hips	Overall Rate of Clinical Success (%)	Mean Follow-up in Months (range, months)	Comments
Radke et al[13]	2004	65	70	-	
Mont et al[14]	2004	45	71	24 (20-39)	
Lieberman[15]	2004	17	82	53 (26-94)	
Aigner et al[16]	2002	45	80	69 (31-120)	
Simank et al[17]	2001	94	69	72	Compared outcome to intertrochanteric osteotomy Excluded patients undergoing corticosteroid therapy
Yoon et al[18]	2001	39	45	-	
Steinberg et al[19]	2001	312	64	(24-168)	Compared outcome by stage versus size of lesion: stage I (72%) and small lesions (86%) fared best
Maniwa et al[20]	2000	26	66	94 (29-164)	Long-term follow-up (mean, 94 months)
Chen et al[21]	2000	27	60	> 24	Conversion to total hip arthroplasty used as end point
Lavernia and Sierra[22]	2000	67	63	> 24	
Bozic et al[23]	1999	54	48	120 (24-196)	Long-term follow-up (mean, 120 months). 100% success in stage IIA sclerotic hips
Simank et al[24]	1999	94	78	72 (18-180)	
Van Laere et al[25]	1998	51	39	24 (6-47)	
Scully et al[26]	1998	98	71	(21-50)	
Iorio et al[27]	1998	33	70	64	End points defined as pain (52% success), collapse (61%), total hip arthroplasty (70%)
Chang et al[28]	1997	84	30	57 (24-165)	
Powell et al[29]	1997	29	66	48	
Mazières et al[30]	1997	20	50	24	Study included only Ficat stage II hips. Outcome evaluated by MRI
Mont et al[31]	1997	79	73	144 (48-216)	Cross-sectional study in patients with corticosteroid-associated osteonecrosis (50% lupus)
Styles and Vichinsky[32]	1996	13	76	44	Sickle cell disease in children
Markel et al[33]	1996	54	35	47 (12-95)	
Holman et al[34]	1995	31	50	> 12	
Smith et al[35]	1995	114	44	40 (24-78)	
Mont et al[12]	1996	1,206	63		Literature review of 23 published studies comparing core decompression to nonsurgical management

entry point for the core decompression is done using a midlateral longitudinal incision and must be made at or just above the level of the lesser trochanter. This entry point presents difficulties, but is necessary to reduce the risk of a stress fracture of the femur. A guidewire is then placed into the osteonecrotic region

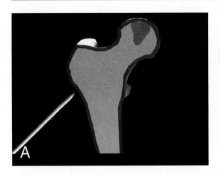
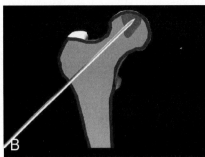

Figure 1 Schematic representation of the percutaneous drilling technique. **A,** The lateral point of entry of the 3.2-mm Steinmann pin is shown. Drilling is performed under fluoroscopic guidance. **B,** The localization of the lesion should be assessed by preoperative MRI. Special attention is given to avoid perforation of the articular cartilage.

of the femoral head under fluoroscopic guidance using AP and lateral views. It is important to avoid the articular surface of the femoral head. If this technique is used in conjunction with a bone graft, a burr is used to remove as much necrotic bone as possible. The core tract then can be grafted with autogenous bone obtained from the greater trochanter or iliac crest with or without the addition of demineralized bone matrix or bone morphogenetic proteins. The size of one core tract can range from 8 to 12 mm depending on the diameter of the patient's femur. A biopsy specimen can be taken from the femoral head to provide a definitive histologic confirmation of osteonecrosis; however, biopsy is rarely necessary because of the high sensitivity and specificity of MRI in detecting this disease. The wound is then surgically closed and protected weight bearing is prescribed for a minimum of 8 weeks after the procedure.

Mont and associates[14] recently described a new technique of core decompression using multiple small drillings with a 3.2-mm Steinmann pin. This technique is based on studies performed in Korea by Kim and associates[41] that showed a lower rate of collapse (14.3%) compared with traditional core decompression methods (45% collapse; $P = 0.03$) 3 years after surgery. In the study by Mont and associates,[14] 80% of stage I hips (24 of 30 hips) had successful outcomes at a mean follow-up of 2 years (range, 20 to 39 months). The procedure is a straightforward technique with low morbidity and no surgical complications. The percutaneous drilling technique follows methods similar to those used in conventional core decompression. Patients are placed supine on either a fracture table or a standard surgical platform. A 3.2-mm Steinmann pin is inserted laterally and percutaneously under fluoroscopic guidance (Figure 1, A). The pin is advanced until it reaches the lateral cortex in the metaphyseal region opposite the superior portion of the lesser trochanter. The femur is penetrated and the pin is advanced through the femoral neck into the femoral head and the site of the lesion (as determined from preoperative radiographs or MRI). Anteroposterior and lateral fluoroscopic views are used while advancing the pin to ensure the correct tract in the medullary canal of the femoral neck. The surgeon performs two passes

through smaller-sized lesions and three passes through larger-sized lesions using one common skin entry point. An effort is made to avoid penetration of the femoral head cartilage when advancing the pin (Figure 1, B). The pin is then removed and the wound is closed with a simple bandage or single nylon suture.

Physical therapy should be encouraged for all patients and should include gait reconditioning with a cane or crutches. Protected weight bearing is important during the immediate postoperative period to facilitate pain control and increase function.

Deconditioning can be prevented by early implementation of isometric strengthening and flexibility and range-of-motion therapy. This plan can progress to include isotonic exercise and nonimpact or low-impact training. Most patients can tolerate aquatic therapy such as water walking or running. Because of the disabling nature of osteonecrosis, the patient should be advised about employment restrictions and access to disability services early in the disease course.

Core decompression is recommended for the treatment of early stage osteonecrosis of the hip. The best results have been observed in precollapse lesions (Ficat stage I and II lesions) that involve less than 30% of the femoral head. Patients who are not candidates for more invasive surgical options may be offered the procedure as a palliative temporary treatment to relieve pain.

Nonvascularized Bone Grafting
The rationale for the use of nonvascularized bone grafting to treat osteonecrosis of the femoral head is to mechanically support the articular cartilage surface to prevent joint col-

lapse and deformity while promoting bone healing.[42] This procedure provides decompression of the femoral head, removal of necrotic bone, and structural support and scaffolding to allow remodeling of subchondral bone. Nonvascularized bone grafting is indicated for patients with postcollapse lesions with less than 2 mm of head depression, or for hips that have been unsuccessfully treated using a core decompression procedure. The efficacy of the technique may depend on intraoperative assessment of the intactness of the articular cartilage and a determination of the presence of bleeding bone after the dead necrotic femoral head bone is removed. Similar to core decompression, the use of growth factors, cytokines, and various synthetic bone graft substitutes can further enhance nonvascularized bone grafting.[43] The results of three different technical approaches for introducing nonvascularized bone graft into the femoral head [42,44-49] are shown in Table 2.

One technique of performing a nonvascularized bone graft involves supplementing the conventional approach of core decompression. A core tract through the femoral head was created that reached the lesion and then the defect was filled with a cortical graft from the tibia, fibula, or ilium.[50] The results of this technique have been quite varied, with success rates ranging from 17% to 90%. Marcus and associates[51] reported satisfactory clinical results in 7 of 11 hips at the time of short-term follow-up (range, 2 to 4 years). Boettcher and associates[52] reported success in 27 of 38 hips (71%) 6 years after nonvascularized tibial strut grafting. A longer-term evaluation of the 38 hips in the study (performed at a mean of 14 years postoperatively) found that only 16 of 56

Table 2 Results of Three Nonvascularized Bone Grafting Techniques

Authors	Year	Number of Hips	Mean Follow-up in Months (range, months)	Overall Clinical Success
Core Tract				
Lieberman et al[44]	2004	17	53 (26-94)	86%
Rijnen et al[45]	2003	28	42 (24-119)	71%
Plakseychuk et al[46]	2003	50	60 (36-96)	36%
Trapdoor Technique				
Mont et al[42]	1998	30	56 (30-60)	58%
Ko et al[47]	1995	14	56 (-)	80%
Lightbulb Technique				
Mont et al[48]	2003	21	48 (36-55)	86%
Rosenwasser et al[49]	1994		144 (120-180)	36%

hips (29%) had a good result. Nelson and Clark[53] performed 52 Phemister bone-grafting procedures in 20 patients and concluded that the technique is not effective after femoral collapse has occurred. Dunn and Grow[54] reported 4 good results in 17 patients (23 hips) treated with nonvascularized bone grafting.

Buckley and associates[55] performed 20 core decompressions with the introduction of corticocancellous bone grafting for stage I or II osteonecrosis of the femoral head. At a mean follow-up of 8 years (range, 2 to 19 years), 18 patients were asymptomatic with no evidence of progression of the necrosis or collapse of the affected segment. Lieberman[15] performed a retrospective evaluation of 15 patients (17 hips) with symptomatic osteonecrosis of the hip. Patients were treated with core decompression combined with an allogenic allograft and 50 mg of partially purified human bone morphogenetic protein. At a mean follow-up of 53 months (range, 26

to 94 months), 14 of 15 hips (93%; 13 patients) with stage IIA disease had clinical success. Three of 17 hips (in 3 patients) had radiographic evidence of disease progression (Ficat and Arlet stages IIA, IIB, and III) of the femoral head and were treated with total hip arthroplasty. No radiographic progression occurred in the three hips with less than one third involvement of the weight-bearing surface.

Another technique of nonvascularized bone grafting involves the use of a chondral window (trapdoor approach). By lifting up a portion of the chondral surface, the underlying lesion is exposed, the necrotic bone is removed, and the cavity is filled with either cancellous and/or cortical bone graft. Meyers[56] reported a 90% good to excellent clinical result at a mean follow-up of 3 years (range, 1 to 9 years). Mont and associates[42] reported an 83% success rate for stage III osteonecrotic hips (20 of 24 hips) treated using the trapdoor technique at a mean follow-up of 56

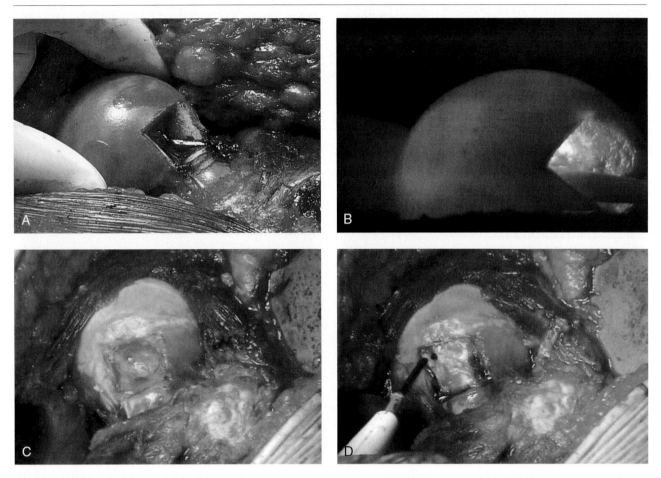

Figure 2 Intraoperative image of bone grafting of the femoral head using the lightbulb technique. **A,** The bone window (trapdoor) at the femoral head-neck junction is shown. **B,** The dead bone is removed from the femoral head (hollow femoral head has the appearance of a light bulb). **C,** The allograft is tightly packed into the cavity with a layered approach. **D,** The trapdoor is replaced and fixed with three 2-mm absorbable pins.

months (range, 30 to 60 months).

Ko and associates[47] treated 13 adolescent patients (14 hips) with severe femoral head osteonecrosis with articular surface collapse using the trapdoor bone grafting technique. Nine patients (10 hips) were simultaneously treated with a containment osteotomy of the femur and acetabulum. At an average follow-up of 4.5 years, seven patients (eight hips) had a good clinical result and two had a fair result. None of the10 hips required hip fusion or total hip arthroplasty at most recent follow-up.

A third approach for introducing nonvascularized bone graft into the femoral head is the so-called lightbulb technique. A bone window (trapdoor) measuring approximately 2 cm in width by 2 cm in length is removed at the femoral head-neck junction using a micro-oscillating saw and osteotomes. This trapdoor segment is saved in normal saline-wrapped gauze for later use. A mushroom-tipped burr is used to curet a cavity in the femoral head using the trapdoor as an entrance; all the dead bone is removed. The allograft is then packed into the cavity with a layered approach and the trapdoor is replaced and fixed with three 2-mm absorbable pins[48] (Figure 2). If the entire femoral head has

dead bone (no bleeding bone encountered), the procedure should be abandoned and a total hip arthroplasty should be performed.

Rosenwasser and associates[49] published the results of long-term follow-up (mean, 12 years; range, 10 to 15 years) of patients treated with cancellous bone graft through a window in the femoral head-neck junction. The débridement of all sclerotic bone was performed using image intensification, and cancellous bone was harvested from the ipsilateral iliac crest and packed tightly into the femoral head to the subchondral plate. Two patients (13%) required revision with total hip arthroplasty.

Mont and associates[48] also described the use of bone grafting through a window at the femoral head-neck junction for the treatment of osteonecrosis of the femoral head. An anterolateral approach to the hip was used in an effort to conserve the blood supply. Bone morphogenetic protein-enriched allograft was used to avoid donor site morbidity. Nineteen patients (21 hips) had a mean follow-up of 48 months (range, 36 to 55 months) after a bone grafting procedure in which the diseased bone was replaced by a bone graft substitute (combination of DBM, processed allograft bone chips, and a thermoplastic carrier). Eighteen of 21 hips (86%) had clinically successful results at the most recent follow-up.

Nonvascularized bone grafting has several advantages for patients with precollapsed and early postcollapsed lesions in which the articular cartilage is relatively undamaged. The current indications for the use of nonvascularized bone grafting include precollapse lesions (Ficat and Arlet stage I and II lesions) and early postcollapse lesions (Ficat and Arlet stage III, crescent sign) with subchondral changes, but with an intact articular surface. The large variation in results using nonvascularized bone grafting may be partly explained by treating patients with this technique outside of strict indications such as those with larger lesions, delaminated cartilage, and severe head collapse. The authors recommend that this procedure be used only in carefully selected patients. **(DVD 22.1)**

Summary

Conventional core decompression and percutaneous drilling techniques, as well as nonvascularized bone grafting, have been shown to be effective alternatives for the treatment of early stage osteonecrosis. Future studies may include the addition of novel growth and differentiation factors to preserve the femoral head. Successful use of these factors may forestall the need for more invasive surgical procedures such as total joint arthroplasty.

References

1. Mont MA, Hungerford DS: Non-traumatic avascular necrosis of the femoral head. *J Bone Joint Surg Am* 1995;77:459-474.

2. Lavernia CJ, Sierra RJ, Grieco FR: Osteonecrosis of the femoral head. *J Am Acad Orthop Surg* 1999;7:250-261.

3. Hungerford DS: Osteonecrosis: Avoiding total hip arthroplasty. *J Arthroplasty* 2002;17:121-124.

4. Aaron RK, Combor DM, Lord CF: Core decompression augmented with human decalcified bone matrix graft for osteonecrosis of the femoral head, in Urbaniak JR, Jones JP (eds): *Osteonecrosis: Etiology, Diagnosis and Treatment.* Rosemont, IL, American Academy of Orthopaedic Surgeons, 1997, pp 301-307.

5. Mont MA, Fairbank AC, Krackow KA, Hungerford DS: Corrective osteotomy for osteonecrosis of the femoral head. *J Bone Joint Surg Am* 1996;78:1032-1038.

6. Nakamura Y, Kumazawa Y, Mitsui H, Toh S, Katano H: Combined rotational osteotomy and vascularized iliac bone graft for advanced osteonecrosis of the femoral head. *J Reconstr Microsurg* 2005;21:101-105.

7. Onodera S, Majima T, Abe Y, Ito H, Matsuno T, Minami A: Transtrochanteric rotational osteotomy for osteonecrosis of the femoral head: Relation between radiographic features and secondary collapse. *J Orthop Sci* 2005;10:367-373.

8. Zhang B, Zhu S, Guo Y: Treatment of ischemic necrosis of femoral head by focal cleaning and bone graft. *Zhongguo Xiu Fu Chong Jian Wai Ke Za Zhi* 2000;14:93-95.

9. Mont MA, Jones LC, Hungerford DS: Survival analysis of hips treated with core decompression or vascularized fibular grafting because of avascular necrosis. *J Bone Joint Surg Am* 2000;82:290-291.

10. Hungerford DS: Bone marrow pressure, venography, and core decompression in isquemic necrosis of the femoral head. *The Hip: Proceedings of the Seventh Open Scientific Meeting of the Hip Society.* St Louis, MO, CV Mosby, 1979, p 218.

11. Ficat RP, Arlet J: Functional investigation of bone under normal conditions, in Hungerford DS (ed): *Ischemia and Necrosis of Bone.* Baltimore, MD, Williams and Wilkins, 1980, pp 29-52.

12. Mont MA, Carbone JJ, Fairbank AC: Core decompression versus nonoperative management for osteonecrosis of the hip. *Clin Orthop Relat Res* 1996;324:169-178.

13. Radke S, Kirschner S, Seipel V, Rader C, Eulert J: Magnetic resonance imaging criteria of successful core decompression in avascular necrosis of the hip. *Skeletal Radiol* 2004;33:519-523.

14. Mont MA, Ragland PS, Etienne G: Core decompression of the femoral head for osteonecrosis using percutaneous multiple small-diameter drilling. *Clin Orthop Relat Res* 2004;429:131-138.

15. Lieberman JR: Core decompression for osteonecrosis of the hip. *Clin Orthop Relat Res* 2004;418:29-33.

16. Aigner N, Schneider W, Eberl V, Knahr K: Core decompression in early stages of femoral head osteonecrosis: An MRI-controlled study. *Int Orthop* 2002;26:31-35.

17. Simank HG, Brocai DR, Brill C, Lukoschek M: Comparison of results of core decompression and intertrochanteric osteotomy for nontraumatic osteonecrosis of the femoral head using Cox regression and survivorship analysis. *J Arthroplasty* 2001;16:790-794.

18. Yoon TR, Song EK, Rowe SM, Park CH: Failure after core decompression in osteonecrosis of the femoral head. *Int Orthop* 2001;24:316-318.

19. Steinberg ME, Larcom PG, Strafford B, et al: Core decompression with bone grafting for osteonecrosis of the femoral head. *Clin Orthop Relat Res* 2001;386:71-78.

20. Maniwa S, Nishikori T, Furukawa S, et al: Evaluation of core decompression for early osteonecrosis of the femoral head. *Arch Orthop Trauma Surg* 2000;120:241-244.

21. Chen CH, Chang JK, Huang KY, Hung SH, Lin GT, Lin SY: Core decompression for osteonecrosis of the femoral head at pre-collapse stage. *Kaohsiung J Med Sci* 2000;16:76-82.

22. Lavernia CJ, Sierra RJ: Core decompression in atraumatic osteonecrosis of the hip. *J Arthroplasty*

2000;15:171-178.

23. Bozic KJ, Zurakowski D, Thornhill TS: Survivorship analysis of hips treated with core decompression for nontraumatic osteonecrosis of the femoral head. *J Bone Joint Surg Am* 1999;81:200-209.

24. Simank HG, Brocai DR, Strauch K, Lukoschek M: Core decompression in osteonecrosis of the femoral head: Risk-factor-dependent outcome evaluation using survivorship analysis. *Int Orthop* 1999;23:154-159.

25. Van Laere C, Mulier M, Simon JP, Stuyck J, Fabry G: Core decompression for avascular necrosis of the femoral head. *Acta Orthop Belg* 1998;64:269-272.

26. Scully SP, Aaron RK, Urbaniak JR: Survival analysis of hips treated with core decompression or vascularized fibular grafting because of avascular necrosis. *J Bone Joint Surg Am* 1998;80:1270-1275.

27. Iorio R, Healy WL, Abramowitz AJ, Pfeifer BA: Clinical outcome and survivorship analysis of core decompression for early osteonecrosis of the femoral head. *J Arthroplasty* 1998;13:34-41.

28. Chang MC, Chen TH, Lo WH: Core decompression in treating ischemic necrosis of the femoral head. *Zhonghua Yi Xue Za Zhi (Taipei)* 1997;60:130-136.

29. Powell ET, Lanzer WL, Mankey MG: Core decompression for early osteonecrosis of the hip in high risk patients. *Clin Orthop Relat Res* 1997;335:181-189.

30. Mazieres B, Marin F, Chiron P, et al: Influence of the volume of osteonecrosis on the outcome of core decompression of the femoral head. *Ann Rheum Dis* 1997;56:747-750.

31. Mont MA, Fairbank AC, Petri M, Hungerford DS: Core decompression for osteonecrosis of the femoral head in systemic lupus erythematosus. *Clin Orthop Relat Res* 1997;334:91-97.

32. Styles LA, Vichinsky EP: Core decompression in avascular necrosis of the hip in sickle-cell disease. *Am J Hematol* 1996;52:103-107.

33. Markel DC, Miskovsky C, Sculco TP, Pellicci PM, Salvati EA: Core decompression for osteonecrosis of the femoral head. *Clin Orthop Relat Res* 1996;323:226-233.

34. Holman AJ, Gardner GC, Richardson ML, Simkin PA: Quantitative magnetic resonance imaging predicts clinical outcome of core decompression for osteonecrosis of the femoral head.

J Rheumatol 1995;22:1929-1933.

35. Smith SW, Fehring TK, Griffin WL, Beaver WB: Core decompression of the osteonecrotic femoral head. *J Bone Joint Surg Am* 1995;77:674-680.

36. Ohzono K, Saito M, Sugano N, Takaoka K, Ono K: The fate of nontraumatic avascular necrosis of the femoral head: A radiologic classification to formulate prognosis. *Clin Orthop Relat Res* 1992;277:73-78.

37. Takatori Y, Kokubo T, Ninomiya S, et al: Avascular necrosis of the femoral head: Natural history and magnetic resonance imaging. *J Bone Joint Surg Br* 1993;75:217-221.

38. Warner JJ, Philip JH, Brodsky GL, Thornhill TS: Studies of nontraumatic osteonecrosis: The role of core decompression in the treatment of nontraumatic osteonecrosis of the femoral head. *Clin Orthop Relat Res* 1987;225:104-127.

39. Hopson CN, Siverhus SW: Ischemic necrosis of the femoral head: Treatment by core decompression. *J Bone Joint Surg Am* 1988;70:1048-1051.

40. Steinberg ME, Brighton CT, Corces A, et al: Osteonecrosis of the femoral head: Results of core decompression and grafting with and without electrical stimulation. *Clin Orthop Relat Res* 1989;249:199-208.

41. Kim Sy: Kim DH, Park IH, et al: Multiple drilling compared with core decompression for the treatment of osteonecrosis of the femoral head. ARCO website. Available at: http://www.arco-intl.org/abstracts/2003%20Abstracts/Kim-MultipleDrilling.htm. Accessed September 27, 2006.

42. Mont MA, Einhorn TA, Sponseller PD, Hungerford DS: The trapdoor procedure using autogenous cortical and cancellous bone grafts for osteonecrosis of the femoral head. *J Bone Joint Surg Br* 1998;80:56-62.

43. Wang CJ, Wang FS, Huang CC, Yang KD, Weng LH, Huang HY: Treatment for osteonecrosis of the femoral head: Comparison of extracorporeal shock waves with core decompression and bone-grafting. *J Bone Joint Surg Am* 2005;87:2380-2387.

44. Lieberman JR, Conduah A, Urist MR: Treatment of osteonecrosis of the femoral head with core decompression and human bone morphogenetic protein. *Clin Orthop Relat Res* 2004;429:139-145.

45. Rijnen WH, Gardeniers JW, Buma P, Yamano K, Slooff TJ, Schreurs BW: Treatment of femoral head osteonecrosis using bone impaction grafting. *Clin Orthop Relat Res* 2003;417:74-83.

46. Plakseychuk AY, Kim SY, Park BC, Varitimidis SE, Rubash HE, Sotereanos DG: Vascularized compared with nonvascularized fibular grafting for the treatment of osteonecrosis of the femoral head. *J Bone Joint Surg Am* 2003;85:589-596.

47. Ko JY, Meyers MH, Wenger DR: "Trapdoor" procedure for osteonecrosis with segmental collapse of the femoral head in teenagers. *J Pediatr Orthop* 1995;15:7-15.

48. Mont MA, Etienne G, Ragland PS: Outcome of nonvascularized bone grafting for osteonecrosis of the femoral head. *Clin Orthop Relat Res* 2003;417:84-92.

49. Rosenwasser MP, Garino JP, Kiernan HA, Michelsen CB: Long term followup of thorough debridement and cancellous bone grafting of the femoral head for avascular necrosis. *Clin Orthop Relat Res* 1994;306:17-27.

50. Kim SY, Kim YG, Kim PT, Ihn JC, Cho BC, Koo KH: Vascularized compared with nonvascularized fibular grafts for large osteonecrotic lesions of the femoral head. *J Bone Joint Surg Am* 2005;87:2012-2018.

51. Marcus ND, Enneking WF, Massam RA: The silent hip in idiopathic aseptic necrosis: Treatment by bone-grafting. *J Bone Joint Surg Am* 1973;55:1351-1366.

52. Boettcher WG, Bonfiglio M, Smith K: Non-traumatic necrosis of the femoral head: II. Experiences in treatment. *J Bone Joint Surg Am* 1970;52:322-329.

53. Nelson LM, Clark CR: Efficacy of phemister bone grafting in nontraumatic aseptic necrosis of the femoral head. *J Arthroplasty* 1993;8:253-258.

54. Dunn AW, Grow T: Aseptic necrosis of the femoral head: Treatment with bone grafts of doubtful value. *Clin Orthop Relat Res* 1977;122:249-254.

55. Buckley PD, Gearen PF, Petty RW: Structural bone-grafting for early atraumatic avascular necrosis of the femoral head. *J Bone Joint Surg Am* 1991;73:1357-1364.

56. Meyers MH: The surgical treatment of osteonecrosis of the femoral head with an osteochondral allograft. *Acta Orthop Belg* 1999;65(suppl 1):66-67.

Advances in Hip Arthroplasty in the Treatment of Osteonecrosis

Thorsten M. Seyler, MD
Quanjun Cui, MD, MS
William M. Mihalko, MD, PhD
Michael A. Mont, MD
Khaled J. Saleh, MD, MSc, FRCSC, FACS

Osteonecrosis of the femoral head is a devastating disease for which many patients will eventually require total hip arthroplasty. Standard total hip arthroplasties have historically had poor results in patients with osteonecrosis. More recently, reports have shown excellent results with second- and third-generation designs that incorporate advances in bearing technology. However, there are still certain subpopulations of patients (those with sickle cell disease, those with systemic lupus erythematosus, and those who have undergone renal transplantation) that have less than optimal results. Other hip arthroplasty alternatives include bipolar hemiarthroplasty, limited femoral resurfacing, and metal-on-metal resurfacing. Bipolar hemiarthroplasty historically and currently has consistently poor results in most studies and should be avoided in patients with osteonecrosis. In multiple reports, limited femoral arthroplasty has demonstrated reasonable midterm and long-term outcomes as a temporizing procedure, with results being less predictable than for standard total hip arthroplasty. Recently, ceramic-on-ceramic and metal-on-metal resurfacing hip arthroplasty has emerged as a viable option that has been used to treat patients with osteonecrosis of the femoral head, and several studies have shown promising short-term outcomes. Overall, however, recent studies have shown more optimal outcomes with hip arthroplasty than resurfacing hip arthroplasty, which makes standard hip replacements, as well as other arthroplasty alternatives, more attractive for young patients with this disease.

Instr Course Lect 2007;56:221-233.

One or more of the authors or the departments with which they are affiliated have received something of value from a commercial or other party related directly or indirectly to the subject of this chapter.

Osteonecrosis is a devastating disease that usually leads to destruction of the hip joint. It typically occurs in young patients who are in the second through fifth decades of life.[1,2] In the early stages of the disease, various treatment alternatives such as core decompression, rotational osteotomy, and vascularized or nonvascularized bone grafting can be used to delay or avoid the need for total hip arthroplasty. Unfortunately, many patients present with late-stage disease (post-collapse) and have few alternatives that allow them to preserve the femoral head. Once the femoral head collapses or arthritis occurs on the acetabular side, the treatment of choice is reconstructive hip replacement.[3] Various types of hip replacement procedures such as limited resurfacing, bipolar hemiarthroplasty, standard total hip arthroplasty, and total resurfacing arthroplasty have been used to treat this patient population.[4]

Historically, the results of standard total hip replacements in patients with osteonecrosis have not been optimal in young patients with other disorders such as rheumatoid arthritis or primary osteoarthritis.[5-8] The poorest results have been found after bipolar hemiarthroplasty, probably because of the use of thin polyethylene, which can lead to extensive wear and subsequent osteolysis.[6,9,10] In addition, various other types of arthroplasty devices

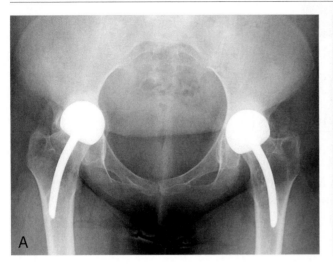
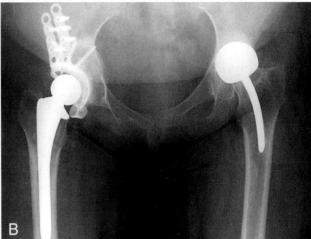

Figure 1 A, Preoperative AP radiograph shows bilateral limited resurfacing with protrusion on the right hip. **B,** Postoperative AP radiograph shows revision total hip arthroplasty has been performed on the right hip.

have been used. There is significant experience with the use of limited femoral resurfacing and renewed interest in metal-on-metal total joint prostheses, including metal-on-metal total resurfacings. Recent advances in prosthesis design, bearing surfaces, and bone ingrowth have led to improved results of reconstructive joint procedures. The selection and criteria for the use of these different devices, new technologies, or surgical techniques are discussed in this chapter.

It is important to make the appropriate choice of treatment for osteonecrosis of the femoral head because this patient population includes a large number of patients who will need to undergo a hip arthroplasty procedure. The true number of patients undergoing total hip arthroplasties annually for the treatment of osteonecrosis in the United States is unknown; however, recent data from both the Canadian Joint Arthroplasty Registry and the Australian National Joint Arthroplasty Registry have demonstrated that the diagnosis of osteonecrosis accounts for 5% of all primary total

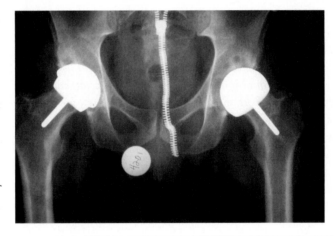

Figure 2 AP radiograph shows a metal-on-metal total hip resurfacing on the right side and a limited femoral resurfacing on the left side.

hip arthroplasties performed annually in those geographic areas.[11,12]

Limited Femoral Head Resurfacing

The high failure rate of total hip arthroplasty in young patients with osteonecrosis of the femoral head has historically made it an unfavorable treatment option (Figure 1). In advanced disease stages, procedures such as core decompression, rotational osteotomies, and nonvascularized and vascularized bone grafting do not have predictable results. In patients with large precollapse lesions and postcollapse disease, an-

other treatment option is femoral head resurfacing arthroplasty. Limited resurfacing (hemiresurfacing) of only the femoral side of the hip joint uses a cemented femoral head prosthesis that is matched in diameter with the native acetabulum (Figure 2). This procedure requires a pristine or relatively undamaged acetabular surface. The potential advantages of hemiresurfacing over total hip arthroplasty are removal of the damaged cartilage, bone stock preservation, lower dislocation rates, delay of a total hip arthroplasty, and easy conversion to hip arthroplasty if necessary.

Table 1
Literature Review of Limited Resurfacing for Osteonecrosis of the Femoral Head

Author(s)	Year	No. of Hips	Procedure	Average Follow-up (Range) [months]	Overall Clinical Success
Cuckler et al[17]	2004	59	Hemiresurfacing	54	68%
Beaulé et al[18]	2004	28	Hemiresurfacing	60 (28-100)	86%
Adili and Trousdale[16]	2003	29	Hemiresurfacing	34 (24-63)	94% (1-year follow-up)
					76% (3-year follow-up)
Beaulé et al[14]	2001	37	Hemiresurfacing	78 (24-216)	79% (5-year follow-up)
					59% (10-year follow-up)
					45% (15-year follow-up)
Mont et al[13]	2001	30	Hemiresurfacing	84 (48-101)	90%
Siguier et al[19]	2001	37	Hemiresurfacing	49 (24-89)	85%
Nelson et al[15]	1997	21	Hemiresurfacing	> 60	82%
Grecula et al[20]	1995	10	Hemiresurfacing	96	70%
Tooke et al[21]	1987	12	Hemiresurfacing	39 (24-62)	92%
Langlais et al[22]	1979	86	Hemiresurfacing	78	85%
Hungerford et al[23]	1998	33	TARA	126 (48-168)	91%
Krackow et al[24]	1993	19	TARA	36 (24-72)	84%
Scott et al[25]	1987	25	TARA	37 (25-60)	88%

TARA = Total articular replacement arthroplasty.

Mont and associates[13] compared the outcome of hemiresurfacing to that of conventional total hip replacement for patients with postcollapse disease. At a mean 7-year follow-up for the hemiresurfacing group and a mean 8-year follow-up for the total hip arthroplasty group, they found that a higher percentage of patients who underwent hemiresurfacing were participating in sports (60% versus 27%). However, more patients who underwent hemiresurfacing had groin pain (20% versus 6%). Overall survivorship was similar in both groups: 90% for the hemiresurfacing group compared with 93% for the total hip arthroplasty group. Beaulé and associates[14] reported on a series of 37 hips followed for a mean of 6.5 years (range, 2 to 18 years) with conversion to total hip arthroplasty as the end point. The overall survival of hemiresurfacing in this study was 79% at 5-year follow-up, 59% at 10-

year follow-up, and 45% at 15-year follow-up. Nelson and associates[15] analyzed 21 hips treated with a custom-cemented titanium femoral component. At a mean follow-up of 6.2 years, the success rate was 82% (14 of 17 hips).

Recently, there have been a few reports detailing the less predictable outcomes and pain relief with resurfacing procedures. Adili and Trousdale[16] reviewed the clinical and radiographic results of 29 consecutive femoral head resurfacing procedures in 28 patients. They found that 17 patients (18 hips, 62%) reported feeling better than they did before surgery, with an overall survivorship of 75.9% at 3 years. At final follow-up, eight hips (27.6%) were converted to a total hip arthroplasty. Cuckler and associates[17] studied 59 hips for a mean follow-up of 4.5 years. They reported that in 16 patients (32%) the resurfacing procedure was considered a failure be-

cause of conversion to total hip arthroplasty or considerable groin pain requiring medication. Conversion of the failed implants to total hip arthroplasty was straightforward, confirming the conservative nature of the procedure. Both of these studies emphasized the unpredictable results obtained with resurfacing procedures.

On the basis of the previously cited reports and the results of the other studies[14-25] listed in Table 1, the following criteria are recommended for identifying appropriate candidates for limited femoral resurfacing: (1) young patients presenting with Ficat and Arlet stage III radiographic disease, (2) lesions with a combined necrotic angle greater than 200° or greater than 30% of femoral head involvement, (3) postcollapse lesions with greater than 2 mm of femoral head depression, and (4) no evidence of acetabular cartilage damage. With careful

Bipolar Hemiarthroplasty

Bipolar hemiarthroplasty has the same indications as hemiresurfacing. It has been designed to decrease the acetabular shear force through the use of an outer free acetabular cup that articulates with the prosthetic femoral head. Bipolar hemiarthroplasty has yielded variable success rates in patients with osteonecrosis of the femoral head, with many previous studies reporting less than optimal success. Although efforts have been made to improve results, hemiarthroplasty requires resection of the femoral neck and violation of the femoral canal, which may complicate future revisions. The most common complication associated with bipolar hemiarthroplasty is protrusio acetabuli.

In a series of 22 patients, Grevitt and Spencer[26] reported good or excellent results (full total hip arthroplasty was avoided) in 21 patients at a mean 40-month follow-up (range, 24 to 27 months). More recently, Chan and Shih[27] compared the outcomes of cementless total hip arthroplasty and hemiarthroplasty in a series of 28 patients with bilateral disease. At a mean 6.4-year follow-up (range, 4 to 12 years), a satisfactory outcome was found in 24 of 28 patients in the hemiarthroplasty group compared with 23 of 28 patients in the cementless total hip arthroplasty group.

Other reports have shown high complication rates in this patient population. Lachiewicz and Desman[9] analyzed 31 bipolar hip arthroplasties performed for osteonecrosis of the femoral head. At a mean 4.6-year follow-up, 48% of the hips had excellent or good results. Sanjay and Moreau[28] reported 17 complications in 21 patients at a mean 4.6-year follow-up (range, 2.1 to 7.0 years). Ito and associates[29] reviewed 48 hips in 35 patients at a mean 11.4-year follow-up and found radiographic failure and/or acetabular degeneration in 42% of patients. Yamano and associates[30] reported the results of 29 cementless press-fit bipolar endoprostheses at a mean 12-year follow-up, with femoral loosening occurring in 6 hips (21%), acetabular protrusio occurring in 5 hips (17%), and osteolysis occurring in 11 hips (38%).

Because of these high failure and complication rates, there has been an overall decrease in the use of bipolar hemiarthroplasty for patients with osteonecrosis of the femoral head. In addition, osteolysis from polyethylene wear has been reported as a late complication in young, active patients probably because the polyethylene liner is often quite thin. Although bipolar hemiarthroplasty may be a reasonable treatment alternative for patients who have undergone renal transplant and have less activity in general,[31] it should not be used in this patient population. A summary of the results of using hemiarthroplasty to treat patients with osteonecrosis of the femoral head[6,9,10,26-35] appears in Table 2.

Standard Total Hip Arthroplasty

Standard total hip arthroplasty predictably provides excellent pain relief and a good functional outcome (Figure 3). However, it sacrifices more host bone and limits future surgical options. The most recent issue with regard to the results of total hip arthroplasty for the treatment of osteonecrosis is the longevity of the prosthesis compared with the longevity reported for other diagnoses such as osteoarthritis and rheumatoid arthritis.[3-5,7,8] Factors that contribute to the high failure rates include relatively young age, long life expectancy, increased body weight, and poor quality of the femoral bone. Some authors have suggested that osteonecrosis of the femoral head itself is not a risk factor for failure of total hip arthroplasty. Historically, there have been poor results, with 30% to 50% failure rates reported with first-generation devices at short-term follow-up. Saito and associates[8] analyzed 29 hips treated with cemented total hip arthroplasty. At a mean 84-month follow-up, the clinical success rate was 52%. Similar results have been reported in studies by Dorr and associates[36] (45% failure rate), Cornell and associates[37] (39% failure rate), and Chandler and associates[7] (57% failure rate). More recently, improved results have been reported with the use of new bearing surfaces, cementing techniques, and new designs, but the results are still inferior to those reported for standard total hip arthroplasty performed for other diagnoses such as osteoarthritis or rheumatoid arthritis.

The results of using cemented standard total hip arthroplasty to treat patients with osteonecrosis of the femoral head vary. Early cementing techniques have had high failure rates, but studies assessing modern cementing methods have reported improved results. Kantor and associates[38] analyzed the results of 28 total hip arthroplasties with second-generation cementing techniques. At a mean 92-month follow-up, the survival rate was 86%. The authors concluded that despite the use of second-generation cementing techniques and improved results, the

Table 2
Literature Review of Bipolar Hemiarthroplasty for Osteonecrosis of the Femoral Head

Author(s)	Year	No. of Hips	Procedure	Average Follow-up (Range) [months]	Overall Clinical Success
Tsumura et al[32]	2005	32	Bipolar hemiarthroplasty	92 (60-180)	86%
Yamano et al[30]	2004	29	Bipolar hemiarthroplasty	144	62%
Lee et al[33]	2004	40	Bipolar hemiarthroplasty	96	95%
Nagai et al[34]	2002	12	Bipolar hemiarthroplasty	144-216	75%
Ito et al[29]	2000	48	Bipolar hemiarthroplasty	137 (84-216)	75%
Chan and Shih[27]	2000	28	Bipolar hemiarthroplasty	77 (48-144)	89%
Sanjay and Moreau[28]	1996	26	Bipolar hemiarthroplasty	55 (25-84)	57%
Grevitt and Spencer[26]	1995	22	Bipolar hemiarthroplasty	40 (24-71)	95%
Murzic and McCollum[31]	1994	32	Bipolar hemiarthroplasty	24-216	88%
Learmonth and Opitz[35]	1993	38	Bipolar hemiarthroplasty	56 (42-72)	87%
Takaoka et al[10]	1992	82	Bipolar hemiarthroplasty	66	86%
Cabanela[6]	1990	23	Bipolar hemiarthroplasty	110	59%
Lachiewicz and Desman[9]	1988	31	Bipolar hemiarthroplasty	55	48%

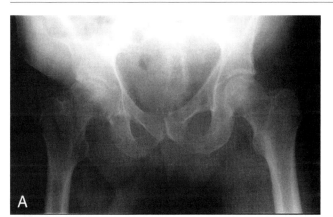

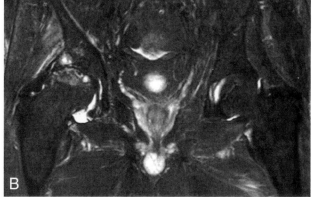

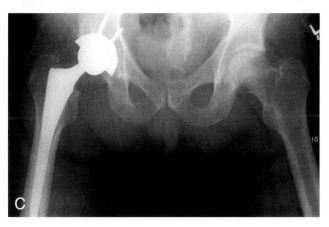

Figure 3 A, Preoperative AP radiograph shows collapse of the femoral head in a patient with osteonecrosis of the right femoral head. **B,** Preoperative MRI scan confirmed the diagnosis. **C,** Postoperative AP radiograph shows that metal-on-polyethylene total hip arthroplasty has been performed.

failure rate was still high. Garino and Steinberg[39] reviewed 123 cemented and hybrid total hip arthroplasties in patients with osteonecrosis. In their series, second-generation cementing techniques resulted in a 96% survival rate at a mean 54-month follow-up (range, 24 to 120 months). These results seem significantly better than previously reported. Recently, Kim and associates[40] prospectively studied the clinical and radiographic outcomes of total hip arthroplasty with so-called third-generation cementing and second-generation cementless total hip arthroplasties in 100 hips with osteonecrosis of the femoral head. At the final 122-month follow-up, they reported a survival rate of 98% in both groups. Radiographically, osteolysis of the femur occurred in 16% of the hips in the group treated with cement and in 24% of the hips in the group treated without cement.

Various reports have demonstrated improved implant fixation and implant longevity using newer designs of cementless total hip arthroplasties. Phillips and associates[41] reported on 20 cementless porous-coated primary total hip arthroplasties performed on 15 patients. At a minimum 24-month follow-up (mean, 62 months), no revisions were performed and one femoral component was loose. However, a high rate of acetabular component wear and osteolysis was radiographically noted and remained one of the major concerns for long-term outcome. Piston and associates[42] reviewed 35 cementless porous-coated total hip arthroplasties in 30 patients. At a mean 90-month follow-up (range, 60 to 120 months), the revision rate was 3% (1 of 30 hips) for the femoral side and 6% (2 of 30 hips) for the acetabular

side, which accounts for an overall failure rate of 6% (2 of 30 hips). All patients returned to a high level of activity postoperatively. Xenakis and associates[43] compared cementless total hip arthroplasties performed on 29 patients with osteonecrosis of the femoral head and on 29 patients with degenerative osteoarthritis. At a mean 7.6-year and 7.1-year follow-up, respectively, only one femoral implant failure occurred in the osteonecrosis group. With an overall survival rate of 96% for cementless total hip arthroplasty, this study demonstrated encouraging clinical results.

The underlying diagnosis associated with osteonecrosis of the femoral head appears to have an impact on implant longevity. Patients in certain subgroups such as those with osteonecrosis secondary to systemic lupus erythematosus, sickle cell disease, or renal transplantation have an increased risk for implant failure. Acurio and Friedman[44] retrospectively reviewed 25 total hip arthroplasties in 25 patients with sickle cell disease and osteonecrosis. At a mean 103-month follow-up (range, 24 to 216 months), 14 of 25 (40%) of the arthroplasties had been revised and 9 other hips (36%) were either radiographically and/or symptomatically loose. The overall complication rate was 49%, and the infection rate 20%. Lieberman and associates[45] reviewed 30 hips in patients with renal transplants and 16 hips in patients on chronic renal dialysis. Patients with renal transplants had generally satisfactory results that were comparable to the results of patients with osteonecrosis without underlying renal disease. However, patients undergoing hip arthroplasty while undergoing long-term renal dialysis demonstrated poor results (81% failure rate). Brinker and associates[5] re-

ported that patients who were younger than 35 years at the time of the total hip arthroplasty had a high failure rate, and the results varied by underlying diagnosis. Patients with systemic lupus erythematosus or an organ transplant had poorer results than those with idiopathic osteonecrosis of the femoral head. In contrast, Huo and associates[46] reported a 94.6% survival probability at 5 years and an 81.8% survival probability at 9 years for patients with osteonecrosis of the femoral head associated with systemic lupus erythematosus. Murzic and McCollum[31] compared cemented total hip arthroplasty, cementless bipolar hemiarthroplasty, and cementless total hip arthroplasty in 46 patients who underwent renal transplantation (77 hips) and had osteonecrosis of the femoral head. With a follow-up ranging from 24 to 216 months, loosening occurred in 46% of the hips treated with cemented total hip arthroplasty, 9% of the hips treated with bipolar hemiarthroplasty, and no hips treated with cementless total hip arthroplasty. The revision rates were 31%, 12.5%, and 0, respectively. Similar results have been reported by Zangger and associates.[47] These authors studied 19 patients with systemic lupus erythematosus and osteonecrosis of the femoral head who underwent 26 total hip arthroplasties. At a minimum follow-up of 24 months, one patient had developed a low-grade prosthetic infection and underwent successful revision, and there was one asymptomatic cup migration, accounting for an overall survival rate of 93%.

The use of ceramic alumina tribology in total hip arthroplasty is now well established (Figure 4). Retrieval studies have demonstrated that the wear rate in stable compo-

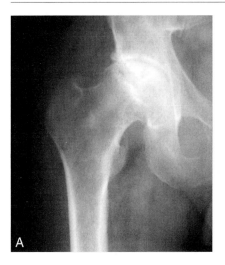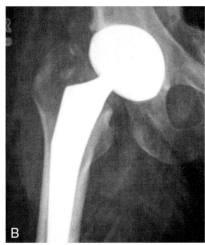

Figure 4   Preoperative **(A)** and postoperative **(B)** AP radiographs of a patient who underwent ceramic-on-ceramic total hip arthroplasty.

nents ranged from 0.025 μm to 2 μm per year. Nich and associates[48] recently reported the long-term results of ceramic-on-ceramic total hip arthroplasty in patients with osteonecrosis. Fifty-two ceramic-on-ceramic total hip arthroplasties were performed in 41 patients with osteonecrosis (mean age, 41 years; age range, 22 to 79 years). At an average 16-year follow-up (range, 11 to 24 years), no osteolysis was observed and no wear was detectable. With revision for aseptic loosening as the end point, the authors reported survival rates of 88.5% for the cup and 100% for the stem at 10-year follow-up. Fye and associates[49] analyzed 72 hips treated with either ceramic-on-ceramic or ceramic-on-polyethylene bearings. At a mean follow-up of 84 months (minimum follow-up, 48 months), the probability of survival for the entire series using revision as the end point was 97% at 11 years. The survival probability decreased to 89% when radiographic failures were included in the analysis. More recently, newer designs such as press-fit metal-backed alumina sockets have shown a better mid-

term outcome. However, long-term outcome studies are needed to further define the role of ceramic-on-ceramic total hip arthroplasty in patients with osteonecrosis of the femoral head.

Better implant designs, new technology, alternative bearings, and advanced surgical technique have shown promising long-term results that may minimize the negative impact of osteonecrosis on implant longevity. Even in patients who are at greater risk for implant failure, newer devices have demonstrated improved implant durability[8,31,39-45,47,49-70] (Table 3).

Metal-on-Metal Resurfacing

Metal-on-metal resurfacing was first introduced in the mid-1960s.[38] The early models of metal-on-metal resurfacing were abandoned because of component loosening and high failure rates.[71] Total hip resurfacing was used to replace both sides of the joint while preserving femoral bone stock. Additionally, the large diameter femoral head that is used permits an increased range of motion with less impingement and lower disloca-

tion rates.[72,73] Recently, there has been an advent in the use of metal-on-metal resurfacing with the development of new technology (Figure 5). Wear particle generation, osteolysis, and subsequent aseptic implant loosening is reduced by the advances in metal-on-metal bearing surfaces (Figure 6).[74-77] In addition, improved cemented fixation of femoral components has shown prolonged durability. The pain relief, function, and patient activity levels achieved using total resurfacing for patients with osteonecrosis are superior to those reported for hemiresurfacing and similar to the results for standard total hip arthroplasty. All these findings have led to an increase in metal-on-polyethylene total hip resurfacings, which have demonstrated low rates of long-term survivorship secondary to high rates of wear generation.

Despite all of the obvious advantages of total hip resurfacing, there are controversies concerning this procedure, including viability of the femoral head,[78] component loosening,[79] femoral neck fractures,[80] and metal ions.[81,82] The general concept that total hip resurfacing can induce femoral head osteonecrosis and subsequent implant failure was rebutted in various histologic studies analyzing the bone in retrieved femoral heads.[78,83-85] With the increasing number of metal-on-metal bearings used clinically, the concerns regarding the levels of metal in serum and urine have also increased.[81,82] Recent studies reported similar levels of cobalt and chromium ions in cohorts of metal-on-metal total hip resurfacings compared with conventional metal-on-metal total hip arthroplasties.[86] An initial peak in cobalt and chromium ion concentration has been detected with the use of newer metal-on-metal total

Table 3
Literature Review of Standard Total Hip Arthroplasty for Patients with Osteonecrosis of the Femoral Head

Author(s)	Year	No. of Hips	Procedure	Follow-up (Range) [months]	Overall Clinical Success
Berend et al[50]	2003	89	THA after failed Bone Grafting	110 (60-180)	82%
Al-Mousawi et al[51]	2002	35	Osteonecrosis secondary to SCD	114 (60-180)	80%
Zangger et al[47]	2000	26	Osteonecrosis secondary to SLE	55 (21-124)	93%
Chen et al[52]	1999	18	Osteonecrosis secondary to SLE	46 (24-85)	100%
Hickman and Lackiewicz[53]	1997	15	Osteonecrosis secondary to SCD	72 (24-144)	67%
Lieberman et al[45]	1995	46	Osteonecrosis and chronic renal failure	54	19%
Murzic and McCollum[31]	1994	77	Osteonecrosis after renal transplantation Cemented/Cementless THA	(24-216)	54%/100%
Moran et al[54]	1993	22	Osteonecrosis secondary to SCD	56	57%
Acurio and Friedman[44]	1992	25	Osteonecrosis secondary to SCD	103 (24-216)	60%
Clarke et al[55]	1989	27	Osteonecrosis secondary to SCD	66	41%
Hanker and Amstutz[56]	1988	8	Osteonecrosis secondary to SCD	78 (24-208)	38%
Schneider and Knahr[57]	2004	57	Cementless THA	(120-168)	82%
Kim et al[40]	2003	100	Cemented/Cementless THA	122	98%/ 98%
Xenakis et al[58]	2001	36	Cementless THA	136 (120-180)	93%
Taylor et al[59]	2001	70	Cementless THA	77	NA
Delank et al[60]	2001	66	Cementless THA	65 (58-94)	93%
Hartley et al[61]	2000	55	Cementless THA	117	79%
Fye et al[49]	1998	72	Cementless THA	84 (> 48)	97%/89%
Stulberg et al[62]	1997	98	Cementless THA	87 (31-134)	75%
Gonzalez et al[63]	1997	40	Cementless THA	58 (24-108)	80%
D'Antonio et al[64]	1997	53	Cementless THA	82 (60-96)	85%
Xenakis et al[43]	1997	29	Cementless THA	91	96%
Kim et al[65]	1995	78	Cementless THA	86 (72-108)	79%
Piston et al[42]	1994	35	Cementless THA	90 (60-120)	94%
Phillips et al[41]	1994	20	Cementless THA	64 (> 24)	95%
Lins et al[66]	1993	37	Cementless THA	48-72	81%
Katz et al[67]	1992	34	Cemented/Cementless THA	46 (24-84)	97%
Fyda et al[68]	2002	53	Cemented THA	> 120	83%
Ortiguera et al[69]	1999	188	Cemented THA	214 (120-304)	82%/50%
Wei et al[70]	1999	22	Revision THA	> 24	82%
Garino and Steinberg[39]	1997	123	Cemented THA	54 (24-120)	96%
Kantor et al[38]	1996	28	Cemented THA	92	86%
Saito et al[8]	1989	29	Cemented THA	84	52%

THA = total hip arthroplasty, SLE = systemic lupus erythematosus, SCD = sickle cell disease, NA=not available

hip resurfacing, followed by a gradual decline during the following 15 months. After a 2-year study period, the bearing has shown excellent wear properties, no radiolucency, and no adverse effects on renal function. There have been various other publications discussing elevated metal ion concentration in patients with metal-on-metal implants, but researchers have concluded that exposure to these elevated metal levels results in theoretic risks.[87,88] Additional studies are needed to elucidate the role of elevated metal ion levels in this patient population.

Grecula and associates[20] compared the outcome of patients younger than 50 years with osteonecrosis of the femoral head who were treated with one of four treatment modalities: standard cemented arthroplasty, total hip articular replacement by internal eccentric shells (THARIES), cementless total hip resurfacing, or cemented titanium femoral surface hemiarthroplasty. Similar degrees of clinical improvement were reported for the four treatments. The 96-month survivorship rates were 70% for cemented titanium femoral surface hemiresurfacing, 15% for cementless total hip resurfacing, 53% for THARIES, and 80% for standard cemented arthroplasty. Even better results have been reported with bone ingrowth total hip arthroplasty (Table 3). More recently, there have been several studies showing promising short-term results with newer devices. Beaulé and associates[18] compared the outcomes of 56 hips treated with metal-on-metal resurfacing arthroplasty with the outcomes of 28 hips treated with hemiresurfacing arthroplasty. The mean age of the patients was 41 years (age range, 16 to 56 years) for the metal-on-metal surface arthroplasty group and 36 years (age range, 22 to 51 years) for the hemiresurfacing group. At 55-month follow-up (range, 24 to 85 months) for the metal-on-metal surface arthroplasty group and 53-month follow-up (range, 25 to 96 months) for the hemiresurfacing group, University of California–Los Angeles hip

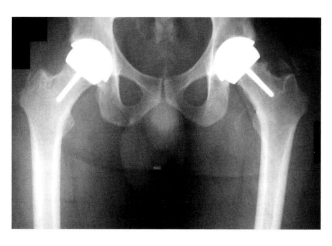

Figure 5 AP radiograph of a patient who underwent bilateral metal-on-metal total hip resurfacing arthroplasty.

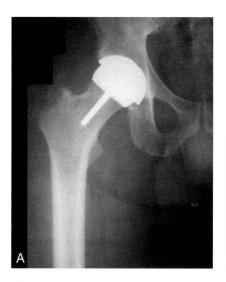
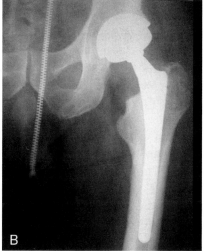

Figure 6 AP radiographs show a patient with a total hip resurfacing arthroplasty **(A)** and a patient with a standard total hip arthroplasty with a large femoral head **(B)**.

Table 4
Literature Review of Metal-on-Metal Resurfacing for Osteonecrosis of the Femoral Head

Author(s)	Year	No. of Hips	Procedure	Average Follow-up (Range) [months]	Overall Clinical Success
Mont et al[91]	2005	41	Metal-on-metal	36 (24-48)	93%
Amstutz et al[89]	2004	36	Metal-on-metal	42 (26-74)	94%
Mohamad et al[90]	2004	12	Metal-on-metal	18 (17-46)	84%
Beaulé et al[18]	2004	56	Metal-on-metal	60 (28-100)	95%
Yoo[92]	2004	40	Metal-on-metal	36 (24-48)	93%
Grecula et al[20]	1995	19	Metal-on-metal	96	53%
Grecula et al[20]	1995	35	Metal-on-metal	96	15%
Dutton et al[93]	1982	42	Metal-on-metal	37	> 76%

scores and Medical Outcome Studies 12-Item Short Form scores for the physical component were significantly better for the metal-on-metal surface arthroplasty group than the hemiresurfacing group. Two metal-on-metal surface replacements failed and were converted to total hip arthroplasties. Amstutz and associates[89] analyzed 400 metal-on-metal total hip arthroplasties done in 355 patients. This large series included 36 hips with osteonecrosis of the femoral head. All femoral head components were cemented. The patients had a mean age of 48 years (age range, 15 to 77 years). At a mean 42-month follow-up (range, 26 to 74 months), the overall survivorship was 94% and most patients had returned to a high level of activity. Twelve hips (3%) had been converted to a total hip arthroplasty, and 7 of those 12 hips (58%) were revised because of loosening of the femoral components. Three hips (25%) were revised for femoral neck fractures. The authors concluded that the most important risk factors for femoral component loosening were large femoral head cysts, low patient height, female gender, and smaller component size in male patients. Mohamad and associates[90] reported early experience with metal-on-metal total hip arthroplasty in 20 hips (19 patients). In this study, osteonecrosis of the femoral head was the diagnosis in 63% of the patients undergoing the procedure. The mean patient age was 43 years (age range, 25 to 58 years), and the mean follow-up was 18 months (range, 7 to 46 months). At final follow-up, 16 of 20 hips (84%) had good or excellent hip scores. Mont and associates[91] reported on 41 hips (37 patients) treated with metal-on-metal total hip arthroplasty for osteone-

crosis. At a mean follow-up of 36 months (range, 24 to 48 months), 38 of 41 hips (93%) had good or excellent results. There was no radiolucency and no component loosening, but heterotopic ossification was reported in three hips (7%).

Although total hip resurfacing may be a bone-preserving alternative for patients with advanced-stage disease and acetabular degeneration, most devices are still under investigation, and long-term outcome studies are necessary before the value of this treatment option can be truly determined. An overview of metal-on-metal studies for osteonecrosis of the femoral head[18,20,89-93] is provided in Table 4.

Summary

Treatment of the late stages of osteonecrosis of the femoral head has been challenging and controversial. There are multiple new devices and emerging new technology that are being proposed for use in patients with osteonecrosis. However, the goals of treatment remain the same and include pain relief, improving function and quality of life, and possibly preservation options for a lifelong treatment plan. Patient selection is important for the outcome, and treatment options depend on factors such as patient's age, underlying disease, and disease stage at presentation. Although hemiresurfacing and total resurfacing procedures are used for young patients with limited involvement of the femoral head, standard total hip arthroplasty may be more appropriate for older patients with significant involvement of the femoral head and acetabulum. The use of alternative bearing surfaces (metal-on-metal, ceramic-on-ceramic, and ceramic on ultra-high molecular weight polyethylene) and improved

surgical techniques provide a new promise for better long-term outcomes than those previously reported.

References

1. Mont MA, Hungerford DS: Nontraumatic avascular necrosis of the femoral head. *J Bone Joint Surg Am* 1995;77:459-474.

2. Assouline-Dayan Y, Chang C, Greenspan A, Shoenfeld Y, Gershwin ME: Pathogenesis and natural history of osteonecrosis. *Semin Arthritis Rheum* 2002;32:94-124.

3. Beaulé PE, Amstutz HC: Management of Ficat stage III and IV osteonecrosis of the hip. *J Am Acad Orthop Surg* 2004;12:96-105.

4. Lieberman JR, Berry DJ, Mont MA, et al: Osteonecrosis of the hip: Management in the 21st century. *Instr Course Lect* 2003;52:337-355.

5. Brinker MR, Rosenberg AG, Kull L, Galante JO: Primary total hip arthroplasty using noncemented porous-coated femoral components in patients with osteonecrosis of the femoral head. *J Arthroplasty* 1994;9:457-468.

6. Cabanela ME: Bipolar versus total hip arthroplasty for avascular necrosis of the femoral head: A comparison. *Clin Orthop Relat Res* 1990;261:59-62.

7. Chandler HP, Reineck FT, Wixson RL, McCarthy JC: Total hip replacement in patients younger than thirty years old: A five-year follow-up study. *J Bone Joint Surg Am* 1981;63:1426-1434.

8. Saito S, Saito M, Nishina T, Ohzono K, Ono K: Long-term results of total hip arthroplasty for osteonecrosis of the femoral head: A comparison with osteoarthritis. *Clin Orthop Relat Res* 1989;244:198-207.

9. Lachiewicz PF, Desman SM: The bipolar endoprosthesis in avascular necrosis of the femoral head. *J Arthroplasty* 1988;3:131-138.

10. Takaoka K, Nishina T, Ohzono K, et al: Bipolar prosthetic replacement for the treatment of avascular necrosis of the femoral head. *Clin Orthop Relat Res* 1992;277:121-127.

11. Canadian Institute for Health Information: *2005 Canadian Joint Replacement Registry Annual Report: Total Hip and Knee Replacements in Canada.*

Available at: http://secure.cihi.ca/cihiweb/dispPage.jsp?cw_page=AR_30_E. Accessed June 2, 2006.

12. Australian Orthopaedic Association National Joint Replacement Registry: 2004 Annual Report. Available at: http://www.dmac.adelaide.edu.au/aoanjrr/documents/aoanjrrreport_2004.pdf. Accessed June 2, 2006.

13. Mont MA, Rajadhyaksha AD, Hungerford DS: Outcomes of limited femoral resurfacing arthroplasty compared with total hip arthroplasty for osteonecrosis of the femoral head. *J Arthroplasty* 2001;16(suppl 1):134-139.

14. Beaule PE, Schmalzried TP, Campbell P, Dorey F, Amstutz HC: Duration of symptoms and outcome of hemiresurfacing for hip osteonecrosis. *Clin Orthop Relat Res* 2001;385:104-117.

15. Nelson CL, Walz BH, Gruenwald JM: Resurfacing of only the femoral head for osteonecrosis: Long-term follow-up study. *J Arthroplasty* 1997;12:736-740.

16. Adili A, Trousdale RT: Femoral head resurfacing for the treatment of osteonecrosis in the young patient. *Clin Orthop Relat Res* 2003;417:93-101.

17. Cuckler JM, Moore KD, Estrada L: Outcome of hemiresurfacing in osteonecrosis of the femoral head. *Clin Orthop Relat Res* 2004;429:146-150.

18. Beaulé PE, Amstutz HC, Le Duff M, Dorey F: Surface arthroplasty for osteonecrosis of the hip: Hemiresurfacing versus metal-on-metal hybrid resurfacing. *J Arthroplasty* 2004;19(suppl 3):54-58.

19. Siguier T, Siguier M, Judet T, Charnley G, Brumpt B: Partial resurfacing arthroplasty of the femoral head in avascular necrosis: Methods, indications, and results. *Clin Orthop Relat Res* 2001;386:85-92.

20. Grecula MJ, Grigoris P, Schmalzried TP, Dorey F, Campbell PA, Amstutz HC: Endoprostheses for osteonecrosis of the femoral head: A comparison of four models in young patients. *Int Orthop* 1995;19:137-143.

21. Tooke SM, Amstutz HC, Delaunay C: Hemiresurfacing for femoral head osteonecrosis. *J Arthroplasty* 1987;2:125-133.

22. Langlais F, Barthas J, Postel M: Adjusted cups for idiopathic necrosis: Radiological results. *Rev Chir Orthop Reparatrice Appar Mot* 1979;65:151-155.

23. Hungerford MW, Mont MA, Scott R, Fiore C, Hungerford DS, Krackow KA: Surface replacement hemiarthroplasty for the treatment of osteonecrosis of the femoral head. *J Bone Joint Surg Am* 1998;80:1656-1664.

24. Krackow KA, Mont MA, Maar DC: Limited femoral endoprosthesis for avascular necrosis of the femoral head. *Orthop Rev* 1993;22:457-463.

25. Scott RD, Urse JS, Schmidt R, Bierbaum BE: Use of TARA hemiarthroplasty in advanced osteonecrosis. *J Arthroplasty* 1987;2:225-232.

26. Grevitt MP, Spencer JD: Avascular necrosis of the hip treated by hemiarthroplasty: Results in renal transplant recipients. *J Arthroplasty* 1995;10:205-211.

27. Chan YS, Shih CH: Bipolar versus total hip arthroplasty for hip osteonecrosis in the same patient. *Clin Orthop Relat Res* 2000;379:169-177.

28. Sanjay BK, Moreau PG: Bipolar hip replacement in sickle cell disease. *Int Orthop* 1996;20:222-226.

29. Ito H, Matsuno T, Kaneda K: Bipolar hemiarthroplasty for osteonecrosis of the femoral head: A 7- to 18-year followup. *Clin Orthop Relat Res* 2000;374:201-211.

30. Yamano K, Atsumi T, Kajwara T: Bipolar endoprosthesis for osteonecrosis of the femoral head: A 12-year follow-up of 29 hips. *ARCO Transactions*, 2004.

31. Murzic WJ, McCollum DE: Hip arthroplasty for osteonecrosis after renal transplantation. *Clin Orthop Relat Res* 1994;299:212-219.

32. Tsumura H, Torisu T, Kaku N, Higashi T: Five- to fifteen-year clinical results and the radiographic evaluation of acetabular changes after bipolar hip arthroplasty for femoral head osteonecrosis. *J Arthroplasty* 2005;20:892-897.

33. Lee SB, Sugano N, Nakata K, Matsui M, Ohzono K: Comparison between bipolar hemiarthroplasty and THA for osteonecrosis of the femoral head. *Clin Orthop Relat Res* 2004;424:161-165.

34. Nagai I, Takatori Y, Kuruta Y, et al: Nonself-centering Bateman bipolar endoprosthesis for nontraumatic osteonecrosis of the femoral head: A 12- to 18-year follow-up study. *J Orthop Sci* 2002;7:74-78.

35. Learmonth ID, Opitz M: Treatment of grade III osteonecrosis of the femoral head with a Charnley/Bicentric hemiarthroplasty. *J R Coll Surg Edinb* 1993;38:311-314.

36. Dorr LD, Takei GK, Conaty JP: Total hip arthroplasties in patients less than forty-five years old. *J Bone Joint Surg Am* 1983;65:474-479.

37. Cornell CN, Salvati EA, Pellicci PM: Long-term follow-up of total hip replacement in patients with osteonecrosis. *Orthop Clin North Am* 1985;16:757-769.

38. Kantor SG, Huo MH, Huk OL, Salvati EA: Cemented total hip arthroplasty in patients with osteonecrosis: A 6-year minimum follow-up study of second-generation cement techniques. *J Arthroplasty* 1996;11:267-271.

39. Garino JP, Steinberg ME: Total hip arthroplasty in patients with avascular necrosis of the femoral head: A 2- to 10-year follow-up. *Clin Orthop Relat Res* 1997;334:108-115.

40. Kim YH, Oh SH, Kim JS, Koo KH: Contemporary total hip arthroplasty with and without cement in patients with osteonecrosis of the femoral head. *J Bone Joint Surg Am* 2003;85:675-681.

41. Phillips FM, Pottenger LA, Finn HA, Vandermolen J: Cementless total hip arthroplasty in patients with steroid-induced avascular necrosis of the hip: A 62-month follow-up study. *Clin Orthop Relat Res* 1994;303:147-154.

42. Piston RW, Engh CA, De Carvalho PI, Suthers K: Osteonecrosis of the femoral head treated with total hip arthroplasty without cement. *J Bone Joint Surg Am* 1994;76:202-214.

43. Xenakis TA, Beris AE, Malizos KK, Koukoubis T, Gelalis J, Soucacos PN: Total hip arthroplasty for avascular necrosis and degenerative osteoarthritis of the hip. *Clin Orthop Relat Res* 1997;341:62-68.

44. Acurio MT, Friedman RJ: Hip arthroplasty in patients with sickle-cell haemoglobinopathy. *J Bone Joint Surg Br* 1992;74:367-371.

45. Lieberman JR, Fuchs MD, Haas SB, et al: Hip arthroplasty in patients with chronic renal failure. *J Arthroplasty* 1995;10:191-195.

46. Huo MH, Salvati EA, Browne MG, Pellicci PM, Sculco TP, Johanson NA: Primary total hip arthroplasty in systemic lupus erythematosus. *J Arthroplasty* 1992;7:51-56.

47. Zangger P, Gladman DD, Urowitz MB, Bogoch ER: Outcome of total hip replacement for avascular necrosis in systemic lupus erythematosus. *J Rheumatol* 2000;27:919-923.

48. Nich C, Sariali el-H, Hannouche D, et al

Long-term results of alumina-on-alumina hip arthroplasty for osteonecrosis. *Clin Orthop Relat Res* 2003;417:102-111.

49. Fye MA, Huo MH, Zatorski LE, Keggi KJ: Total hip arthroplasty performed without cement in patients with femoral head osteonecrosis who are less than 50 years old. *J Arthroplasty* 1998;13:876-881.

50. Berend KR, Gunneson E, Urbaniak JR, Vail TP: Hip arthroplasty after failed free vascularized fibular grafting for osteonecrosis in young patients. *J Arthroplasty* 2003;18:411-419.

51. Al-Mousawi F, Malki A, Al-Aradi A, Al-Bagali M, Al-Sadadi A, Booz MM: Total hip replacement in sickle cell disease. *Int Orthop* 2002;26:157-161.

52. Chen YW, Chang JK, Huang KY, Lin GT, Lin SY, Huang CY: Hip arthroplasty for osteonecrosis in patients with systemic lupus erythematosus. *Kaohsiung J Med Sci* 1999;15:697-703.

53. Hickman JM, Lachiewicz PF: Results and complications of total hip arthroplasties in patients with sickle-cell hemoglobinopathies: Role of cementless components. *J Arthroplasty* 1997;12:420-425.

54. Moran MC, Huo MH, Garvin KL, Pellicci PM, Salvati EA: Total hip arthroplasty in sickle cell hemoglobinopathy. *Clin Orthop Relat Res* 1993;294:140-148.

55. Clarke HJ, Jinnah RH, Brooker AF, Michaelson JD: Total replacement of the hip for avascular necrosis in sickle cell disease. *J Bone Joint Surg Br* 1989;71:465-470.

56. Hanker GJ, Amstutz HC: Osteonecrosis of the hip in the sickle-cell diseases: Treatment and complications. *J Bone Joint Surg Am* 1988;70:499-506.

57. Schneider W, Knahr K: Total hip replacement in younger patients: Survival rate after avascular necrosis of the femoral head. *Acta Orthop Scand* 2004;75:142-146.

58. Xenakis TA, Gelalis J, Koukoubis TA, Zaharis KC, Soucacos PN: Cementless hip arthroplasty in the treatment of patients with femoral head necrosis. *Clin Orthop Relat Res* 2001;386:93-99.

59. Taylor AH, Shannon M, Whitehouse SL, Lee MB, Learmonth ID: Harris-Galante cementless acetabular replacement in avascular necrosis. *J Bone Joint Surg Br* 2001;83:177-182.

60. Delank KS, Drees P, Eckardt A, Heine J: Results of the uncemented total hip arthroplasty in avascular necrosis of the femoral head. *Z Orthop Ihre Grenzgeb* 2001;139:525-530.

61. Hartley WT, McAuley JP, Culpepper WJ, Engh CA Jr, Engh CA Sr: Osteonecrosis of the femoral head treated with cementless total hip arthroplasty. *J Bone Joint Surg Am* 2000;82:1408-1413.

62. Stulberg BN, Singer R, Goldner J, Stulberg J: Uncemented total hip arthroplasty in osteonecrosis: A 2- to 10-year evaluation. *Clin Orthop Relat Res* 1997;334:116-123.

63. Gonzalez MH, Ortinau ET, Buonanno W, Prieto J: Cementless total hip arthroplasty in patients with advanced avascular necrosis. *J South Orthop Assoc* 1997;6:162-168.

64. D'Antonio JA, Capello WN, Manley MT, Feinberg J: Hydroxyapatite coated implants: Total hip arthroplasty in the young patient and patients with avascular necrosis. *Clin Orthop Relat Res* 1997;344:124-138.

65. Kim YH, Oh JH, Oh SH: Cementless total hip arthroplasty in patients with osteonecrosis of the femoral head. *Clin Orthop Relat Res* 1995;320:73-84.

66. Lins RE, Barnes BC, Callaghan JJ, Mair SD, McCollum DE: Evaluation of uncemented total hip arthroplasty in patients with avascular necrosis of the femoral head. *Clin Orthop Relat Res* 1993;297:168-173.

67. Katz RL, Bourne RB, Rorabeck CH, McGee H: Total hip arthroplasty in patients with avascular necrosis of the hip: Follow-up observations on cementless and cemented operations Clin Orthop Relat Res 1992;281:145-151.

68. Fyda TM, Callaghan JJ, Olejniczak J, Johnston RC: Minimum ten-year follow-up of cemented total hip replacement in patients with osteonecrosis of the femoral head.*Iowa Orthop J* 2002;22-8-19

69. Ortiguera CJ, Pulliam IT, Cabanela ME: Total hip arthroplasty for osteonecrosis: Matched-pair analysis of 188 hips with long-term follow-up. *J Arthroplasty* 1999;14:21-28

70. Wei SY, Klimkiewicz JJ, Steinberg ME: Revision total hip arthroplasty in patients with avascular necrosis. *Orthopedics* 1999;22:747-757.

71. Amstutz HC, Grigoris P, Dorey FJ: Evolution and future of surface replacement of the hip. *J Orthop Sci* 1998;3:169-186.

72. Cuckler JM, Moore KD, Lombardi AV Jr, McPherson E, Emerson R: Large versus small femoral heads in metal-on-metal total hip arthroplasty. *J Arthroplasty* 2004;19(suppl 3):41-44.

73. Crowninshield RD, Maloney WJ, Wentz DH, Humphrey SM, Blanchard CR: Biomechanics of large femoral heads: What they do and don't do. *Clin Orthop Relat Res* 2004;429:102-107.

74. Dorr LD, Long WT: Metal-on-metal: Articulations for the new millennium. *Instr Course Lect* 2005;54:177-182.

75. Schmalzried TP, Peters PC, Maurer BT, Bragdon CR, Harris WH: Long-duration metal-on-metal total hip arthroplasties with low wear of the articulating surfaces. *J Arthroplasty* 1996;11:322-331.

76. Sieber HP, Rieker CB, Kottig P: Analysis of 118 second-generation metal-on-metal retrieved hip implants. *J Bone Joint Surg Br* 1999;81:46-50.

77. Campbell P, Urban RM, Catelas I, Skipor AK, Schmalzried TP: Autopsy analysis thirty years after metal-on-metal total hip replacement: A case report. *J Bone Joint Surg Am* 2003;85:2218-2222.

78. Little CP, Ruiz AL, Harding IJ, et al: Osteonecrosis in retrieved femoral heads after failed resurfacing arthroplasty of the hip. *J Bone Joint Surg Br* 2005;87:320-323.

79. Beaule PE, Le Duff M, Campbell P, Dorey FJ, Park SH, Amstutz HC: Metal-on-metal surface arthroplasty with a cemented femoral component: A 7-10 year follow-up study. *J Arthroplasty* 2004;19(suppl 3):17-22.

80. Amstutz HC, Campbell PA, Le Duff MJ: Fracture of the neck of the femur after surface arthroplasty of the hip. *J Bone Joint Surg Am* 2004;86-A:1874-1877.

81. MacDonald SJ: Metal-on-metal total hip arthroplasty: The concerns. *Clin Orthop Relat Res* 2004;429:86-93.

82. Tharani R, Dorey FJ, Schmalzried TP: The risk of cancer following total hip or knee arthroplasty. *J Bone Joint Surg Am* 2001;83:774-780.

83. Campbell P, Mirra J, Amstutz HC: Viability of femoral heads treated with resurfacing arthroplasty. *J Arthroplasty* 2000;15:120-122.

84. Howie DW, Cornish BL, Vernon-Roberts B: The viability of the femoral head after resurfacing hip arthroplasty in humans. *Clin Orthop Relat Res* 1993;291:171-184.

85. Bradley GW, Freeman MA, Revell PA: Resurfacing arthroplasty: Femoral head viability. *Clin Orthop Relat Res* 1987;220:137-141.

86. Back DL, Young DA, Shimmin AJ: How

do serum cobalt and chromium levels change after metal-on-metal hip resurfacing? *Clin Orthop Relat Res* 2005;438:177-181.

87. MacDonald SJ: Can a safe level for metal ions in patients with metal-on-metal total hip arthroplasties be determined? *J Arthroplasty* 2004;19(suppl 3):71-77.

88. MacDonald SJ, Brodner W, Jacobs JJ: A consensus paper on metal ions in metal-on-metal hip arthroplasties. *J Arthroplasty* 2004;19(suppl 3):12-16.

89. Amstutz HC, Beaule PE, Dorey FJ, Le Duff MJ, Campbell PA, Gruen TA: Metal-on-metal hybrid surface arthroplasty: Two to six-year follow-up study. *J Bone Joint Surg Am* 2004;86:28-39.

90. Mohamad JA, Kwan MK, Merican AM, et al: Early results of metal on metal articulation total hip arthroplasty in young patients. *Med J Malaysia* 2004;59:3-7.

91. Mont MA, Ragland PS, Marulanda GA, Delanois RE, Seyler TM: Use of metal-on-metal resurfacing arthroplasty for avascular necrosis of the hip. *ARCO Transactions*, 2005.

92. Yoo TC: Results of metal-on-metal resurfacing for avascular necrosis of the femoral head. *ARCO Transactions*, 2005.

93. Dutton RO, Amstutz HC, Thomas BJ, Hedley AK: Tharies surface replacement for osteonecrosis of the femoral head. *J Bone Joint Surg Am* 1982;64:1225-1237.

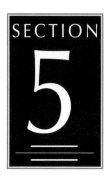

SECTION 5

Spine

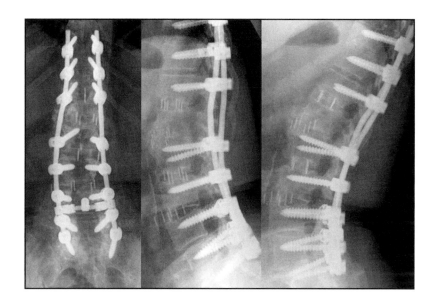

Update on Cervical Artificial Disk Replacement

Paul A. Anderson, MD
Rick C. Sasso, MD
K. Daniel Riew, MD

Abstract

Cervical disk arthroplasty, one of the emerging motion-sparing technologies, is currently undergoing evaluation in the United States as an alternative to arthrodesis for the treatment of cervical radiculopathy and myelopathy. With both arthrodesis and arthroplasty, the primary surgical goal is thorough decompression of neurocompressive pathology—directly by removal of osteophyte and disk and indirectly by disk distraction. There is, however, one principal difference between arthrodesis and arthroplasty. With a solid fusion, resorption of osteophytes (in accordance with Wolff's law) further enhances decompression. In contrast, osteophyte resorption will not occur with motion-preserving arthroplasty. There are many challenges when deciding between arthrodesis and arthroplasty. Prosthetic performance demands exacting implantation techniques to ensure correct placement, thus placing increasing demands on special instrumentation and surgical skills. It is also important to understand the tribology (the study of prosthetic lubrication, wear, and biologic effects) of disk arthroplasty and to be familiar with currently available information regarding kinematics, basic science, testing, and early clinical results.

Instr Course Lect 2007;56:237-246

The primary rationale for disk arthroplasty is motion preservation, with the theoretic advantage of avoiding adjacent segment degeneration. It is believed that motion preservation allows fewer activity restrictions and earlier return to activities, including work and driving.

Rationale for Disk Arthroplasty
Adjacent-Level Degeneration

There is general consensus that degeneration occurs in segments adjacent to fusion. However, no study has definitively established that this adjacent-level degeneration is primarily caused by the adverse mechanical effect of fusion versus the natural history of degenerative disk disease.

Numerous studies have demonstrated the incidence of adjacent level degeneration following arthro-deses. Baba and associates[1] examined 106 patients following anterior fusion for myeloradiculopathy over an average of 8.6 years. Overall, 25% of patients had progressive neurologic changes at adjacent levels; 17 of these patients required additional surgery. As expected, patients who underwent multilevel arthrodesis had a greater chance of adjacent-level degeneration. Gore and Sepic[2,3] similarly reported short- and long-term follow-up of anterior cervical diskectomy and arthrodesis. At 5-year follow-up, 18 of 37 patients had symptoms at adjacent levels. The authors compared these patients with a cohort of asymptomatic patients who were followed over the same period and found no differences in radiographic evidence of deterioration, except for increased osteophyte formation.[4] Gore and Sepic did not comment on whether there were any changes in symptoms. In reporting their 21-year results, Gore and Sepic noted that 16 of 50 patients at 10-year follow-up had new onset of symptoms related to adjacent-level disease, half of whom required further surgery.[3] Based on these long-term data, they recommended that this patient population be informed of the significant chance of revision surgery at long-term follow-up.

The most often cited article on adjacent-level disease is by Hilibrand and associates,[5] who analyzed the results of Bohlman's surgical cases. They reported long-term follow-up in 374 patients at 2 to 21 years after anterior cervical diskectomy and arthrodesis. The annual incidence of symptomatic, adjacent-level degenerative disease was 2.9%, and the prevalence at 10-year follow-up was 25.9%. In contrast to the findings of Baba and associates,[1] single-level fusions, especially at C5-6 or C6-7, were associated with a greater risk of symptomatic degeneration than multilevel fusions. Patients who had a three-level arthrodesis from C4 to C7 had the lowest risk of requiring additional surgery. The authors, therefore, concluded that the risk for adjacent-level disease is not increased in patients who undergo longer fusions. As expected, patients with preoperative disease at adjacent levels were more likely to have symptomatic adjacent-level disease postoperatively. Consequently, the authors suggested that adjacent-level degeneration more likely resulted from the natural history of spondylosis as opposed to the increased stresses of multilevel fusions.

To determine whether the indication for the procedure had an effect on adjacent-level degeneration, Goffin and associates[6] compared the 5-year follow-up results of cohorts who underwent arthrodeses for degeneration and trauma. They found that 85% of both groups had postoperative evidence of progressive radiographic deterioration and that there was no difference between the groups based on the index indication. These findings imply that the etiology of the adjacent-level degen-

eration may have been mechanically related to the fusion rather than the natural history of spondylosis. Thus, there appears to be an 85% incidence of radiographic degenerative changes and a 25% incidence of new symptomatic radiculopathy in patients who undergo anterior fusion.

In an effort to determine the natural history of spondylosis, Gore and associates[7] determined the incidence of cervical degeneration in 200 asymptomatic patients. They found that significant degenerative changes were common in patients older than 50 years. By age 60 years, 95% of men and 65% of women had degenerative changes. In a follow-up study, significant degenerative changes were found in most patients, but surprisingly 15% had now developed pain.[8] This finding suggests that degenerative disk disease is common and symptomatic disease occurs in the absence of fusion. With the limitations of these studies, conflicting data, and the lack of adequate controlled studies, no conclusions can be drawn regarding the mechanical versus biologic etiology of degenerative disk disease. Nevertheless, the high incidence of adjacent-level degeneration has provided a justifiable reason to develop new technologies to limit disk deterioration.

Viscoelasticity

The intervertebral disk functions as a shock absorber based on the viscoelastic properties of its collagen and proteoglycan molecular structure. Proteoglycans, in particular, absorb water molecules, creating a large matrix of negative charges that repel under load. Loss of this viscoelastic property by fusion is therefore believed to be a major factor leading to adjacent-level degeneration. However, none of the cur-

rently available prostheses allow viscoelasticity comparable to that provided by the normal disk. Furthermore, LeHuec and associates[9] compared the ability of a metal-polymer and metal-on-metal lumbar prosthesis to absorb impulse and vibrational load. Despite an order of magnitude difference in elastic properties between the two implants, no difference in the shock-absorbing effect was noted. Similarly, Dahl and associates[10] compared a simulated fusion with cervical artificial disks having different elastic properties. They found significant difference between all arthroplasties and fusion. However, no differences were found among arthroplasties with different elasticities. Thus, any motion-sparing device appeared to be protective of adjacent segments compared with fusion under impulse and vibrational stresses.

Maintenance of Motion

Loss of overall range of motion following fusion is poorly documented and, in fact, is rarely reported by patients with successful pain relief. Although 7° to 10° of motion at the surgical level has been reported following cervical arthroplasty, no evidence of functional impairment has been reported.[11,12] Most patients having arthroplasty do not require immobilization and therefore regain overall motion faster than patients treated with fusion.

The pattern of motion in normal individuals and patients who underwent fusion or arthroplasty was studied by Goffin and associates.[13] Using video fluoroscopy and digital processing, the patients who underwent fusion were noted to have asynchronous (jerky) motion at adjacent segments, whereas motion in patients who underwent arthroplasty was similar to that of normal asymptomatic individuals.

Perioperative Morbidity

Because arthroplasty generally does not require postoperative immobilization, return to function, including work and driving, can theoretically occur much earlier than in patients who undergo arthrodesis. Furthermore, complications related to fusion, such as hardware failure and pseudarthrosis, are avoided. Anderson and associates[14] compared revision rates in 1,229 patients who underwent cervical arthroplasty or arthrodesis and found that in the 580 patients who underwent arthrodesis, 4.8% had revisions by 2 years postoperatively, whereas only 2.9% of the 649 patients who underwent arthroplasty had revisions. These data suggest that symptomatic adjacent-level degeneration may be decreased by arthroplasty because significantly fewer patients who undergo arthroplasty require revisions to treat adjacent-level degeneration.

Mitigation of Fusion Effects by Arthroplasty

Dmitriev and associates[15] compared the biomechanical effects on adjacent segments for cervical disk arthroplasty and fusion and found that significant increases in intradiskal pressures occurred at both the cranial and caudal levels. Puttlitz and associates[16] performed a similar analysis and found that motion at adjacent levels after arthroplasty mimicked that of the normal functional unit, including coupled motion. DiAngelo and associates[17,18] also found that motion normalized to the intact segment after arthroplasty and that increased range of motion was seen after fusion. These results are similar to those reported for lumbar arthroplasty and indicate that cervical arthroplasty normalizes

the adverse biomechanical consequences of fusion. The findings of these basic investigations have been confirmed by postoperative human kinematic studies.

Sasso and Rouleau[19] studied cervical motion in 22 patients enrolled in a prospective, randomized clinical trial. Radiographic data, including flexion, extension, and neutral lateral radiographs, were obtained preoperatively and at regular postoperative intervals for up to 24 months. Cervical vertebral bodies were tracked on digital radiographs using quantitative motion analysis software to calculate the functional spinal unit motion parameters. The anterior-posterior translation during flexion-extension activities remained unchanged for the disk replacement group (8.3% preoperatively, 8.4% at 6 months, and 8.2% at 12 months) for the level above the disk. In contrast, the anterior-posterior translation increased for the level above the fusion (8.5% preoperatively, 12.4% at 6 months, and 11.0% at 12 months). This increase was dramatic for some patients who underwent fusion, but was not uniformly noted. At 6-month follow-up, the increase in translation was significantly greater for patients who underwent fusion ($P < 0.02$) than for those who received a disk replacement. Pickett and associates[20] performed a similar analysis and found that the center of rotation following arthroplasty was similar to the center of rotation that was present preoperatively. The importance of these clinical and biomechanical findings in reducing the risk of adjacent-level degeneration is unknown at this time.

Design Considerations
Kinematics
One of the primary goals of cervical disk replacement is to reproduce

normal kinematics. Normal range of motion in the subaxial cervical spine is 10° to 20° of flexion-extension, 5° to 15° of lateral bending, and 5° to 10° of rotation. Additionally, coupled motions are present, including anterior-posterior translation during flexion and extension and axial rotation during lateral bending. Also, the instantaneous axis of rotation in flexion-extension is located inferior to the caudal end plate and is relatively posterior in the vertebral body. This position changes during motion as a result of combined angulation and translation. In flexion-extension, there is 1 to 2 mm of anterior translation. Current implant designs differ in how well these normal mechanics are reproduced.

Cervical disk replacements can be classified as unconstrained, semiconstrained, and constrained, depending on how they mimic normal kinematics. Unconstrained devices allow coupled translation with angulation. Two types of unconstrained designs are available: a three-piece device in which the center or nuclear core can translate forward or backward and a device with saddle joints. A semiconstrained prosthesis allows coupled motion in some directions (flexion-extension), but has a fixed center of rotation in other directions (lateral bending). The Prestige ST Artificial Cervical Disc and the Prestige LP Cervical Disc (Medtronic, Minneapolis, MN), both with a ball and trough design, are examples of semiconstrained prostheses. A constrained device has a constant center of rotation and a ball and socket design that does not allow anterior-posterior translation. The clinical effects of the differences in prostheses designs are unknown. Theoretically, an important distinction between constrained and unconstrained designs is a change in balance of loads between the disk and facets, especially in extension. When the spine is in flexion, the facets "unshingle" and are less active in constraining the motion of the functional spine unit. However, when the spine is in extension, the facets "shingle" and become more involved in constraining the motion. Thus, with a constrained facet joint and a constrained disk joint, binding or limited motion (also known as "kinematic conflict") would be expected because one joint works against the other. This conflict would give rise to decreased motion or increased stress on the system and would potentially reduce motion.

DiAngelo and associates[17] investigated constrained and unconstrained designs in human cadaver spines to compare the motion of the harvested spine and the implanted spine. The results demonstrated that the unconstrained device mimicked normal mechanics, whereas the semiconstrained device failed to reproduce normal motion in extension. Both devices should achieve greater than normal segmental motion, which occurs in ± 15° in flexion/extension.

Materials

The most likely mode of failure is wear of the bearing surface, which is largely determined by the materials used. Current cervical disk replacements are made from materials similar to those used for joint arthroplasty, including cobalt-chromium-molybdenum alloy, stainless steel, and ultra high-density molecular weight polyethylene. Additionally, because lower load occurs in the spine than in joints such as the knee, other materials have been used for cervical disk replacements, includ-

ing titanium, polyurethane, and titanium carbide, the latter of which has the advantage of much better imaging quality.

Bone Fixation

Biologic fixation to bone is important for the long-term function of the prosthesis. A variety of stabilization and surface treatments are used. Cervical prostheses are initially stabilized to prevent expulsion or displacement into the spinal canal with screws, keels, ridges, and specially machined cavities. Surface treatments include titanium plasma spray with calcium phosphate and cinctured beads. Bone ingrowth into the Porous Coated Motion (PCM) Artificial Cervical Disc (Cervitech, Rockaway, NJ) and the Bryan Cervical Disc System (Medtronic) appears to be satisfactory. McAfee and associates[21] evaluated bone ingrowth in the PCM device and found a 40% to 50% rate of incorporation in a nonhuman primate model. In human explants, Jensen and associates[22] reported a 32% rate of bone ingrowth with Bryan Cervical Disc System explants.

Testing of Cervical Devices

Seven cervical disk prostheses are currently undergoing clinical testing in the United States (Figure 1). The basic design parameters of each of these prostheses are provided in Table 1. Extensive preclinical and clinical testing of new motion-sparing devices such as cervical disk prostheses are required to ensure safety and efficacy. Cervical disk prostheses are intended for use in patients who are younger than those who undergo arthroplasties for appendicular joints; therefore, long-term wear characteristics are a major concern. In total hip and knee arthroplasty implantations, younger,

more active patients experience a much higher failure rate. During testing, the response of the implant to the host as well as the response of the host to the implant should be measured. Clinical testing of efficacy should also be conducted via rigorous randomized controlled trials that measure the primary outcome variables of pain, neurologic function, and functional outcomes.

Mechanical Testing

All components initially should be tested for fatigue. Because of the large number of cycles required (a minimum of 10 million) for fatigue testing, this is done on a simulator. Unlike hip and knee implants for which protocols are well established and have a track record of predicting long-term function, spine simulators are undergoing evolution. Simulator wear results for the Bryan and Prestige cervical prostheses have been reported.[23,24] At 10 million cycles, a mean volume loss for the Bryan disk was 0.76%. Failure occurred when end plates contacted each other at 39 million cycles. The wear debris consisted of large elliptical particles with a mean ferret diameter of 3.89 μm and aspect ratio of 1.38. The Prestige metal-on-metal disk had less wear than the Bryan disk (0.19% at 20 million cycles); a linear wear rate of 0.18 mm^3 per 1 million cycles was reported.

Inflammatory Reaction

Wear particles are bioactive and under certain conditions can induce a significant inflammatory response, resulting in failure and loosening of the device. In the spine, additional concerns arise because of the location of the devices adjacent to vascular, visceral, and neurologic structures. Devices are tested for their

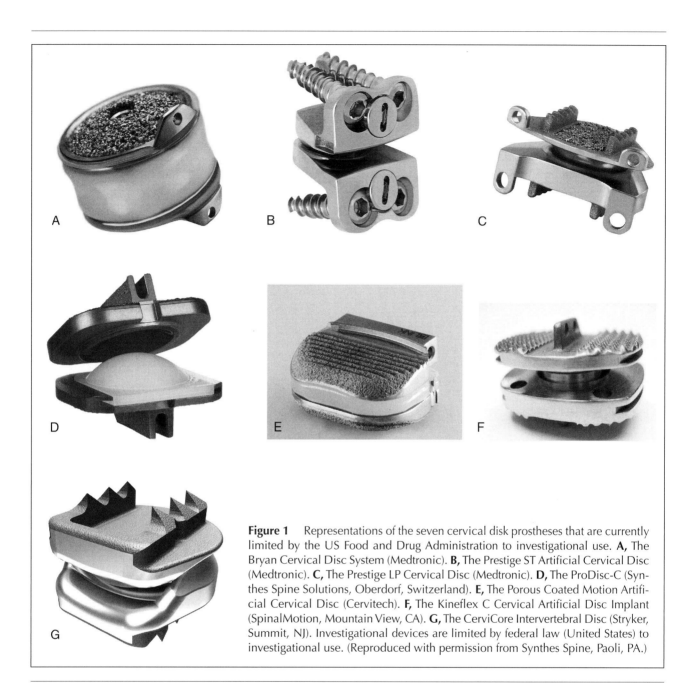

Figure 1 Representations of the seven cervical disk prostheses that are currently limited by the US Food and Drug Administration to investigational use. **A,** The Bryan Cervical Disc System (Medtronic). **B,** The Prestige ST Artificial Cervical Disc (Medtronic). **C,** The Prestige LP Cervical Disc (Medtronic). **D,** The ProDisc-C (Synthes Spine Solutions, Oberdorf, Switzerland). **E,** The Porous Coated Motion Artificial Cervical Disc (Cervitech). **F,** The Kineflex C Cervical Artificial Disc Implant (SpinalMotion, Mountain View, CA). **G,** The CerviCore Intervertebral Disc (Stryker, Summit, NJ). Investigational devices are limited by federal law (United States) to investigational use. (Reproduced with permission from Synthes Spine, Paoli, PA.)

inflammatory properties in two manners: in a rabbit laminectomy defect model in which large amounts of wear debris are installed directly into the epidural space, and by implantation in a suitable animal. McAfee and associates[21] reported minimal change in the dura mater and no effect on the neuronal elements of polyethylene particles for the PCM prosthesis.

Placement of the device in the cervical spine in animals allows for analysis of responses of the implant to the host and the host to the implant. This type of analysis is limited, however, by time and cost considerations as well as by an unequal biomechanical environment in humans. Anderson and associates[23] assessed the Bryan disk in goats and reported that debris was observed in 8 of 11 specimens, but only

a minimal inflammatory response was observed in the periprosthetic tissue. No toxic effects were noted in the neural elements, draining lymph nodes, or distant sites such as liver and spleen.

Retrieval Studies

Retrieval analysis of implants from humans is important to understand the in vivo biologic reaction of the

Table 1

Cervical Disk Prostheses in US Food and Drug Administration Investigations (2005)

Prosthesis	Material	Bearing Surface	Articulation(s)		US Food and Drug Administration (FDA) Status	Bone Ingrowth	Fixation
			No.	Type			
Bryan Cervical Disc System (Medtronic)	Titanium alloy Polyurethane	Metal-on-polymer	2	Three piece Nuclear core	Completed enrollment	Titanium shards	Mortise
Prestige ST Artificial Cervical Disc (Medtronic)	Stainless steel	Metal-on-metal	1	Ball and trough	Completed enrollment	Grit blast	Screws
Prestige LP Cervical Disc (Medtronic)	Titanium ceramic composite	Metal-on-metal	1	Ball and trough	Completed enrollment	Titanium plasma spray	Rails
ProDisc-C (Synthes Spine Solutions)	Cobalt-chromium-molybdenum-polyethylene	Metal-on-polymer	1	Ball and socket	Completed enrollment	Titanium plasma spray	Keel
Porous Coated Motion (PCM) Artificial Cervical Disc (Cervitech)	Cobalt-chromium-molybdenum-polyethylene	Metal-on-polymer	1	Ball and socket	In FDA trial	Titanium plasma spray using calcium phosphates	Surface ridges or screws
Kineflex C Cervical Artificial Disc Implant (Spinal-Motion)	Cobalt-chromium-molybdenum	Metal-on-metal	2	Three piece Nuclear core	In FDA trial	Unconstrained	Keel
CerviCore Intervertebral Disc (Stryker)	Cobalt-chromium-molybdenum	Metal-on-metal	1	Saddle	In FDA trial	Unconstrained	Rails

implant and the potential implications of wear. These results can help validate preclinical testing in simulators and animal models. Anderson and associates[24] reported retrievals of 11 Bryan disks and 3 Prestige disks because of infection, failure to relieve initial symptoms, and adjacent segment degeneration. None of the devices had mechanical failure. The prosthetic wear patterns of the Prestige disk were similar to those observed in simulators. However, the amount of wear was less than one tenth of that predicted, based on 1 million cycles per year. In both brands/types of prostheses, revision was achieved relatively easily without corpectomy. The polyurethane nucleus of the Bryan disk was assessed chemically with spectroscopy and chromatography. After implantation of up to 11 months, no oxidation was observed, and the molecular weight of the polymer was similar to that of a control implant. No observable changes in the surface were present and all nuclei were dimensionally normal, without evidence of loss from wear. These results were reassuring, indicating that the prosthesis, at least in the short term, was durable and had wear rates much less than those predicted by design and reported in testing protocols.

Indications

In the United States, the indications for surgery in Investigational Device Exemption studies are radiculopathy or myelopathy at a single level between C3 and C7; the contraindications are osteoporosis, instability of more than 3 mm, moderate or severe facet arthritis, or a history of infection. The intent is to use an arthroplasty as an alternative to an arthrodesis. The results of using the Bryan disk at two levels was reported in Europe, with slightly better outcomes than when used at a single level, but this device has not been tested in a randomized controlled study in which it is compared with fusion.[11] Another study reported the successful treatment of levels adjacent to a prior fusion.[25] Concerns regarding the treatment of myelopathy using arthroplasty have been raised because maintaining motion may be a disadvantage to neural recovery. In one report, satisfactory outcomes have been reported in a small number of patients treated with the Bryan disk.[26]

Clinical Outcomes

Reports of early clinical experience with disk arthroplasty devices have been uniformly favorable. Studies have shown that the outcomes of cervical arthroplasty are at least as good, if not better, than arthrodesis. Although it is certainly possible that long-term clinical results will also be favorable, good short-term outcomes do not necessarily predict good long-term outcomes. For example, the early results of lumbar cage fusions showed excellent clinical results and led to an increase in the use of lumbar cages; however, the popularity of such procedures has significantly diminished over the past several years. It is entirely possible that the use of cervical disk arthroplasty may undergo a similar evolution.

Goffin and associates[11,27] reported the results of a multicenter European study. For both single-level and bilevel arthroplasty, 90% of patients had excellent, good, or fair results at 2 years postoperatively. Lafuente and associates[28] evaluated 46 consecutive patients who underwent disk arthroplasty using the Bryan device and reported a highly statistically significant difference between preoperative and 12-month postoperative scores for the Visual Analog Scale (VAS), the Medical Outcomes Study Short Form 36-Item Health Survey (SF-36), and the Neck Disability Index (NDI). Two patients (4.3%) were found to have a bony ankylosis of the disk arthroplasty.

Duggal and associates[29] reported on the results of 26 patients undergoing one- and two-level Bryan disk replacement for radiculopathy and/or myelopathy. They found that motion was preserved (mean range of motion, 7.8°) at up to 24 months postoperatively. Postoperative NDI scores were significantly improved and there was a trend toward improvement of the SF-36 physical component score.

Bertagnoli and associates[30] reported on 16 patients with cervical spondylosis who prospectively underwent cervical arthroplasty using the ProDisc-C (Synthes Spine Solutions). There were 12 single-level and 4 two-level procedures; a total of 20 artificial disks were implanted. At a maximum follow-up of 12 months, Oswestry Disability Index and VAS scores were significantly improved. The arthroplasty levels had motion from 4° to 12° postoperatively and no complications were noted.

The Prestige disk has undergone several modifications. The Prestige I disk, which was used for the treatment of adjacent-level degeneration, demonstrated excellent outcomes and a satisfactory range of motion in 14 of the original 14 patients.[31] The Prestige II added bone ingrowth surfaces, a lower profile, and a trough to allow coupled motions. Porchet and Metcalf[32] reported the results of a prospective randomized controlled multicenter study in which NDI and SF-36 scores were measured preoperatively and for up to 24 months postoperatively. In comparison to patients who underwent fusion, all of the outcome measures showed equivalency at up to 24 months postoperatively. Radiographic analysis revealed preservation of motion for all prostheses.

Pimenta and associates[33] reported the results of an uncontrolled study of the PCM Artificial Cervical Disc. Fifty-three patients underwent 83 arthroplasties, and outcomes were measured using the VAS, NDI, and the Treatment Intensity Gradient Test. Scores for all of these measures improved postoperatively. The authors noted one complication in which a device migrated 4 mm. This complication was kept under observation without any further treatment. At up to 3-month follow-up, 90% of the patients had good to excellent results using Odom's criteria.

Myelopathy

Thus far, results for the treatment of myelopathy appear satisfactory, but data are limited because the results of randomized controlled studies have not been reported. Concerns when using arthroplasty for this condition have been raised because preservation of motion may have an adverse effect on spinal cord recovery. Sekhon[26] reported a case series of nine patients with cervical spondylotic myelopathy who were treated with anterior decompression and reconstruction with the Bryan disk. Follow-up ranged from 1 to 17 months. On average, the Nurick grade improved by 0.72 and Oswestry NDI scores improved by 51.4 points. Improvement in cervical lordosis was noted in 29% of the patients. No complications were reported.

Summary and Critique of Clinical Data

When examining these cervical arthroplasty studies, it is important to be aware that there may be significant placebo effects associated with the clinical outcome measures. Any patient who received the disk in a nonrandomized or randomized study knew that they had been treated with the new study device. Virtually all of these patients were pleased that they received this new device.

On the other hand, in the randomized trials, most of the patients who underwent arthrodesis were disappointed that they were not in the arthroplasty group. This realization has the potential for setting different expectations for the surgical procedure, which might ultimately affect the postoperative clinical outcome measures. Whether this theoretic critique is actually valid remains to be determined and would require a study in which patients are blinded to their treatment, even postoperatively.

It should be noted that most of these studies only reported short-term results, some with only a 3-month follow-up. It remains to be determined whether the early enthusiasm for artificial cervical disks will be borne out by long-term studies. Despite these concerns, the data from prospective, randomized clinical trials of cervical prostheses in the United States suggest that artificial cervical disk replacements, in general, produce outcomes similar to those of anterior fusions, but maintain motion across the disk space.

Complications

Few complications of cervical disk arthroplasty have been reported. Perioperative complications included a possibly higher rate of hematoma (epidural and retropharyngeal) and infections.[24] Technical complications that have been anecdotally reported have included reports of vertebral body fracture during implantation and early dislodgement requiring reoperation.

Adverse inflammatory reactions with osteolysis have not been observed. Paravertebral ossification of unknown etiology has been reported to occur in up to 5% of patients.[11,34] It has been demonstrated, however, that treatment with anti-inflammatory agents may decrease this tendency.[34] Failure of clinical improvement is the most common cause for reoperation,[24] and often results from incomplete removal of compressive pathology posterior to the uncinate process. Arthroplasty requires more aggressive decompression because maintenance of motion will not result in bony remolding such as occurs following fusion. Neurologic complications have been rarely reported.

Summary

Cervical disk arthroplasty was developed to maintain motion hypothetically to reduce the risk of future adjacent-level degeneration. Other advantages are believed to be earlier return to activity and reduced surgical morbidity. Seven devices are currently undergoing US Food and Drug Administration investigation. The differences in materials, design, and implantation techniques on device performance are unknown. Preclinical testing for durability, stability, bony ingrowth, and inflammatory reactions shows that current designs are meeting established criteria for success.

Early follow-up of human studies are encouraging, demonstrating outcomes comparable to those of fusion, with the added advantage of motion preservation. Reported complications are few and manageable and have not resulted in catastrophic neural injury. The rate of revision has also been low. Longer follow-up is needed to determine whether these devices can function well over time and to determine long-term implant to host and host to implant reactions.

References

1. Baba H, Furusawa N, Imura S, Kawahara N, Tsuchiya H, Tomita K: Late radiographic findings after anterior cervical fusion for spondylotic myeloradiculopathy. *Spine* 1993;18:2167-2173.

2. Gore DR, Sepic SB: Anterior cervical fusion for degenerated or protruded discs: A review of one hundred forty-six patients. *Spine* 1984;9:667-671.

3. Gore DR, Sepic SB: Anterior discectomy and fusion for painful cervical disc disease: A report of 50 patients with an average follow-up of 21 years. *Spine* 1998;23:2047-2051.

4. Gore DR, Gardner GM, Sepic SB, Murray MP: Roentgenographic findings following anterior cervical fusion. *Skeletal Radiol* 1986;15:556-559.

5. Hilibrand AS, Carlson GD, Palumbo MA, Jones PK, Bohlman HH: Radiculopathy and myelopathy at segments adjacent to the site of a previous anterior cervical arthrodesis. *J Bone Joint Surg Am* 1999;81:519-528.

6. Goffin J, Geusens E, Vantomme N, et al: Long-term follow-up after interbody fusion of the cervical spine. *J Spinal Disord Tech* 2004;17:79-85.

7. Gore DR, Sepic SB, Gardner GM: Roentgenographic findings of the cervical spine in asymptomatic people. *Spine* 1986;11:521-524.

8. Gore DR: Roentgenographic findings in the cervical spine in asymptomatic persons: A ten-year follow-up. *Spine* 2001;26:2463-2466.

9. LeHuec JC, Kiaer T, Friesem T, Mathews H, Liu M, Eisermann L: Shock absorption in lumbar disc prosthesis: A preliminary mechanical study. *J Spinal Disord Tech* 2003;16:346-351.

10. Dahl MC, Rouleau JP, Papadopoulos SM, Nuckley RP, Ching RP: A dynamic characteristic comparison of the intact, fused, and prosthetic replaced cervical disc, in *Proceedings of the 5th Combined Meeting of the Orthopaedic Research Societies*, Banff, Alberta, Canada, July 1, 2004.

11. Goffin J, Van Calenbergh F, van Loon J, et al: Intermediate follow-up after treatment of degenerative disc disease with the Bryan cervical disc prosthesis: Single-level and bi-level. *Spine* 2003;28:2673-2678.

12. Bertagnoli R, Duggal N, Pickett GE, et al: Cervical total disc replacement: Part II. Clinical results. *Orthop Clin North Am* 2005;36:355-362.

13. Goffin J, Komistek R, Mahfouz H, Wong D, Macht D: In vivo kinematics of normal, degenerative, fused and

disk-replaced cervical spines, in *Proceedings of the 2003 Annual Meeting*. Rosemont, IL, American Academy of Orthopaedic Surgeons, 2003, pp 473-474.

14. Anderson PA, Sasso R, Riew KD, Metcalf NH: Reoperation rates of cervical arthroplasty versus arthrodesis. *Spine J* 2005;5:S76-S77.

15. Dmitriev AE, Cunningham BW, Hu N, Sell G, Vigna F, McAfee PC: Adjacent level intradiscal pressure and segmental kinematics following a cervical total disc arthroplasty: An in vitro human cadaveric model. *Spine* 2005;30:1165-1172.

16. Puttlitz CM, Rousseau MA, Xu Z, Hu S, Tay BK, Lotz JC: Intervertebral disc replacement maintains cervical spine kinetics. *Spine* 2004;29:2809-2814.

17. DiAngelo DJ, Roberston JT, Metcalf NH, McVay BJ, Davis RC: Biomechanical testing of an artificial cervical joint and an anterior cervical plate. *J Spinal Disord Tech* 2003;16:314-323.

18. DiAngelo DJ, Foley KT, Morrow BR, et al: In vitro biomechanics of cervical disc arthroplasty with the ProDisc-C total disc implant. *Neurosurg Focus* 2004;17:E7.

19. Sasso R, Rouleau JP: Kinematics of a cervical disc prosthesis. *Spine J* 2005;5:S87.

20. Pickett GE, Rouleau JP, Duggal N: Kinematic analysis of the cervical spine following implantation of an artificial cervical disc. *Spine* 2005;30:1949-1954.

21. McAfee PC, Cunningham BW, Orbegoso CM, Sefter JC, Dmitriev AE, Fedder IL: Analysis of porous ingrowth in intervertebral disc prostheses: A nonhuman primate model. *Spine* 2003;28:332-340.

22. Jensen WK, Anderson PA, Rouleau JP: Bone ingrowth in retrieved Bryan Cervical Disc prostheses. *Spine* 2005;30:2497-2502.

23. Anderson PA, Rouleau JP, Bryan VE, Carlson CS: Wear analysis of the Bryan Cervical Disc prosthesis. *Spine* 2003;28:S186-S194.

24. Anderson PA, Rouleau JP, Toth JM, Riew KD: A comparison of simulator-tested and retrieved cervical disc prostheses: Invited submission from the Joint Section Meeting on Disorders of the Spine and Peripheral Nerves, March 2004. *J Neurosurg Spine* 2004;1:202-210.

25. Sekhon LH: Reversal of anterior cervical fusion with a cervical arthroplasty prosthesis. *J Spinal Disord Tech* 2005;18:S125-S128.

26. Sekhon LH: Cervical arthroplasty in the management of spondylotic myelopathy. *J Spinal Disord Tech* 2003;16:307-313.

27. Goffin J, Casey A, Kehr P, et al: Preliminary clinical experience with the Bryan cervical disc prosthesis. *Neurosurgery* 2002;51:840-845.

28. Lafuente J, Casey AT, Petzold A, Brew S: The Bryan cervical disc prosthesis as an alternative to arthrodesis in the treatment of cervical spondylosis. *J Bone Joint Surg Br* 2005;87:508-512.

29. Duggal N, Pickett GE, Mitsis DK, Keller JL: Early clinical and biomechanical results following cervical arthroplasty. *Neurosurg Focus* 2004;17:E9.

30. Bertagnoli R, Yue JJ, Pfeiffer F, et al: Early results after ProDisc-C cervical disc replacement. *J Neurosurg Spine* 2005;2:403-410.

31. Wigfield CC, Gill SS, Nelson RJ, Metcalf NH, Robertson JT: The new Frenchay artificial cervical joint: Results from a two-year pilot study. *Spine* 2002;27:2446-2452.

32. Porchet F, Metcalf NH: Clinical outcomes with the Prestige II cervical disc: Preliminary results from a prospective randomized clinical trial. *Neurosurg Focus* 2004;17:E6.

33. Pimenta L, McAfee PC, Cappuccino A, Bellera FP, Link HD: Clinical experience with the new artificial cervical PCM (Cervitech) disc. *Spine J* 2004;4:315S-321S.

34. Heller J, Goffin J: Classification of paravertebral ossification after insertion of the Bryan cervical disc prosthesis, in *Proceedings of the 31st Annual Meeting of the Cervical Spine Research Society*. Cervical Spine Research Society, 2003.

Pedicle Screw Fixation (T1, T2, and T3)

Michael D. Daubs, MD
Yongjung J. Kim, MD
Lawrence G. Lenke, MD

Abstract

The indications for thoracic pedicle screw fixation have expanded over the past decade. Thoracic pedicle screws are now being used in the treatment of degenerative, traumatic, neoplastic, congenital, and developmental disorders. The pedicles of T1, T2, and T3 are typically large and ovoid in shape and amenable to pedicle screw fixation in most instances. The placement of thoracic pedicle screws requires knowledge of the topographic and deep bony anatomy of the thoracic spine as well as an appreciation of the surrounding visceral structures at risk. With strict adherence to the surgical techniques of insertion, thoracic pedicle screw fixation is a safe and effective method of stabilization. It offers several advantages over other forms of fixation, especially in the upper thoracic spine where the options are limited.

Instr Course Lect 2007;56:247-255.

The use of thoracic pedicle screw fixation in patients requiring spinal surgery has expanded over the past decade. Most spinal surgeons currently consider the placement of pedicle screws into the lumbar spine routine. However, placement of pedicle screws into the thoracic spine is still considered a challenge, and the potential risk of major neurologic and vascular complications, although rare, has caused many surgeons to

avoid the technique. Pedicle screws offer distinct advantages over other forms of fixation. Theoretically, pedicle screws provide a form of three-column fixation that allows for greater control in the sagittal, coronal, and rotational planes, resulting in greater stability. They are now commonly used in the treatment of degenerative and traumatic disorders. In the treatment of scoliosis, thoracic pedicle screws have improved the three-dimensional curve correction, decreased the rates of curve progression, and resulted in higher fusion rates.[1-7] Biomechanically, pedicle screws have been shown to provide stronger fixation when compared with hooks,[8] the

more traditional form of fixation of the thoracic region.

Several clinical studies have been published evaluating the complications of thoracic screw insertion. The largest study reported a malposition rate of 1.5% and a neurologic complication rate of 0.8%.[5] Kim and associates[7] reported moderate cortical perforation of the pedicle in 6.2% of 3,204 thoracic screws placed, of which 1.7% violated the medial wall. Despite the perforations, there were no reported neurologic complications or need for revisions. At the senior author's institution, more than 10,000 thoracic pedicle screws have now been inserted as an alternative to wire and hook fixation with no neurologic, vascular, or visceral complications. With a thorough knowledge of the thoracic spine anatomy and the surrounding structures, pedicle screw fixation can be safely used.

Relevant Anatomy

In the thoracic spine, three anatomic characteristics of the pedicle affect the size and position of the screw: transverse pedicle diameter, angle of the pedicle trajectory, and length of the pedicle trajectory. These measurements vary throughout the

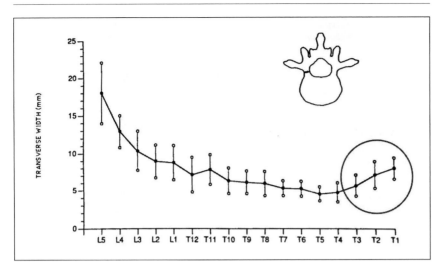

Figure 1 Graph displaying the transverse pedicle widths from T1 to L5. The T1-T3 pedicles are on average significantly wider in diameter than the midthoracic pedicles. (Reproduced with permission from Zindrick MR, Wiltse LL, Doornik A, et al: Analysis of the morphometric characteristics of the thoracic and lumbar pedicles. *Spine* 1987;12:160-166.)

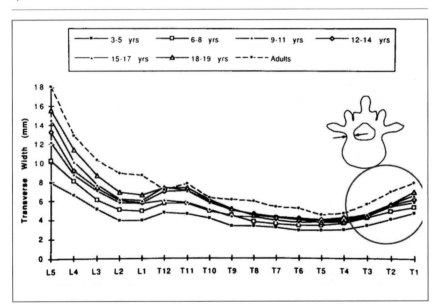

Figure 2 Graph displaying the mean transverse pedicle widths from pediatric age (3 to 5 years) to adulthood (> 20 years). The pedicle width increases with age until adulthood but throughout ages it remains consistently larger at T1, T2, and T3 than the pedicles in the midthoracic spine. (Reproduced with permission from Zindrick MR, Knight GW, Sartori MJ, et al: Pedicle morphology of the immature spine. *Spine* 2000;25:2726-2735.)

length of the thoracic spine. From T1 to T3, the pedicle width decreases fairly dramatically[9] (Figure 1). The width is approximately 8.0 mm at T1, 6.5 mm at T2, and 5.0 mm at T3.[9,10] In the immature spine, the pedicle widths are smaller and increase with age.[11] In the 3- to 5-year age group, the mean width is 4.8 mm at T1, 4.0 mm at T2, and 3.4 mm at T3 (Figure 2). The shape is consistently oval in the upper tho-

racic spine.[11] The average screw diameter used at T1-T3 is 6.0 mm. The pedicle wall is two to three times thicker on the medial side than on the lateral side at all levels.[12] The angle of the trajectory in the transverse plane is approximately 25° convergent for T1 and T2 and decreases to approximately 15° at T3 (Figure 3).[9-11,13] The trajectory in the sagittal angle is approximately 15° caudad.[9-11,13] The length of the pedicle trajectory varies with the age and size of the patient. In 3- to 5-year-old patients, the pedicle trajectory is approximately 22 mm and increases 70% to the adult length of approximately 36 mm.[11] Another important anatomic landmark is the distance from the dorsal lamina to the pedicle isthmus. A cadaver study has demonstrated this average distance to be 12 mm (YJ Kim, MD, LG Lenke, MD, G Cheh, MD, KD Riew, MD, Southampton, Bermuda, unpublished data presented at the 11th International Meeting on Advanced Spine Technologies, 2004).

Thoracic pedicle dimensions vary with each individual. In most patients, the pedicles are large enough for screw fixation, and screws are routinely used in pediatric as well as older adult patients. Even in patients with small pedicles, it has been shown that screws 80% to 115% of the size of the outer pedicle diameter can be safely inserted through gradual plastic deformation with a probe and bone tap[14] (S Suk, MD, JH Lee, MD, Boston MA, unpublished data presented at the 3rd Intermeeting of the Societe Internationale de Recherches Orthopedique et de Traumatologie, 1994). The use of pedicle screws in patients with scoliosis was initially believed to be too dangerous because of the abnormal anatomy. The pedicle morphology in patients with scoliotic spines has now been extensively studied. No significant difference has been found when comparing scoliotic vertebrae and normal vertebrae in the thoracic spine in relation to the angle or length of the pedicle trajectory.[13] As the spine becomes more rotated in patients with severe deformity, there is no change in the angle of the pedicle trajectory to the corresponding vertebral body, but there is a change in spatial orientation to the floor. Therefore, although the surgeon has to adjust for the proper angle of insertion, the anatomic landmarks are constant. In adolescent patients with idiopathic scoliosis (average age, 15.5 years) who were evaluated with CT scans, no correlation of pedicle size to age, Risser grade, curve magnitude, or the amount of segmental axial rotation was reported.[15] There is a significant decrease in the width of the concave pedicles compared with the convex side in patients with thoracic scoliosis.[13]

Thoracic pedicles have recently been morphologically classified.

The system of classification is stratified on the basis of ease of pedicle screw insertion (Figure 4). A type A pedicle has a large cancellous channel, a type B pedicle has a small cancellous channel, a type C pedicle has a cortical channel, and a type D pedicle has an absent channel (slit pedicle). In type C pedicles, intraosseous screw insertion is possible with gradual dilation with the pedicle probe and taps. In type D pedicles, screws are placed juxtapedicular along the lateral pedicle wall into the vertebral body (Figure 5). Most upper thoracic pedicles

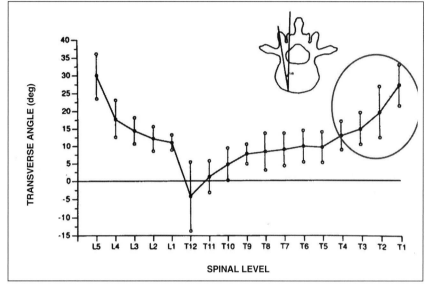

Figure 3   Graph displaying the mean transverse angle of the pedicles from T1 to L5. The angle is extremely convergent at T1 to T3. (Reproduced with permission from Zindrick MR, Wiltse LL, Doornik A, et al: Analysis of the morphometric characteristics of the thoracic and lumbar pedicles. *Spine* 1987;12:160-166.)

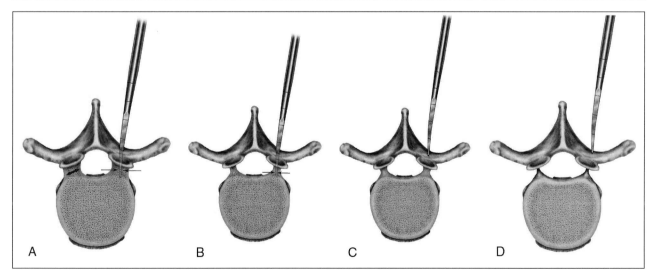

Figure 4   Illustration of the pedicle classification system. **A,** Type A has a large cancellous channel. **B,** Type B has a small cancellous channel. **C,** Type C has a thin cortical channel with absent cancellous bone. **D,** Type D has an absent pedicle channel (slit pedicle). The level of difficulty of pedicle screw insertion increases from type A to D.

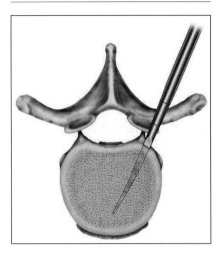

Figure 5 Illustration of a type D pedicle in which the pedicle probe has been inserted along the lateral wall of the pedicle and into the vertebral body in a juxtapedicular fashion.

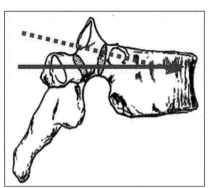

Figure 6 Illustration of the anatomic (*dashed line*) and the straightforward (*solid line*) trajectories for thoracic pedicle insertion.

(T1, T2, and T3) will be either type A or B pedicles. However, if scoliosis is present, the concave pedicles may be type C or D.

Structures at Risk

The placement of pedicle screws in the thoracic spine requires a discrete knowledge of the three-dimensional anatomy. Understanding the surface landmarks as well as the deep bony anatomy is essential to correctly identify the pedicle entrance and the proper insertion trajectory. The "safe zone" around the pedicle is extremely small. There is no epidural space between the thoracic pedicle and the dura. The average distance from the pedicle to the nerve root has been determined to be approximately 2.0 mm superiorly and inferiorly at T1 and T2 and 2.8 mm at T3.[16] However, the nerve roots in the thoracic spine exit more horizontally at high angles (120° at T1) compared with the lumbar spine, where they run longitudinally along the medial pedicle wall.[16] Medially, the spinal cord is insulated by the epidural and subarachnoid spaces,

which may explain why breaches in the medial pedicle wall are rarely symptomatic except in instances of gross violation with severe encroachment of the spinal canal. Directly lateral to the pedicle in the upper thoracic spine is the rib. Beyond the rib head is the pleural cavity. Structures anterior to the vertebral body at T1, T2, and T3 include the esophagus, thoracic duct, and sympathetic ganglion. The aorta is present in 30% of patients anteriorly on the left at T3.[17]

Technique

Several pedicle screw insertion techniques have been described: freehand, fluoroscopically-assisted, computer-assisted, and open lamina.[5,6,18-25] The computer-assisted techniques have been developed to improve the accuracy of screw placement, but their ease of use is variable.[19-24] The open-lamina technique has been shown to also improve accuracy. The best technique combines accuracy and ease of use and uses methods and instruments familiar to most spinal surgeons. The freehand technique satisfies these requirements and for this reason is the preferred technique.

Freehand Technique

The freehand technique is based on the insertion techniques used in the lumbar spine. It uses the same instruments (pedicle probe and pedicle sound) used for lumbar pedicle screw insertion and also relies on the knowledge of anatomic landmarks. It is based on three important principles: (1) the correct anatomic starting point, (2) the correct trajectory, and (3) the intraosseous feel while probing the pathway down the pedicle into the vertebral body. It requires a thorough knowledge of the topical landmarks of the pedicle and the underlying bony anatomy to extrapolate the proper three-dimensional pathway. Two approaches have been described: the anatomic approach and the straightforward approach (Figure 6). With the straightforward approach, the sagittal trajectory of the screw parallels the superior end plate of the vertebral body (Figure 6). In the anatomic approach, the screw trajectory follows the anatomic axis of the pedicle, which is 15° caudad in the sagittal plane. The straightforward approach has a 39% increase in maximum insertional technique and a 27% increase in pullout strength compared with the anatomic approach.[26] The increase in fixation strength with the straightforward approach is believed to be a result of improved engagement of the superior cortex of the pedicle and compact cancellous bone along the superior end plate of the vertebral body. The straightforward approach is recommended for most patients, whereas the anatomic approach should be reserved for salvage purposes only.[26]

The technique begins with a meticulous exposure of the posterior elements. The spine is exposed to the tips of the transverse processes bilaterally. The facet joints are then cleared of soft tissue using a combination of cautery and curettage. With an osteotome, the inferior 5 mm of the inferior facet is removed, and the exposed cartilage is scraped from the superior facet surface. The inferior portion of the facet is not removed from the most cephalad level of the construct to avoid disruption of the facet joint.

The starting points for the pedicles at T1, T2, and T3 are shown in Figure 7. At all three levels, the cephalad-caudad starting point is the midpoint of the transverse process. The mediolateral starting point is slightly medial to the lateral border of the superior facet. The more lateral starting point allows for the more convergent transverse trajectory of the pedicles at T1, T2, and T3. Once the starting point is located, a high-speed cortical burr is used to create a posterior cortical breach of approximately 5 mm in depth. A "blush" may be seen that indicates entrance into the cancellous bone at the base of the pedicle; it may not be seen with smaller type B or type C pedicles because of the limited cancellous space. The thoracic gearshift probe (2-mm blunt-tipped, slightly curved) (Figure 8) is placed at the base of the pedicle and gently used to search for the cancellous "soft spot" at the entrance of the pedicle. The gearshift is initially pointed laterally to avoid medial wall perforation. The pressure used for the probe is slightly greater than what is typically used in the lumbar spine. The small 2-mm tip allows the probe to slide down the cancellous channel of the pedicle even if it is extremely small. With extremely small type C pedicles, the ventral surface of the lamina can be gently palpated while sloping down into the pedicle in a funnel-like fashion.

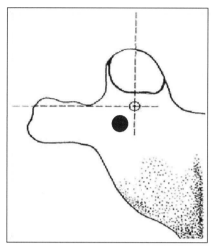

Figure 7 Illustration of the starting point (*black dot*) for insertion of thoracic pedicle screws into T1, T2, and T3. The horizontal dashed line represents the superior edge of the transverse process. The vertical dashed line represents the midpoint of the facet joint. The cephalad-caudad landmark is the midpoint of the transverse process. The mediolateral landmark is just lateral to the midpoint (vertical dashed line) of the facet joint. The lateral starting point allows for the angle of convergence of the pedicles at T1-T3. A starting point medial to the midpoint of the superior facet should be avoided.

This is a helpful step in identifying the pedicle entrance in small pedicles and is frequently used as a confirmatory step for all thoracic pedicles. Once the probe is started, it is inserted 15 to 20 mm just beyond the medially located spinal canal (Figure 9). The gearshift is then removed and the tip is then pointed medially and carefully placed into the base of the hole and advanced 20 to 25 mm. The probe is then rotated 180° to widen the channel for the pedicle screw. It is important to feel bone the entire length of the pedicle and into the body. The probing should be smooth, and consistent pressure should be applied. Any sudden advancement suggests a pedicle wall or vertebral body viola-

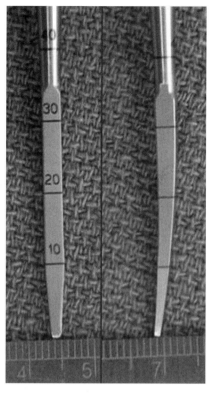

Figure 8 Photograph showing two views of the tip of the gearshift pedicle probe. It is slightly curved and blunt tipped with marked measurement lines to determine the depth of insertion. (Reproduced with permission from Kim YJ, Lenke LG, Bridwell KH, Cho YS, Riew KD: Free hand pedicle screw placement in the thoracic spine: Is it safe? *Spine* 2004;29:333-342.)

tion. The anterior and lateral cortices of the vertebral bodies are weak and can be easily penetrated by the probe. If a sudden advancement does occur, it should be evaluated immediately to avoid complications and possibly salvage the pedicle for fixation.

The gearshift probe is then removed, and the hole is visualized to ensure that only blood and no cerebrospinal fluid is present. Excessive bleeding may indicate a medial wall perforation and secondary epidural bleeding. The flexible ball-tipped sounding probe is then used to palpate the four walls of the pedicle

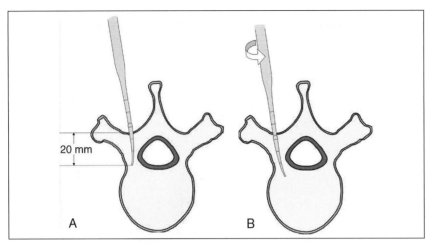

Figure 9 Illustration showing the technique for insertion of the pedicle probe. **A,** The probe is initially started with the curve pointed laterally until it reaches a depth of 20 mm. **B,** It is then reinserted and directed medially into the pedicle and into the vertebral body. (Reproduced with permission from Kim YJ, Lenke LG, Bridwell KH, Cho YS, Riew KD: Free hand pedicle screw placement in the thoracic spine: Is it safe? *Spine* 2004;29:333-342.)

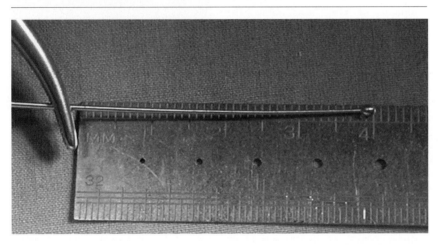

Figure 10 Photograph of the pedicle sounding device. Once the pedicle has been successfully probed, the sounding device is inserted to determine the depth of the pedicle tract and appropriate screw length. (Reproduced with permission from Kim YJ, Lenke LG, Bridwell KH, Cho YS, Riew KD: Free hand pedicle screw placement in the thoracic spine: Is it safe? *Spine* 2004;29:333-342.)

(medial, lateral, superior, and inferior) and the anterior floor. While probing with the sound, the proximal 10 to 15 mm of the channel should be carefully palpated, which is the area of the pedicle isthmus and the location of most pedicle wall perforations. If a perforation is identified, it is possible to carefully redirect the pedicle probe down a new path. If the pedicle is not salvageable, bone wax is placed in the hole to avoid bleeding.

Next, the pedicle tract is tapped with a tap that is 1.0 mm smaller in diameter than the planned screw diameter. If there is resistance to the tap, a tap that is one size smaller should be used to make another attempt. Once tapped, the sounding probe is again used to palpate the bony ridges of the four walls of the pedicle and the floor. With the sounding probe in position at the proper depth, a hemostat is clamped on the probe at the corresponding entrance of the pedicle tract, marking the appropriate length for the screw (Figure 10). The length of the marked probe is compared with the screw length to ensure accuracy of length. The screw is then inserted slowly by hand using the same trajectory as the pedicle probe that was inserted. The slow insertion allows for the viscoelastic expansion of the pedicle walls. At T1, T2, and T3, the typical screw diameter used is 5.0 to 6.0 mm, although larger screws can be placed depending on the individual pedicle size. The typical length of screw used at these levels is 25 to 35 mm.

There are unique challenges of proximal thoracic pedicle screw insertion. Because the upper level of the thoracic spine is kyphotic, the kyphotic angle can make it difficult to gain the correct sagittal trajectory without interference from the skull and the paraspinal muscles. The lateral wound and muscles can also interfere with the convergent trajectory (25°) needed for screw insertion in the upper thoracic spine. Placing halo skull traction with the patient's neck in a slightly flexed position can reduce the kyphotic angle and ease screw placement.

The transition from cervical to thoracic instrumentation can also be problematic, depending on the system used. Lateral mass screws are typically used at C6 and above, and pedicle screws are typically used at C7 and below. The transition is from the more mediolateral mass fixation points to the laterally placed pedicle screws of the upper thoracic spine. It is best to place the rod medially in

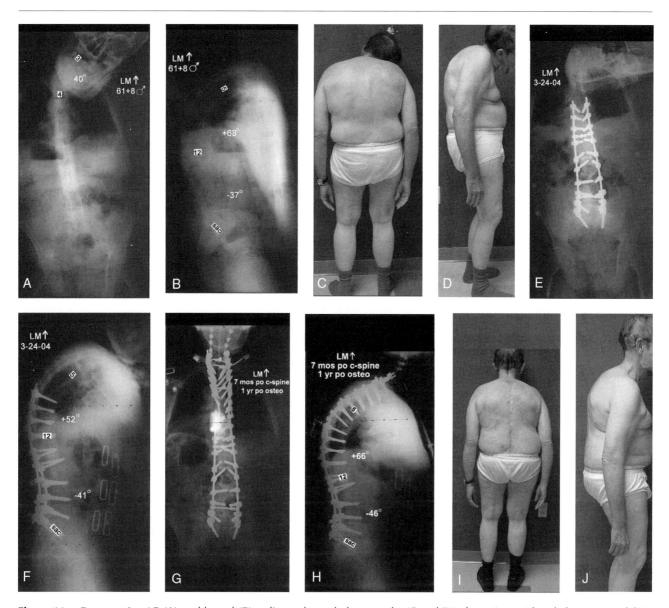

Figure 11   Preoperative AP (**A**) and lateral (**B**) radiographs and photographs (**C** and **D**) of a patient with ankylosing spondylitis with a chronic kyphotic deformity of the thoracolumbar spine secondary to a chronic L1 fracture; the patient also had a severe angular deformity of the cervical spine. Postoperative AP (**E**) and lateral (**F**) radiographs show that the thoracolumbar deformity was initially corrected with a pedicle subtraction osteotomy at L2 followed by a posterior arthrodesis with instrumentation from T9 to the sacrum using a 5.5-mm rod. The patient was placed in cervical traction following the thoracolumbar procedure and 5 months later the cervical deformity was addressed. AP (**G**) and lateral (**H**) radiographs and photographs (**I** and **J**) obtained 1 year postoperatively show that lateral mass fixation was used in the cervical spine with a 3.2-mm rod, which attached to a 4.5-mm rod in the upper thoracic spine and finally into the previously placed 5.5-mm rod.

the upper thoracic spine. The typical cervical rod construct is 3.5 mm, and the typical upper thoracic rod construct is 4.5 mm to 6.35 mm. The ideal transition is from a 3.5-mm rod in the cervical spine to a 4.5-mm rod in the proximal thoracic spine to a 5.5-mm rod in the lower thoracic spine (Figure 11). Tapered and screw-in rods are available for this purpose. Dominoes are helpful, but they can be bulky and can impede arthrodesis. If dominoes are used bilaterally, they should be placed at different levels to reduce the chance of pseudarthrosis.

After screw placement, plain radiography or fluoroscopic imaging should be used to assess screw position. Evaluation of thoracic screw position with plain radiography has been extensively studied and has been found to be accurate when compared with CT.[27] Currently, 1% to 2% of pedicle screws are readjusted or removed as a result of intraoperative radiographic findings. It can be difficult to adequately image the upper thoracic spine. Proper preoperative positioning and skull traction both can aid this process.

Pedicle Salvage

If a pedicle breach is found while probing with the sounding device, the pedicle can be salvaged by redirecting the pedicle probe and changing the insertion trajectory. The same degree of caution should be used as the probe is inserted and advanced. Once the new tract is successfully made, the sound is again used to assess the floor and the walls of the new tract. A Kirschner wire can be used to direct a cannulated tap down the new tract if available. If there is any question as to the integrity of the anterior wall of the vertebral body, a Kirschner wire should not be used to avoid advancement of the wire beyond the body wall. After tapping, a screw is carefully directed down the new trajectory. If this technique is unsuccessful, changing to the anatomic trajectory (Figure 6) and repeating the steps of insertion is another option. One study reported that the anatomic trajectory achieved 62% of maximal insertional torque during the salvage of a failed/violated pedicle and provided adequate fixation in the salvage situation.[26]

If the pedicle cannot be salvaged, juxtapedicular screw placement is possible (Figure 5). The starting point is slightly more lateral on the transverse process, and the medial angulation is greater. The pedicle probe is aimed along the lateral wall of the pedicle and aimed medially into the vertebral body at the junc-

tion of the pedicle and vertebral body. The purchase is weaker, but still stronger than hook fixation. If screws cannot be placed and the lamina is intact, hooks or sublaminar wires can be used.

Complications

There are few published reports on complications associated with the use of thoracic pedicle screws. Suk and associates[5] reported their experience with the placement of 4,600 thoracic screws. Using plain AP and lateral radiographic analysis, 1.5% of the thoracic screws were determined to be malpositioned. The malpositioning was lateral in 27% of instances, medial in 6%, superior in 18%, and inferior in 49%. There was one instance of neurologic injury with transient paraparesis resulting from a medial pedicle wall violation. Other reported complications included pedicle fracture (0.24%), screw loosening (0.76%), and infections (1.9%).

Liljenqvist and associates[3] assessed the placement of 120 thoracic pedicle screws using CT. The overall rate of cortical penetration was 25%, with 8.3% of the screws penetrating medially, 14.2% penetrating laterally, and 2.5% penetrating inferiorly. There were no neurologic complications reported. Three screws placed laterally were found to be in close proximity to the aorta.

Kim and associates[6] reported on the safety and reliability of the freehand technique as described previously. More than 3,200 screws were placed by two surgeons and random CT was used to evaluate the placement of 577 screws. Of these, more than 250 were placed at the T1, T2, and T3 level. When evaluating all of the screws placed, 36 (6.9%) were inserted with moderate cortical perforation of which 9 (1.8%) were medial. There were no neurologic, vas-

cular, or visceral complications reported at up to 10-year follow-up.

A few case reports have been published of vascular injuries related to thoracic pedicle screws. Heini and associates[28] reported a case of fatal cardiac tamponade resulting from an injury to the right coronary artery by a Kirschner wire used during screw insertion. Papin and associates[29] reported the unusual clinical symptoms of abdominal pain, mild lower extremity weakness, tremor, thermoalgic discrimination loss, and imbalance related to spinal cord compression from a medially placed thoracic pedicle screw. The symptoms resolved after the screw was removed.

Complication Avoidance

The experience with lumbar pedicle screw placement has shown that most complications occur during the initial learning phase, but dramatically decrease as surgical experience improves.[30] Thoracic screw insertion is no different. The key to avoiding major complications is to use the most familiar and comfortable technique of insertion consistent with the surgeon's personal training. Regardless of the specific method used, there are several key steps to reducing complications. Obtaining intraoperative radiographs on the operating room table is important. AP and lateral radiographs provide an accurate, on-table position of the vertebrae, especially in the sagittal plane. Meticulous exposure of the bony landmarks of the posterior elements and a blood-free surface are also important. By exposing the transverse process, the lamina, the pars interarticularis, and the base of the superior articular process, the entrance point of the pedicle can be accurately identified. Expert knowledge of the topographic anatomic landmarks is essential to understanding the correct three-dimensional trajectory into the pedicle and ensuring accurate placement. Once the screws are inserted, plain radiographs or fluoroscopic images should be obtained to ensure intraosseous placement.

The freehand technique as described previously relies on well-learned methods used in the lumbar spine. The instruments for pedicle probing, tapping, and sounding are the same, as is the reliance on topographic landmarks. With this technique, few major complications have been reported, and the rate of malpositioning is low.

Summary

Pedicle screw fixation in the upper thoracic spine is a safe and effective form of stabilization. It offers advantages over other forms of fixation in the treatment of a variety of spinal disorders. The technique requires expert knowledge of the surface and deep anatomy of the thoracic spine and a thorough awareness of the possible pitfalls. With strict adherence to the surgical methods of insertion, the complication rates are low and similar to those for other forms of fixation.

References

1. Suk SI, Lee CK, Kim WJ, Chung YJ, Park YB: Segmental pedicle screw fixation in the treatment of thoracic idiopathic scoliosis. *Spine* 1995;20:1399-1405.

2. Hamill CL, Lenke LG, Bridwell KH, Chapman MP, Blanke K, Baldus C: The use of pedicle screw fixation to improve correction in the lumbar spine of patients with idiopathic scoliosis: Is it warranted? *Spine* 1996;21:1241-1249.

3. Liljenqvist UR, Halm HF, Link TM: Pedicle screw instrumentation of the thoracic spine in idiopathic scoliosis. *Spine* 1997;22:2239-2245.

4. Halm H, Niemeyer T, Link T, Liljenqvist U: Segmental pedicle screw instrumentation in idiopathic thoracolumbar and lumbar scoliosis. *Eur Spine J* 2000;9:192-197.

5. Suk Si, Kim WJ, Lee SM, Kim JH, Chung ER, Lee JH: Thoracic pedicle screw fixation in spinal deformities: Are they really safe? *Spine* 2001;26:2049-2057.

6. Kim YJ, Lenke LG, Bridwell KH, Cho YS, Riew KD: Free hand pedicle screw placement in the thoracic spine: Is it safe? *Spine* 2004;29:333-342.

7. Kim YJ, Lenke LG, Cho SK, Bridwell KH, Sides B, Blanke K: Comparative analysis of pedicle screw versus hook instrumentation in posterior spinal fusion of adolescent idiopathic scoliosis. *Spine* 2004;29:2040-2048.

8. Hackenberg L, Link T, Liljenqvist U: Axial and tangential fixation strength of pedicle screws versus hooks in the thoracic spine in relation to bone mineral density. *Spine* 2002;27:937-942.

9. Zindrick MR, Wiltse LL, Doornik A, et al: Analysis of the morphometric characteristics of the thoracic and lumbar pedicles. *Spine* 1987;12:160-166.

10. Stanescu S, Ebraheim NA, Yeasting R, et al: Morphometric evaluation of the cervico-thoracic junction. *Spine* 1994;19:2082-2088.

11. Zindrick MR, Knight GW, Sartori MJ, et al: Pedicle morphology of the immature spine. *Spine* 2000;25:2726-2735.

12. Kothe R, O'Holleran JD, Liu W, Panjabi MM: Internal architecture of the thoracic pedicle: An anatomical study. *Spine* 1996;21:264-270.

13. Parent S, Labelle H, Skalli W, de Guise J: Thoracic pedicle morphometry in vertebrae from scoliotic spines. *Spine* 2004;29:239-248.

14. Misenhimer GR, Peek RD, Wiltse LL, Rothman SL, Widell EH Jr: Anatomic analysis of pedicle cortical and cancellous diameter as related to screw size. *Spine* 1989;14:367-372.

15. O'Brien MF, Lenke LG, Mardjetko S, et al: Pedicle morphology, in thoracic adolescent idiopathic scoliosis. *Spine* 2000;25:2285-2293.

16. Ebraheim NA, Jabaly G, Rongming X, Yesting RA: Anatomic relations of the thoracic pedicle to the adjacent neural structures. *Spine* 1997;22:1553-1557.

17. Bailey AS, Stanescu S, Yeasting RA, et al: Anatomic relationships of the cervicothoracic junction. *Spine* 1995;20:1431-1439.

18. Belmont PJ, Klemme WR, Dhawan A, et al: In vivo accuracy of thoracic pedicle screws. *Spine* 2001;26:2340-2346.

19. Kim KD, Johnson PJ, Bloch BS, et al: Computer assisted thoracic pedicle screw placement: An in vitro feasibility study. *Spine* 2001;26:360-364.

20. Amiot LP, Labelle H, De Guise JA, et al: Computer-assisted pedicle screw fixation: A feasibility study. *Spine* 1995;20:1208-1212.

21. Amiot LP, Lang K, Putsier M, et al: Comparative results between conventional and computer assisted pedicle screw installation in the thoracic, lumbar and sacral spine. *Spine* 2000;25:606-614.

22. Choi WW, Breen BA, Levi AD: Computer-assisted fluoroscopic targeting system for pedicle screw insertion. *Neurosurgery* 2000;47:872-878.

23. Kothe R, Matthias Strauss J, Deuretzbacher G, Hemmi T, Lorenzen M, Wiesner L: Computer navigation of parapedicular screw fixation in the thoracic spine: A cadaver study. *Spine* 2001;26:E496-E501.

24. Youkilis AS, Quint DJ, McGillicuddy JE, et al: Stereotactic navigation for placement of pedicle screw in the thoracic spine. *Neurosurgery* 2001;48:771-778.

25. Xu R, Ebraheim NA, Ou Y, Yeasting RA: Anatomic consideration of pedicle screw placement in the thoracic spine: Roy-Camille technique versus open lamina technique. *Spine* 1998;23:1065-1068.

26. Lehman RA, Kuklo TR: Use of the anatomic trajectory for thoracic pedicle screw salvage after failure/violation using the straight-forward technique: A biomechanical analysis. *Spine* 2003;28:2072-2077.

27. Kim YJ, Lenke LG, Cheh G, Riew KD: Evaluation of pedicle screw placement in the deformed spine using intraoperative plain radiographs: A comparison with computerized tomography. *Spine* 2005;30:2084-2088.

28. Heini P, Scholl E, Wyler D, et al: Fatal cardiac tamponade associated with posterior spinal instrumentation: A case report. *Spine* 1998;23:2226-2230.

29. Papin P, Arlet V, Marchesi D, et al: Unusual presentation of spinal cord compression related to misplaced pedicle screws in thoracic scoliosis. *Eur Spine J* 1999;8:156-159.

30. Gertzbein SD, Robbins SE: Accuracy of pedicular screw placement in vivo. *Spine* 1990;15:11-14.

Spine Surgery for Lumbar Degenerative Disease in Elderly and Osteoporotic Patients

Robert A. Hart, MD, MA
Michael A. Prendergast, BA

Abstract

Elderly patients with lumbar spine degenerative disease present significant challenges regarding surgical decision making and management. Because osteoporosis is a particularly prevalent comorbidity in the elderly population, it must be a concern in all elderly patients with degenerative disease of the lumbar spine. Careful attention to surgical indications and surgical technique is always required for the successful treatment of this challenging patient population.

Instr Course Lect 2007;56:257-272.

The rate of spinal stenosis surgery in the United States for patients older than 65 years has shown an eightfold increase over a 14-year period, and given the ongoing aging of the American population this trend is likely to continue.[1] This trend likely reflects several factors, including surgeons' increased ability to safely care for these patients as well as the increasing expectations of elderly patients regarding activity levels. Elective spinal surgery, especially surgical fusion, presents unique challenges to surgeons with respect to decision making, surgical technique, and perioperative care.

Every organ system manifests specific changes with aging, resulting in demonstrably higher surgical morbidity and mortality among elderly patients.[2] The effect of osteoporosis is a fundamental concern for spine surgeons planning spine fusion procedures in elderly patients. The spine surgeon must be informed regarding specific surgical risk factors and work to develop an appropriate treatment plan that accommodates the specific needs of elderly and osteoporotic patients.

Physiologic Concerns in the Elderly Patient

The elderly patient has several unique considerations, including medical comorbidities, nutritional status, reduced activity demands, and osteoporosis. These factors must be kept in mind and appropriately addressed during all phases of surgical management to optimize outcome.

Cardiac assessment should include obtaining a history of myocardial infarction, congestive heart failure, and arrhythmias. Goldman and associates[3] developed a cardiac risk assessment scale that identified several factors related to occurrence of perioperative cardiac complications. Particularly worrisome risk factors include an S3 gallop or jugular venous distension, myocardial infarction within the prior 6 months, nonsinus rhythm or premature atrial contractions, and more than five premature ventricular contractions per minute. These factors are weighted to assign a patient to one of four cardiac risk categories, a procedure that has been widely adopted among anesthesiologists.

Respiratory status also should be carefully evaluated in the elderly patient. Preoperative chest radiographs in patients older than 70 years should probably be ordered routinely, even without a more specific indication, to avoid complications and delays in treatment.[4] During the clinical evaluation, it is important to determine whether the patient has experienced

Table 1
Preoperative Assessment in Elderly Patients

Organ System	Possible Tests
Cardiac	Echocardiography Stress thallium test Exercise stress test Angiography
Pulmonary	Resting O_2 saturation Arterial blood gases Forced expiratory volume in 1 second Forced vital capacity
Renal	Serum area nitrogen Creatinine clearance
Nutrition/health status	Hematocrit Total protein Albumin
Musculoskeletal	Plain radiographs DEXA scan Quantitative CT

exercise intolerance, chronic cough, or unexplained dyspnea and to look for physical findings such as wheezes or rhonchi. An assessment of arterial blood gases is useful in evaluating for hypoxia or hypercarbia.[5,6] Incentive spirometry (especially forced expiratory volume in 1 second and forced vital capacity) should be considered for patients with a history of smoking or chronic obstructive pulmonary disease and those undergoing anterior thoracic or upper abdominal spinal surgery.[5,7,8]

Renal status is another important medical consideration in the elderly surgical patient. During surgery, patients older than 65 years undergo more dramatic changes in renal function than younger patients.[9-11] Renal status can be assessed using functions such as the Cockroft-Gault equation $((([140–age] \times \text{weight (kg)})/ (72 \times \text{serum creatinine}))$ because it corrects for the false elevation of the serum creatinine level, which can occur with a reduction of muscle mass in elderly patients.[12]

Nonsteroidal anti-inflammatory drugs (NSAIDs) are commonly used by elderly patients. These agents have multiple potential negative impacts, especially with respect to kidney function, gastrointestinal bleeding, and bone healing, and must be a source of concern.[13,14] NSAIDs should be avoided in patients undergoing spine fusion, especially during the early inflammatory phase of fusion when the effects of NSAIDs appear to have the greatest impact on bone healing.[15]

Oral bisphosphonates are also commonly used to treat osteoporosis in elderly patients. Although these agents appear to have minimal effect on creatinine clearance,[16] some have been shown to adversely affect bone healing in animal models, depending on the size of the fusion mass and animal model used.[17-20] Discontinuation of oral bisphosphonates before surgery and throughout the perioperative period is prudent until more definitive evidence is available.

Nutritional status is another concern in elderly patients and may be difficult to ascertain through history taking.[21] Assessment of the elderly patient with laboratory data such as total protein, serum albumin, and C-reactive protein levels should be part of the preoperative workup. A well-balanced diet complemented with oral supplements can be used to provide additional calories to correct nutritional deficits preoperatively. Vitamin D (400 to 800 IU/day) and calcium (1,200 mg/day) are also important nutrients for the maintenance of skeletal health in elderly patients[22] (Table 1).

Osteoporosis

Osteoporosis is a major health concern among the elderly population in the United States, with the condition diagnosed in approximately 10 million people and an estimated 44 million people at risk.[22] Although 80% of these patients are women, a significant number of men are also affected.[22,23,24] The financial burden to the medical system because of osteoporotic fractures exceeds $20 billion.[25]

At the biochemical level, bone is composed of an organic and a mineral component. Osteoid, the organic component, is composed of collagen and other proteins, whereas the mineral component is hydroxyapatite (HA). At a cellular level, remodeling depends on the balance between bone formation by osteoblasts and bone resorption by osteoclasts. At a microstructural level, bone is organized into cortical and trabecular bone.

Cortical bone is formed of interconnected cylinders organized around haversian canals, whereas trabecular bone is constructed as a densely interconnected lattice. The greater surface area in trabecular bone results in a higher turnover rate than in cortical bone. Bone loss thus occurs more rapidly in trabecular bone, with replacement of the normal trabecular lattice by thinner and ultimately discontinuous spicules in the disease state referred to as osteoporosis.[26]

Osteoporosis is a metabolic bone disorder that results in decreased bone mineral density. The biochemical composition and microscopic structure of osteoporotic bone are normal, but the volume density of bone is substantially reduced. A reduction of more than 2.5 standard deviations of the bone mineral density of a young adult roughly corresponds to values below 0.8 to 0.9 g/cm^2, depending on gender.[27] This decreased structural density adversely affects the mechanical properties of bone.[28]

Postmenopausal osteoporosis occurs within 10 to 20 years after the onset of menopause and is related to the loss of estrogen, resulting in excess bone resorption, particularly within trabecular bone.[29-31] Senile osteoporosis occurs in men and women and is a result of multisystem, age-related changes in the regulation of overall calcium, vitamin D, and other nutrients.[29] The specific changes in bone resorption and formation are less well defined than for postmenopausal osteoporosis, although both cortical and trabecular bone appear to be affected.[31]

Currently, two methods are used clinically to evaluate bone density. Dual energy x-ray absorptiometry (DEXA) measures bone density by area (g/cm^2). This test is simple, accurate, and carries a low radiation dose. It is also well tolerated, with a procedure duration of 10 to 15 minutes. Quantitative CT scanning is a measurement of volume density (g/cm^3) calculated via cross-sectional images of a vertebral body. The precision of this test is excellent, although it can be compromised by patient positioning and movement. However, the relatively small increase in accuracy of this test over DEXA scanning may not justify the greater expense, greater level of patient discomfort, and exposure of the patient to a greater radiation dose.[32] Osteophyte formation and calcification in the degenerative spine may reduce the accuracy of spinal DEXA scans, a limitation that is usually avoidable by using DEXA scanning of the proximal femur.[33]

Concerns regarding patients with osteoporosis undergoing spinal fusion surgery depend on the underlying pathology and the extent of surgery planned. Specific concerns of hardware failure, adjacent segment fracture, and the possibility of an increased nonunion rate all must be considered in this patient population.

Degenerative Lumbar Spinal Stenosis

Degenerative lumbar spinal stenosis, a common disorder of the elderly population, is an acquired condition resulting from osteoarthritis of the intervertebral disk and the facet joints as well as hypertrophy of the ligamentum flavum.[32,34,35] Most commonly, injury or degenerative changes within the disk initiate a cycle of degeneration of the three-joint complex of the spinal motion segment; however, in some patients, the degenerative process appears to start in the facet joints.[34,36] Progression of the degeneration leads to osteophyte formation at the facet joints, calcification and hypertrophy of the ligamentum flavum, intervertebral disk prolapse, and disk osteophyte formation.[34] All of these features may diminish the room available for the lumbar nerve roots in the central canal, the lateral recess, and the neural foramina.

The classic presentation of patients with lumbar spinal stenosis is neurogenic claudication, which refers to pain in the lower extremities brought on by activity. Although symptoms can be unilateral or bilateral, they are usually asymmetric. Pain is classically described as being exacerbated by activity and by positions of extension of the lumbar spine, with relief occurring following cessation of activity or forward flexion. Reduced pain with activities such as walking uphill or riding a stationary bicycle, which induce flexion of the lumbar spine, may sometimes help distinguish this symptom from vascular claudication.[36] With flexion of the spine, the diameter of the canal is increased and the ligamentum flavum is flat-tened, which is offered as an explanation of the postural relief of symptoms.[37]

The pathogenesis of these symptoms is not completely understood but is likely the result of mechanical compression of the lumbar nerve roots and consequent compromise of the neural blood supply.[36,38] Compression at more than one spinal level has been shown in animal models to produce venous congestion and insufficient arterial inflow, creating a relatively ischemic environment within the neural elements between the areas of congestion.[36,38] Compromised autonomic innervation of the lower limbs may inhibit the appropriate vasodilation response to increased muscle use, which may partially account for similarities in clinical appearance to vascular claudication.[38]

Most patients present with a normal motor examination.[36] Patients with long-standing and severe stenosis may ultimately experience lower extremity weakness or neurogenic bowel and bladder dysfunction.[36] Deep tendon reflexes are often reduced in elderly patients, especially at the Achilles tendon.[39] In addition to a neurologic examination, distal pulses and hip range of motion should also be assessed (Figure 1).

Imaging of the spine in patients suspected of having lumbar spinal stenosis should begin with plain radiographs, including dynamic flexion and extension lateral views. Additional imaging may include MRI and CT with or without myelography.[36,37] Although these studies provide detail regarding the location and extent of stenosis, it is important to remember that the severity of stenosis noted on imaging studies often does not correlate with the severity of symptoms and that stenosis

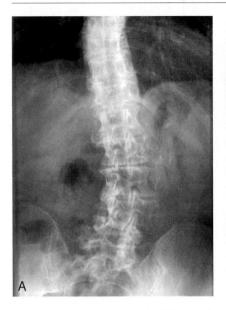 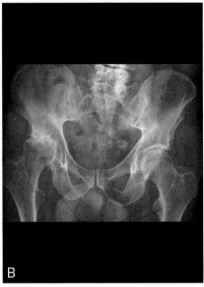 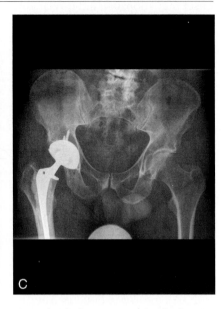

Figure 1   A, AP radiograph of the lumbar spine of a 74-year-old man with low back pain and right lower extremity thigh pain. Physical examination revealed stiffness and pain with range of motion of the right hip. **B,** AP pelvis radiograph demonstrating severe degenerative arthritis of the right hip joint. **C,** AP pelvis radiograph obtained 5 years after right total hip replacement. Patient obtained excellent relief of right lower extremity pain, and excellent pain relief was maintained over the duration of follow-up. No procedure to the lumbar spine has been performed to date.

is not a radiographic diagnosis but a clinical diagnosis.[35,40]

Electromyography is most often normal, especially in the early course of the disease, but it can be helpful in ruling out peripheral neuropathy resulting from other causes such as diabetes.[41] Selective nerve root blocks, facet infections, and sacroiliac joint injections may not only be therapeutic, but also are helpful diagnostically in localizing the source of a patient's pain, which can remain unclear even after a thorough clinical and radiographic assessment.[42,43]

Treatment of patients without neurologic deficits should generally begin nonsurgically and progress to surgical options only after more conservative measures have failed. Nonsurgical treatment options include NSAIDs, lumbar flexion and abdominal strengthening exercises, braces, and epidural injections.[44] In general, surgery is indicated for pa-

tients with severe functional compromise and those with persistently troubling symptoms despite efforts at nonsurgical treatment.

Fundamental to the successful surgical treatment of a stenotic segment is decompression, which is accomplished by a thorough removal of all structures contributing to the neurologic compression.[43] Generally, the type of decompression performed will depend on the anatomic site of stenosis and the patient's symptoms. If instability in the form of spondylolisthesis or scoliosis is not demonstrated preoperatively, fusion is generally recommended only when laminectomy is accompanied by greater than 50% resection of both facets or complete facetectomy on one side.[45,46]

Elderly patients often present with central spinal canal stenosis in addition to lateral and foraminal narrowing. Complete laminectomy often provides better neurologic de-

compression than fenestrated laminotomies or limited access procedures, which may fail to address all locations of compression.[47] In at least one clinical study, single-level laminectomies have been associated with diminished outcomes, which suggests that all levels of radiographic stenosis should be decompressed, unless the clinical assessment definitively indicates a specific spinal level.[51,52]

Medicare database studies have shown a correlation between increasing age and the risk of postoperative complications.[48,49] Deyo and associates[48-50] found a complication rate of 14.6% in patients between the ages of 65 and 74 years that increased to 17.7% in patients older than 75 years, with increased complication rates noted for patients undergoing fusion procedures. Such studies, however, do not allow an assessment of specific risk factors, and the age effect noted likely in part reflects the increased rate of associated medical comorbidities in the elderly patient population.

Age alone should not preclude lumbar spinal surgery, although comorbid conditions such as diabetes and heart disease must be discussed with patients because these conditions have been shown to affect surgical outcomes.[51,52] Recently Ragab and associates[53] studied 118 patients older than 70 years, including 21 patients older than 80 years, who were treated for stenosis with decompression alone or decompression and fusion. They described successful outcomes in 109 patients (92%), including 68 of 73 patients (93%) who were treated with decompression alone, which is consistent with the results reported for clinical series that include younger patients.[43,52,53] These authors emphasized the need for close intraoperative monitoring and aggressive fluid management in elderly patients.[53]

To improve the chance of success in patients with medical comorbidities, patients must be optimized medically and educated appropriately before undergoing surgery. One study found that an individual patient's own assessment of personal health and cardiovascular status was the most powerful predictor of success.[54] Other medical comorbidities have also been shown to affect outcomes. For example, Arinzon and associates[55] compared outcomes for 62 diabetic and nondiabetic patients older than 65 years who underwent decompression for spinal stenosis. Although most patients in both groups achieved successful pain relief, nondiabetic patients reported better overall satisfaction, showed more improvement in activities of daily living, required less revision surgery, and experienced fewer perioperative complications. It is impor-

tant to recognize that complications do not always compromise clinical outcomes, as suggested in a retrospective study by Benz and associates,[56] which found that despite a 40% complication rate in laminectomy patients older than 70 years, an overall satisfaction rate of 71% was reported.

Degenerative Lumbar Spondylolisthesis

Degenerative lumbar spondylolisthesis occurs when osteoarthritis of the facet joints leads to anterior displacement of the cranial vertebral body relative to the caudal adjacent vertebrae, which occurs most frequently at the L4-L5 level. Compromise of the vertebral canal results, often worsening preexisting stenosis caused by degenerative disease. More commonly seen in women than men, degenerative spondylolisthesis is a disease of older adults, seldom seen in those younger than 50 years, and perhaps affecting up to 10% of women older than 60 years.[57,58]

Although patients with degenerative lumbar spondylolisthesis report symptoms of lumbar stenosis at higher rates than patients with similar degrees of stenosis but without accompanying spondylolisthesis, many also report back pain.[59,60] Degenerative lumbar spondylolisthesis rarely exceeds 30% of vertebral body width, although slip progression may occur in up to 30% of untreated patients.[59,60] Plain radiography is usually sufficient to determine the nature of the spondylolisthesis and the slip grade.[58,61] MRI or CT with myelography can help evaluate associated compression of the neurologic elements and help screen for other potential causes of back pain in elderly patients, such as vertebral body compression frac-

tures or infectious diskitis.[58,62]

As for patients with stenosis, nonsurgical interventions, including NSAIDs, epidural medications, and lumbar flexibility and strengthening exercises, may be appropriate for patients without neurologic deficit and relatively recent symptom onset.[57] Surgery is an option for patients with severe or persistent symptoms that interfere significantly with quality of life and are refractory to nonsurgical treatment.[59]

Surgical options include decompression alone or decompression combined with a fusion procedure; the fusion procedure may be performed with or without instrumentation. Fusion can be accomplished in several ways, but most commonly is performed via posterior fusion with or without pedicle screw instrumentation. The best available evidence suggests that decompression with arthrodesis results in better clinical outcomes than decompression alone in patients with degenerative spondylolisthesis.[63-67] Despite this evidence, although use of pedicle screw–based instrumentation clearly increases the rate of successful fusion, it is less clearly beneficial in terms of clinical outcome.

Patients with relatively stable spondylolisthesis can be safely treated via laminectomy without fusion.[68] However, the subgroup of patients with degenerative spondylolisthesis that does not benefit from fusion has not been clearly defined. An evidence-based medicine approach, therefore, favors including fusion as a routine part of surgical treatment of these patients.[45,59,69,70] However, current clinical practice does not appear uniform in regard to addition of fusion for these patients.[71] As in patients with lumbar stenosis, the overall risk of compli-

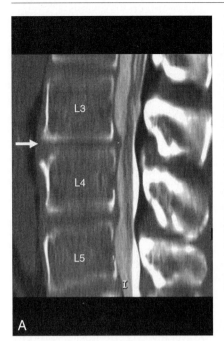
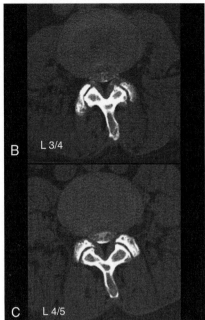
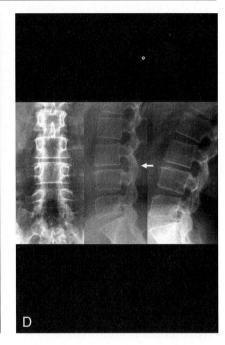

Figure 2   **A,** Sagittal CT myelogram of a 68-year-old woman with neurogenic claudication. A grade I degenerative spondylolisthesis is present the L3-4 disk space (*arrow*). Transverse cuts through the CT myelogram show marked central and lateral recess stenosis at the L3-4 (**B**) and L4-5 disk spaces (**C**). Note relatively coronal orientation of the facet joints at L4-5 with increased sagittal orientation at the L3-4 facet joint. **D,** AP (*left*) and lateral flexion (*center*) and extension (*right*) radiographs obtained 3 years postoperatively following laminectomies of L3, L4, and L5, with posterior facet fusion at L3-4. Note obliteration of the facet joint at L3-4 on the lateral flexion view (*arrow*) and the absence of motion at the L3-4 disk space between the flexion and extension views. The patient had excellent relief of lower extremity pain at 3-year follow-up.

cations, morbidity, and mortality increase with age, and including fusion has been shown to further increase surgical duration and complication rates.[48,49]

When fusion is performed, many authors recommend including instrumentation to improve fusion rates and reduce postoperative activity limitations.[45,59,67] However, avoiding instrumentation is also a reasonable option, particularly when facets are oriented in a relatively coronal plane and segmental instability is limited[45] (Figure 2). It must also be recognized that pedicle screw–based instrumentation is less effective in patients with severe osteoporosis.[72,73] Recently, however, long-term follow-up has suggested that uninstrumented fusion patients with nonunion do ultimately require higher rates of reintervention than patients who gain solid fusion.[65]

Degenerative Scoliosis

Degenerative scoliosis is an acquired disorder of adult patients for which there is no gender preference. It is a distinct diagnosis from that of patients with idiopathic scoliosis who develop secondary spinal degenerative disease because patients with true degenerative scoliosis develop de novo rotational deformity of the spine during the adult years. Patients with degenerative scoliosis typically present with symptoms similar to those of patients with degenerative lumbar stenosis, but often report back pain and may also experience problems with spinal alignment.[74] Patients with symptomatic degenerative scoliosis may have severe functional limitations, especially when sagittal plane imbalance is present.[75,76]

The pathophysiology of degenerative scoliosis is similar to that of lumbar stenosis, but appears to result when there is asymmetric degeneration of the facet joints and disk, resulting in a rotatory effect.[77] The relationship between osteoporosis and degenerative scoliosis is unclear, although the diagnoses often coexist.[78] Vertebral compression fractures can certainly produce sagittal plane and coronal plane deformities, although osteoporosis has not been definitively shown to be a risk factor for development or progression of degenerative scoliosis.[78-80] Severe rotation of the apical vertebrae, a Cobb angle of 30° or more, lateral vertebral translation of 6 mm or more, or a position of L5 above the intercrestal line have all been discussed as features that are predictive of curve progression in patients with degenerative lumbar scoliosis.[81-83]

The choice and success of non-surgical treatment modalities depends on the type and extent of the deformity, the severity of the stenosis, and the presence of lateral listhesis.[82] In addition to physical therapy and medical treatments, use of spinal orthoses also may be an option. Although bracing generally will not prevent progression of degenerative curves, it may alleviate symptoms of back pain in some patients.[82] Whenever orthotic devices are used in elderly patients, care must be taken to pad bony prominences well to avoid skin breakdown.[81]

Surgical treatment may or may not be appropriate for patients with degenerative scoliosis, depending on the patient's presentation, health status, and expectations from surgery.[77,84] As with degenerative spondylolisthesis, there are conflicting reports regarding the need for spinal stabilization as an adjunct to decompressive surgery in this patient population.[77,84,85] Although the quality of clinical evidence to support the addition of fusion in patients with scoliosis is not as high as in those with degenerative spondylolisthesis, there are several clinical presentations that should generally not be treated by decompression alone, including significant sagittal plane imbalance, lateral listhesis of 5 mm or greater, and patients requiring wide decompression because of associated central canal stenosis.[81-84]

Elderly patients with severe scoliotic curves are not always suitable candidates for the large reconstructive fusion procedures required to treat spinal deformity. It is therefore tempting in patients without severe scoliotic

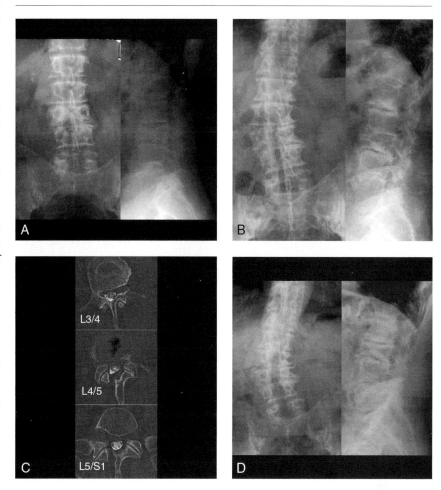

Figure 3 **A,** AP (*left*) and lateral (*right*) radiographs of a 74-year-old man with low back pain. Nearly normal alignment with axial degenerative disease was noted. A long-standing compression fracture of L3 is present. **B,** AP (*left*) and lateral (*right*) radiographs obtained 10 years later of the same patient. A degenerative scoliosis measuring 18° from the L1 to L4 levels has developed. By this time, the patient had undergone a right-sided foraminotomies at L3-4, L4-5, and L5-S1 for radicular leg pain, but remained symptomatic despite this intervention. **C,** CT myelograms through the L3-4 (*top*), L4-5 (*center*), and L5-S1 (*bottom*) disk spaces demonstrate moderate central spinal stenosis despite prior foraminotomies. **D,** AP (*left*) and lateral (*right*) radiographs obtained 2 years after a central laminectomy from L2 to L5 without fusion. Despite the absence of lateral lithiasis or spondylolisthesis on preoperative radiographs, the patient's degenerative scoliosis progressed to 26°. Although some relief of lower extremity symptoms occurred, the patient remained symptomatic and was dissatisfied with the outcome.

curves, significant lateral listhesis, or spinal decompensation to limit surgery to laminectomy or laminotomy alone without fusion.[82] It should be emphasized, however, that there is a lack of specific information regarding the success of decompression without fusion in this patient population, and

the scoliotic curves of some patients will progress following laminectomy despite the absence of these risk factors (Figure 3).

When fusion is elected, the length and location of fusion will vary depending on the patient's presentation. Treatment of mild defor-

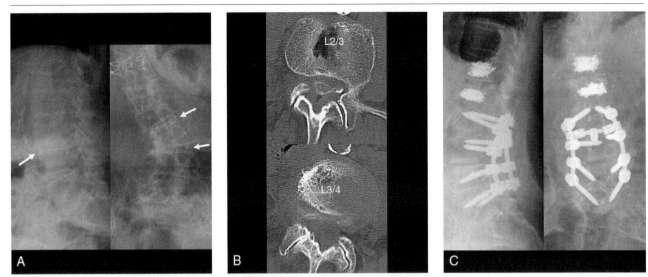

Figure 4   **A,** AP (*left*) and lateral (*right*) radiographs of the lumbar spine of an 86-year-old woman with symptoms of bilateral neurogenic claudication, relatively limited issues of back pain, and severe activity restriction. The patient had no significant medical comorbidities. Note the lateral listhesis at both the L2-3 and L3-4 disk spaces (*arrow*) in the AP view and the anterolisthesis at the L3-4 disk space on the lateral view (*double arrow*). **B,** CT myelograms through the L2-3 (*top*) and L3-4 (*bottom*) disk spaces demonstrate a complete block at the L3-4 level, with a near-complete block at the L2-3 level. **C,** AP (*left*) and lateral (*right*) radiographs after posterior laminectomy and fusion with segmental instrumentation from L2 to L5 using iliac crest bone graft. Prophylactic vertebroplasties of the T12 and L1 vertebrae were performed to prevent adjacent level fractures. At 2-year follow-up, the patient had excellent recovery of functional activities, with near-complete resolution of lower extremity symptoms.

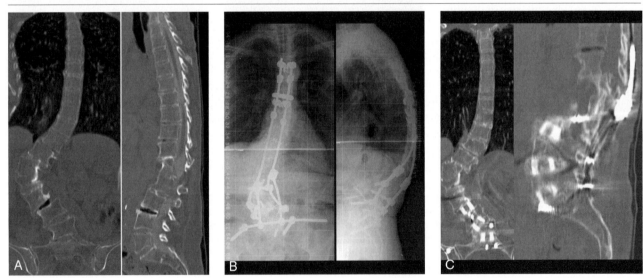

Figure 5   **A,** Sagittal (*left*) and coronal (*right*) reconstructions of postmyelography CT of a 78-year-old woman who had severe degenerative scoliosis of the lumbar spine and was incapacitated by back and leg pain. Although these are not upright images, note the apparent maintenance of both sagittal and coronal balance that was clinically confirmed in this patient. In addition, the CT scan demonstrated that autofusion had occurred from T12 to L3 with severe degenerative disease and lateral lithiasis noted at L3-4 and L4-5; coronal plane deformity and degeneration of the L5-S1 disk space was also noted. **B,** AP (*left*) and lateral (*right*) plain radiographs obtained at 2 years postoperatively demonstrate maintenance of spinal balance with minimal correction through the lumbar curve. Pelvic fixation was used because of the long thoracolumbar fusion and the need to fuse across the L5-S1 disk space. Graft was used in the posterolateral fusion harvested from the left iliac crest during placement of the iliac bolt. On the opposite side, a transiliac bar was placed extending through the right S1 pedicle screw. Vertical cross-extenders were then connected by dominoes to posterior rods extending from T4 to L5. Anterior interbody fusions were performed as a first-stage procedure via a midline retroperoneal approach from L3 to S1, with structural allograft rings filled with autologous bone graft. **C,** Coronal (*left*) and sagittal (*right*) CT reconstructions obtained 2 years postoperatively demonstrate complete consolidation of the anterior interbody grafts at all three levels. The patient had excellent pain relief and recovery of activity after undergoing this procedure.

mities with a coronally and sagittally balanced spine generally can be achieved with decompression and fusion with limited curve correction using instrumentation between the end vertebrae of the Cobb angle. In the senior author's experience, many elderly patients do not require fusion across the lumbosacral junction (Figure 4). Patients with sagittal imbalance, primary lumbar curves larger than 30°, painful lumbosacral fractional curves, or L5-S1 spondylolisthesis may, however, require fusion of the L5-S1 disk space. When fusion to the sacrum is elected, augmentation of sacral pedicle screws with a secondary point of fixation and structural interbody grafting at the L5-S1 disk is important for patients with constructs extending above the thoracolumbar junction. An anterior interbody fusion may be elected in order to better correct sagittal imbalance, for patients requiring fusion over more than three disk spaces, or as a means of increasing fusion rates in patients requiring fusion at the L5-S1 interspace. If anterior lumbar diskectomy and fusion is planned, a midline approach to L3-S1 is better tolerated than the traditional open lateral retroperitoneal (flank) approach with isolated posterior or posterior interbody fusion performed as needed above the L3 level[86] (Figure 5).

When spine surgery is elected in the elderly patient population, efforts to limit the extent of surgery are appropriate, provided the surgical option chosen retains the potential to successfully meet the clinical needs of the patient. Examples of limited surgical approaches include the use of posterior or transforaminal lumbar interbody fusions or transpsoas lateral interbody fusion in favor of anterior approaches[87,88] (Figure 6). In patients with less cen-

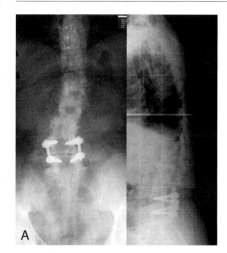
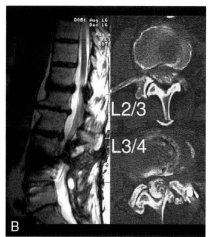
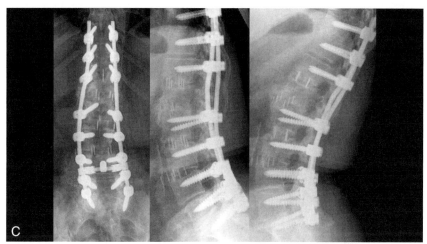

Figure 6 **A,** AP (*left*) and lateral (*right*) radiographs of a 67-year-old woman who had laminectomy and fusion of L4-5 1 year earlier demonstrate severe degenerative disease cranial to the fusion with coronal plane listhesis and lumbar kyphosis. The patient continued to have axial back pain and lumbar radiculopathy, which were likely the result of incomplete treatment of the presenting surgical pathology. **B,** Sagittal plane MRI and CT myelograms at L2-3 (*left*) and L3-4 (*right*) demonstrate persistent lateral recess and foraminal stenosis. **C,** AP (*left*) and lateral flexion (*center*) and extension (*right*) radiographs obtained after T12 to S1 fusion with percutaneous transpsoas approach was performed at the L1-2, L2-3, and L3-4 disk spaces. T12-L1 diskectomy and fusion was performed through a mini-open approach. Bone morphogenetic protein was used for the anterior interbody fusion. By 8-month follow-up, interbody fusions were nearly consolidated and the patient was fully recovered with excellent relief of axial back pain and leg symptoms.

tral canal stenosis, the use of an extended paraspinal (Wiltse) approach may help limit denervation and devascularization of the paraspinal musculature.[89,90]

In patients who require extended constructs for correction and stabilization, attention must be given to spinal balance and load sharing among implants, especially in the presence of osteoporosis. In such patients, significant loads can be placed on mechanically compromised points of fixation and can lead to implant or adjacent segment failure.

Table 2
Methods for Improving Fixation and Reducing Implant Loads in Patients With Osteoporosis*

Method	Citation	Caveat
Increase pedicle screw size	Brantley et al[118] Hirano et al[119]	Larger screws may not increase purchase and may increase risk of pedicle fracture
Conical screws	Ono et al[112] Kwok et al[113]	Loose fixation if backed out
Undertapping or self-tapping screws	Halvorson et al[72]	Possibility of pedicle screw malposition or pedicle fracture
"Up and in" screw orientation	Ruland et al[123] Ono et al[112] McKinley et al[124] Youssef et al[125]	Pullout at end of construct can result in neurologic injury
Pediculolaminar fixation	Hilibrand et al[101] Chiba et al[99] Halvorson et al[72]Hasegawa et al[102] Tan et al[103] Butler et al[107] Hu[93]	Increased volume of instrumentation Requires some soft tissue disruption at ends of construct
Injectable fillers	Zindrick et al[126] Sarzier et al[127] Lotz et al[129] Wuisman et al[130] Pfeifer et al[134]	Potential for late infection around PMMA Off-label use of cement Potential for cement extravasation
Coated screws	Sanden et al[135, 136] Hasegawa et al[102]	Potential for loosening as coating resorbs
Expandable screws	Cook et al[114,117] McKoy and An[116]	Potential for screw expansion through end plate or lateral wall May be difficult to remove following ingrowth
Interbody grafting	Polikeit et al[97] Lowe et al[96] Hackenberg et al[98]	Requires additional surgery Vascular risk anteriorly Neurologic risk posteriorly
Adjacent segment augmentation	Hu[93] Kostuik and Shapiro[106]	Off-label cement use Potential to reduce nutrition supply to disk Potential for cement extravasation

*Citations supporting the use of each method and potential concerns are also listed.

Considerations for Instrumentation of the Osteoporotic Spine

Although the mechanical compromise of osteoporotic bone is well known, evidence has demonstrated that spinal instrumentation in patients with osteoporosis can be done with relative safety and effectiveness.[91,92] However, it must be recognized that in the presence of osteoporosis, the mechanical strength of each point of fixation is reduced. For example, the pullout strength, cutout torque, and maximum insertional torque for pedicle screws have all been shown to correlate with bone mineral density and are significantly decreased in osteoporotic vertebrae.[72,73] Therefore, in patients with osteoporosis, careful attention to principles that optimize the strength and minimize loading of individual points of fixation is required[74,93,94] (Table 2).

Minimizing Loads at Individual Fixation Points

Minimizing implant loads at indi- vidual points of fixation can be accomplished in several ways. Using multiple points of fixation, obtaining adequate sagittal balance, interbody structural support, accepting lesser degrees of coronal deformity correction, and using accessory means of fixation at individual levels all will reduce pedicle screw or hook loading.[74,93,94] In certain patients, protecting sacral pedicle screws with additional fixation either within the sacrum or at the pelvis should be considered at the end of a long construct.

Using multiple points of fixation, such as segmental pedicle screws, reduces the load applied to individual screws and increases the stiffness of the overall construct. A similar principle applies to hooks or wires, although these implants generally require longer constructs than pedicle screws to provide adequate fixation.[93,95] One disadvantage of using segmental pedicle screw fixation is that the space occupied by the implants can reduce the room available for bone graft.

Sagittal imbalance caused by instrumentation with insufficient lumbar lordosis can result in forward tilt of the head and trunk anterior to the sacrum and pelvis. This can contribute significantly to instrument strains, especially at the cranial and caudal ends of a construct. Efforts to improve sagittal balance are, therefore, important not only to improve patient outcomes, but also from the standpoint of reducing the potential for hardware failure. Shortening of the posterior column may be required to accomplish this, either through aggressive loosening of facet joints and removal of interspinous ligaments or in patients with severe sagittal imbalance, via Smith-Petersen or pedicle subtraction osteotomy techniques. The use of interbody grafting will also help maintain lordosis and reduce loads on posterior instrumentation through load sharing.

Several principles are important in optimizing outcomes of interbody graft placement, specifically in patients with osteoporosis. Careful technique is required to avoid removal of the bony end plate, which provides the greatest mechanical resistance to implant subsidence. Choosing an appropriately sized implant is also important because smaller implants may not engage enough cortical surface and are thus more susceptible to subsidence into the osteoporotic vertebral body.[96,97] Posterior interbody fusion techniques, such as transforaminal lumbar interbody fusion and posterior lumbar interbody fusion, provide surgeons with additional options that may avoid the need for an anterior operation while still providing anterior column support and can be combined with posterior osteotomy techniques to help restore and maintain lordosis.[88,98]

Although sagittal plane balance is important to reduce implant loading, it may be beneficial to accept less correction of coronal deformity in elderly patients with osteoporosis. Whereas maximizing coronal plane balance correction is typically a goal of spinal deformity surgery, in the presence of osteoporosis the strength of bone anchors may not allow strong compression/distraction or vertebral rotation forces to be applied.[74,93,94] Clinical outcomes in elderly patients are strongly related to achieving sagittal balance and obtaining a solid fusion.

Augmenting pedicle screw fixation at individual segments with offset sublaminar hooks or sublaminar wires also reduces the load at individual screws.[99,100] Sublaminar

hooks have been shown to increase pullout strength, construct stiffness, reduce pedicle screw bending moments, and absorb some of the construct strain, especially in significantly osteoporotic bone.[72,99,101-103] Although load sharing can also be considered a means of augmenting fixation at individual vertebrae, the load-sharing effect also reduces loading resulting from the primary fixation devices, which is especially valuable at the cranial and caudal ends of instrumentation constructs.

Supplementary fixation below S1 sacral pedicle screws at the caudal end of long constructs is an important means of reducing pseudarthrosis rates at the L5-S1 disk space.[104,105] Sacral alar screws, S2 pedicle screws, transsacral bars, iliac bolts, and the Galveston iliac rodding technique all can be used effectively.[82] The addition of structural interbody grafting at L5-S1, although it does not necessarily improve the mechanical situation, is an important consideration from the standpoint of increasing the bone surface area available for fusion and thereby increasing fusion rates.

Avoiding Failure of Adjacent Vertebral Segments

Failure of the cranial adjacent segment can occur acutely as a result of vertebral body fracture or loss of implant fixation, or as a longer term complication caused by degeneration of the adjacent motion segment. Avoiding failure of adjacent vertebral segments is also important and may be a particular challenge in longer fusion constructs in elderly patients and those with osteoporosis. Despite this challenge, guidelines for choice of fusion end points remain incompletely defined. In general, ending a fusion of most of the lumbar spine at T12 or L1

should be avoided, particularly in patients with osteoporosis.[106] Most of these constructs should be extended to T9 or T10 to delay or avoid junctional breakdown.

Patients with prior fusion of the thoracic spine or clinically significant deformity in this region should have instrumentation and fusion of remaining unfused segments extending to the upper thoracic spine.[93,107] It is generally not recommended to stop a fusion within a region of kyphosis, such as the midthoracic spine, to avoid excess loading to the cranialmost implants and vertebrae. Augmentation of fixation at the cranial segments with sublaminar wires or the addition of a cranial offset hook is also a potentially useful means of protecting pedicle screws.[74,108]

Consideration should also be given to the prophylactic augmentation of vertebrae adjacent to long fusion constructs through procedures such as vertebroplasty or kyphoplasty, particularly for areas of high mechanical stress such as the thoracolumbar junction. Augmentation of the top instrumented segment and the first cranial adjacent vertebrae is probably most important because these are the most common sites of postoperative vertebral fracture.

Maximizing Strength of Individual Anchor Points

Several studies have demonstrated a direct correlation between bone mineral density and screw pullout forces, with substantially reduced pullout forces noted in osteoporotic bone.[72,73,108-111] Improving the bone-implant interface is fundamental to optimize pedicle screw fixation in osteoporotic bone.[94] Several techniques and devices have been developed that enhance the strength of the interface between bone and pedicle screws, which is generally regarded as the "weakest link" in overall construct stability. These techniques include specific pedicle screw designs, careful pilot hole preparation, optimizing screw orientation, and enhancement with fillers and coatings.

Several unique pedicle screw designs have been described for use in osteoporotic bone. Conical screws, which better approximate pedicle morphometry, have been shown to increase pullout resistance in osteoporotic bone.[112,113] It should be noted, however, that conical screws lose a significant portion of their strength when backed out by even a half turn, which may limit their ability to accommodate rod contour by backing out the screw.[112]

Expandable screws offer additional improvement in pullout strength in severely osteoporotic bone.[114-116] Clinical series using these devices, which include 21 patients with osteoporosis, demonstrated radiographic evidence of fusion in 86% of patients.[114,117] One concern with such implants is that increasing screw diameter could fracture the pedicle, placing the adjacent nerve root at risk.[118] As a guideline, final screw diameters should not exceed 70% of the outer diameter of the pedicle when the bone mineral density is less than 0.7 g/cm^2.[119]

In patients with osteoporosis, undertapping or avoiding tapping of the pilot hole altogether before screw insertion does help improve screw fixation, especially in the lumbar spine.[72,120] Careful evaluation of final screw position in such patients is critical, however, because some tactile feedback during pilot hole preparation is lost, and pedicle fracture can occur during screw placement.[121,122]

Screw orientation also should be optimized in patients with osteoporosis. Screw triangulation via a medial orientation takes advantage of the bone mass between the converging screws for fixation, rather than only that bone lying between threads of a single screw, and has been shown to improve pullout strength in osteoporotic bone.[112,123] Similarly, screws oriented caudal or parallel relative to the vertebral end plate, as opposed to a cranial orientation, avoid increased bending moments at the screw hub in normal vertebrae, and use of this technique is also prudent in osteoporotic bone.[124,125]

Injectable cements of several types have been shown to substantially increase the pullout strength of screw fixation in osteoporotic bone.[74,109,126-133] However, cement extravasation can potentially injure surrounding structures, and permanent cements such as polymethylmethacrylate represent a potential locus for late infection.[74,109] In addition, these techniques currently are considered an off-label use of bone cement. These concerns may be avoided by insertion of cancellous bone chips into the pedicle screw hole before screw insertion, although vertebral body strength is not enhanced by this technique.[110,134]

HA-coated screws have been shown to increase pullout forces, presumably by increasing both the contact surface area as well as the frictional coefficient at the bone-implant interface.[135-137] Hasegawa and associates[137] demonstrated that HA-coated screws had greater pullout force than screws without HA coating specifically in an osteoporotic model. The mechanical behavior of these implants over time as resorption of the HA coating occurs has not been studied, however.

Summary

The elderly patient with lumbar spine degenerative disease presents significant challenges regarding surgical decision making and management. Even the presence of medical comorbidities need not always exclude the elderly patient from elective spine surgery. Both surgeon and patient, however, must be aware of how age and comorbid conditions may affect perioperative management and ultimate clinical outcome.

Osteoporosis is a particularly prevalent comorbidity in the elderly population. The potential presence of osteoporosis, thus, must be a concern in all elderly patients with degenerative disease of the lumbar spine. Several options are available to the spine surgeon that can improve implant fixation and potentially improve outcomes in this patient group. Careful assessment of patients for surgical indications and attention to surgical technique are critical for successful treatment of this challenging patient population.

References

1. Ciol MA, Deyo RA, Howell E, Kreif S: An assessment of surgery for spinal stenosis: Time trends, geographic variations, complications, and reoperations. *J Am Geriatr Soc* 1996;44:285-290.

2. Watters JM, McClaran JC: The elderly surgical patient, in Wilmore DW (ed): *American College of Surgeons: Care of the Surgical Patient, Vol I.* New York, NY, Scientific American, 1991, pp 1-31.

3. Goldman L, Caldera CL, Nussbaum SR, et al: Multifactorial index of cardiac risk in noncardiac surgical procedures. *N Engl J Med* 1977;297:845-850.

4. Tornebrandt K, Fletcher R: Pre-operative chest x-rays in elderly patients. *Anaesthesia* 1982;37:901-902.

5. Smetana GW: Preoperative pulmonary evaluation. *N Engl J Med* 1999;340:937-944.

6. Nunn JF, Milledge JS, Chen D, Dore C:

Respiratory criteria of fitness for surgery and anaesthesia. *Anaesthesia* 1988;43:543-551.

7. Joehl RJ: Preoperative evaluation: Pulmonary, cardiac, renal dysfunction and comorbidities. *Surg Clin North Am* 2005;85:1061-1073.

8. Milledge JS, Nunn JF: Criteria of fitness for anaesthesia in patients with chronic obstructive lung disease. *BMJ* 1975;3:670-673.

9. Older P, Smith R: Experience with the preoperative invasive measurement of haemodynamic, respiratory and renal function in 100 elderly patients scheduled for major abdominal surgery. *Anaesth Intensive Care* 1988;16:389-395.

10. Kumle B, Boldt J, Piper S, Schmidt C, Suttner S, Salopek S: The influence of different intravascular volume replacement regimens on renal function in the elderly. *Anesth Analg* 1999;89:1124-1130.

11. Boldt J, Brenner T, Lang J, Kumle B, Isgro F: Kidney-specific proteins in elderly patients undergoing cardiac surgery with cardiopulmonary bypass. *Anesth Analg* 2003;97:1582-1589.

12. Beliveau MM, Multach M: Perioperative care for the elderly patient. *Med Clin North Am* 2003;87:273-289.

13. Niccoli L, Bellino S, Cantini F: Renal tolerability of three commonly employed non-steroidal anti-inflammatory drugs in elderly patients with osteoarthritis. *Clin Exp Rheumatol* 2002;20:201-207.

14. Thaller J, Walker M, Kline AJ, Anderson DG: The effect of non-steroidal anti-inflammatory agents on spinal fusion. *Orthopedics* 2005;28:299-303.

15. Riew KD, Long J, Rhee J, et al: Time dependent inhibitory effects of indomethacin on spinal fusion. *J Bone Joint Surg Am* 2003;85:632-634.

16. Linnebur SA, Milchak JL: Assessment of oral bisphosphonate use in elderly patients with varying degrees of kidney function. *Am J Geriatr Pharmacother* 2004;2:213-218.

17. Huang RC, Khan SN, Sandhu HS, et al: Alendronate inhibits spine fusion in a rat model. *Spine* 2005;30:2516-2522.

18. Xue Q, Li H, Zou X, et al: The influence of alendronate treatment and bone graft volume on posterior lateral spine fusion in a porcine model. *Spine* 2005;30:1116-1121.

19. Xue Q, Li H, Zou X, et al: Healing properties of allograft from

alendronate-treated animal in lumbar spine interbody cage fusion. *Eur Spine J* 2005;14:222-226.

20. Lehman RA Jr, Kuklo TR, Freedman BA, Cowart JR, Mense MG, Riew KD: The effect of alendronate sodium on spinal fusion: a rabbit model. *Spine J* 2004;4:36-43.

21. Nourhashemi F, Andrieu S, Rauzy O, et al: Nutrition support and aging in preoperative nutrition. *Curr Opin Clin Nutr Metab Care* 1999;2:87-92.

22. Fast Facts on Osteoporosis. Web site of the National Osteoporosis Foundation. Available at: http://www.NOF.org/statistics. Accessed November 18, 2005.

23. Cummings SR, Melton LJ: Epidemiology and outcomes of osteoporotic fractures. *Lancet* 2002;359:1761-1767.

24. Cauley JA, Fullman RL, Stone KL, et al: Factors associated with the lumbar spine and proximal femur bone mineral density in older men. *Osteoporos Int* 2005;16:1525-1537.

25. Melton LJ: Epidemiology of spinal osteoporosis. *Spine* 1997;22(suppl 24):2S-11S.

26. Lee CA, Einhorn TA: The bone organ system: Form and function, in Feldman MR, Kelsey J (eds): *Osteoporosis*, ed 2. San Diego, CA, Academic Press, 2001, pp 3-30.

27. Wahner HW: Use of densitometry in management of osteoporosis, in Marcus R, Feldman D, Kelsey J (eds): *Osteoporosis*, San Diego, CA, Academic Press, 1996, pp 1055-1072.

28. Einhorn TA: The structural properties of normal and osteoporotic bone. *Instr Course Lect* 2003;52:533-539.

29. Kahanovitz N: Osteoporosis and fusion. *Instr Course Lect* 1992;41:231-233.

30. Khoska S, Riggs BL, Melton LJ: Clinical spectrum of osteoporosis, in Riggs BL, Melton LJ (eds): *Osteoporosis: Etiology Diagnosis and Management*, ed 2. Philadelphia, PA, Lippincott-Raven, 1995, pp 205-223.

31. Riggs BL, Melton LJ: Involutional osteoporosis. *N Engl J Med* 1986;314:1676-1684.

32. Kirkaldy-Willis WH, Paine KW, Cauchoix J, McIvor G: Lumbar spinal stenosis. *Clin Orthop Relat Res* 1974;99:30-50.

33. Lane JM, Gardner MJ, Lin JT, van der Meulen MC, Myers E: The aging spine: New technologies and therapeutics for the osteoporotic spine. *Eur Spine J* 2003;12(suppl 2):S147-S154.

34. Benoist M: Natural history of the aging spine. *Eur Spine J* 2003;12(suppl 2):S86-S89.

35. Szpalski M, Gunzburg R: Lumbar spinal stenosis in the elderly: An overview. *Eur Spine J* 2003;12(suppl 2):S170-S175.

36. Arbit E, Pannullo S: Lumbar stenosis: A clinical review. *Clin Orthop Relat Res* 2001;384:137-143.

37. Kurz LT, Dvorak J: Clinical radiologic and electrodiagnostic diagnosis of degenerative lumbar stenosis, in Wiesel SW, Weinstein JN, Herkowitz H, Dvorak J, Bell G (eds): *The Lumbar Spine*, ed 2. Philadelphia, PA, WB Saunders, 1996, p 731.

38. Porter RW: Pathophysiology of neurogenic claudication, in Wiesel SW, Weinstein JN, Herkowitz H, Dvorak J, Bell G (eds): *The Lumbar Spine*, ed 2. Philadelphia, PA, WB Saunders, 1996, p 717.

39. Baloh RW, Ying SH, Jacobson KM: A longitudinal study of gait and balance dysfunction in normal older adults. *Arch Neurol* 2003;60:835-839.

40. Boden SD, Davis DO, Dina TS, Patronas NJ, Wiesel SW: Abnormal magnetic resonance scans of the lumbar spine in asymptomatic subjects. *J Bone Joint Surg Am* 1990;72:403-408.

41. Carlson N, Carlson H: Electrodiagnostic studies, in Bernstein J (ed): *Musculoskeletal Medicine*. Rosemont, IL, American Academy of Orthopedic Surgeons, 2003, pp 409-417.

42. Deen HG, Fenton DS, Lamer TJ: Minimally invasive procedures for disorders of the lumbar spine. *Mayo Clin Proc* 2003;78:1249-1256.

43. Sengupta DK, Herkowitz HN: Lumbar spinal stenosis: Treatment strategies and indications for surgery. *Orthop Clin North Am* 2003;34:281-295.

44. Gunzburg R, Szpalski M: The conservative surgical treatment of lumbar spinal stenosis in the elderly. *Eur Spine J* 2003;12(suppl 2):S176-S180.

45. Postacchini F: Surgical management of lumbar spinal stenosis. *Spine* 1999;24:1043-1047.

46. White AA, Panjabi MM (eds): The problem of instability in the human spine: A systematic approach, in *Clinical Biomechanics or the Spine*. Philadelphia, PA, Lippincott, 1990.

47. Epstein NE, Epstein JE: Surgery for spinal stenosis, in Wiesel SW, Weinstein JN, Herkowitz H, Dvorak J, Bell G (eds):

The Lumbar Spine, ed 2. Philadelphia, PA, WB Saunders, 1996, p 737.

48. Deyo RA, Cherkin DC, Loeser JD, Bigos SJ, Ciol MA: Morbidity and mortality in association with operations on the lumbar spine. *J Bone Joint Surg Am* 1992;74:536-543.

49. Deyo RA, Ciol MA, Cherkin DC, Loeser JD, Bigos SJ: Lumbar spinal fusion: A cohort study of complications, reoperations, and resource use in the Medicare population. *Spine* 1993;18:1463-1470.

50. Malter AD, McNeney B, Loeser JD, Deyo RA: 5-year reoperation rates after different types of lumbar spine surgery. *Spine* 1998;23:814-820.

51. Postacchine F: Classification and treatment, in Weinstein JN, Wiesel SW (eds): *The Lumbar Spine*. Philadelphia, PA, WB Saunders, 1990, p 605.

52. Katz JN, Lipson SJ, Larson MG, McInnes JM, Fossel AH, Liang MH: The outcome of decompressive laminectomy for degenerative lumbar stenosis. *J Bone Joint Surg Am* 1991;73:809-816.

53. Ragab AA, Fye MA, Bohlman HH: Surgery of the lumbar spine for spinal stenosis in 118 patients 70 years of age or older. *Spine* 2003;28:348-353.

54. Katz JN, Stucki G, Lipson SJ, Fossel AH, Grobler LJ, Weinstein JN: Predictors of surgical outcome in degenerative lumbar spinal stenosis. *Spine* 1999;24:2229-2233.

55. Arinzon Z, Adunsky A, Fidelman Z, Gepstein R: Outcomes of decompression surgery for lumbar spinal stenosis in elderly diabetic patients. *Eur Spine J* 2004;13:32-37.

56. Benz RJ, Ibrahim ZG, Afshar P, Garfin SR: Predicting complications in elderly patients undergoing lumbar decompression. *Clin Orthop Relat Res* 2001;384:116-121.

57. Balderston RA, Vaccaro AR: Surgical treatment of adult degenerative spondylolisthesis, in Wiesel SW, Weinstein JN, Herkowitz H, Dvorak J, Bell G (eds): *The Lumbar Spine*, ed 2. Philadelphia, PA, WB Saunders, 1996, p 701.

58. Wiltse LL, Newman PH, Macnab I: Classification of spondylosis and spondylolisthesis. *Clin Orthop Relat Res* 1976;117:23-29.

59. Bassewitz H, Herkowitz H: Lumbar stenosis with spondylolisthesis. *Clin Orthop Relat Res* 2001;384:54-60.

60. Rosenberg NJ: Degenerative

spondylolisthesis: Surgical treatment. *Clin Orthop Relat Res* 1976;117:112-120.

61. Meyerding HW: Spondylolisthesis. *Surg Gynecol Obstet* 1932;54:371-379.

62. Phillips FM, Pfeifer BA, Lieberman IH, Kerr EJ, Choi IS, Pazianos AG: Minimally invasive treatments of osteoporotic vertebral compression fractures: Vertebroplasty and kyphoplasty. *Instr Course Lect* 2003;52:559-567.

63. Herkowitz HN, Kurz LT: Degenerative lumbar spondylolisthesis with spinal stenosis. *J Bone Joint Surg Am* 1991;73:802-808.

64. Bjarke Christensen F, Stender Hansen ES, Laursen M, Thomsen K, Bunger CE: Long-term functional outcome of pedicle screw instrumentation as a support for posterolateral spinal fusion: A randomized clinical study with 5-year followup. *Spine* 2002;27:1269-1277.

65. Fischgrund JS, Mackay M, Herkowitz HN, Brower R, Montgomery D, Kurz L: Degenerative lumbar spondylolisthesis with spinal stenosis: A prospective, randomized study comparing decompressive laminectomy and arthrodesis with and without spinal instrumentation. *Spine* 1997;22:2807-2812.

66. Thomsen K, Christiensen FB, Eiskjær SP, Hansen ES, Fruensgaard S, Bunger CE: The effect of pedicle screw instrumentation on functional outcome and fusion rates in posterolateral lumbar spine fusion: A prospective, randomized clinical study. *Spine* 1997;22:2813-2822.

67. Mardjetko SM, Connolly PJ, Shott S: Degenerative lumbar spondylolisthesis: A meta-analysis of literature 1970-1993. *Spine* 1994;19(suppl 20):2256S-2265S.

68. Herron LD, Trippi AC: L4-5 degenerative spondylolisthesis: the results of treatment by decompressive laminectomy without fusion. *Spine* 1989;14:534-538.

69. Guyatt G, Rennie D: *Users' Guide to the Medical Literature*. Chicago, IL, American Medical Association Press, 2004.

70. Sackett DL, Straus SE, Richardson WS, Rosenberg W, Haynes RB: *Evidence Based Medicine*. London, UK, Churchill Livingstone, 2000.

71. Irwin ZN, Hilibrand A, Gustavel M, et al: Variations in surgical decision making for degenerative spinal disorders: Part I. Lumbar spine. *Spine* 2005;30:2208-2213.

72. Halvorson TL, Kelley LA, Thomas KA, Whitecloud TS, Cook SD: Effects of bone mineral density on pedicle screw fixation. *Spine* 1994;19:2415-2420.

73. Okuyama K, Sato K, Abe E, Inaba H, Shimada Y, Murai H: Stability of transpedicle screwing for the osteoporotic spine. *Spine* 1993;18:2240-2245.

74. Glassman SD, Alegre GM: Adult spinal deformity in the osteoporotic spine: Options and pitfalls. *Instr Course Lect* 2003;52:579-588.

75. Schwab F, Dubey A, Pagala M, Gamez L, Farcy JP: Adult scoliosis: A health assessment analysis by SF-36. *Spine* 2003;28:602-606.

76. Jackson RP, Simmons EH, Stripinis D: Incidence and severity of back pain in adult idiopathic scoliosis. *Spine* 1983;8:749-756.

77. Lonstein J: Adult scoliosis, in Bradford D, Lonstein J, Ogilvie T, Winter R (eds): *Moe's Textbook of Scoliosis and Other Spinal Disorders*, ed 2. Philadelphia, PA, WB Saunders, 1987.

78. Healey JH, Lane JM: Structural scoliosis in osteoporotic women. *Clin Orthop Relat Res* 1985;195:216-223.

79. Robin GC, Span Y, Steinberg R, Makin M, Menczel J: Scoliosis in the elderly: A follow-up study. *Spine* 1982;7:355-361.

80. Korovessis P, Piperos G, Sidiropoulos P, Dimas A: Adult idiopathic lumbar scoliosis: A formula for prediction of progression and review of the literature. *Spine* 1994;19:1926-1932.

81. Balderston RA, Albert TJ: Adult Scoliosis: Evaluation and decision making, in Wiesel SW, Weinstein JN, Herkowitz H, Dvorak J, Bell G (eds): *The Lumbar Spine*, ed 2. Philadelphia, PA, WB Saunders, 1996, p 1118.

82. Gupta MC: Degenerative scoliosis: Options for surgical management. *Orthop Clin North Am* 2003;34:269-279.

83. Pritchett JW, Bortel DT: Degenerative symptomatic lumbar scoliosis. *Spine* 1993;18:700-703.

84. Benner B, Ehni G: Degenerative lumbar scoliosis. *Spine* 1979;4:548-552.

85. San Martino A, D'Andria FM, San Martino C: The surgical treatment of nerve root compression caused by scoliosis of the lumbar spine. *Spine* 1983;8:261-265.

86. Esses SI, Botsford DJ: Surgical anatomy and operative approaches to the sacrum, in Frymoyer JW (ed): *The Adult Spine: Principles and Practice*. New York, NY, Raven Press, 1991, pp 2104-2105.

87. Lippman CR, Spence CA, Youssef AS, Cahill DW: Correction of adult scoliosis via a posterior-only approach. *Neurosurg*

Focus 2003;14:e5.

88. Potter BK, Freedman BA, Verwiebe EG, Hall JM, Polly DW Jr, Kuklo TR: Transforaminal lumbar interbody fusion: clinical and radiographic results and complications in 100 consecutive patients. *J Spinal Disord Tech* 2005;18:337-346.

89. Wiltse LL: The paraspinal sacrospinal-splitting approach to the lumbar spine. *Clin Orthop Relat Res* 1973;91:48-57.

90. Wiltse LL, Spencer CW: New uses and refinements of the paraspinal approach to the lumbar spine. *Spine* 1988;13:696-706.

91. Kumano K, Hirabayashi S, Ogawa Y, Aota Y: Pedicle screws and bone mineral density. *Spine* 1994;19:1157-1161.

92. McAfee PC, Farey ID, Sutterlin CE, Gurr KR, Warden KE, Cunningham BW: Device related osteoporosis with spinal instrumentation. *Spine* 1989;14:919-926.

93. Hu SS: Internal fixation in the osteoporotic spine. *Spine* 1997;22(suppl 43):43S-48S.

94. Hettwer WH, Hart RA: Principles of instrumentation in the osteoporotic spine: An overview. *Advances in Osteoporotic Fracture Management* 2004;3:1-7.

95. Hart R, Hettwer W, Liu Q, Prem S: Mechanical stiffness of segmental versus nonsegmental pedicle screw constructs: The effect of cross-links. *Spine* 2006;31:E35-E38.

96. Lowe TG, Hashim S, Wilson LA, et al: A biomechanical study of regional endplate strength and cage morphology as it relates to structural interbody support. *Spine* 2004;29:2389-2394.

97. Polikeit A, Ferguson SJ, Nolte LP, Orr TE: Factors influencing stresses in the lumbar spine after the insertion of intervertebral cages: Finite element analysis. *Eur Spine J* 2003;12:413-420.

98. Hackenberg L, Halm H, Bullman V, Volker V, Schneider M, Liljenqvist U: Transforaminal lumbar interbody fusion: A safe technique with satisfactory three to five year results. *Eur Spine J* 2005;14:551-558.

99. Chiba M, McLain RF, Yerby SA, Moseley TA, Smith TS, Benson DR: Short-segment pedicle screw fixation: Biomechanical analysis of supplemental hook fixation. *Spine* 1996;21:288-294.

100. Yerby SA, Ehteshami JR, McLain RF: Offset laminar hooks decrease bending moments of pedicle screws during in situ contouring. *Spine* 1997;22:376-381.

101. Hilibrand AS, Moore DC, Graziano GP: The role of pediculolaminar fixation in compromised pedicle bone. *Spine* 1996;21:445-451.

102. Hasegawa K, Takahashi HE, Uchiyama S, et al: An experimental study of a combination of method using a pedicle screw and laminar hook for the osteoporotic spine. *Spine* 1997;22:958-962.

103. Tan JS, Kwon BK, Dvorak MF, Fisher CG, Oxland TR: Pedicle screw motion in the osteoporotic spine after augmentation with laminar hooks, sublaminar wires, or calcium phosphate cement: A comparative analysis. *Spine* 2004;29:1723-1730.

104. Islam NC, Wood KB, Transfeldt EE, et al: Extension of fusion to the pelvis in idiopathic scoliosis. *Spine* 2001;26:166-173.

105. Alegre GM, Gupta MC, Bay BK, Smith TS, Laubach JE: S1 Screw bending moment with posterior spinal instrumentation across the lumbosacral junction after unilateral iliac crest harvest. *Spine* 2001;26:1950-1955.

106. Kostuik JP, Shapiro MB: Open surgical treatment of osteoporotic fractures and deformity of the spine. *Instr Course Lect* 2003;52:569-578.

107. Butler TE, Asher MA, Jayaraman G, Nunley PD, Robinson RG: The strength and stiffness of thoracic implant anchors in osteoporotic spines. *Spine* 1994;19:1956-1962.

108. Coe JD, Warden KE, Herzig MA, McAfee PC: Influence of bone mineral density on the fixation of thoracolumbar implants: A comparative study of transpedicular screws, laminar hooks, and spinous process wires. *Spine* 1990;15:902-907.

109. Soshi S, Shiba R, Kondo H, Murota K: An experimental study on transpedicular screw fixation in relation to osteoporosis in the lumbar spine. *Spine* 1991;16:1335-1341.

110. Breeze SW, Doherty BJ, Noble PS, LeBlanc A, Heggeness MH: A biomechanical study of anterior thoracolumbar screw fixation. *Spine* 1998;23:1829-1831.

111. Eysel P, Schwitalle M, Oberstein A, Rompe JD, Hopf C, Kullmer K: Preoperative estimation of screw fixation strength in vertebral bodies. *Spine* 1998;23:174-180.

112. Ono A, Brown MD, Latta LL, Milne EL, Holmes DC: Triangulated pedicle screw

construct and pullout strength of conical and cylindrical screws. *J Spinal Disord* 2001;14:323-329.

113. Kwok AW, Finkelstein JA, Woodside T, Hearn T, Hu RW: Insertional torque and pullout strengths of conical and cylindrical pedicle screw in cadaveric bone. *Spine* 1996;21:2429-2434.

114. Cook SD, Salkeld SL, Whitecloud TS III, Barbera J: Biomechanical evaluation and preliminary clinical experience with an expansive pedicle screw design. *J Spinal Disord* 2000;13:230-236.

115. Cook SD, Salkeld SL, Stanley T, Faciane A, Miller SD: Biomechanical study of pedicle screw fixation in severely osteoporotic bone. *Spine J* 2004;4:402-408.

116. McKoy BE, An YH: An expandable anchor for fixation in osteoporotic bone. *J Orthop Res* 2001;19:545-547.

117. Cook SD, Barbera J, Rubi M, Salkeld SL, Whitecloud TS III: Lumbosacral fixation using expandable pedicle screws. An alternative in reoperation and osteoporosis. *Spine J* 2001;1:109-114.

118. Brantley AG, Mayfield JK, Koeneman JB, Clark KR: The effects of pedicle screw fit. *Spine* 1994;19:1752-1758.

119. Hirano T, Hasegawa K, Washio T, Hara T, Takahashi H: Fracture risk during pedicle screw insertion in osteoporotic spine. *J Spinal Disord* 1998;11:493-497.

120. Carmouche JJ, Molinari RW, Gerlinger T, Devine J, Patience T: Effects of pilot hole preparation technique on pedicle screw fixation in different regions of the osteoporotic thoracic and lumbar spine. *J Neurosurg Spine* 2005;3:364-370.

121. Ozawa T, Takahashi K, Yamagata M, et al: Insertional torque of the lumbar pedicle screw during surgery. *J Orthop Sci* 2005;10:133-136.

122. Okuyama K, Abe E, Suzuki T, Tamura Y, Chiba M, Sato K: Can insertional torque predict screw loosening and related failures? *Spine* 2000;25:858-864.

123. Ruland CM, McAfee PC, Warden KE, Cunningham BW: Triangulation of pedicular instrumentation: A biomechanical analysis. *Spine* 1991;16(6 Suppl):S270-S276.

124. McKinley TO, McLain RF, Yerby SA, Sharkey NA, Sarigul-Klijin N, Smith TS: Characteristics of pedicle screw loading: effect of surgical techniques on intravertebral and intrapedicular bending moments. *Spine* 1999;24:18-24.

125. Youssef JA, McKinley TO, Yerby SA, McLain RF: Characteristics of pedicle screw loading: Effect of sagittal insertion angle on intrapedicular bending moments. *Spine* 1999;24:1077-1081.

126. Zindrick MR, Wiltse LL, Widell EH, et al: A biomechanical study of intrapeduncular screw fixation in the lumbosacral spine. *Clin Orthop Relat Res* 1986;203:99-112.

127. Sarzier JS, Evans AJ, Cahill DW: Increased pedicle screw pullout strength with vertebroplasty augmentation in osteoporotic spines. *J Neurosurg* 2002;96:309-312.

128. Hernigou P, Duparc F: Rib graft or cement to enhance screw fixation in anterior vertebral bodies. *J Spinal Disord* 1996;9:322-325.

129. Lotz JC, Hu SS, Chiu DFM, Yu M, Colliou O, Poser RD: Carbonated apatite cement augmentation of pedicle screw fixation in the lumbar spine. *Spine* 1997;22:2716-2723.

130. Wuisman PI, Van Dijk M, Staal H, Van Royen BJ: Augmentation of pedicle screws with calcium apatite cement in patients with severe progression of osteoporotic spinal deformities: An innovative technique. *Eur Spine J* 2000;9:528-533.

131. Bai B, Kummer FJ, Spivak J: Augmentation of anterior vertebral body screw fixation by an injectable, biodegradable calcium phosphate bone substitute. *Spine* 2001;26:2679-2683.

132. Yerby SA, Toh E, McLain RF: Revision of failed pedicles screws using hydroxyapatite cement: A biomechanical analysis. *Spine* 1998;23:1657-1661.

133. Taniwaki Y, Takemasa R, Tani T, Mizobuchi H, Yamamoto H: Enhancement of pedicle screw stability using calcium phosphate cement in osteoporotic vertebrae: In vivo biomechanical study. *J Orthop Sci* 2003;8:408-414.

134. Pfeifer BA, Krag MH, Johnson C: Repair of failed transpedicle screw fixation. *Spine* 1994;19:350-353.

135. Sanden B, Olerud C, Larsson S: Hydroxyapatite coating enhances fixation of loaded pedicle screws: A mechanical in vivo study in sheep. *Eur Spine J* 2001;10:334-339.

136. Sanden B, Olerud C, Johansson C, Larsson S: Improved bone-screw interface with hydroxyapatite coating. *Spine* 2001;26:2673-2678.

137. Hasegawa T, Inufusa A, Imai Y, Mikawa Y, Lim TH, An HS: Hydroxyapatite-coating of pedicle screws improves resistance against pull-out force in the osteoporotic canine lumbar spine model: A pilot study. *Spine J* 2005;5:239-243.

Minimally Invasive Techniques for the Treatment of Osteoporotic Vertebral Fractures

Neil A. Manson, MD, FRCSC

Frank M. Phillips, MD

Abstract

Osteoporotic vertebral compression fractures are a leading cause of disability and morbidity in the elderly. The consequences of these fractures include pain, progressive vertebral collapse with resultant spinal kyphosis, and systemic manifestations. Nonsurgical measures have proved unsuccessful in a portion of this population and for this group, minimally invasive vertebral augmentation can be beneficial. Vertebroplasty is designed to address vertebral fracture pain. It involves percutaneous injection of polymethylmethacrylate (PMMA) directly into a fractured vertebral body with the goals of pain relief and prevention of further collapse of the fractured vertebra. Kyphoplasty is designed to address the kyphotic deformity as well as the fracture pain. It involves the percutaneous insertion of an inflatable bone tamp into a fractured vertebral body. Bone tamp inflation works to elevate the end plates and create a cavity to be filled with PMMA with the goals of pain relief, restoration of vertebral body height, and reduced kyphotic deformity. Optimizing surgical technique can improve outcomes and decrease complication rates, and decrease radiation exposure to the patient and surgical team. Obtaining a biopsy prior to cement injection has proved efficacious and may result in the diagnosis of occult pathology underlying a seemingly routine vertebral fracture. As competence and surgical success are acquired, the indications will continue to expand to encompass more challenging pathologies. Recently, vertebral augmentation during spinal decompression and instrumented fusion for burst fracture with neurologic insult has been reported to be successful.

Instr Course Lect 2007;56:273-285.

The National Osteoporosis Foundation has estimated that more than 100 million people worldwide are at risk for the development of fragility fractures secondary to osteoporosis. In the United States, the lifetime risk of fractures of the spine, hip, and distal part of the radius is up to 40% for women and 13% for men older than 50 years. This leads to an estimated 700,000 osteoporotic vertebral body compression fractures each year, of which more than one third become chronically painful.[1] Vertebral compression fractures occur in 20% of people older than 70 years and in 16% of postmenopausal women.[2] Not surprisingly, vertebral compression fractures account for a large portion of the more than $17 billion of annual direct costs associated with osteoporotic fractures in the United States.[3]

Osteoporotic Vertebral Fractures

Osteoporotic vertebral compression fractures are a leading cause of disability and morbidity in the elderly.[4-6] The consequences of these fractures include pain, progressive vertebral collapse with resultant spinal kyphosis, and systemic manifestations.

The pain associated with acute vertebral compression fractures may be incapacitating. In several patients, the pain subsides over a period of weeks or months, but it is not uncommon for the pain to become chronic.[7] Chronic pain after vertebral fracture may result from (1) incomplete vertebral healing with progressive osseous collapse, (2) altered spine kinematics as a consequence of spinal deformity, or (3) the development of a pseudarthrosis at the involved vertebra. Chronic pain associated with vertebral compression fractures often leads to impaired quality of life and depression.[7,8]

Kyphotic deformity in the osteoporotic spine may also create a biomechanical environment favoring additional fractures. The kyphotic deformity shifts the patient's center of gravity anteriorly, creating greater flexion bending moments around the apex of the kyphosis, which increase the kyphotic angulation further and promote additional fractures.[9-12] Clinical natural history studies have shown that the risk of a new vertebral fracture in the first year after an incident of vertebral compression fracture increases 5 to 25 times above baseline,[13-15] with the vertebra adjacent to the previously fractured level at particular risk.[16,17] Many patients with fractures and kyphosis become less active because they fear falls and new fractures. This inactivity in turn leads to accelerated osteoporosis and muscle deconditioning.[7] Because of the kyphotic deformity, paraspinal muscles must exert more force to maintain an erect posture. This prolonged exertion can cause backaches and muscle fatigue. Extreme kyphosis places unusual amounts of strain on the ligaments and other soft tissues. Pressure on the lower rib cage near the pelvic rim can produce substantial loin pain and tenderness.[18] Prevention of progressive kyphotic deformity or correction of existing deformity may therefore be important both to reduce the risk of fracture at adjacent levels and to prevent the consequences of spinal kyphosis.

Vertebral compression fractures have been shown to adversely affect quality of life, physical function, mental health, and survival.[7,8,19-22] These effects are related to the severity of the spinal deformity and are partly independent of pain.[7,19] In recent years, researchers have highlighted the impaired pulmonary function that is associated with osteoporotic vertebral compression fractures and spinal deformity.[23,24] Leech and associates[23] reported a 9% decrease in pulmonary vital capacity for each thoracic vertebral fracture. Kyphosis can lead to reduced abdominal space with poor appetite and resultant nutritional problems.[7,25] By shifting the patient's center of gravity forward, kyphotic deformity not only increases the risk of additional fractures,[26] but also may lead to poor balance, which increases the risk of accidental falls.[10,27] In addition to the morbidity associated with vertebral compression fractures, there is an increased mortality rate for older women with vertebral compression fractures compared with that for age-matched controls, as found in a prospective study.[28] The mortality rate was related to pulmonary problems, and it increased with the number of vertebrae fractured.

Nonsurgical Management

Traditionally, acute vertebral compression fractures have been treated nonsurgically except in rare instances in which the fracture is associated with neurologic compromise or advanced spinal instability. In fact, an unknown number of vertebral compression fractures produce no or only slight symptoms and are not seen for acute medical attention. Nonsurgical measures for some symptomatic vertebral compression fractures fail as a result of intolerable pain, deformity, loss of function, or a combination thereof. Open spinal surgery in patients with osteoporosis is fraught with complications because these patients are often of advanced age and frequently have comorbidities and because of the difficulty of securing fixation in osteoporotic bone. Thus, in the past, most patients with painful vertebral compression fractures have been treated with bed rest, analgesic medications, bracing, antiosteoporotic drugs, or some combination thereof.[18,29-31] Although these treatments can be successful, anti-inflammatory and narcotic medications are often poorly tolerated by elderly patients and may predispose them to confusion, an increased risk of falls, and gastrointestinal side effects. Bed rest can lead to an overall physiologic deconditioning and acceleration of bone loss. Bracing is typically poorly tolerated by older patients, is expensive, and may further restrict diaphragmatic excursion. Furthermore, none of these treatments reduces the fracture or corrects the spinal deformity.

Minimally Invasive Interventions

Orthopaedic fracture care emphasizes restoration of anatomy, correction of deformity, and preservation of function. The treatment of osteoporotic vertebral compression fractures ideally should address both the fracture-related pain and the kyphotic deformity. In addition, this should be accomplished without subjecting the elderly patient to inordinate risks or surgical trauma. Vertebroplasty and kyphoplasty are two minimally invasive surgical interventions offering promising results for this patient population.

Definitions

Vertebroplasty Percutaneous injection of a bone filler, typically polymethylmethacrylate (PMMA), directly into a fractured vertebral body with use of fluoroscopic guidance. The goals of vertebroplasty are pain relief and prevention of further collapse of the fractured vertebra. It may be possible to achieve some postural reduction of certain fractures.

Kyphoplasty Percutaneous insertion of an inflatable bone tamp into a fractured vertebral body with use of fluoroscopic guidance. Inflation of the bone tamp elevates the end plates to restore the vertebral body closer to its original height while creating a cavity to be filled with bone void filler, usually PMMA. The goals of kyphoplasty are pain relief, restoration of vertebral body height, and reduction of kyphotic deformity.

Indications

Vertebroplasty and kyphoplasty are indicated for the treatment of painful osteoporotic vertebral fractures, painful vertebrae due to metastasis, multiple myeloma, Kümmell disease, and painful vertebral hemangioma.[32-38] In addition, kyphoplasty may be indicated to correct severe and progressive kyphosis resulting from a vertebral compression fracture.[32,36,39]

The contraindications to both procedures include systemic pathologic conditions such as sepsis, prolonged bleeding times, or cardiopulmonary conditions that preclude the safe completion of the operations. Relative contraindications include vertebral bodies with deficient posterior cortices and neurologic signs or symptoms related to the vertebral fracture. Certain burst or vertebra plana fracture configurations pose technical challenges, and the feasibility of vertebroplasty or kyphoplasty should be cautiously assessed. Treating more than three vertebral levels in one surgical setting is not advocated because of the potential for deleterious cardiopulmonary effects related to PMMA monomer and/or fat or PMMA embolization to the lungs.

The benefits of prophylactic reinforcement of vertebrae "at risk" for fracture remain unproven. Finite element modeling suggested a high potential for complications given the volume of PMMA required for a vertebroplasty to successfully reinforce a vertebra at risk for fracture.[40]

Outcomes and Complications

Vertebroplasty Reports on the outcomes of vertebroplasty have suggested that most patients experience partial or complete pain relief within 72 hours after the procedure.[18,41-49] As reported in the literature, 60% to 100% of patients overall have noted decreased pain after vertebroplasty,[44,48] and improved functional levels and a reduced need for analgesic medication have been reported as well.[46,48,50-53] Zoarski and associates[54] administered the Musculoskeletal Outcomes Data Evaluation and Management Systems (MODEMS) scale before and at 2 weeks after vertebroplasty in 30 patients and found improvement in all four modules of the scale (treatment score, pain and disability, physical function, and mental function). Similarly, improvement in the Nottingham Health Profile scores have been observed after vertebroplasty.[42] Grados and associates,[55] in a longer-term follow-up study in which 25 of 40 patients were evaluated at a mean of 48 months after treatment of osteoporotic vertebral compression fractures with vertebroplasty, reported that the mean score for pain, as measured on a 100-point visual analog scale, decreased from 80 before the vertebroplasty to 37 one month after it. These results remained stable over time, with a pain score of 34 at the time of final follow-up. Published reports have noted a low complication rate after vertebroplasty. Most complications result from extravertebral leakage of PMMA causing spinal cord or nerve root compression or pulmonary embolism.[18,41-49]

Disease-specific questionnaires have further validated the success of vertebroplasty. Using the Roland-Morris Disability Questionnaire, Trout and associates[56] noted decreased pain and disability at 1 week after vertebroplasty, with maintenance of the pain relief at 1 year, in 113 patients who had a total of 164 vertebral fractures. McKiernan and associates[57] thought that the Osteoporosis Quality of Life Questionnaire, with the responses marked on a visual analog scale, was the best tool for evaluating health-related quality-of-life issues in osteoporotic women with back pain caused by vertebral compression fractures. Their prospective evaluation of 46 patients (66 vertebral compression fractures) demonstrated marked improvement in all factors at 1 day after the vertebroplasty with persistence of, although a slight decrease in, the benefit at 6 months. Larger prospective cohort evaluations confirmed these outcomes, demonstrating decreases in pain and analgesic use and improvements in mobility.[58,59] These studies did not show any clinically relevant complications. This suggests an improvement in the understanding and execution of this technique since earlier reports.

The limitations of the vertebroplasty technique are related to the inability of the procedure to correct spinal deformity and the risk of extravertebral PMMA extravasation during injection. During vertebroplasty, low-viscosity PMMA is injected under high pressure directly into cancellous bone. This makes it difficult to control PMMA flow into the vertebral body, creating the risk of extravasation outside of the vertebral body.[60] Extravertebral extravasation of PMMA regularly occurs during vertebroplasty, with reported leak rates of up to 65%.[42] The rate of extravasation has been noted to be higher in patients with metastases or hemangiomas than in patients with osteoporosis.[49,60]

Proponents of vertebroplasty have reported infrequent clinical sequelae of extravertebral leakage of PMMA. Cortet and associates[42] reported extravertebral PMMA in association with 13 of 20 vertebrae that had been treated with vertebroplasty because of an osteoporotic fracture. PMMA leaked into the paravertebral soft tissues in six instances, into the epidural space in three, into the disk space in three, and into the lumbar venous plexus in one. No adverse events were observed. Cyteval and associates[43] noted extravertebral PMMA in 8 of 20 patients treated with vertebroplasty, with leakage into the intervertebral disk in 5 patients, into the neural foramen in 2, and into the lumbar venous plexus in 1. Again, no adverse clinical events were observed. Chiras and associates[41] reported that 4% of patients who had undergone vertebroplasty had radiculopathy that was likely related to intraforaminal PMMA leakage. In a recent study, 3 of 35 patients treated with vertebroplasty had extravasation of PMMA into the epidural space, necessitating open surgical decompression in 2 of the patients.[61] Ryu and associates[62] reported a 26.5% rate of epidural PMMA leakage following 347 vertebroplasties and concluded that the prevalence of epidural leakage depended on the amount of PMMA injected. Use of a PMMA injector tool also increased the prevalence of epidural leakage, whereas the position of the needle tip in the vertebral body did not pre-

dict leakage. In summary, despite the substantial prevalence of extravertebral extravasation of PMMA during vertebroplasty, the risk of clinically relevant complications has been reported to be low.

It has been recommended that, to reduce extravertebral leakage of PMMA, studies with intravertebral injections of contrast medium be performed before injection of the PMMA in an attempt to predict potential egress of the PMMA from the vertebral body. Theoretically, extravasation of contrast medium signals the potential for subsequent extravasation of PMMA and thus indicates the need to redirect the needle and repeat the injection of the contrast material until no extravasation is observed. Lower volumes and higher viscosity of PMMA may also be warranted to avoid leakage. McGraw and associates[63] found that intraosseous venography predicted the subsequent flow of PMMA during vertebroplasty in 83% of patients. Gaughen and associates[64] reported that 22 of 42 vertebrae demonstrated PMMA extravasation during vertebroplasty, and venograms had showed correlative extravasation in 14 of the 22 vertebrae. However, the authors concluded that venography did not improve the effectiveness or safety of vertebroplasty performed by experienced physicians. Using intravertebral injections of contrast medium, Phillips and associates[65] showed that rates of transcortical and intravenous leakage of the contrast medium were higher for vertebroplasty than for kyphoplasty. Others have argued that intravertebral injections of contrast medium are not useful and that discontinuing the PMMA injection once the PMMA leaks out of the vertebral body or fills the perivertebral veins

remains the best technique for reducing the risk of complications.

The pressurized injection of PMMA during vertebroplasty has also raised concerns about embolization of the PMMA, unreacted PMMA monomer, or bone marrow to the lungs through the venous system.[66] Occasional instances of symptomatic and lethal PMMA pulmonary embolism following vertebroplasty have been reported.[50,67-69]

Groen and associates[70] revisited the vertebral venous system, emphasizing its large volume; numerous valveless connections with cranial, spinal, thoracic, abdominal, and subcutaneous veins; and open connections to the vertebral body and its bone marrow. Because of these characteristics, there is a risk of extrusion of marrow and fat from the vertebral body during a forced external increase of intravertebral pressure. This risk of fat or marrow embolism is present during the PMMA injection in vertebroplasty and also during the balloon inflation in kyphoplasty. Also, PMMA extravasation through this venous system can be expected, particularly with the increased pressures and the more fluid PMMA mixture required during vertebroplasty.[70] Complications including hypotension,[49] pulmonary embolism,[71,72] pulmonary PMMA embolism,[50,68,73,74] adult respiratory distress syndrome,[49] cerebral PMMA embolism,[75] intravascular extension of polymethylmethacrylate,[76] and PMMA toxicity[77] have been reported. An understanding of the pathomechanics, clinical indicators, and optimal technique for vertebroplasty is crucial, despite the low rate of these complications.

Kyphoplasty Early results suggest that kyphoplasty can provide excellent pain relief, improve the height of the collapsed vertebral body, and reduce spinal kyphosis.[29,49,60,78-82] Because kyphoplasty was first reported in 2000, the literature on this procedure is less extensive than that on vertebroplasty. Garfin and Reilley[83] reported the initial multicenter experience with kyphoplasty, in which 2,194 vertebral fractures in 1,439 patients were treated between 1998 and 2000. Ninety percent of the patients reported pain relief within 2 weeks after the procedure. Four neurologic complications were reported in this series; all occurred in the first 50 patients treated, and all were directly attributable to surgeon error and breach of technique. Three instances of postoperative paraparesis were related to insertion of an instrument through the medial pedicle wall, and one epidural hematoma requiring surgical decompression was in a patient who was being treated with anticoagulants. The serious adverse event rate was 0.2% per fracture.

In the study by Wong and associates,[60] 80 of 85 patients reported good to excellent pain relief after kyphoplasty. As experience with kyphoplasty has increased, it has become apparent that the intravertebral cavity created by the inflatable bone tamp allows placement of more viscous, partially cured PMMA. In a prospectively followed cohort of patients treated with kyphoplasty, Lieberman and associates[81] observed improvement in the postoperative scores for physical function, role limitations because of physical health, vitality, mental health, and social function on the Short Form-36 questionnaire. Of 70 vertebral fractures that were treated, five were associated with a clinically irrelevant PMMA leak. The PMMA entered the epidural space in one instance, the disk space in two, and the paraspinal tissues in three. No major

systemic complications or neurologic injuries occurred. In a study of 29 patients treated with kyphoplasty, Phillips and associates[39] reported a decrease in the mean visual analog pain score from 8.6 preoperatively to 2.6 at 1 week postoperatively to 0.6 at 1 year postoperatively. PMMA leaks without apparent clinical consequence occurred at 6 of 61 vertebral levels, with no instances of leakage into the spinal canal.

In addition to pain relief, kyphoplasty affords the opportunity to restore vertebral body height and thereby improve spinal sagittal balance. In an ex vivo study, Belkoff and associates[78] showed a 97% reversal of deformity with kyphoplasty and a 30% reversal with vertebroplasty. Lieberman and associates[81] reported that height was increased (by a mean of 46.8%) in 70% of 70 fractured vertebrae treated with kyphoplasty. Wong and associates[60] similarly noted increased vertebral body height after kyphoplasty. Phillips and associates[84] reported on a series of 40 patients treated with kyphoplasty. In the patients who had reducible fractures, local kyphosis decreased by a mean of 14°. The ability to reduce kyphosis is thought to be a major benefit of kyphoplasty.

The complications of kyphoplasty mirror those discussed regarding vertebroplasty. There are concerns about embolic events initiated by the intravertebral pressure changes caused by inflation of the bone tamp rather than the PMMA injection. Extravasation of PMMA also continues to be a concern, but the rate is lower given the low pressure and increased viscosity during the injection. Complications related to the hardware and balloon rupture have been reported.[32,80] However, subsequent evaluations of larger groups treated with kyphoplasty

support the earlier findings of successful management of both pain and deformity with low complication rates.[85-87] Majd and associates[86] found an 89% rate of clinical success in 360 patients, and Ledlie and Renfro[87] reported radiographic evidence of success in 100 patients.

In an attempt to improve the reliability and extent of fracture reduction, one might consider performing kyphoplasty soon after the fracture. Our experience suggests that, in selected patients, it is easier to elevate the end plates and restore vertebral body height when the kyphoplasty is performed within 1 month after the fracture than when it is performed several months after the fracture. The appropriate duration of nonsurgical treatment of a vertebral fracture before kyphoplasty is considered has not been established. It seems reasonable that patients presenting with an acute vertebral compression fracture and substantial kyphosis might be best managed with earlier intervention in an attempt to maximize improvement in spinal sagittal alignment. This may be particularly important at the thoracolumbar junction, where there is a tendency for the development of kyphosis. However, the efficacy of early intervention has not been elucidated.

Elderly patients with osteoporotic burst fractures and concomitant spinal stenosis can be extremely difficult to treat. Surgical decompression with instrumentation and fusion across the fractured segment is associated with a substantial risk of the instrumentation failing in the osteoporotic bone. Recently, Singh and associates[88] reported the benefits of vertebral augmentation in conjunction with laminectomy to manage this clinical dilemma. Of 25 patients with lumbar spinal stenosis and osteoporotic vertebral fractures (39 fractures) in their series, 9 required concomitant instrumentation for the treatment of spondylolisthesis at the decompressed level. Twenty of the 25 patients demonstrated a good or excellent result. Complications were observed in five patients. Others have reported similar successes with the management of burst fractures that presented without neurologic deterioration.[33,89,90] The ability of kyphoplasty combined with posterior instrumentation to restore vertebral height and spinal alignment following thoracic and lumbar burst fractures was validated in a cadaver model.[91] Unfortunately, the rates of PMMA extravasation secondary to the disruption of the cortical osseous walls of the vertebrae may be a reason for concern, in particular because loss of the integrity of the posterior wall places the neural elements at risk. However, although the use of kyphoplasty for this injury profile is not without risks, the potential to relieve symptoms and provide structural improvement is promising. Presently, there is insufficient information to fully understand the role of PMMA augmentation in the treatment of osteoporotic vertebral burst fractures.

Subsequent Vertebral Fracture After Vertebroplasty and Kyphoplasty

It remains unclear whether subsequent vertebral fractures are related to the natural progression of osteoporosis or are a consequence of augmentation with bone PMMA.[92] A natural history study of 2,725 women with a mean age of 74 years demonstrated a cumulative incidence of new vertebral fractures of 6.6% in the first year.[26] The incidence of second vertebral fractures

in the first year after an initial vertebral fracture was 19%. Only 23% of these second fractures were symptomatic; thus, 5% of women with an untreated compression fracture are expected to sustain a symptomatic subsequent vertebral fracture within 1 year.

The rate of vertebral fracture following vertebroplasty has been reported to be between 12% and 52%, depending on the duration and nature of the follow-up.[55,93] Two thirds of these fractures were identified at levels adjacent to the vertebroplasty and the remainder, at remote levels.[93] Grados and associates[55] reported that the odds ratio of a vertebral fracture occurring in the vicinity of a PMMA-augmented vertebra was 2.27 compared with an odds ratio of 1.44 for a vertebral fracture occurring in the vicinity of a cementless fractured vertebra. This equates to a 57% greater risk of fracture adjacent to a vertebroplasty.

The rate of vertebral fracture following kyphoplasty is 19% to 29%, again depending on the duration and nature of the follow-up. Fribourg and associates[94] documented a subsequent fracture rate of 26%, with 63% of the fractures occurring at adjacent levels. These adjacent-level fractures occurred within 60 days after the kyphoplasty. Thereafter, the fracture incidence mirrored that found in the natural history study previously described,[26] and adjacent-level fractures no longer predominated. Fribourg and associates suggested that patients should be informed of this fracture risk in the early postoperative period.

Harrop and associates[95] found a subsequent vertebral fracture in 23% of 115 patients treated with kyphoplasty. Although no correlation was found between recurrent frac-

tures and age, bone density, T score, gender, or number of augmented levels, stratification by osteoporosis type (primary versus steroid-induced) delineated patients at increased risk. A subsequent fracture was observed in 49% of patients with steroid-induced osteoporosis compared with only 11% of those with primary osteoporosis. Steroid-induced osteoporosis, rather than the kyphoplasty, was thought to be a greater risk factor predicting subsequent fractures. In the only prospective controlled study of kyphoplasty of which we are aware, Kasperk and associates[96] confirmed the nonsignificant differences in the rate of subsequent fractures, at both 6 and 12 months, between patients treated with kyphoplasty and those managed medically.[97] The correction of biomechanical variables following kyphoplasty should work to counteract subsequent fractures.[12] Thus, the concern regarding subsequent vertebral fracture following PMMA augmentation persists but is unconfirmed.

Advantages

Vertebroplasty The advantages of this technique are its simplicity and its ability to relieve pain. The procedure is typically performed with the use of local anesthesia and intravenous sedation. The avoidance of general anesthesia for frail, elderly patients is advantageous. The procedure is straightforward to perform and requires little special equipment. This can equate to faster procedure times and lower costs.

Kyphoplasty The advantages of this technique are deformity correction and relief of pain. Fracture reduction and correction of kyphotic deformity can be achieved with use of specialized instrumentation. It has been hypothesized that restoration of spinal alignment improves the functional capacity of the respiratory, cardiac, gastrointestinal, and musculoskeletal systems. Decreased PMMA extravasation resulting from low-pressure injection of more viscous PMMA reduces complications. Kyphoplasty is more costly than vertebroplasty.

Surgical Technique

Before proceeding with either intervention, the physician must confirm that the back pain is caused by a vertebral compression fracture. This requires careful correlation of the patient's history and findings on clinical examination with radiographic documentation of an acute or unhealed vertebral compression fracture. The possibility of secondary osteoporosis or a malignant tumor producing the back pain must be considered. Degenerative spinal disorders may also present with kyphosis and back pain. A thorough neurologic examination is essential to rule out neurologic compromise. Pain radiating around the trunk in a dermatomal manner may accompany vertebral compression fractures. Pulmonary function should be evaluated in patients in whom advanced kyphosis may have led to respiratory difficulty.

Preoperative planning includes making radiographs to define the fracture geometry and for surgical planning. Lateral radiographs are particularly useful for planning the trajectory for any percutaneous procedure. MRI is typically used to evaluate the acuity of the fracture. When MRI is contraindicated, nuclear bone scans may help the physician to estimate the acuity of the fracture. Osseous edema is readily seen on MRI and can indicate an acute fracture as well as help rule out a tumor or infection. Malignant

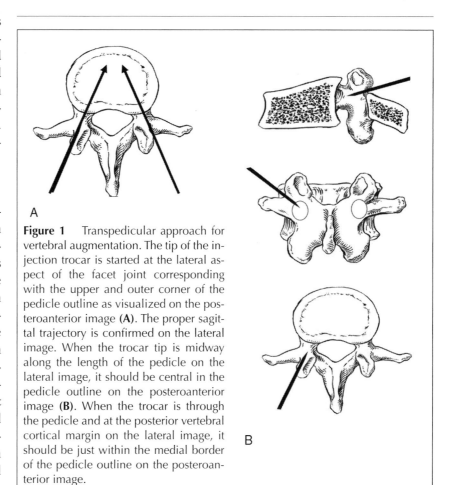

Figure 1 Transpedicular approach for vertebral augmentation. The tip of the injection trocar is started at the lateral aspect of the facet joint corresponding with the upper and outer corner of the pedicle outline as visualized on the posteroanterior image (**A**). The proper sagittal trajectory is confirmed on the lateral image. When the trocar tip is midway along the length of the pedicle on the lateral image, it should be central in the pedicle outline on the posteroanterior image (**B**). When the trocar is through the pedicle and at the posterior vertebral cortical margin on the lateral image, it should be just within the medial border of the pedicle outline on the posteroanterior image.

diseases causing vertebral compression fracture are usually associated with an ill-defined margin, enhancement with gadolinium, and pedicle involvement as well as a paravertebral soft-tissue mass.[98] Sagittal MRI with short tau inversion recovery (STIR) sequences highlight the marrow edema changes associated with acute fractures, and STIR MRI has proved to be useful in determining the acuity of a vertebral compression fracture.

To perform either of the procedures, the patient is positioned prone on the operating room table or in the radiology suite on a spinal frame with cushioned bolsters. Attention to patient positioning and bolster support on the procedure table can provide postural fracture re-

duction, thus improving the chance of correcting kyphosis. Local anesthesia with intravenous conscious sedation (more common for vertebroplasty) or general anesthesia (more common for kyphoplasty) may be used. Local anesthesia may be preferable for patients with medical illness. Fluoroscopy is used throughout the procedure, and we prefer simultaneous biplanar fluoroscopy.

Typically, the transpedicular approach is used in the lumbar spine. The tip of the injection trocar is started at the outer aspect of the pedicle as visualized on the posteroanterior image, and the proper sagittal trajectory is confirmed on the lateral image (Figure 1). When the trocar tip is midway along the length

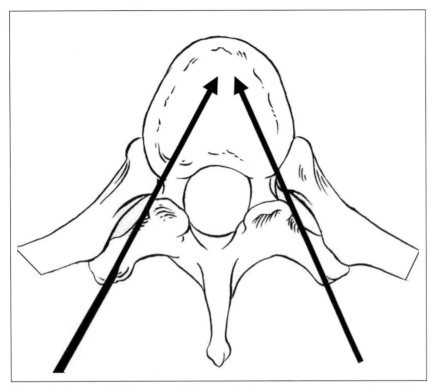

Figure 2 Extrapedicular approach for vertebral augmentation. The starting point is craniolateral toward the costovertebral joint. Contact is made with the neck of the rib or transverse process. The needle is advanced along the neck of the rib, passed under the transverse process, and passed through the ligament complex of the costovertebral joint until the lateral pedicle wall is reached. The needle is then advanced into the vertebral body.

of the pedicle on the lateral image, it should be central in the pedicle outline on the posteroanterior image. When the trocar is through the pedicle and at the posterior vertebral cortical margin on the lateral image, it should be just within the medial border of the pedicle outline on the posteroanterior image. For vertebroplasty, the trocar is advanced until the tip is at the junction of the anterior and middle thirds of the vertebral body. For kyphoplasty, the positioning trocar is exchanged for a working cannula over a guidewire. The cannula is positioned near the posterior margin of the vertebral body while the working instruments are advanced anteriorly until they are 3 mm from the anterior border of the vertebral body.[32]

The extrapedicular approach is commonly used in the thoracic spine because of the smaller pedicle diameter and a less medially angulated pedicle trajectory. The starting point is craniolateral toward the costovertebral joint (Figure 2). Contact is made with the neck of the rib or transverse process. The needle is advanced along the neck of the rib, passed under the transverse process, and passed through the ligament complex of the costovertebral joint until the lateral pedicle wall is reached. The projection of the tip of the needle should be at the upper and outer circumference of the pedicle as seen on the posteroanterior image. On the lateral image, the tip of the needle should be projected between the pedicle margins and an-

terior to the facet joints. Only after the posterior vertebral wall has been passed on the lateral image should the tip of the needle cross the medial pedicle wall on the posteroanterior image. Strict adherence to these landmarks is mandatory to avoid spinal perforation.[32,99] Boszczyk and associates[99] used this technique to perform kyphoplasty at levels from T2 to T8 and noted precise introduction of the tools in all 55 vertebrae, despite the narrow pedicle diameter.

A unipedicular rather than a bipedicular technique has been suggested to decrease risks associated with cannulation, surgical time, radiation exposure, and cost. The unipedicular technique for both vertebroplasty and kyphoplasty has been shown to restore strength, stiffness, and height as well as the bipedicular technique in a cadaver model.[100,101] Lateral wedging was not observed. Using a finite-element model, Liebschner and associates[102] found that, although unipedicular PMMA injection restored stiffness, a mediallateral bending motion (toggle) toward the untreated side with application of a uniform compressive load was created. This finding has not been confirmed in clinical trials.

Performance of a vertebral body bone biopsy should be considered. When a trephine needle was used before PMMA injection, adequate tissue was obtained for analysis from 67% to 100% of the samples.[36,99] Togawa and associates[103] obtained biopsy specimens from 178 vertebrae and identified possible osteomalacia in 21% of them, with another four confirming an occult or unconfirmed plasma cell dyscrasia. Togawa and associates advocated performance of a biopsy during each first-time vertebral augmentation procedure so as not to miss occult lesions.

Vertebroplasty After proper needle placement and biopsy, PMMA is injected through a cannula into the vertebral body. The PMMA should be of a consistency that minimizes filling pressures and yet prevents leakage. The judicious use of fluoroscopic imaging throughout the procedure is paramount to the success and safety of a vertebroplasty. The procedure is completed when imaging demonstrates adequate vertebral filling or when extravasation of the PMMA is identified.

Kyphoplasty After proper needle placement and biopsy, the inflatable balloon tamp (KyphX Inflatable Bone Tamp; Kyphon, Sunnyvale, California) is inserted through the cannula and expanded under visual (fluoroscopic) and volume and pressure (digital manometer) controls. The bone tamp is inflated until fracture reduction is achieved, the maximal pressure or volume of the balloon is reached, or contact occurs with the cortical wall. The balloon is then deflated and removed. Partially cured PMMA can then be introduced through the cannula under low pressure to fill the void created by the balloon tamp. The volume of the PMMA should approximate that of the intravertebral cavity. Volumes from 3.5 to 8.5 mL have been observed.[36] Again, the judicious use of fluoroscopic imaging throughout the procedure is paramount. To our knowledge, no one has quantified PMMA viscosity to define an optimal injection. **(DVD 27.1)**

Biomaterials

To date, most vertebroplasty and kyphoplasty procedures have been performed with use of PMMA to augment the fractured vertebral body. The mechanism of pain relief by these procedures is uncertain and may be related to PMMA "stabilization" of the fractured vertebral body or deafferentation related to heating of nerve endings as the PMMA cures. The optimal PMMA volume required to relieve pain and restore strength and stiffness is unknown. In an ex vivo study of experimental osteoporotic compression fractures, injection of 2 mL of PMMA (with barium sulfate) restored vertebral strength (the ability of the vertebral body to bear load) to prefracture levels, whereas 4 to 8 mL of PMMA was required to restore stiffness (resistance to micromotion).[104]

For many years, PMMA has been commonly used around joint prostheses, to fill long bone defects, and to reconstruct the spinal column.[105-107] Potential problems with PMMA include the exothermic reaction during the curing process, when temperatures may reach 100°C and cause thermal damage to adjacent structures; cardiopulmonary toxicity of the unreacted monomer; and the lack of long-term biointegration of the PMMA. A repair process, including primitive mesenchymal cell proliferation, neovascularization, resorption of dead bone, and new bone formation, was found to be absent in a histopathologic assessment following PMMA augmentation of vertebral fractures.[108]

The ideal biomaterial for vertebral augmentation would be radiolucent and nontoxic, would have handling characteristics that allow easy injection, would undergo a gradual transition from a viscous to a solid state with low exothermic temperatures, and would have adequate compressive strength to stabilize the fractured vertebral body. An osteoconductive, biodegradable material, which is replaced by host bone, may be advantageous; however, the ability of osteoporotic bone to remodel and replace a biodegradable material with host bone of adequate quality is uncertain and must be studied before such materials are considered for clinical use. Several alternate biomaterials, including carbonated apatite,[109] bioactive PMMA,[110] and calcium phosphate,[111,112] have been shown to substantially improve compressive strength and load to failure of vertebral bodies. A more extensive understanding of the toxicity profiles and long-term stability of these materials is essential.

Radiation

As the number of minimally invasive techniques to treat spine disorders, and the number of vertebroplasties and kyphoplasty procedures in particular, increases, the use of radiographic guidance in the operating room increases as well. Concerns regarding the radiation exposure to both the patient and the surgeon have been raised.

Boszczyk and associates[113] monitored the radiation exposure to the patients during 60 kyphoplasty procedures guided with biplanar fluoroscopy to treat 104 vertebrae. Exposure times per level during lateral plane imaging were noted to be 2.2 minutes for a single level and 1.7 minutes for a multiple-level session. Exposure times per level during anteroposterior plane imaging were noted to be 1.6 minutes for a single level and 1.1 minutes for a multiple-level session. Imaging times in the lateral plane consistently remained above those in the anteroposterior plane. Entrance skin doses ranged from 0.05 to 1.43 Gy with average values of 0.68 Gy in the lateral plane and 0.32 Gy in the anteroposterior plane. Calculated effective dose values averaged 4.28 mSv with a maximum of 10.14 mSv. In light of a baseline risk of cancer death of 20% to 25%, the postulated increase in lifetime cancer risk after a single kyphoplasty procedure was 0.02% to 0.06%.

Harstall and associates[114] monitored the radiation exposure to the surgeon during 32 vertebroplasty procedures performed with use of a single fluoroscopic unit to image in two planes to treat 136 vertebrae. The average surgical time was 56.2 minutes, and an average of 4.25 vertebrae were augmented. The average exposure time was 2.23 minutes per augmented vertebra. Measurements at the thyroid gland, eye lens equivalent, left and right hands, left arm, and back demonstrated radiation doses per augmented level of 0.052, 0.020, 0.107, 0.049, 0.084, and 0.002 mSv, respectively. Extrapolated radiation doses per year were troubling. Eight percent of the maximum allowed annual dose for the eye lens is expected with this procedure alone. Although the annual morbidity risk for thyroid exposure was calculated to be 0.025%, representing a low to medium 1-year risk, the lifetime risk was considered to be high to very high.

Average whole-body doses are variable and have been calculated to be between 1.44 mSv per level and 96 mSv per patient.[115,116] Theocharopoulos and associates[116] concluded that 90% of the surgeon's effective radiation dose and cancer risk was attributed to kyphoplasty and vertebroplasty procedures, with another 8% attributed to other spine procedures, at their center. Certain intraoperative techniques reduce radiation exposure time. Biplanar fluoroscopy eliminates the unnecessary exposure time required for repositioning of equipment. Surgeon-

controlled foot pedals to direct fluoroscopy time streamlined surgical flow. In one study, whenever feasible with regard to fluoroscopic visualization, the PMMA was injected into as many as three adjacent vertebrae simultaneously.[113] Pulsed fluoroscopic operation at 4 pulses/s, positioning of the radiograph tube under the patient table, and use of lead sheets on the patient and a lead apron, lead collar, and goggles by the surgeon further minimize radiation exposure.[114,115] If these measures are followed, exposure levels will be sufficiently low to permit the safe performance of more than 6,700 vertebroplasty procedures by a single surgeon per year.[115]

Summary

Minimally invasive surgical techniques are being used with increasing frequency to manage vertebral compression fractures. Alleviation of fracture pain and optimization of comorbid factors aggravated by these fractures have been demonstrated after use of these techniques. Both vertebroplasty and kyphoplasty demonstrate distinct advantages. Complications do occur during both procedures, but they can be minimized through meticulous surgical technique and surgeon experience. Greater understanding of the histopathologic, biomechanical, and clinical factors involved in these techniques will provide even greater successes in the future.

References

1. Riggs BL, Melton LJ III: The worldwide problem of osteoporosis: Insights afforded by epidemiology. *Bone* 1995;17(5 Suppl):505S-511S.

2. Cohen LD: Fractures of the osteoporotic spine. *Orthop Clin North Am* 1990;21:143-150.

3. National Osteoporosis Foundation: *America's Bone Health: The State of Osteoporosis and Low Bone Mass in Our Nation.* Washington, DC, 2002.

4. Iqbal MM, Sobhan T: Osteoporosis: A review. *Mo Med* 2002;99:19-24.

5. Johnell O: Advances in osteoporosis: Better identification of risk factors can reduce morbidity and mortality. *J Intern Med* 1996;239:299-304.

6. Verbrugge LM, Lepkowski JM, Imanaka Y: Comorbidity and its impact on disability. *Milbank Q* 1989;67:450-484.

7. Silverman SL: The clinical consequences of vertebral compression fracture. *Bone* 1992;13(Suppl 2):S27-S31.

8. Gold DT: The clinical impact of vertebral fractures: Quality of life in women with osteoporosis. *Bone* 1996;18(3 Suppl):185S-189S.

9. Belmont PJ Jr, Polly DW Jr, Cunningham BW, Klemme WR: The effects of hook pattern and kyphotic angulation on mechanical strength and apical rod strain in a long-segment posterior construct using a synthetic model. *Spine* 2001;26:627-635.

10. White AA III, Panjabi MM, Thomas CL: The clinical biomechanics of kyphotic deformities. *Clin Orthop Relat Res* 1977;128:8-17.

11. Gaitanis IN, Carandang G, Phillips FM, et al: Restoring geometric and loading alignment of the thoracic spine with a vertebral compression fracture: Effects of balloon (bone tamp) inflation and spinal extension. *Spine J* 2005;5:45-54.

12. Yuan HA, Brown CW, Phillips FM: Osteoporotic spinal deformity: A biomechanical rationale for the clinical consequences and treatment of vertebral body compression fractures. *J Spinal Disord Tech* 2004;17:236-242.

13. Nevitt MC, Ettinger B, Black DM, et al: The association of radiographically detected vertebral fractures with back pain and function: A prospective study. *Ann Intern Med* 1998;128:793-800.

14. Nevitt MC, Thompson DE, Black DM, et al: Effect of alendronate on limited-activity days and bed-disability days caused by back pain in postmenopausal women with existing vertebral fractures. Fracture Intervention Trial Research Group. *Arch Intern Med* 2000;160:77-85.

15. Wasnich RD: Vertebral fracture epidemiology. *Bone* 1996;18(3 Suppl):179S-183S.

16. Haczynski J, Jakimiuk A: Vertebral fractures: A hidden problem of osteoporosis. *Med Sci Monit* 2001;7:1108-1117.

17. Ross PD, Davis JW, Epstein RS, Wasnich RD: Pre-existing fractures and bone mass predict vertebral fracture incidence in women. *Ann Intern Med* 1991;114:919-923.

18. Rapado A: General management of vertebral fractures. *Bone* 1996;18(3 Suppl):191S-196S.

19. Gold D, Lyles K: Fractures: Effects on quality of life, in Bilezikian JP, Glowacki J, Rosen CJ (eds): *The Aging Skeleton*. San Diego, CA, Academic Press, 1999.

20. Leidig G, Minne HW, Sauer P, et al: A study of complaints and their relation to vertebral destruction in patients with osteoporosis. *Bone Miner* 1990;8:217-229.

21. Lyles KW, Gold DT, Shipp KM, Pieper CF, Martinez S, Mulhausen PL: Association of osteoporotic vertebral compression fractures with impaired functional status. *Am J Med* 1993;94:595-601.

22. Pluijm SM, Tromp AM, Smit JH, Deeg DJ, Lips P: Consequences of vertebral deformities in older men and women. *J Bone Miner Res* 2000;15:1564-1572.

23. Leech JA, Dulberg C, Kellie S, Pattee L, Gay J: Relationship of lung function to severity of osteoporosis in women. *Am Rev Respir Dis* 1990;141:68-71.

24. Schlaich C, Minne HW, Bruckner T, et al: Reduced pulmonary function in patients with spinal osteoporotic fractures. *Osteoporos Int* 1998;8:261-267.

25. Ross PD, Davis JW, Epstein RS, Wasnich RD: Pain and disability associated with new vertebral fractures and other spinal conditions. *J Clin Epidemiol* 1994;47:231-239.

26. Lindsay R, Silverman SL, Cooper C, et al: Risk of new vertebral fracture in the year following a fracture. *JAMA* 2001;285:320-323.

27. Keller TS, Harrison DE, Colloca CJ, Harrison DD, Janik TJ: Prediction of osteoporotic spinal deformity. *Spine* 2003;28:455-462.

28. Kado DM, Browner WS, Palermo L, Nevitt MC, Genant HK, Cummings SR: Vertebral fractures and mortality in older women: A prospective study. Study of Osteoporotic Fractures Research Group. *Arch Intern Med* 1999;159:1215-1220.

29. Eck JC, Hodges SD, Humphreys SC: Vertebroplasty: A new treatment strategy for osteoporotic compression fractures. *Am J Orthop* 2002;31:123-128.

30. Lukert BP: Vertebral compression fractures: How to manage pain, avoid disability. *Geriatrics* 1994;49:22-26.

31. Meunier PJ, Delmas PD, Eastell R, et al: Diagnosis and management of osteoporosis in postmenopausal women: Clinical guidelines. International Committee for Osteoporosis Clinical Guidelines. *Clin Ther* 1999;21:1025-1044.

32. Spivak JM, Johnson MG: Percutaneous treatment of vertebral body pathology. *J Am Acad Orthop Surg* 2005;13:6-17.

33. Boszczyk BM, Bierschneider M, Schmid K, Grillhosl A, Robert B, Jaksche H: Microsurgical interlaminar vertebro- and kyphoplasty for severe osteoporotic fractures. *J Neurosurg* 2004;100:32-37.

34. Cortet B, Cotten A, Deprez X, et al: [Value of vertebroplasty combined with surgical decompression in the treatment of aggressive spinal angioma. Apropos of 3 cases]. *Rev Rhum Ed Fr* 1994;61:16-22.

35. Cotten A, Duquesnoy B: Vertebroplasty: Current data and future potential. *Rev Rhum Engl Ed* 1997;64:645-649.

36. Gaitanis IN, Hadjipavlou AG, Katonis PG, Tzermiadianos MN, Pasku DS, Patwardhan AG: Balloon kyphoplasty for the treatment of pathological vertebral compressive fractures. *Eur Spine J* 2005;14:250-260.

37. Galibert P, Deramond H: [Percutaneous acrylic vertebroplasty as a treatment of vertebral angioma as well as painful and debilitating diseases]. *Chirurgie* 1990;116:326-335.

38. Ide C, Gangi A, Rimmelin A, et al: Vertebral haemangiomas with spinal cord compression: The place of preoperative percutaneous vertebroplasty with methyl methacrylate. *Neuroradiology* 1996;38:585-589.

39. Phillips FM, Ho E, Campbell-Hupp M, McNally T, Todd Wetzel F, Gupta P: Early radiographic and clinical results of balloon kyphoplasty for the treatment of osteoporotic vertebral compression fractures. *Spine* 2003;28:2260-2267.

40. Sun K, Liebschner MA: Biomechanics of prophylactic vertebral reinforcement. *Spine* 2004;29:1428-1435.

41. Chiras J, Depriester C, Weill A, Sola-Martinez MT, Deramond H: [Percutaneous vertebral surgery. Technics and indications]. *J Neuroradiol* 1997;24:45-59.

42. Cortet B, Cotten A, Boutry N, et al: Percutaneous vertebroplasty in the treatment of osteoporotic vertebral compression fractures: An open prospective study. *J Rheumatol* 1999;26:2222-2228.

43. Cyteval C, Sarrabere MP, Roux JO, et al: Acute osteoporotic vertebral collapse: Open study on percutaneous injection of acrylic surgical cement in 20 patients. *AJR Am J Roentgenol* 1999;173:1685-1690.

44. Gangi A, Kastler BA, Dietemann JL: Percutaneous vertebroplasty guided by a combination of CT and fluoroscopy. *AJNR Am J Neuroradiol* 1994;15:83-86.

45. Hardouin P, Grados F, Cotton A, Cortet B: Should percutaneous vertebroplasty be used to treat osteoporotic fractures? An update. *Joint Bone Spine* 2001;68:216-221.

46. Jensen ME, Evans AJ, Mathis JM, Kallmes DF, Cloft HJ, Dion JE: Percutaneous polymethylmethacrylate vertebroplasty in the treatment of osteoporotic vertebral body compression fractures: Technical aspects. *AJNR Am J Neuroradiol* 1997;18:1897-1904.

47. Lapras C, Mottolese C, Deruty R, Lapras C Jr, Remond J, Duquesnel J: [Percutaneous injection of methyl-metacrylate in osteoporosis and severe vertebral osteolysis (Galibert's technic)]. *Ann Chir* 1989;43:371-376.

48. Mathis JM, Petri M, Naff N: Percutaneous vertebroplasty treatment of steroid-induced osteoporotic compression fractures. *Arthritis Rheum* 1998;41:171-175.

49. Watts NB, Harris ST, Genant HK: Treatment of painful osteoporotic vertebral fractures with percutaneous vertebroplasty or kyphoplasty. *Osteoporos Int* 2001;12:429-437.

50. Amar AP, Larsen DW, Esnaashari N, Albuquerque FC, Lavine SD, Teitelbaum GP: Percutaneous transpedicular polymethylmethacrylate vertebroplasty for the treatment of spinal compression fractures. *Neurosurgery* 2001;49:1105-1115.

51. Kim AK, Jensen ME, Dion JE, Schweickert PA, Kaufmann TJ, Kallmes DF: Unilateral transpedicular percutaneous vertebroplasty: Initial experience. *Radiology* 2002;222:737-741.

52. Martin JB, Jean B, Sugiu K, et al: Vertebroplasty: Clinical experience and follow-up results. *Bone* 1999;25(2 Suppl):11S-15S.

53. Tsou IY, Goh PY, Peh WC, Goh LA, Chee TS: Percutaneous vertebroplasty in the management of osteoporotic vertebral

compression fractures: Initial experience. *Ann Acad Med Singapore* 2002;31:15-20.

54. Zoarski GH, Snow P, Olan WJ, et al: Percutaneous vertebroplasty for osteoporotic compression fractures: Quantitative prospective evaluation of long-term outcomes. *J Vasc Interv Radiol* 2002;13:139-148.

55. Grados F, Depriester C, Cayrolle G, Hardy N, Deramond H, Fardellone P: Long-term observations of vertebral osteoporotic fractures treated by percutaneous vertebroplasty. *Rheumatology (Oxford)* 2000;39:1410-1414.

56. Trout AT, Kallmes DF, Gray LA, et al: Evaluation of vertebroplasty with a validated outcome measure: The Roland-Morris Disability Questionnaire. *AJNR Am J Neuroradiol* 2005;26:2652-2657.

57. McKiernan F, Faciszewski T, Jensen R: Quality of life following vertebroplasty. *J Bone Joint Surg Am* 2004;86:2600-2606.

58. Do HM, Kim BS, Marcellus ML, Curtis L, Marks MP: Prospective analysis of clinical outcomes after percutaneous vertebroplasty for painful osteoporotic vertebral body fractures. *AJNR Am J Neuroradiol* 2005;26:1623-1628.

59. Kobayashi K, Shimoyama K, Nakamura K, Murata K: Percutaneous vertebroplasty immediately relieves pain of osteoporotic vertebral compression fractures and prevents prolonged immobilization of patients. *Eur Radiol* 2005;15:360-367.

60. Wong W, Reiley M, Garfin S: Vertebroplasty/ kyphoplasty. *J Wom Imag* 2000;2:117-124.

61. Moreland DB, Landi MK, Grand W: Vertebroplasty: Techniques to avoid complications. *Spine J* 2001;1:66-71.

62. Ryu KS, Park CK, Kim MC, Kang JK: Dose-dependent epidural leakage of polymethylmethacrylate after percutaneous vertebroplasty in patients with osteoporotic vertebral compression fractures. *J Neurosurg* 2002;96(1 Suppl):56-61.

63. McGraw JK, Heatwole EV, Strnad BT, Silber JS, Patzilk SB, Boorstein JM: Predictive value of intraosseous venography before percutaneous vertebroplasty. *J Vasc Interv Radiol* 2002;13:149-153.

64. Gaughen JR Jr, Jensen ME, Schweickert PA, Kaufmann TJ, Marx WF, Kallmes DF: Relevance of antecedent venography in percutaneous vertebroplasty for the treatment of osteoporotic compression fractures. *AJNR Am J Neuroradiol* 2002;23:594-600.

65. Phillips FM, Todd Wetzel F, Lieberman I, Campbell-Hupp M: An in vivo comparison of the potential for extravertebral cement leak after vertebroplasty and kyphoplasty. *Spine* 2002;27:2173-2179.

66. Aebli N, Krebs J, Davis G, Walton M, Williams MJ, Theis JC: Fat embolism and acute hypotension during vertebroplasty: An experimental study in sheep. *Spine* 2002;27:460-466.

67. Levine SA, Perin LA, Hayes D, Hayes WS: An evidence-based evaluation of percutaneous vertebroplasty. *Manag Care* 2000;9:56-60, 63.

68. Padovani B, Kasriel O, Brunner P, Paretti-Viton P: Pulmonary embolism caused by acrylic cement: A rare complication of percutaneous vertebroplasty. *AJNR Am J Neuroradiol* 1999;20:375-377.

69. Perrin C, Jullien V, Padovani B, Blaive B: [Percutaneous vertebroplasty complicated by pulmonary embolus of acrylic cement]. *Rev Mal Respir* 1999;16:215-217.

70. Groen RJ, du Toit DF, Phillips FM, et al: Anatomical and pathological considerations in percutaneous vertebroplasty and kyphoplasty: A reappraisal of the vertebral venous system. *Spine* 2004;29:1465-1471.

71. Chen HL, Wong CS, Ho ST, Chang FL, Hsu CH, Wu CT: A lethal pulmonary embolism during percutaneous vertebroplasty. *Anesth Analg* 2002;95:1060-1062.

72. Tozzi P, Abdelmoumene Y, Corno AF, Gersbach PA, Hoogewoud HM, von Segesser LK: Management of pulmonary embolism during acrylic vertebroplasty. *Ann Thorac Surg* 2002;74:1706-1708.

73. Bernhard J, Heini PF, Villiger PM: Asymptomatic diffuse pulmonary embolism caused by acrylic cement: An unusual complication of percutaneous vertebroplasty. *Ann Rheum Dis* 2003;62:85-86.

74. Jang JS, Lee SH, Jung SK: Pulmonary embolism of polymethylmethacrylate after percutaneous vertebroplasty: A report of three cases. *Spine* 2002;27:E416-E418.

75. Scroop R, Eskridge J, Britz GW: Paradoxical cerebral arterial embolization of cement during intraoperative vertebroplasty: Case report. *AJNR Am J Neuroradiol* 2002;23:868-870.

76. Wenger M, Markwalder TM: Surgically controlled, transpedicular methyl methacrylate vertebroplasty with fluoroscopic guidance. *Acta Neurochir (Wien)* 1999;141:625-631.

77. Lane JM, Johnson CE, Khan SN, Girardi FP, Cammisa FP Jr: Minimally invasive options for the treatment of osteoporotic vertebral compression fractures. *Orthop Clin North Am* 2002;33:431-438.

78. Belkoff SM, Mathis JM, Fenton DC, Scribner RM, Reiley ME, Talmadge K: An ex vivo biomechanical evaluation of an inflatable bone tamp used in the treatment of compression fracture. *Spine* 2001;26:151-156.

79. Garfin S, Reiley M, Wong W: Vertebroplasty and kyphoplasty, in Savitz MH, Chiu JC, Yueng AT (eds): *The Practice of Minimally Invasive Spinal Technique*. Richmond, VA, AAMISMS Education, 2000.

80. Garfin SR, Yuan HA, Reiley MA: New technologies in spine: Kyphoplasty and vertebroplasty for the treatment of painful osteoporotic compression fractures. *Spine* 2001;26:1511-1515.

81. Lieberman IH, Dudeney S, Reinhardt MK, Bell G: Initial outcome and efficacy of "kyphoplasty" in the treatment of painful osteoporotic vertebral compression fractures. *Spine* 2001;26:1631-1638.

82. Theodorou DJ, Theodorou SJ, Duncan TD, Garfin SR, Wong WH: Percutaneous balloon kyphoplasty for the correction of spinal deformity in painful vertebral body compression fractures. *Clin Imaging* 2002;26:1-5.

83. Garfin S, Reilley MA: Minimally invasive treatment of osteoporotic vertebral body compression fracture. *Spine J* 2002;2:76-80.

84. Phillips F, Ho E, Campbell-Hupp M, McNally T, Todd Wetzel F, Gupta P: Early clinical and radiographic results of kyphoplasty for the treatment of osteopenic vertebral compression fractures. *Eur Spine J* 2001;10(Suppl 1):S7.

85. Atalay B, Caner H, Gokce C, Atinors N: Kyphoplasty: 2 years of experience in a neurosurgery department. *Surg Neurol* 2005;64(Suppl 2):S72-S76.

86. Majd ME, Farley S, Holt RT: Preliminary outcomes and efficacy of the first 360 consecutive kyphoplasties for the treatment of painful osteoporotic vertebral compression fractures. *Spine J* 2005;5:244-255.

87. Ledlie JT, Renfro MB: Decreases in the number and severity of morphometrically

defined vertebral body deformities after kyphoplasty. *Neurosurg Focus* 2005;18:e4.

88. Singh K, Heller JG, Samartzis D, et al: Open vertebral cement augmentation combined with lumbar decompression for the operative management of thoracolumbar stenosis secondary to osteoporotic burst fractures. *J Spinal Disord Tech* 2005;18:413-419.

89. Boszczyk B, Bierschneider M, Potulski M, Robert B, Vastmans J, Jaksche H: [Extended kyphoplasty indications for stabilization of osteoporotic vertebral compression fractures]. *Unfallchirurg* 2002;105:952-957.

90. Chen JF, Lee ST: Percutaneous vertebroplasty for treatment of thoracolumbar spine bursting fracture. *Surg Neurol* 2004;62:494-500.

91. Verlaan JJ, van de Kraats EB, Oner FC, van Walsum T, Niessen WJ, Dhert WJ: The reduction of endplate fractures during balloon vertebroplasty: A detailed radiological analysis of the treatment of burst fractures using pedicle screws, balloon vertebroplasty, and calcium phosphate cement. *Spine* 2005;30:1840-1845.

92. Villarraga ML, Bellezza AJ, Harrigan TP, Cripton PA, Kurtz SM, Edidin AA: The biomechanical effects of kyphoplasty on treated and adjacent nontreated vertebral bodies. *J Spinal Disord Tech* 2005;18:84-91.

93. Uppin AA, Hirsch JA, Centenera LV, Pfiefer BA, Pazianos AG, Choi IS: Occurrence of new vertebral body fracture after percutaneous vertebroplasty in patients with osteoporosis. *Radiology* 2003;226:119-124.

94. Fribourg D, Tang C, Sra P, Delamarter R, Bae H: Incidence of subsequent vertebral fracture after kyphoplasty. *Spine* 2004;29:2270-2277.

95. Harrop JS, Prpa B, Reinhardt MK, Lieberman I: Primary and secondary osteoporosis' incidence of subsequent vertebral compression fractures after kyphoplasty. *Spine* 2004;29:2120-2125.

96. Kasperk C, Hillmeier J, Noldge G, et al: Treatment of painful vertebral fractures by kyphoplasty in patients with primary osteoporosis: A prospective nonrandomized controlled study. *J Bone Miner Res* 2005;20:604-612.

97. Grafe IA, Da Fonseca K, Hillmeier J, et al: Reduction of pain and fracture incidence after kyphoplasty: 1-year outcomes of a prospective controlled trial of patients with primary osteoporosis. *Osteoporos Int* 2005;16:2005-2012.

98. Shih TT, Huang KM, Li YW: Solitary vertebral collapse: Distinction between benign and malignant causes using MR patterns. *J Magn Reson Imaging* 1999;9:635-642.

99. Boszczyk BM, Bierschneider M, Hauck S, Beisse R, Potulski M, Jaksche H: Transcostovertebral kyphoplasty of the mid and high thoracic spine. *Eur Spine J* 2005;14:992-999.

100. Steinmann J, Tingey CT, Cruz G, Dai Q: Biomechanical comparison of unipedicular versus bipedicular kyphoplasty. *Spine* 2005;30:201-205.

101. Tohmeh AG, Mathis JM, Fenton DC, Levine AM, Belkoff SM: Biomechanical efficacy of unipedicular versus bipedicular vertebroplasty for the management of osteoporotic compression fractures. *Spine* 1999;24:1772-1776.

102. Liebschner MA, Rosenberg WS, Keaveny TM: Effects of bone cement volume and distribution on vertebral stiffness after vertebroplasty. *Spine* 2001;26:1547-1554.

103. Togawa D, Lieberman IH, Bauer TW, Reinhardt MK, Kayanja MM: Histological evaluation of biopsies obtained from vertebral compression fractures: Unsuspected myeloma and osteomalacia. *Spine* 2005;30:781-786.

104. Belkoff SM, Mathis JM, Jasper LE, Deramond H: The biomechanics of vertebroplasty: The effect of cement volume on mechanical behavior. *Spine* 2001;26:1537-1541.

105. Bauer TW, Schils J: The pathology of total joint arthroplasty: I. Mechanisms of implant fixation. *Skeletal Radiol* 1999;28:423-432.

106. Jang JS, Lee SH, Rhee CH, Lee SH: Polymethylmethacrylate-augmented screw fixation for stabilization in metastatic spinal tumors: Technical note. *J Neurosurg* 2002;96(1 Suppl):131-134.

107. Wada T, Kaya M, Nagoya S, et al: Complications associated with bone cementing for the treatment of giant cell tumors of bone. *J Orthop Sci* 2002;7:194-198.

108. Huang K-Y, Yan JJ, Lin RM: Histopathologic findings of retrieved specimens of vertebroplasty with polymethylmethacrylate cement: Case control study. *Spine* 2005;30:E585-E588.

109. Schildhauer TA, Bennett AP, Wright TM, Lane JM, O'Leary PF: Intravertebral body reconstruction with an injectable in situ-setting carbonated apatite: Biomechanical evaluation of a minimally invasive technique. *J Orthop Res* 1999;17:67-72.

110. Belkoff SM, Mathis JM, Erbe EM, Fenton DC: Biomechanical evaluation of a new bone cement for use in vertebroplasty. *Spine* 2000;25:1061-1064.

111. Barr JD, Barr MS, Lemley TJ, McCann RM: Percutaneous vertebroplasty for pain relief and spinal stabilization. *Spine* 2000;25:923-928.

112. Lim TH, Brebach GT, Renner SM, et al: Biomechanical evaluation of an injectable calcium phosphate cement for vertebroplasty. *Spine* 2002;27:1297-1302.

113. Boszczyk BM, Bierschneider M, Panzer S, et al: Fluoroscopic radiation exposure of the kyphoplasty patient. *Eur Spine J* 2006;15:347-355.

114. Harstall R, Heini PF, Mini RL, Orler R: Radiation exposure to the surgeon during fluoroscopically assisted percutaneous vertebroplasty: A prospective study. *Spine* 2005;30:1893-1898.

115. Kruger R, Faciszewski T: Radiation dose reduction to medical staff during vertebroplasty: A review of techniques and methods to mitigate occupational dose. *Spine* 2003;28:1608-1613.

116. Theocharopoulos N, Perisinakis K, Damilakis J, Papadokostakis G, Hadjipavlou A, Gourtsoyiannis N: Occupational exposure from common fluoroscopic projections used in orthopaedic surgery. *J Bone Joint Surg Am* 2003;85:1698-1703.

Radiculopathy and the Herniated Lumbar Disk: Controversies Regarding Pathophysiology and Management

John M. Rhee, MD
Michael K. Schaufele, MD
William A. Abdu, MD, MS

Abstract

Lumbar disk herniation is one of the most common problems encountered in orthopaedic practice. Despite the frequency of its occurrence, however, much about lumbar disk herniation is poorly understood. It is important to review the basic and clinical science underlying the pathophysiology and treatment, surgical and nonsurgical, of this disorder.

Instr Course Lect 2007;56:287-299.

Lumbar disk herniations remain among the most common diagnoses encountered in clinical spine practice. The incidence of symptomatic lumbar disk herniations in the American population has been estimated to be 1% to 2%,[1] for which approximately 200,000 lumbar diskectomies are performed annually.[2] Yet despite the frequency with which lumbar disk herniation occurs, there is substantial controversy regarding its pathophysiology and treatment. For example, from the standpoint of basic science, mounting evidence suggests that biochemical factors—in addition to the mechanical effects of the disk material on the nerve root—underlie the development of symptomatic radiculopathy, but those factors remain to be clearly elucidated. On the clinical end of the spectrum, large (fivefold to fifteenfold) variations[3] in the rates of lumbar surgery in geographically adjacent areas suggest radical heterogeneity in the application of surgical criteria to this diagnosis. In this chapter, the available basic science regarding the anatomy and pathophysiology of lumbar disk herniations is examined as well as the clinical evidence supporting nonsurgical compared with surgical management of this common, yet surprisingly poorly understood, orthopaedic disorder.

Anatomy of Lumbar Disk Herniation

Structurally, the lumbar disk has three components: the anulus fibrosus, which forms the circumferential rim of the disk; the nucleus pulposus, which comprises its central core; and the cartilaginous end plates on the adjacent vertebral bodies. The anulus fibrosus has a multilayer lamellar architecture made of collagen fibers. Within each layer, the collagen is oriented at approximately 30° to the horizontal. Each successive layer is oriented at 30° to the horizontal in the opposite direction, leading to a "crisscross" type pattern. This composition allows the anulus fibrosus, and in particular the outer anulus fibrosus, which has the highest tensile modulus, to resist torsional, axial, and tensile loads. The nucleus pulposus provides resistance to axial compression and is the principal determinant of disk height because of its unique composition consisting of large, highly charged proteoglycan macromolecules within a collagen matrix. These macromolecules are hydrophilic and are contained within the confines of the anulus fibrosus peripherally and the end plates above and below. Thus, imbibed water causes the nucleus to swell and to generate large hydrostatic pressures within the disk. A healthy nucleus consists of approximately 70% water. The nucleus also contains a cellular component of both fibroblast-like and chondrocyte-like cells. These cells maintain the matrix in which they exist, and they also receive metabolic nutrients that diffuse through the matrix.

The intervertebral disk is anatomically unique for several reasons. First, it is mostly avascular—it is the largest avascular structure in the body. Blood vessels lie on the surface of the anulus fibrosus but penetrate only a very short distance into the outer portions of the anulus fibrosus. Similarly, blood vessels from the vertebral body lie against the cartilaginous end plates but do not enter the central regions of the disk. As a result, disk cells derive their nutrition from diffusion through the end plates and connective tissue transport from one part of the matrix to the other. Second, the disk is only minimally innervated. Nerve endings are present only on the surface of the disk, and they penetrate a very short distance into the outer anulus fibrosus. The normal inner anulus fibrosus and nucleus completely lack innervation. In contrast, the posterior and anterior longitudinal ligaments are innervated. The anterior longitudinal ligament receives nerve branches from the segmental ventral ramus and sympathetic trunk. The posterior longitudinal ligament is innervated by a branch of the dorsal root ganglion known as the sinuvertebral nerve. Experimental studies of patients undergoing diskectomy with local anesthetic have demonstrated that surgical stimulation of the posterior longitudinal ligament can cause low back pain.[4] Thus, stimulation of the sinuvertebral nerve may be one mediator of the low back pain component associated with lumbar disk hernia-

tions and annular tears.

The terminology used to describe the spectrum of lumbar disk herniations varies and is often confusing; however, when properly applied, it provides useful descriptive information. One useful method of classifying disk herniations is according to whether the herniated fragments are "contained" or "noncontained" by the anulus fibrosus.[5] A protrusion is a focal bulging of nuclear material contained by the anulus fibrosus (that is, the annular fibers remain continuous and attached to the vertebral bodies). Subannular extrusions occur when the anulus fibrosus remains intact but the fragment has migrated behind the body either above or below the disk while maintaining continuity with the disk. Transannular extruded disk herniations occur when the fragments have ruptured through the anulus fibrosus but maintain continuity with the disk space of origin. A sequestration arises when the material has not only broken through the anulus fibrosus but has also migrated away from the disk space of origin and is no longer in contact with it. Any of the three components of the intervertebral disk (the nucleus, anulus fibrosus, or end plate), alone or in combination, may be the offending material when a disk herniates.

Pathophysiology of Lumbar Disk Herniation

The origins of the modern era of lumbar disk surgery can be traced to the seminal work of Mixter and Barr[6] 70 years ago. Those authors found that sciatic pain could be relieved by removing herniated disk material compressing a nerve root. Logically, the association was made between lumbar disk herniation and the clinical entity of sciatica. That finding led to the general assump-

tion that mechanical compression of the nerve root is the primary pathogenic factor inducing radiculopathy. Several lines of evidence support this notion. First, the structure of the nerve root renders it relatively poorly resistant to compression. Like peripheral nerves, nerve roots have an endoneurium. However, the layers equivalent to the perineurium and epineurium are cerebrospinal fluid and dural lining, respectively. Thus, the nerve root is a comparatively delicate structure that is not well insulated to resist compressive forces. Second, because nerve roots are tethered to the vertebral body at their takeoff from the common dural sac and to the subjacent pedicle within the foramen by ligamentous attachments, a disk herniation ventral to the root is poised to generate high tensile forces. The situation is analogous to the tension generated in a bowstring by the pull of an archer's hand. Third, animal models of cauda equina compression have demonstrated that compression of a nerve root impairs its nutrition. In a series of experiments, Olmarker and associates[7,8] showed that mechanical compression on nerve roots within the porcine cauda equina led to decreased nutrient delivery by reducing both blood flow and nutrient diffusion from cerebrospinal fluid. Histologically, compressed nerve roots demonstrate evidence of intraneural edema, which can directly lead to nerve fibrosis and injury. Alternatively, intraneural edema can secondarily lead to an intraneural "compartment syndrome," as pressures within the nerve root overcome perfusion pressures, resulting in nerve root ischemia and injury.[9]

Although this and other studies suggest that the mechanical effect of a herniated disk is the main factor in the genesis of radiculopathy, other lines of evidence indicate that mechanical compression alone may not be a sufficient cause for the radiculopathy associated with herniated disks. First, MRI studies have shown that nerve root compression is often asymptomatic (Figure 1). Boden and associates[10] found that, in a group of people who had never had radicular pain, 20% of those under the age of 60 years and 36% of those over the age of 60 years had evidence of a herniated disk on MRI. Second, other reports have suggested that, although irritated nerve roots demonstrate susceptibility to mechanical compression, normal (nonsensitized) roots do not. Smyth and Wright[11] found that, when sutures placed around nerve roots at the time of surgery were tugged postoperatively, only those roots that had been noted at surgery to be compressed by a herniated disk generated a radicular pain response. When there had been no intraoperative evidence of root compression by a herniated disk, tugging on the suture and creating tension in the root postoperatively did not elicit radicular symptoms. Kuslich and associates[4] performed lumbar diskectomy, using local anesthesia, on awake patients and found that surgical stimulation of compressed roots caused pain 90% of the time, whereas manipulation of normal roots provoked pain only 9% of the time. These observations suggest that a nerve root needs to be sensitized to be mechanically susceptible and that mechanical compression alone is not the sine qua non of radiculopathy.

A growing body of evidence has implicated bioactive molecules within the disk as important in sensitizing nerve roots and participating in the pathogenesis of radiculopathy. Olmarker and associates[12] re-

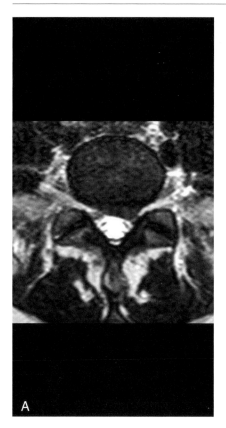
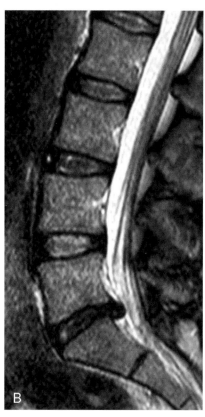

Figure 1 Asymptomatic posterolateral disk herniation in a 45-year-old woman with pain in the right leg. She had absolutely no symptoms in the left leg, despite the axial **(A)** and sagittal **(B)** T2-weighted MRIs demonstrating an extruded left L5-S1 disk herniation. Asymptomatic disk herniations are not uncommon, underlying the need to treat symptoms rather than MRI findings per se.

ported that, when autogenous nucleus pulposus was applied to the porcine cauda equina, physiologic and anatomic evidence suggestive of radiculopathy was noted, even in the absence of any nerve root compression. Compared with control animals in which autologous fat had been applied epidurally, those in which nucleus pulposus had been applied demonstrated a decrease in nerve conduction velocity and histologic evidence of nerve fiber degeneration (axonal swelling and demyelination). This study suggested that nuclear material could itself lead to neural injury in the absence of mechanical compression. Authors of later studies attempted to deter-

mine whether the observed changes in nerve structure and electrophysiology correlated with a clinical syndrome of radiculopathy. In one such study, rats underwent laminectomy and were randomized to one of three groups: (1) incision of the disk such that nuclear contents could come into contact with, but not displace, the nerve root; (2) displacement of the nerve root by placement of a pin into the vertebral body that deflected the course of the root but no incision of the disk; or (3) incision of the disk and displacement of the nerve root with the vertebral body pin.[13] Only the animals that had both disk incision and root displacement displayed behaviors consistent with pain and radiculopathy.

The picture emerging is that disk herniation-associated radiculopathy is both a biochemical and a mechanical disorder. Several bioactive molecules known to be present in the nucleus pulposus, including interleukins and other inflammatory factors,[14-16] have been purported to be biochemical "sensitizers" capable of making nerve roots susceptible to the mechanical effect of the herniated mass. Tumor necrosis factor-α (TNF-α) has received considerable attention in this regard. In the porcine model, TNF-α caused reductions in nerve conduction velocity similar to those seen with autologous nucleus pulposus, whereas interleukin 1β (IL-1β) and interferon gamma (INF-γ) did not.[17] Furthermore, TNF-α inhibition with infliximab (a monoclonal antibody to TNF-α) blocked the pain behaviors noted above after the performance of disk incision and root displacement in rats.[18] Overall, the roles of TNF-α and other bioactive agents in herniated disk-associated radiculopathy remain poorly undiagnosed.

Epidemiology and Natural History

Various studies have shown that the lifetime prevalence of a major episode of low back pain ranges from 60% to 80%, but only 10% of these episodes are accompanied by sciatica. Sciatica lasting longer than 2 weeks is even less common, with a lifetime prevalence of 1.6%.[19] The highest prevalence (23.7 per 100 persons) is in individuals between the ages of 45 and 64 years.[20] A sedentary lifestyle, frequent driving, chronic cough, pregnancy, smoking, and frequent lifting of heavy objects are considered risk factors.[19,21,22]

It is commonly agreed that lumbar disk herniation has a favorable natural history (that is, the clinical course of the disease without therapeutic intervention). Hakelius[23] examined essentially a natural history cohort, in that the patients were treated with only bed rest and a corset for 2 months, and he observed a marked reduction in pain and improvement in function over time: 80% of the patients had major improvements after 6 weeks; 90%, after 12 weeks; and 93%, after 24 weeks. Other studies have revealed less favorable results in that, although most patients without surgical treatment had improvement, 30% had persistent pain and restrictions at work and leisure activities after 1 year.[24] Most disk herniations diminish in size over time, with 80% decreasing by more than 50% in one study.[25] Larger disk herniations tend to regress more, most likely because of their higher water content. A positive correlation has been noted between regression of lumbar disk herniations and resolution of symptoms,[25,26] and regression is thought to occur as the herniated tissue dehydrates and immunologic responses help to resorb the disk material. In terms of motor function, Hakelius did not find a significant advantage to surgical treatment of patients with stable motor deficits (excluding those with cauda equina syndrome): 45% of such patients had improvement with nonsurgical treatment, and 53% had improvement after surgery.

Evidence Regarding Nonsurgical Treatment

Currently accepted indications for nonsurgical treatment of lumbar disk herniations include the absence of a progressive neurologic deficit or cauda equina syndrome. Thus, nonsurgical treatment is the initial "default" pathway for most patients with lumbar radiculopathy due to disk herniation. It is not clear, however, whether nonsurgical treatment offers improvement over the natural history of the disorder. Although there have been numerous studies of nonsurgical treatments of low back pain, there have been few randomized controlled trials specifically comparing the various nonsurgical regimens (physical therapy, medications, traction, manipulation, immobilization, and spinal injections) with the natural history (no treatment at all). However, predictors of favorable outcomes of nonsurgical care have been reported to include a negative result on the crossed straight leg-raising test, absence of leg pain with spinal extension, absence of stenosis on imaging studies, favorable response to steroids, return of neurologic deficits within 12 weeks, a motivated physically fit patient with more than 12 years of education, no workers' compensation claim, and a normal psychological profile.[27] Nonsurgical treatment of noncontained disk herniations may also have a favorable outcome.[28]

Medications

Commonly used medications for pain associated with lumbar disk herniations include nonsteroidal anti-inflammatory drugs, corticosteroids, muscle relaxants, and opioid pain medications. Nonsteroidal anti-inflammatory drugs have been shown to be helpful for the management of acute low back pain,[29] but a meta-analysis of the literature demonstrated that they had no benefit in the treatment of radiculopathy compared with controls (odds ratio = 0.99).[30] Corticosteroids are administered orally or by injection. Although oral steroids are commonly prescribed in clinical practice, only one study on their use for the treatment of lumbosacral radicular pain was found.[31] In that study, dexamethasone was not superior to a placebo for either early or long-term relief of lumbosacral radicular pain, but it helped patients who had presented with a positive result on the straight leg raising test. The use of intramuscular corticosteroid injections for acute sciatica was examined in two randomized controlled trials. One trial showed no benefit (odds ratio = 0.8),[32] and the other trial showed a modest benefit (odds ratio = 2.0).[33] We are not aware of any randomized clinical trials that tested the effectiveness of opioid analgesics for patients with lumbar disk herniations, although such analgesics are commonly used in clinical practice for the treatment of acute and chronic radiculopathies. Muscle relaxants have been shown to be effective for the treatment of acute low back pain,[34] but we found no data from well-controlled studies of their use for pain associated with lumbar disk herniations. Antiepileptics such as gabapentin and tricyclic antidepressants such as amitriptyline are commonly used to treat the neuropathic pain component associated with lumbar disk herniations. Again, we are not aware of any controlled trials of the use of those medications for patients who have lumbar disk herniation with radiculopathy, but one open, uncontrolled trial of lamotrigine showed a significant improvement in patients with chronic sciatica ($P < 0.05$).[35]

Physical Medicine

When a patient has incapacitating pain, a period of bed rest is often unavoidable. Immobilization presumably diminishes inflammation around an irritated nerve root. However, there are no data to suggest that bed rest alters the natural history of lumbar disk herniations or improves outcomes. Because of the potentially harmful effects of prolonged bed rest, it is best to advise patients to limit bed rest to a short term only and to resume activities as soon as possible.[36] Bracing is another method of immobilizing the lumbar spine, but there is a lack of good evidence to support the use of braces and corsets for patients with lumbar disk herniations. These devices have not been shown to be effective for primary or secondary prevention of low back pain; however, the Cochrane review found "limited" evidence favoring lumbar supports compared with no treatment.[37]

Traction remains of unproven benefit in the treatment of lumbar disk herniations. A meta-analysis of pooled data from four randomized controlled trials showed some benefit of traction therapy compared with a placebo (odds ratio = 1.2).[38] In one controlled trial, traction with physical therapy resulted in a greater reduction in the sizes of disk herniations than did physical therapy alone.[39] Vertebral axial decompression (VAX-D) therapy was developed according to the principles of traction and is popular among chiropractors. One randomized clinical trial, in which one of the authors was the medical director for a VAX-D manufacturer, demonstrated greater than 50% relief of chronic low back pain in 68.4% of patients treated with VAX-D therapy compared with 0% of patients treated with transcutaneous electrical nerve stimulation.[40] However, we are not aware of any studies of VAX-D therapy for patients with isolated lumbar disk herniation. The Cochrane Review in 2005 concluded that "traction is probably not effective" on the

basis of the finding that neither continuous nor intermittent traction was more effective for decreasing pain, disability, or work absence than were placebo, sham, or other treatments of patients with low back pain, with or without sciatica.[41]

Physical therapy in general has not been proven to be beneficial for patients with acute low back pain, but it may be helpful for those with chronic low back pain.[42] We are not aware of any randomized trials examining the outcomes of physical therapy alone for the treatment of lumbar radiculopathy. Active exercises are more appropriate than passive modalities, particularly for patients with subacute or chronic pain.[27] Hofstee and associates[43] showed that bed rest and physiotherapy are not more effective for the treatment of acute sciatica than is continuation of activities of daily living. McKenzie therapy is commonly advocated for treatment of lumbar disk herniations. However, in one study on the management of low back pain, there was no difference among the results of McKenzie therapy, manipulation, and providing the patient with an educational booklet.[44] Another common physical therapy technique involves the spectrum of lumbar stabilization exercises. Although randomized trials have not been performed, to our knowledge, outcomes of nonsurgical treatment have been better in studies employing active lumbar stabilization exercises[45] than they were in older controlled trials that used passive treatment modalities.[46]

Acupuncture is another physical medicine modality that might be applied to the treatment of lumbar disk herniations. Although anecdotal stories of success are extant in popular culture, the available literature has not demonstrated the efficacy of acupuncture in treating low back pain.[47] Manipulation and chiropractic are similarly unproven. Burton and associates[48] compared chemonucleolysis with manipulation in the treatment of symptomatic lumbar disk herniations in a controlled trial. After 12 months, there was no significant difference in overall outcome between the treatments, but manipulation did result in a greater decrease in back pain and disability during the first weeks. At a minimum, manipulation is relatively unlikely to cause harm: it has been estimated that less than 1 in 3.7 million treatments with spinal manipulation results in clinical worsening of disk herniation.[49] Other modalities that are commonly used in clinical practice include massage therapy, transcutaneous electrical nerve stimulation, and biofeedback. These methods have not been evaluated for the treatment of lumbar disk herniations and radiculopathy in well-controlled trials. Cognitive behavioral therapy has shown efficacy for the treatment of chronic low back pain,[50] but we are not aware of any studies of its effectiveness for patients with lumbar disk herniation.

Epidural Steroid Injections

Epidural steroid injections have been used for decades for the treatment of spinal pain, particularly radiculopathy. In a review of four older randomized trials, epidural steroid injections were found to be more beneficial than the control treatment, especially with respect to short-term outcomes, for the treatment of acute radiculopathy (odds ratio = 2.2).[38] A more recent study of interlaminar epidural steroid injections demonstrated a transient decrease in sciatic symptoms at 3 weeks but no sustained benefits in

terms of pain relief, function, or avoidance of surgery.[51] Epidural steroid injections also do not appear to change the rate at which lumbar disk herniations regress.[52]

Fluoroscopically guided transforaminal injection techniques, which have the theoretical advantage of delivering the injectate to the site of the disk herniation in the anterior epidural space, have been more commonly used in modern studies. Although the traditional, more dorsal interlaminar approaches may allow the injectate to flow to the site of the lesion by seeping around the thecal sac and into the ventral epidural space, a transforaminal route is presumably more reliable for delivering the steroid to the affected area, where the herniated disk comes into contact with the nerve root. One study showed transforaminal injections to be superior to trigger-point injections, with "successful" outcomes following 84% of the former procedures and 48% of the latter.[53] Other studies have suggested that transforaminal epidural steroid injections may actually change the natural history of radiculopathy by decreasing the need for surgery. In one study of 55 patients with lumbar radiculopathy who were all considered surgical candidates, 71% of those who received a steroid nerve-root injection and 33% of those who received a control injection of local anesthetic only decided not to have surgery.[54] Another study compared pain scores on a visual analog scale and the need for surgery between patients who had received transforaminal steroid injections and those who had received interlaminar epidural steroid injections.[55] The patients treated with the transforaminal injections had a 46% reduction in the pain score, and 10% went on to need surgery. In contrast, the pa-

tients treated with the interlaminar injections had a 19% reduction in the pain score, and 25% required surgery. These findings indicated that the short-term outcomes were better following transforaminal injections.

It is impossible to directly compare the literature on outcomes of surgical diskectomy with reports on outcomes of epidural injections because of the numerous differences in surgical technique (open, "minimally invasive," microdiskectomy, and aggressive disk-space curettage); injection technique (transforaminal or interlaminar, fluoroscopically guided or not); dose, timing, and type of steroid delivered; and patient selection criteria (in many studies, those with severe pain or progressive neurologic deficits were not considered candidates for nonsurgical treatment). In a recent study that provided level I evidence, 100 patients who had had failure of 6 weeks of noninvasive treatment of a disk herniation measuring at least 25% of the cross-sectional area of the spinal canal were randomized to be treated with interlaminar epidural injections or surgical diskectomy.[56] The success rates, which were 92% to 98% in the surgically treated group and 42% to 56% in the group treated with epidural injection, were significantly different. Twenty-seven patients crossed over from the epidural injection group to the surgical group because of persistent pain, but their outcomes were not adversely affected by the delay in surgery because of the trial of the epidural injection. Whether the transforaminal approach would have led to better outcomes of the epidural injections remains unclear, but, on the basis of this study, surgery appears to be more effective than injections, at least in patients with large disk herniations. Although informative, this finding does not change the commonly accepted indications for surgery, as surgery is associated with not only greater benefit but also with higher risk than epidural injections. Data from the United States National Institutes of Health-funded multicenter randomized trial comparing surgical with nonsurgical treatment of lumbar disk herniations, spinal stenosis, and spondylolisthesis (the Spine Patient Outcome Research Trial [SPORT] study) will hopefully provide clearer guidelines when they become available.

Novel Treatments

On the basis of the understanding that the mechanisms underlying herniated disk-associated radiculopathy are both biochemical and mechanical, novel treatments have been developed to attenuate biochemical sensitization of the nerve root by factors within the nucleus pulposus. As mentioned previously, TNF-α appears to play a role in the pathogenesis of radiculopathy associated with disk herniations. In a very small pilot trial in which 10 patients received a single intravenous injection of infliximab (a monoclonal antibody to TNF-α) for treatment of acute sciatica (lasting 2 to 12 weeks) due to disk herniation, 8 patients had no leg pain at 12 months, compared with 43% of a historical control population who had received saline solution nerve root blocks.[57] However, when a subsequent randomized controlled trial was performed by the same authors on the basis of these promising pilot data, they noted no difference in the reduction of leg pain or the need for surgery at 3 months between patients who had received a single dose of infliximab and controls.[58] Other authors reported success with medical ozone injections into the disk and around the nerve root,[59] although the

study lacked a control group treated without ozone. Various percutaneous, intradiskal treatments, such as electrothermal disk decompression, percutaneous disk decompression, and nucleoplasty, have been developed and marketed by manufacturers. However, the efficacy of these methods is yet to be demonstrated in properly controlled trials.

Overview of Nonsurgical Treatment

The available literature indicates that effective nonsurgical treatments of lumbar disk herniations include observation only as the condition has a favorable natural history, and probably epidural steroid injection, at least for short-term relief. Intramuscular injections of steroids may provide some benefit. Nonsteroidal anti-inflammatory drugs are effective for low back pain only, and traction is probably not effective. There are insufficient data to provide recommendations regarding the role of oral steroids, physical therapy, transcutaneous electrical stimulation, corsets, and manual therapy. On the horizon are medications to suppress reactive nerve root inflammation and medications to inhibit cytokine production, which may improve the pharmacologic treatment options for lumbar disk herniations.

Evidence Regarding Surgical Treatment

Despite the facts that more than $90 billion per year is spent on the management of spine conditions and more than seven decades have passed since Mixter and Barr reported on the surgical management of disk herniations, there remains little level I evidence regarding the effectiveness of surgery for symptomatic lumbar disk herniations. Although many retrospective studies have

suggested a benefit, these studies have the common weakness of inadequate design. The lack of level I data leads to widespread uncertainty with regard to the selection of patients for surgery, as reflected in the varied rates of disk excision surgery: there was a nearly twentyfold difference between high and low surgery rate regions in an otherwise controlled population analysis in the United States.[60,61] However, these statements should not be misconstrued as a condemnation of diskectomy surgery. Much to the contrary, under the right circumstances, surgery clearly "works" very well: any surgeon who has seen a patient suffer for months before surgery and then wake up from a diskectomy with immediate relief of leg pain, numbness, and weakness can attest to that fact. Instead, the question that remains unanswered by the available literature is that, given that not every patient has an excellent result from surgery, surgery has the potential for complications, and the natural history of lumbar disk herniation tends to be favorable in most patients, when and in whom should surgery be recommended?

Neurologic Variables

Although one might expect surgery to be superior to nonsurgical care of patients with stable neurologic deficits, this has not been supported by the available literature. Hakelius,[23] Weber,[46] the Maine Lumbar Spine Study,[60] and Saal[27,45] demonstrated that stable radicular weakness resolves equally well regardless of treatment. In a more recent pilot study of 60 patients with stable paresis associated with lumbar disk herniation, Dubourg and associates[62] also found no difference between neurologic recovery following surgical management and that following medical management. This finding is in contrast to the situation for a patient with a progressive neurologic deficit and cauda equina syndrome, for whom, the evidence suggests, urgent decompression provides the best functional improvement.[63]

Surgical Volume

Increased surgical volume has been correlated with improved outcomes of several operations, including joint arthroplasty, cardiac surgery, and cancer surgery, suggesting that a surgeon's experience and skill as well as the hospital's overall experience play important roles in outcomes. Paradoxically, the same may not be true for lumbar diskectomy. The Maine Lumbar Spine Study showed that patients who had surgery in the highest utilization regions actually had worse outcomes than those treated in the lowest utilization area.[64] The authors concluded that these paradoxically inferior results may be related to the application of more stringent criteria for surgery in regions with lower surgical rates and expanded indications beyond what might be considered the standard in the higher rate regions. Thus, patient selection and patient factors may have a greater influence than surgical technique on the results of spine surgery, for which the indications are not as clear-cut as they are for the types of surgery listed above.

Anatomic Features of the Herniation

Although the size of a disk herniation correlates poorly with pain, there is evidence to suggest that other anatomic characteristics of the herniated disk may be predictive of clinical outcome following diskectomy. In one study,[65] patients who had extruded disk fragments with a

largely intact anulus fibrosus and those who had extruded fragments contained within an intact anulus fibrosus had the best postoperative outcome scores and the lowest reherniation rates. The scores were poorer for those who had extruded disk fragments with a massive annular defect as well as for those who had no identifiable fragment within an intact anulus fibrosus. Those with a massive annular defect had the highest rate of reherniation, whereas those without identifiable fragments had a high rate of persistent symptoms postoperatively despite the absence of clear structural abnormalities to account for them. This last group of patients had a clinical profile (for example, with regard to compensation status and psychometric abnormalities) that was similar to that of patients with chronic low back pain: both had pain behavior that was out of proportion to the anatomic pathologic findings.

Contrary to popular opinion, the size of a disk herniation does not appear to correlate with the need for eventual surgical intervention. Natural history studies[27,66-68] have shown that the largest disk herniations actually demonstrate the greatest degree of resorption, whereas contained herniations demonstrate the least. Thus, the disk abnormality that seems to be best suited for surgery—a large extruded fragment—also has the greatest likelihood of natural regression; this means that size cannot be used reliably as a criterion for surgery.

Variations in Surgical Technique

Although various surgical techniques have been used to decompress symptomatic nerves, the data suggest that the choice of surgical technique is less critical to a good

outcome than proponents of various techniques have suggested.[69] To date, there has been no proven difference in outcomes regardless of whether the root is decompressed by means of a traditional ("large incision") laminotomy-diskectomy, an endoscopic diskectomy, or a microdiskectomy (Figure 2).

The optimal amount of disk that should be removed during surgery is not clear. Although it has been established that the primary goal of surgery is neural decompression, competing considerations remain: too little removal seemingly raises the specter of increased recurrence, whereas too much removal raises concerns about accelerated disk degeneration and increased back pain. The available evidence, based largely on case reports and retrospective studies, suggests no benefit to more aggressive disk removal in terms of recurrence; to the contrary, it may be deleterious with respect to the later development of back pain.[70-73] Lumbar disk herniations recur at about equal rates (approximately 5%) regardless of treatment, and neither surgical intervention nor medical management can prevent reherniation.

Patient Factors Affecting Surgical Outcome

Although traditionally, spinal research has focused on physician-determined outcomes—such as a physician's assessment of relief of symptoms (for example, according to Odom's criteria),[74] radiographic evidence of a successful fusion, and the magnitude of deformity correction—it has become increasingly evident that the most useful measure of a given operation's success is whether the patient perceives it to be successful, regardless of what the physician-determined outcomes

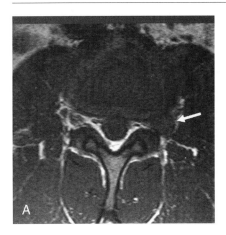 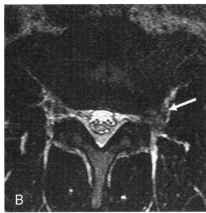 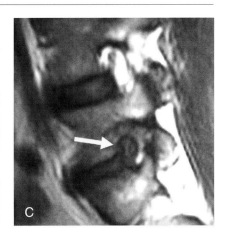

Figure 2 Axial T1-weighted (**A**) and T2-weighted (**B**) MRI scans of a patient with an extraforaminal disk herniation (arrows). This type of herniation is more readily removed by an extraforaminal approach rather than from inside the spinal canal. Extraforaminal herniations are often better seen on T1-weighted images and are more likely to be missed on T2-weighted images. Posterolateral disk herniations, in contrast, are generally well demonstrated on T2-weighted images (see Figure 1). **C,** The sagittal T1-weighted image of a different patient demonstrates that the exiting nerve root is pinned cephalad against the undersurface of the pedicle by the foraminal portion of the disk herniation.

may demonstrate. The patient's perception of successful treatment, in turn, appears to be influenced at least as much by psychosocial and other patient factors as it is by the specific type of disk lesion or the design and execution of a proper operation by the treating surgeon. Patient-reported health surveys, which allow self-evaluation of function, are useful tools for assessing these patient factors preoperatively and postoperatively.[75-77] The health surveys include both condition-specific surveys, such as the Roland-Morris Disability Questionnaire and the Oswestry Disability Index (ODI), and the commonly used general health survey, the Short Form-36 (SF-36).[78-80] Although the outcomes measured by the SF-36 are not specific to the spine, it is useful for measuring the outcomes of spine surgery because spinal disorders have been shown to impart a substantial negative effect on self-reported physical function. As demonstrated in one study by the Physical Component Score (PCS) of the SF-36, spinal stenosis had a greater

negative effect on physical function than all other medical conditions studied with use of the SF-36,[81] including cancer, chronic obstructive pulmonary disease, and congestive heart failure.

Studies of self-reported health surveys have identified several patient factors with significant effects on patient-determined outcomes after spine surgery. In one such study, smoking had a significant negative effect ($P < 0.05$) on self-reported function at baseline as measured by all eight subscales of the SF-36.[82] One year after spinal surgery, smokers did not have significant improvement in the scores on any subscale of the SF-36, whereas their non-smoking counterparts had significantly improved scores on six subscales ($P < 0.05$). In another study, a low education level was an independent predictor of poor self-reported function at baseline as measured with both the condition-specific ODI and the SF-36 general health survey.[83] It was also noted that the major drivers of physical function as measured by the SF-36 and ODI were psychoso-

cial variables rather than traditional medical conditions. In addition to low education level, these other variables included poor self-reported health, work and disability status, legal status, body mass index, and smoking. In a related study, self-reported health was also found to be an independent predictor of functional outcome following surgery.[84] Of 1833 patients who had undergone surgical intervention for lumbar disk herniation, those reporting "good" health and "poor" health both had improvement following surgical intervention. However, there was a significant difference ($P < 0.05$) between the groups with respect to scores on the SF-36 bodily pain and physical function components as well as the ODI scores, with those reporting good health faring better. Other studies have also demonstrated a negative effect of patient factors such as depression, frequent headaches, compensation status, low education level, and unemployment on both the ODI and the PCS of the SF-36.[85]

Taken together, these studies

demonstrate that proper selection of patients for lumbar diskectomy should include a thorough assessment of patient factors as such factors have important effects on function and on the response to treatment independent of the specifics regarding the disk lesion. Identifying these factors can assist providers and patients in decision-making as well as guide reasonable expectations from surgery. In certain patient populations, the effect of low back problems may be a greater reflection of psychosocial distress than anatomic dysfunction, which may explain why the traditional surgical model of treating spinal problems fails in many patients. If patients and surgeons are not aware of this association between patient factors and functional outcome, both may be disappointed with the results.

Medical Comorbidities Affecting Surgical Outcome

The presence of comorbidities also has a significant effect on surgical outcomes. In one study, the presence of four comorbidities was noted to significantly ($P < 0.05$) and independently lower the improvement in the ODI score by almost five points and the improvement in the SF-36 score by more than four points at 1 year after lumbar spine surgery.[86] In another study, of 15,974 patients, obesity had a negative influence on self-reported function, as measured by both the SF-36 and the ODI, and obese patients reported a greater degree of pain than nonobese patients.[87]

Surgical Compared With Nonsurgical Treatment

There is a dearth of level I evidence comparing surgical with nonsurgical management of lumbar disk herniations. In 1983, Weber's classic work,

"Lumbar Disc Herniation. A Controlled, Prospective Study with Ten Years of Observation,"[46] included a randomized trial (the first randomized trial in spinal surgery) in which 60 patients had surgery and 66 continued to be treated with conservative measures. Weber found that those treated with surgery had a significantly better result at 1 year postoperatively ($P < 0.05$). At 4 years postoperatively, the surgically treated patients had a trend toward better results, but that difference was not present at 10 years. The surgically treated patients had far fewer relapses than the nonsurgically treated group in the first 4 years. Motor weakness improved equally in both groups, as did sensory dysfunction. Thirty-five percent of the patients, equally distributed in the two groups, had demonstrable sensory dysfunction 10 years after the hospitalization for the herniated lumbar intervertebral disk. Although it was a breakthrough study, it did have flaws. Not all of the patients were randomized: 67 additional patients had "symptoms and signs that beyond doubt required surgical therapy" and 87 others were treated "conservatively as there was no indication for operative intervention." Furthermore, a large number of nonsurgically treated patients crossed over into the surgical group, the study lacked adequate statistical power, the outcome assessment was not blinded, and the outcome measurement was relatively insensitive.[88]

More recently, the Maine Lumbar Spine Study, an observational (nonrandomized) study of 507 patients (with follow-up data available for 400 of them), compared the 10-year results of surgical and nonsurgical treatment.[60] As would be expected with an observational study,

the surgically treated patients had had worse baseline symptoms and functional status than the nonsurgically treated patients. Despite that fact, over the 10-year period, the proportion of patients who reported that their low back pain and leg pain were greatly decreased or completely gone was larger in the surgically treated group than in the nonsurgically treated group (56% compared with 40%, $P = 0.006$), and more surgically treated patients than nonsurgically treated patients were satisfied with their current status (71% compared with 56%, $P = 0.002$). The greatest improvement in the surgically treated group occurred in the first 2 years after the operation. There was smaller but continued improvement in both groups through the 10-year period.

Overview of Surgery for Lumbar Disk Herniations

Regardless of treatment, lumbar disk herniations usually have a favorable natural history with improvement over time, but it may take 1 to 2 years for functional improvement to plateau. In the absence of a cauda equina syndrome or progressive weakness, the best indication for surgical management is refractory radicular pain. Surgical decision-making should not be based on the size of the disk herniation, as large extruded herniations tend to resolve more predictably, or on either stable motor weakness or numbness, as the ultimate resolution of weakness and sensory deficits is similar following either nonsurgical or surgical management, although surgery hastens the process. When intractable radicular pain is the strict indication for surgery, surgical intervention provides substantial and more rapid pain relief than does nonsurgical treatment.

The specific method of surgical intervention probably contributes little to the overall success of the intervention as long as the root is properly decompressed.

The treatment should be chosen by the patient—after proper education through a process of shared decision-making—rather than reflect the "surgical signature" of the surgeon. Health surveys can provide additional assessment of psychosocial comorbidities that are not otherwise evident during the usual clinical evaluation. Such comorbidities should be identified preoperatively as they are not likely to resolve with surgical intervention but may have greater impact than the diskal pathoanatomy on the ultimate outcome.

Summary
Both mechanical and biomechanical factors play roles in the development of lumbar radiculopathy with disk herniation. In most instances, symptoms resolve with time. Nonsurgical treatments such as physical therapy, medications, and spinal injections may provide symptom relief, but none have been demonstrated to conclusively alter the natural history of the condition. When pain persists despite time and conservative care, surgical decompression of the nerve root provides predictable relief of radicular leg pain.

References

1. Deyo RA, Tsui-Wu YJ: Descriptive epidemiology of low-back pain and its related medical care in the United States. *Spine* 1987;12:264-268.

2. Taylor VM, Deyo RA, Cherkin DC, Kreuter W: Low back pain hospitalization: Recent United States trends and regional variations. *Spine* 1994;19:1207-1213.

3. Atlas SJ, Deyo RA, Keller RB, et al: The Maine Lumbar Spine Study, Part II: 1-year outcomes of surgical and nonsurgical management of sciatica. *Spine* 1996;21:1777-1786.

4. Kuslich SD, Ulstrom CL, Michael CJ: The tissue origin of low back pain and sciatica: A report of pain response to tissue stimulation during operations on the lumbar spine using local anesthesia. *Orthop Clin North Am* 1991;22:181-187.

5. McCulloch JA, Young PH: Pathophysiology and clinical syndromes in lumbar disc herniation, in McCulloch JA, Young PH (eds): *Essentials of Spinal Microsurgery*. Philadelphia, PA, Lippincott-Raven, 1998, pp 219-247.

6. Mixter WJ, Barr JS: Rupture of the intervertebral disk with involvement of the spinal canal. *N Engl J Med* 1934;211:210-215.

7. Olmarker K, Rydevik B, Holm S, Bagge U: Effects of experimental graded compression on blood flow in spinal nerve roots: A vital microscopic study on the porcine cauda equina. *J Orthop Res* 1989;7:817-823.

8. Olmarker K, Rydevik B, Hansson T, Holm S: Compression-induced changes of the nutritional supply to the porcine cauda equina. *J Spinal Disord* 1990;3:25-29.

9. Rydevik BL, Myers RR, Powell HC: Pressure increase in the dorsal root ganglion following mechanical compression: Closed compartment syndrome in nerve roots. *Spine* 1989;14:574-576.

10. Boden SD, Davis DO, Dina TS, Patronas NJ, Wiesel SW: Abnormal magnetic-resonance scans of the lumbar spine in asymptomatic subjects: A prospective investigation. *J Bone Joint Surg Am* 1990;72:403-408.

11. Smyth MJ, Wright V: Sciatica and the intervertebral disc: An experimental study. *J Bone Joint Surg Am* 1958;40:1401-1418.

12. Olmarker K, Rydevik B, Nordborg C: Autologous nucleus pulposus induces neurophysiologic and histologic changes in porcine cauda equina nerve roots. *Spine* 1993;18:1425-1432.

13. Olmarker K, Larsson K: Tumor necrosis factor alpha and nucleus-pulposus-induced nerve root injury. *Spine* 1998;23:2538-2544.

14. Brisby H, Byrod G, Olmarker K, Miller VM, Aoki Y, Rydevik B: Nitric oxide as a mediator of nucleus pulposus-induced effects on spinal nerve roots. *J Orthop Res* 2000;18:815-820.

15. Kang JD, Georgescu HI, McIntyre-Larkin L, Stefanovic-Racic M, Donaldson WF III, Evans CH: Herniated lumbar intervertebral discs spontaneously produce matrix metalloproteinases, nitric oxide, interleukin-6, and prostaglandin E2. *Spine* 1996;21:271-277.

16. Miyamoto H, Saura R, Doita M, Kurosaka M, Mizuno K: The role of cyclooxygenase-2 in lumbar disc herniation. *Spine* 2002;27:2477-2483.

17. Aoki Y, Rydevik B, Kikuchi S, Olmarker K: Local application of disc-related cytokines on spinal nerve roots. *Spine* 2002;27:1614-1617.

18. Murata Y, Olmarker K, Takahashi I, Takahashi K, Rydevik B: Effects of selective tumor necrosis factor-alpha inhibition to pain-behavioral changes caused by nucleus pulposus-induced damage to the spinal nerve in rats. *Neurosci Lett* 2005;382:148-152.

19. Kelsey JL, White AA III: Epidemiology and impact of low-back pain. *Spine* 1980;5:133-142.

20. Praemer A, Furner S, Rice DP: *Musculoskeletal Conditions in the United States*, ed 2. Rosemont, IL, American Academy of Orthopaedic Surgeons, 1999.

21. Kelsey JL: An epidemiological study of the relationship between occupations and acute herniated lumbar intervertebral discs. *Int J Epidemiol* 1975;4:197-205.

22. Kelsey JL, Githens PB, O'Conner T, et al: Acute prolapsed lumbar intervertebral disc: An epidemiologic study with special reference to driving automobiles and cigarette smoking. *Spine* 1984;9:608-613.

23. Hakelius A: Prognosis in sciatica: A clinical follow-up of surgical and non-surgical treatment. *Acta Orthop Scand Suppl* 1970;129:1-76.

24. Weber H: The natural history of disc herniation and the influence of intervention. *Spine* 1994;19:2234-2238.

25. Saal JA, Saal JS, Herzog RJ: The natural history of lumbar intervertebral disc extrusions treated nonoperatively. *Spine* 1990;15:683-686.

26. Bush K, Cowan N, Katz DE, Gishen P: The natural history of sciatica associated with disc pathology: A prospective study with clinical and independent radiologic follow-up. *Spine* 1992;17:1205-1212.

27. Saal JA: Natural history and nonoperative treatment of lumbar disc herniation. *Spine* 1996;21(24 suppl):2S-9S.

28. Ito T, Takano Y, Yuasa N: Types of lumbar herniated disc and clinical course. *Spine* 2001;26:648-651.

29. van Tulder MW, Scholten RJ, Koes BW, Deyo RA: Nonsteroidal anti-inflammatory drugs for low back pain: A systematic review within the framework of the Cochrane Collaboration Back Review Group. *Spine* 2000;25:2501-2513.

30. Vroomen PC, De Krom MC, Slofstra PD, Knottnerus JA: Conservative treatment of sciatica: A systematic review. *J Spinal Disord* 2000;13:463-469.

31. Haimovic IC, Beresford HR: Dexamethasone is not superior to placebo for treating lumbosacral radicular pain. *Neurology* 1986;36:1593-1594.

32. Porsman O, Friis H: Prolapsed lumbar disc treated with intramuscularly administered dexamethasonephosphate: A prospectively planned, double-blind, controlled clinical trial in 52 patients. *Scand J Rheumatol* 1979;8:142-144.

33. Hofferberth B, Gottschaldt M, Grass H, Buttner K: [The usefulness of dexamethasonephosphate in the conservative treatment of lumbar pain—a double-blind study]. *Arch Psychiatr Nervenkr* 1982;231:359-367

34. van Tulder MW, Touray T, Furlan AD, Solway S, Bouter LM, Cochrane Back Review Group: Muscle relaxants for nonspecific low back pain: A systematic review within the framework of the Cochrane Collaboration. *Spine* 2003;28:1978-1992.

35. Eisenberg E, Damunni G, Hoffer E, Baum Y, Krivoy N: Lamotrigine for intractable sciatica: Correlation between dose, plasma concentration and analgesia. *Eur J Pain* 2003;7:485-491.

36. Hagen KB, Hilde G, Jamtvedt G, Winnem MF: The Cochrane review of bed rest for acute low back pain and sciatica. *Spine* 2000;25:2932-2939.

37. Van Tulder MW, Jellema P, van Poppel MN, Nachemson AL, Bouter LM: Lumbar supports for prevention and treatment of low back pain. *Cochrane Database Syst Rev* 2000;3:CD001823.

38. Vroomen PC, de Krom MC, Slofstra PD, Knottnerus JA: Conservative treatment of sciatica: a systematic review. *J Spinal Disord* 2000;13:463-469.

39. Ozturk B, Gunduz OH, Ozoran K, Bostanoglu S: Effect of continuous lumbar traction on the size of herniated disc material in lumbar disc herniation. *Rheumatol Int* 2006;26:622-626.

40. Sherry E, Kitchener P, Smart R: A prospective randomized controlled study of VAX-D and TENS for the treatment of chronic low back pain. *Neurol Res* 2001;23:780-784.

41. Clarke JA, van Tulder MW, Blomberg SE, de Vet HC, van der Heijden GJ, Bronfort G: Traction for low-back pain with or without sciatica. *Cochrane Database Syst Rev* 2005;4:CD003010.

42. van Tulder MW, Malmivaara A, Esmail R, Koes BW: Exercise therapy for low back pain. *Cochrane Database Syst Rev* 2000;2:CD000335.

43. Hofstee DJ, Gijtenbeek JM, Hoogland PH, et al: Westeinde sciatica trial: Randomized controlled study of bed rest and physiotherapy for acute sciatica. *J Neurosurg* 2002;96(1 Suppl):45-49.

44. Cherkin DC, Deyo RA, Battie M, Street J, Barlow W: A comparison of physical therapy, chiropractic manipulation, and provision of an educational booklet for the treatment of patients with low back pain. *N Engl J Med* 1998;339:1021-1029.

45. Saal JA, Saal JS: Nonoperative treatment of herniated lumbar intervertebral disc with radiculopathy: An outcome study. *Spine* 1989;14:431-437.

46. Weber H: Lumbar disc herniation. A controlled, prospective study with ten years of observation. *Spine* 1983;8:131-140.

47. van Tulder MW, Cherkin DC, Berman B, Lao L, Koes BW: The effectiveness of acupuncture in the management of acute and chronic low back pain: A systematic review within the framework of the Cochrane Collaboration Back Review Group. *Spine* 1999;24:1113-1123.

48. Burton AK, Tillotson KM, Cleary J: Single-blind randomised controlled trial of chemonucleolysis and manipulation in the treatment of symptomatic lumbar disc herniation. *Eur Spine J* 2000;9:202-207.

49. Oliphant D: Safety of spinal manipulation in the treatment of lumbar disk herniations: A systematic review and risk assessment. *J Manipulative Physiol Ther* 2004;27:197-210.

50. van Tulder MW, Ostelo R, Vlaeyen JW, Linton SJ, Morley SJ, Assendelft WJ: Behavioral treatment for chronic low back pain: A systematic review within the framework of the Cochrane Back Review Group. *Spine* 2000;25:2688-2699.

51. Arden NK, Price C, Reading I, et al; WEST Study Group.: A multicentre randomized controlled trial of epidural corticosteroid injections for sciatica: The WEST study. *Rheumatology (Oxford)* 2005;44:1399-1406.

52. Buttermann GR: Lumbar disc herniation regression after successful epidural steroid injection. *J Spinal Disord Tech* 2002;15:469-476.

53. Vad VB, Bhat AL, Lutz GE, Cammisa F: Transforaminal epidural steroid injections in lumbosacral radiculopathy: A prospective randomized study. *Spine* 2002;27:11-16.

54. Riew KD, Yin Y, Gilula L, et al: The effect of nerve-root injections on the need for operative treatment of lumbar radicular pain: A prospective, randomized, controlled, double-blind study. *J Bone Joint Surg Am* 2000;82:1589-1593.

55. Schaufele M, Hatch L: Interlaminar versus transforaminal epidural injections in the treatment of symptomatic lumbar intervertebral disc herniations. *Arch Phys Med Rehabil* 2002;83:1661.

56. Buttermann GR: Treatment of lumbar disc herniation: epidural steroid injection compared with discectomy: A prospective, randomized study. *J Bone Joint Surg Am* 2004;86:670-679.

57. Korhonen T, Karppinen J, Malmivaara A, et al: Efficacy of infliximab for disc herniation-induced sciatica: One-year follow-up. *Spine* 2004;29:2115-2119.

58. Korhonen T, Karppinen J, Paimela L, et al: The treatment of disc herniation-induced sciatica with infliximab: Results of a randomized, controlled, 3-month follow-up study. *Spine* 2005;30:2724-2728.

59. Andreula CF, Simonetti L, De Santis F, Agati R, Ricci R, Leonardi M: Minimally invasive oxygen-ozone therapy for lumbar disk herniation. *AJNR Am J Neuroradiol* 2003;24:996-1000.

60. Atlas SJ, Keller RB, Wu YA, Deyo RA, Singer DE: Long-term outcomes of surgical and nonsurgical management of sciatica secondary to a lumbar disc herniation: 10 year results from the Maine Lumbar Spine Study. *Spine* 2005;30:927-935.

61. Weinstein JN, Birkmeyer JD: *The Dartmouth Atlas of Musculoskeletal Health Care*. Chicago, IL, American Hospital Association Press, 2000.

62. Dubourg G, Rozenberg S, Fautrel B, et al: A pilot study on the recovery from paresis after lumbar disc herniation. *Spine* 2002;27:1426-1431.

63. Ahn UM, Ahn NU, Buchowski JM, Garrett ES, Sieber AN, Kostuik JP:

Cauda equina syndrome secondary to lumbar disc herniation: A meta-analysis of surgical outcomes. *Spine* 2000;25:1515-1522.

64. Keller RB, Atlas SJ, Singer DE, et al: The Maine Lumbar Spine Study, Part 1: Background and concepts. *Spine* 1996;21:1769-1776.

65. Carragee EJ, Han MY, Suen PW, Kim D: Clinical outcomes after lumbar discectomy for sciatica: The effects of fragment type and anular competence. *J Bone Joint Surg Am* 2003;85:102-108.

66. Bush K, Cowan N, Katz DE, Gishen P: The natural history of sciatica associated with disc pathology: A prospective study with clinical and independent radiologic follow-up. *Spine* 1992;17:1205-1212.

67. Reyentovich A, Abdu WA: Multiple independent, sequential, and spontaneously resolving lumbar intervertebral disc herniations: A case report. *Spine* 2002;27:549-553.

68. Ahn SH, Ahn MW, Byun WM: Effect of the transligamentous extension of lumbar disc herniations on their regression and the clinical outcome of sciatica. *Spine* 2000;25:475-480.

69. Gibson JN, Grant IC, Waddell G: The Cochrane review of surgery for lumbar disc prolapse and degenerative lumbar spondylosis. *Spine* 1999;24:1820-1832.

70. Faulhauer K, Manicke C: Fragment excision versus conventional disc removal in the microsurgical treatment of herniated lumbar disc. *Acta Neurochir (Wien)* 1995;133:107-111.

71. Spengler DM: Lumbar discectomy. Results with limited disc excision and selective foraminotomy. *Spine* 1982;7:604-607.

72. Striffeler H, Groger U, Reulen HJ:

"Standard" microsurgical lumbar discectomy vs. "conservative" microsurgical discectomy: A preliminary study. *Acta Neurochir (Wien)* 1991;112:62-64.

73. Balderston RA, Gilyard GG, Jones AA, et al: The treatment of lumbar disc herniation: Simple fragment excision versus disc space curettage. *J Spinal Disord* 1991;4:22-25.

74. Odom GL, Finney W, Woodhall B: Cervical disk lesions. *JAMA* 1958;166:23-28.

75. Nelson EC, Batalden PB, Homa K, et al: Microsystems in health care: Part 2. Creating a rich information environment. *Jt Comm J Qual Saf* 2003;29:5-15.

76. Nelson EC, Batalden PB, Huber TP, et al: Microsystems in health care: Part 1. Learning from high-performing front-line clinical units. *Jt Comm J Qual Improv* 2002;28:472-493.

77. Weinstein JN, Brown PW, Hanscom B, Walsh T, Nelson EC: Designing an ambulatory clinical practice for outcomes improvement: From vision to reality—the Spine Center at Dartmouth-Hitchcock, year one. *Qual Manag Health Care* 2000;8:1-20.

78. Roland M, Morris R: A study of the natural history of back pain. Part I: Development of a reliable and sensitive measure of disability in low-back pain. *Spine* 1983;8:141-144.

79. Fairbank JC, Couper J, Davies JB, O'Brien JP: The Oswestry low back pain questionnaire. *Physiotherapy* 1980;66:271-273.

80. Ware JE Jr: SF-36 health survey update. *Spine* 2000;25:3130-3139.

81. Fanuele JC, Birkmeyer NJ, Abdu WA, Tosteson TD, Weinstein JN: The impact of spinal problems on the health status of

patients: Have we underestimated the effect? *Spine* 2000;25:1509-1514.

82. Vogt MT, Hanscom B, Lauerman WC, Kang JD: Influence of smoking on the health status of spinal patients: The National Spine Network database. *Spine* 2002;27:313-319.

83. Abdu WA, Weinstein JN, Hanscom B, Fanuele J: The impact of education on the health status of lumbar spine patients. Read at the Annual Meeting of the North American Spine Society; 2001 Oct 31-Nov 3; Seattle, WA.

84. Abdu W, Mitchell B, Hanscom B, Weinstein J: Self-reported health as a predictor of lumbar surgical outcomes. Read at the Annual Meeting of the International Society for the Study of the Lumbar Spine; 2004 May 30-June 5; Porto, Portugal.

85. Slover J, Abdu WA, Hanscom B, Lurie J, Weinstein JN: Can condition-specific health surveys be specific to spine disease? An analysis of the effect of comorbidities on baseline condition-specific and general health survey scores. *Spine* 2006;31:1265-1271.

86. Slover J, Abdu W, Hanscom B, Lurie J, Weinstein J: The impact of comorbidities on the change in SF- 36 and Oswestry scores following lumbar spine surgery. *Spine* 2006;31:1974-1980.

87. Fanuele JC, Abdu WA, Hanscom B, Weinstein JN: Association between obesity and functional status in patients with spine disease. *Spine* 2002;27:306-312.

88. Bessette L, Liang MH, Lew RA, Weinstein JN: Classics in Spine: Surgery literature revisited. *Spine* 1996;21:259-263.

Thorough Decompression of the Posterior Cervical Foramen

Ronald A. Lehman, Jr, MD
K. Daniel Riew, MD

Abstract

Regardless of the approach to the cervical spine, it is clear that surgical outcome is directly related to surgical technique. Posterior decompressions must be thorough and complete because laminoforaminotomies provide an excellent means of decompressing foraminal pathology. One of the distinct advantages of posterior laminoforaminotomy is that it offers direct visualization, exposure, and decompression of the nerve root without performing a fusion. A posterior laminoforaminotomy is the preferred approach for patients with a soft lateral disk herniation, for those at increased risk for nonunion, or those for whom an anterior procedure would not be optimal. To perform a thorough decompression and prevent iatrogenic instability and neurologic deficits, however, surgeons must be familiar with the anatomy of the foramen as well as the compressive pathology. Several issues must be addressed before performing a posterior laminoforaminotomy, namely, the absence of instability and junctional kyphosis, and the proper identification of the offending pathology.

Instr Course Lect 2007;56:301-309.

As surgical treatment of the spine has advanced, it has become evident that there are a variety of procedures for addressing cervical spine pathology. The use of a certain approach or procedure is often based on the training and personal preference of the operating surgeon.[1] To provide the highest level of care, accomplished spine surgeons should be able to offer patients a variety of approaches depending on the circumstances. Ideally, operating surgeons will choose the best procedure depending on the pathology, their ability, and the patient's desires.

Early surgical interventions for cervical disk pathology were often aggressive posterior approaches, using laminectomies, dural incisions, and dentate ligament resection to access the offending pathology. Fager[2] initially described the use of transdural excision of disk fragments using direct visualization of the spinal cord. The predecessor to the modern laminoforaminotomy was described by Scoville[3] and others.[2,4,5] With the popularity of anterior fusions of the cervical spine, these procedures have largely overtaken posterior or dorsal approaches as the preferred procedures to address cervical pathology.[6-8] However, several authors have described success with the use of the posterior laminoforaminotomy.[9-11] Henderson and associates[12] described relief of 96% of arm pain in a series of 736 patients (846 operated cases). Zeidman and Ducker[13] showed a similar success rate, with 97% of the patients in their series of 172 laminoforaminotomies showing improvement in their radicular pain. Additionally, Herkowitz[11] showed, in a prospective comparison of anterior and posterior approaches, that there was no significant difference between the two approaches.

Advantages and Disadvantages of Posterior Laminoforaminotomies

One of the distinct advantages of posterior laminoforaminotomy is that it offers direct visualization, exposure, and decompression of the nerve root without performing a fusion.[14-16] Fusion complications are not insignificant and include plate and implant failures, dislodgement, graft-site morbidity, and pseudarthrosis. In addition, depending on the technique used, the intervertebral disk space is often not violated. This procedure offers ideal access for posterolateral sequestrations and paramedian disk protrusions without violation of the entire disk space. Another advantage of the posterior-only procedure is that it obviates the risks to the anterior soft-tissue structures. The use of topically placed steroids intraoperatively, although controversial, may help with immediate postoperative pain. Furthermore, postoperative immobilization is entirely optional and for patient comfort only. Finally, from a purely economic standpoint, a laminoforaminotomy costs less than an anterior diskectomy/ decompression and fusion.[17]

Despite all of the advantages of posterior laminoforaminotomy, there are several disadvantages. Some of the more dreaded complications include dural injuries, cerebrospinal fluid fistulas, air emboli, pneumocephali, and bilateral subdural hematoma formations.[18] The structural integrity of the facet is also of concern during the decompression of the nerve root. Several authors have described the importance of limiting the resection of the facet to less than 50% to decrease the risk of segmental instability.[19-21] Additionally, a 10% risk of worsening radiculopathy and/or postoperative paresthesias has been reported, along with potential injury to the spinal cord and/or nerve root.[22] The risk of wound infection is also higher in posterior cervical procedures versus anterior procedures. Other concerns with both anterior and posterior procedures at any level include wrong-site surgery and missed pathology.

Indications

A posterior laminoforaminotomy is the preferred approach for patients with a soft lateral disk herniation, for those at increased risk for nonunion, or those for whom an anterior procedure would not be optimal (patients with a short neck or pathology cephalad to C3 or caudad to T1).[23] Patients who exhibit reproducible symptoms with a Spurling's maneuver that improve with neck flexion are ideal candidates for a posterior laminoforaminotomy. Spurling's maneuver involves extending and laterally rotating the patient's neck to the side of symptomatology. If this maneuver reproduces the pain, and is subsequently relieved with contralateral rotation and neck pain, the test is positive. In extension, the nerve is pincered between the posterior uncinate and the superior articular facet. In flexion, the foramen enlarges in size such that the posterior facet no longer causes as much compression, a situation similar to what happens after a laminoforaminotomy. If the symptoms do not improve with neck flexion, they are believed to be less likely to respond to a posterior approach; therefore, an anterior procedure is recommended.

Another relative indication for a laminoforaminotomy is in a patient with a lateral disk herniation that impinges upon the nerve root, either in the axilla or out laterally. Although it is possible to resect disk herniations at the lateral third of the disk space, it is recommended that these herniations be addressed anteriorly. Additionally, the anterior approach is recommended for patients who exhibit constant, severe numbness or weakness (less than grade four out of five [4/5] motor strength) because it often takes weeks to months for such deficits to resolve. Following a posterior laminoforaminotomy, if the patient fails to improve, it is often difficult to determine if the failure is the result of a permanent nerve injury to the root or an inadequate decompression. This is especially true in patients with radiculopathy resulting from spondylotic uncinate spurs, for which resection through a laminoforaminotomy approach is not recommended. In contrast, with an anterior approach, direct decompression of the entire foramen can be achieved by resecting the uncinate and disk material past the lateral margin of the pedicle, which can ensure that the persistent numbness is caused by the original injury and not by an inadequate decompression. An added benefit of the anterior approach is that the arthrodesis will decrease nerve root irritation secondary to motion, and this may aid in the neurologic recovery.

Preoperative Considerations

During the preoperative planning of a posterior laminoforaminotomy, several factors must be addressed. The issue of preoperative instability must be assessed with flexion and extension views of the cervical spine. Additionally, the presence of junctional kyphosis must be evaluated to prevent progression or iatrogenic sagittal plane deformity postoperatively. Junctional kyphosis is depicted by measuring the vertebrae above and below the area of pathology. If there is loss of normal cervical lordosis, then there is radiographic evidence of kyphosis. Instability is defined as > 3.5 mm of listhesis of two adjacent vertebrae or is seen when the spinous processes 'splay' on lateral flexion/extension views. Additionally, surgeons must be certain to correctly identify the offending pathology with the proper use of preoperative imaging modalities.

Anesthesia

In the past several years, laminoforaminotomies have been performed with local anesthesia and with minimally invasive techniques.[24] Tomaras and associates[25] described performing this procedure under local anesthesia in 200 patients, with 92.8% showing good to excellent results. This has been postulated to decrease the risk of neurologic injury because patients are not subjected to the physiologic insult that occurs with general anesthetic agents.[26] The surgeon is allowed to assess the patient in an awake state to determine if their symptoms have improved after decompression. In general, however, it is recommended that these procedures be performed with the patient under general anesthesia.

Positioning

Positioning for posterior cervical procedures is just as critical as it is for anterior procedures. Several described positions include the lateral decubitus, the prone reverse-Trendelenburg (Concorde), and the seated position. The use of the seated position has been associated with several complications, including an increased risk for air embolus and cardiovascular compromise. Air emboli, if present, can be managed with a central cardiac catheter placement and an atrial catheter to remove the emboli as necessary. If an embolus is detected, venous bleeding is coagulated, the wound packed, and the patient placed into the left

lateral decubitus position.[20] This position allows the air to be trapped in the right atrium. However, in their review of 736 patients, Henderson and associates[12] reported no occurrences of emboli, and in their series of 172 patients, Zeidman and Ducker[13] reported only four instances of embolic phenomena, all without clinical sequelae. The risk appears to be higher when patients are placed in the seated rather than the prone position. The benefit of the prone Concorde position is that it decreases venous engorgement, providing a drier surgical field.

The prone position is recommended for these procedures using the Jackson frame (Orthopaedic Systems, Union City, CA) (Figure 1). The shoulders are taped down just as is done for anterior procedures. Care is taken to make sure that one shoulder is not pulled asymmetrically to prevent an iatrogenic coronal plane deformity if an arthrodesis is being performed. Bolsters are placed just underneath the clavicle and Gardner-Wells tongs with bivector traction are used to allow positioning of the neck in either flexion or extension. The position is checked before draping to ensure that the neck can be placed into an adequate amount of flexion and extension. Foraminotomies are best accomplished with the neck in maximal flexion, which unshingles the facets and exposes the underlying superior articular facet. If the neck is not adequately flexed during a foraminotomy, a large amount of the overhanging inferior articular facet must be resected to expose the underlying superior facet, which may weaken the structure and lead to a fracture. More commonly, this makes it difficult to place a lateral mass screw in patients who require decompression as well as a fusion. If

the patient requires a fusion, the neck must be placed in an extended position. To extend the neck, the weight from the lower (flexion) rope is changed to the upper (extension) rope. The advantage of using bivector tong traction is that surgeons can easily alter the position of the neck intraoperatively. Fixed head holders such as Mayfield tongs require that an assistant crawl under the table to reposition the head holder.

The head of the Jackson frame is placed on the top rung of the table, whereas the foot of the frame is placed on the bottom rung. The patient is placed in a modified knee-chest position with the legs supported in a sling, and the chest and anterior iliac crest supported by bolsters that allow the visceral contents to hang free. A buttocks strap is placed over padding to keep the patient secured on the table. The table is then tilted in a reverse Trendelenburg position to decrease the blood flow into the surgical field. An airflow warming blanket is placed on the ventral surface of the patient to keep the core temperature warm throughout the procedure. Because heat rises and because the greatest heat loss occurs on the ventral surface of the body, a ventral heating blanket works effectively to maintain core temperature.

Foraminal Stenosis and the Anatomy of the Foramen

Before performing a foraminotomy, surgeons must have a thorough understanding of the etiology of the compression as well as the anatomic boundaries of the foramen. Although this may seem trivial and obvious, many surgeons do not have such a thorough understanding.

The anterior wall of the foramen is the uncovertebral joint and the

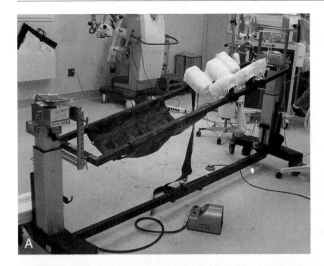

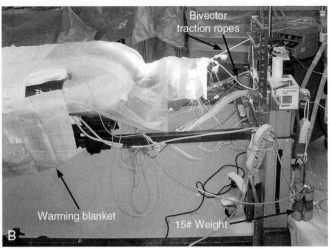

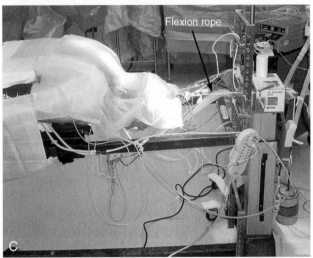

Figure 1 **A,** Operating room photograph shows the full Jackson frame setup with three bolsters and a sling for the leg. The foot of the bed is at the bottom rung, the head of the bed is at the top rung, and the table is placed into a reverse Trendelenburg position. **B,** Operating room photograph show that bivector traction is used with two traction ropes, one of which goes over a bar and acts as the extension rope. **C,** The flexion rope goes straight through the center hole. The top bolster is placed just underneath the clavicle such that if both ropes come undone, the chin rests on the bolster and the head cannot fall farther.

lateral disk (Figure 2). The posterior wall is the superior articular facet of the caudal vertebral segment (the superior facet of C6 at the C5-6 foramen). The cranial and caudal borders of the foramen are the pedicles of the respective vertebrae. The medial and lateral borders of the foramen are the medial and lateral borders of the pedicles, and the width of the foramen is only as wide as those pedicles. Therefore, to thoroughly decompress the entire foramen, the dorsal aspect of the foramen must be unrooted from the medial border of the pedicle laterally until the lateral border of the pedicle can be felt.

Anteriorly, foraminal compression can occur from uncovertebral spurs or a lateral disk herniation. Posteriorly, foraminal stenosis can occur from hypertrophic facets. This condition more commonly occurs between the second through the fourth cervical levels than at the lower cervical levels. It is rare for loss of disk height to be so severe that compression between the pedicles in the cranial-caudal direction occurs. Therefore, when decompressing the foramen from a posterior approach, the neuroforamen needs to be decompressed only in the anteroposterior direction. This is accomplished

by resecting the medial 50% of the superior articular facet. Burring down the uncovertebral joint posteriorly can be accomplished; however, care must be taken to ensure that there is minimal nerve root retraction while protecting the root from injury by the burr. Additionally, as surgeons progress ventrally, lateral to the neuroforamen, the vertebral artery lies anterior to the root and is at risk. Consequently, resection of the superior articular facet and removal of only soft disks are recommended, but only if the hypertrophied uncinate is easily accessible and can be safely resected.

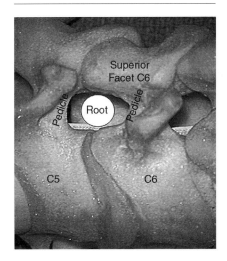

Figure 2   Model representation showing borders of the foramen. The foramen is bordered by the superior facet posteriorly, the posterior uncinate (not visible on this figure) and disk space anteriorly, and the pedicles superiorly and inferiorly. Notice that the root only comes into contact with the superior facet of C6 and not the inferior facet of C5.

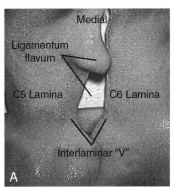

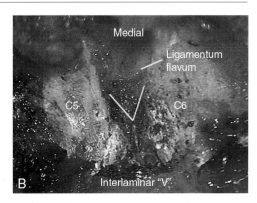

Figure 3   A, Model representation showing the interlaminar V. B, Intraoperative photograph showing the interlaminar V, which is a good starting point for the decompression because it defines the juncture between the lamina and the facet, as well as the lateral mass. In addition, the medial wall of the pedicle lies just below the interlaminar V.

Technique for Posterior Laminoforaminotomy

There are various techniques for performing a posterior lamino-foraminotomy, including open, endoscopic, and microscopically assisted procedures to access the spine. For a single-level foraminotomy, a 3- to 4-cm incision can be made just off the midline. Subperiosteal dissection is carried down to expose the junction between the lamina and the medial aspect of the facet while preserving the facet capsule. The cranial and caudal laminae overlap at this point and form the facet joint. This overlapping point makes a V-shaped point and, hence, is called the interlaminar V (Figure 3). When performing a foraminotomy, it is imperative that the full extent of the facet is delineated because the desired goal is to resect only the medial 50% (or less) of the facet joint. If removal of more than 50% of the facet joint occurs, it can lead to in-

stability with the potential for post-foraminotomy kyphosis, especially if the procedure is being performed bilaterally.[27]

Step 1

For ease of description, the technique for performing a foraminotomy at the C5-6 level is outlined. The decompression is started by identifying the interlaminar V between C5 and C6. An estimate is made as to where the C6 pedicle is located and where the cranial aspect of the C6 superior facet lies under the C5 facet. Care is taken to make sure that the neck is maximally flexed to minimize the facet resection (Figure 4, A). The medial 40% or so of the C5 inferior facet is then burred off (Figure 4, B and C). The assistant provides constant irrigation using a 30- to 50-mL syringe with an 18-gauge angiocatheter. The irrigation washes away bone dust, allowing better visualization, and also decreases the risk of heat-induced necrosis from the high-speed burr. The burring is done so as to expose the cranial border of the underlying C6 facet (Figure 4, D). This burring is done rapidly because the underly-

ing C6 facet protects the neural elements from the burr. Up to this point, no neural decompression has occurred because the inferior facet of C5 does not come into contact with the root; it merely covers the superior facet of C6, which is the dorsal cover of the root.

Step 2

The next step is to remove the dorsal cover of the foramen (the C6 superior facet up to the lateral aspect of the pedicle) with a high-speed burr. The basic principle behind posterior decompression surgery is to indirectly decompress the nerve root by resecting the posterior compressive structures and allow the nerve root to "float" away from the offending ventral pathology. As a result, a simple keyhole foraminotomy can sometimes be inadequate in a patient with a large anterior uncinate spur. In such patients, the unresected lamina, medial to the foramen, can prevent the root from migrating posteriorly away from the anterior pathology (Figure 5); therefore, resecting a part of the cranial and caudal laminae such that the root is fully decompressed from its

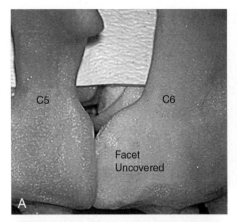

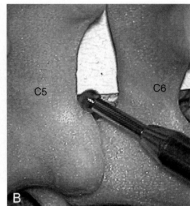

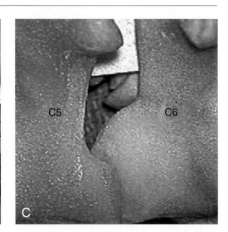

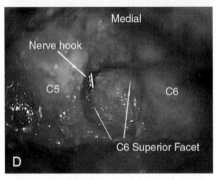

Figure 4 **A,** Model representation showing that flexing the neck uncovers the C6 facet so that a minimal amount of C5 facet needs to be resected to expose the cranial border of C6. **B,** The starting point of the burr is just cranial to the interlaminar V. **C,** The lateral aspect of the C5 lamina and the medial caudal aspect of the C5 facet has been removed. **D,** Intraoperative photograph showing that this procedure exposes the cranial border of the C6 facet, which is outlined by the small nerve hook.

origin in the spinal cord to the lateral margin of the neuroforamen is recommended. Starting with the lateral aspect of the C6 lamina, the C6 facet is carefully burred just cranial to the C6 pedicle. A mediolateral light brushing technique is used. Because the facet is tilted medial to lateral at about 30°, the burr has to be placed deeper into the facet as it is progressing farther laterally. Once the estimated lateral border of the pedicle is reached, burring is done in a cranial-caudal direction until the cranial border of the facet is reached. The resected portion of the facet then detaches (Figure 6). A 2-mm microcuret is used to detach this piece from the underlying soft tissues and remove it with a pituitary rongeur. It is common to tear one of the epidural veins at this point. Bipolar electrocautery is used to achieve hemostasis. Hemostatic agents (FloSeal,

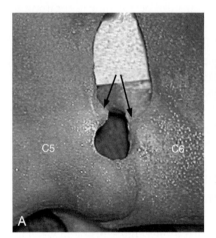

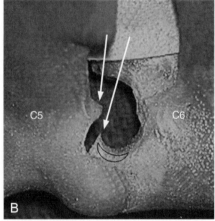

Figure 5 **A,** Model representation showing that a simple keyhole foraminotomy does not decompress the lateral aspect of the lamina or the medial aspect of the C5 facet, which can result in root impingement (*arrows*). **B,** In addition, a small foraminotomy can leave a sickle-shaped decompression (*outlined*) with a sharp point to the superomedial aspect of C6 that can continue to impinge on the root (*arrows*).

Baxter Healthcare, Deerfield, IL or Gelfoam, Pharmacia-Upjohn, Kalamazoo, MI) are also helpful during the procedure to control epidural venous bleeding.

A common mistake when performing a foraminotomy occurs when surgeons fail to visualize the cranial border of the superior facet. A burr hole is then made in the cau-

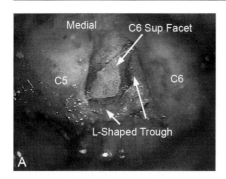
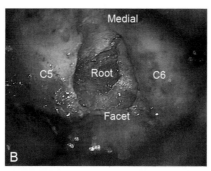

Figure 6   A, Intraoperative photograph showing that after the superior facet of C6 is exposed, a mediolateral trough and a cranial caudal trough are made. **B,** Intraoperative photograph showing that the superior facet is then removed to expose a thin rim of bone just cranial to the C6 pedicle, which can be removed with a high-speed burr or Kerrison rongeur.

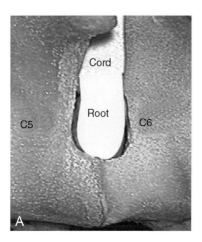
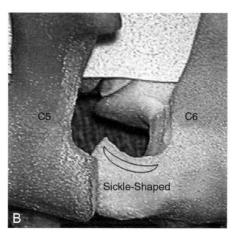

Figure 7   A, Model representation showing that care must be taken not to leave a sickle-shaped C6 facet, which can remain if care is not taken to expose the superior facet of C6 and if the undersurface of C5 is not palpated at the conclusion of the decompression. **B,** Model representation showing that the sickle-shaped decompression (*outlined*) is only visible with the facets distracted apart.

dal portion of the facet, and the root is visualized, but surgeons may fail to realize that the cranial border of the facet has not been resected. The remaining facet is shaped like a sickle, with a cranial spike of bone that can still impinge on the nerve root. In performing the decompression, it is important to make sure that no such sickle-shaped bone is left behind (Figure 7). Therefore, after removing the resected C6 facet, the undersurface of the C5 facet should be palpated to ensure that a part of

the C6 facet does not remain.

Perhaps the most common concern regarding laminoforaminotomies has to do with the lateral extent of the decompression. To adequately decompress the foramen, the dorsal aspect of the entire width of the foramen must be resected. As stated previously, the lateral margin of the foramen is the lateral wall of the pedicles; therefore, once the entire superior facet is resected to the lateral margin of the pedicles, the decompression is complete. If an ade-

quate amount of the facet has been resected laterally, surgeons should be able to palpate the lateral margin of the pedicle using a small probe (Figure 8). In addition, the cranial border of the caudal pedicle should be palpated (C6 pedicle at the C5-6 level) to ensure that there is no overhang or "shelf" of lamina that can still impinge on the root. If overhang remains, this should be resected with a high-speed burr or a 1-mm Kerrison rongeur, which allows the root to migrate posteriorly without impediment.

Foraminotomy for Disk Herniation
When performing a foraminotomy for disk herniation, the exposure is identical to that described for the standard foraminotomy used for cervical spondylosis and uncinate hypertrophy. The main difference is that the nerve root must be manipulated to expose the herniated fragment, which lies ventral to the nerve root itself. The easiest way to accomplish this is to burr down the cranial aspect of the caudal pedicle. The cranial portion (2 to 3 mm) of the pedicle needs to be burred flush with the vertebral body, allowing retraction of the nerve root caudally without injuring the nerve root. Additionally, this allows for easier retraction of the nerve and extrication of the disk fragment. The use of microinstruments, a 1-mm Kerrison punch, a 3-mm round (or a 2-mm acorn-shaped) burr, and micronerve hooks are ideal to free the disk fragment. It is important to probe cranially and caudally to ensure all of the fragments have been obtained.

Although infrequent, drains can be used if there has been excessive bleeding during the procedure or other concerns about postoperative bleeding exist. The wound is closed

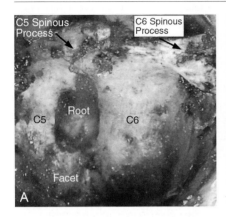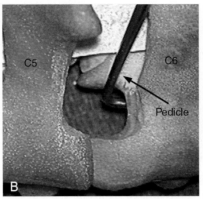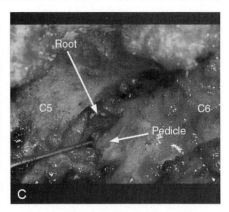

Figure 8 **A,** Intraoperative photograph of a completed foraminotomy. **B,** Model representation showing that the lateral margin of the pedicle wall (*arrow*) should be palpated at the conclusion of the procedure to ensure that the entire foramen has been decompressed. **C,** Intraoperative photograph showing a small nerve hook palpating the lateral margin of the C6 pedicle (*small arrow*). Part of the cranial aspect of this pedicle has been burred down flush with the posterior vertebral body, which allows easy access to the undersurface of the root (*large arrow*).

in multiple layers. No immobilization is used postoperatively and range-of-motion exercises are started immediately.

Mini-Open Posterior Foraminotomy

Additional techniques include the use of a tubular, endoscopic system, which allows muscle preservation and smaller incisions. Adamson[28] used a minimally invasive technique to treat 100 patients and reported that all patients rapidly returned to full activities. The author speculated that the rapid return to function was a testament to maintaining the muscular attachments to the spinous processes and avoiding subperiosteal stripping.

When patients present with pathology at one or two levels on the same side, mini-open procedures using a tubular retractor system are recommended. A paramedian incision is made approximately 1.5 to 2 cm off the midline, and a dilating tubular retractor system is used that allows for less mechanical trauma to the muscles and soft tissues. The procedure is done under fluoroscopic control. The neck is extended

to decrease the interlaminar space so as to minimize the exposure of the spinal cord. A guidewire pin is placed onto the medial aspect of the facet to be decompressed. Care must be taken to prevent placement too medial (which would injure the spinal cord) and too lateral (which would make the decompression difficult). A lateral fluoroscopic image is then obtained. Although anterior-posterior images are not required, they can be obtained to make sure that the mediolateral starting point is correct. A dilator is then gently placed over the guidewire under image guidance. Care is taken to prevent ventral migration of the pin into the spinal cord. Sequentially larger dilators are then placed over the initial dilator. Once a dilator with a diameter greater than 1 cm has made bony contact, a "wanding" motion is used to clear off a space on top of the facet and also to "feel" the facet and the lamina. Care must be taken to prevent intrusion into the interlaminar space into the spinal cord, although it is much less likely with the neck in extension and with a 1-cm diameter dilator. A 2-cm diameter retractor is recommended.

Once this retractor is in place, microscopic visualization is used to perform the procedure.

Although tubular retractors have the theoretic advantage of a muscle-splitting approach that may decrease postoperative pain, there are distinct disadvantages and risks as well. First, the use of tubular retractors results in a limited field of view. If an endoscope (instead of a microscope) is used, an additional loss of three-dimensional perspective occurs, which can result in surgeons getting "lost" and performing decompressions that are inadequate, misplaced, or overly aggressive, resulting in instability. It is therefore imperative to identify the interlaminar V formed by the overlapping laminae once subperiosteal dissection and hemostasis have been obtained. After identifying this important landmark, the foraminotomy can be completed as described previously.

A second major disadvantage of using tubular retractors is that the guide pin and tubular retractors have to be placed blindly onto the facet, risking injury to the spinal cord. A third disadvantage is that there is limited room in the tube to use tools such as high-speed burrs. In addition, the burrs have to be grasped higher in the stem, resulting in some loss of control. The burr tip will tend to rattle more, which increases the likelihood of complications. A fourth disadvantage is that using tubular retractors requires fluoroscopic guidance, which exposes both the patient and the surgeon to radiation. In addition, decompression cannot be achieved at any level that cannot be visualized by fluoroscopy, which typically means any level below C6.

Because of limited visualization, difficulty with localization, and increased potential for complications, it is recommended that only surgeons who are experts at open laminoforaminotomies attempt to use tubular retractors.

Summary

Laminoforaminotomies provide an excellent means of decompressing foraminal pathology. However, to perform a thorough decompression and prevent iatrogenic instability and neurologic deficits, surgeons must be thoroughly familiar with the anatomy of the foramen as well as the compressive pathology.

References

1. Epstein JA: The surgical management of cervical spinal stenosis, spondylosis, and myeloradiculopathy by means of the posterior approach. *Spine* 1988;13:864-869.

2. Fager CA: Posterior surgical tactics for the neurological syndromes of cervical disc and spondylotic lesions. *Clin Neurosurg* 1978;25:218-244.

3. Scoville WB: Cervical disc: Classifications, indication and approaches with special reference to posterior keyhole operation, in An HS, Samartzis

D (eds): *Cervical Spondylosis*. New York, NY, Raven Press, 1981, pp 155-167.

4. Fager CA: Posterolateral approach to ruptured median and paramedian cervical disk. *Surg Neurol* 1983;20:443-452.

5. Epstein J, Lavine LS, Aronson HA, Epstein BS: Cervical spondylotic radiculopathy: The syndrome of foraminal constriction treated by foraminotomy and the removal of osteophytes. *Clin Orthop Relat Res* 1965;40:113-122.

6. Bailey R, Bagdley SK: Stabilization of the cervical spine by an anterior fusion. *J Bone Joint Surg Am* 1960;42:565-594.

7. Cloward R: The anterior approach for removal of ruptured cervical disks. *J Neurosurg* 1958;15:602-617.

8. Robinson R, Smith G: Anterolateral cervical disc removal and interbody fusion for cervical disc syndrome. *Bull Johns Hopkins Hosp* 1955;96:223-224.

9. Aldrich F: Posterolateral microdiscectomy for cervical monoradiculopathy caused by posterolateral soft cervical disc sequestration. *J Neurosurg* 1990;72:370-377.

10. Murphey F, Simmons JC: Ruptured cervical disc: Experience with 250 cases. *Am Surg* 1966;32:83-88.

11. Herkowitz H: Surgical management of cervical soft disc herniation: A comparison between the anterior and posterior approach. *Spine* 1990;15:1026-1030.

12. Henderson CM, Hennessy RG, Shuey HM Jr, Shackelford EG: Posterior-lateral foraminotomy as an exclusive operative technique for cervical radiculopathy: A review of 846 consecutively operated cases. *Neurosurgery* 1983;13:504-512.

13. Zeidman SM, Ducker TB: Posterior cervical laminoforaminotomy for radiculopathy: Review of 172 cases. *Neurosurgery* 1993;33:356-362.

14. Albert TJ, Murrell SE: Surgical management of cervical radiculopathy. *J Am Acad Orthop Surg* 1999;7:368-376.

15. Fessler RG, Khoo LT: Minimally invasive cervical microendoscopic foraminotomy: An initial clinical experience. *Neurosurgery* 2002;51:S37-45.

16. Fager CA: Management of cervical disc lesions and spondylosis by posterior approaches. *Clin Neurosurg*

1977;24:488-507.

17. Parker WD: Cervical laminoforaminotomy. *J Neurosurg* 2002;96:254.

18. Epstein N: A review of laminoforaminotomy for the management of lateral and foraminal cervical disc herniations or spurs. *Surg Neurol* 2002;57:226-234.

19. Raynor R: Cervical facetectomy and its effect on spine strength. *J Neurosurg* 1985;63:278-282.

20. Epstein NE: A review of laminoforaminotomy for the management of lateral and foraminal cervical disc herniations or spurs. *Surg Neurol* 2002;57:226-233.

21. Ebraheim NA, Xu R, Bhatti RA, Yeasting RA: The projection of the cervical disc and uncinate process on the posterior aspect of the cervical spine. *Surg Neurol* 1999;51:363-367.

22. Williams RW: Microcervical foraminotomy: A surgical alternative for intractable radicular pain. *Spine* 1983;8:708-716.

23. Brodsky A: Management of radiculopathy secondary to acute cervical disc degeneration and spondylosis by the posterior approach, in The Cervical Spine Research Society (eds): *The Cervical Spine*, ed 2. Philadelphia, PA, Lippincott, 1983, pp 395-402.

24. Witzmann A, Hejazi N, Krasznai L: Posterior cervical foraminotomy: A follow-up study of 67 surgically treated patients with compressive radiculopathy. *Neurosurg Rev* 2000;23:213-217.

25. Tomaras CR, Blacklock JB, Parker WD, Harper RL: Outpatient surgical treatment of cervical radiculopathy. *J Neurosurg* 1997;87:41-43.

26. Nygaard OP, Romner B, Thoner J, Due-Tonnessen B: Local anesthesia in posterior cervical surgery. *Anesthesiology* 1997;86:242-243.

27. Zdeblick TA, Abitbol JJ, Kunz DN, McCabe RP, Garfin S: Cervical stability after sequential capsule resection. *Spine* 1993;18:2005-2008.

28. Adamson TE: Microendoscopic posterior cervical laminoforaminotomy for unilateral radiculopathy: Results of a new technique in 100 cases. *J Neurosurg* 2001;95:51-57.

C1 Lateral Screws and C2 Pedicle/Pars Screws

Rick C. Sasso, MD

Abstract

A variety of techniques exist for fixation of the upper cervical spine. The development of universal posterior cervical screw-rod instrumentation systems has resulted in recent interest in new and stable segmental fixation into C1 and C2. The C1 lateral mass is a safe and robust anchor point; however, the anatomic corridor to access the screw entry portal is unfamiliar. Understanding the C1 bony landmarks and the course and relationship of the soft-tissue structures (such as the vertebral artery and the C2 nerve root) is critically important. Alternative techniques for achieving segmental screw fixation into C2 are being developed. With polyaxial screw heads and lateral offset connectors, screw anchors can be driven into the most sturdy and safest aspects of C2 without concern for the position of the longitudinal rod.

Instr Course Lect 2007;56:311-317.

Historically, anchors into C1 have been limited by the inability to fasten a stable longitudinal structure to connect anchors attached to adjacent vertebrae. Although Magerl originally placed screws into the lateral mass of C1, he was unable to rigidly couple them to a fixation device into C2. Thus, he originated a transarticular screw technique across the C1-C2 facet joint that bears his name.[1] This transarticular screw was a huge advance over the traditional wire/cable techniques of atlantoaxial stabilization.[2] Biomechanically, transarticular

The author or the departments with which he is affiliated has received something of value from a commercial or other party related directly or indirectly to the subject of this chapter.

screws are much more stable under shear and rotational loads compared with wire/cable constructs, and postoperative halo immobilization is not required. Extremely high fusion rates are achieved without the morbidity of halos. Magerl screws, however, do have several disadvantages and carry the distinction of being the most dangerous screw that a spine surgeon can implant. The C1-C2 articulation must be perfectly reduced before attempting transarticular screw insertion, and it is impossible to obtain the steep cranial trajectory in many patients with a fixed cervicothoracic kyphosis. Biplane fluoroscopy is required intraoperatively, and preoperative parasagittal CT reconstructions are mandatory to assess for a high-riding vertebral artery groove in C2, which precludes transarticular screw

implantation in up to 20% of patients. Bilateral vertebral artery injury has proven lethal.

The introduction of universal polyaxial screw/rod instrumentation for the posterior cervical spine has finally allowed surgeons to individually anchor into C1 and C2, provide stability as strong as that of transarticular screws, provide the versatility of incorporating the occiput and the subaxial cervical spine easily into the construct, and allow for safer and less difficult screw insertion. The lateral mass of C1 is a strong and safe anchor point for a screw and may be used to provide additional fixation points in occipitocervical constructs, thus increasing resistance to construct failure in the cervical spine without increasing the number of cervical levels fused. With traditional plate/screw occipitocervical constructs, C1 was entirely bypassed or relatively weak cables were passed under the C1 posterior arch and crimped through the plate holes.

There has been considerable confusion in the literature regarding screws placed into the C2 vertebra from a posterior approach.[3] The distinction between C2 pedicle screws and C2 pars interarticularis screws hinges on the anatomic definitions of the true pedicle and pars interar-

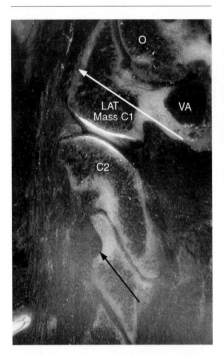

Figure 1 Anatomic specimen of the parasagittal occipitocervical junction through the lateral mass of C1 (Lat Mass C1). The long arrow shows the path of the screw through the C1 lateral mass. O is the occipital condyle, and C2 is the superior articular process of C2. VA is the vertebral artery in the groove along the cephalad aspect of the C1 posterior arch. The short arrow shows the path of the screw through the C3 lateral mass.

ticularis. C2 screws may be coupled to C1 lateral mass screws to achieve atlantoaxial stabilization.

C1 Lateral Mass Screws

The atlantoaxial joint is challenging to stabilize because of the unique characteristics of the C1 and C2 vertebrae. The anatomic differences between C1 and C2 and the remainder of the subaxial cervical spine require individual strategies for screw insertion. The lateral mass of C1 is not analogous to the lateral mass of the subaxial vertebrae. Therefore, C1 lateral mass screws are distinct from the standard lateral mass screws inserted from C3 to C7 (Figure 1).

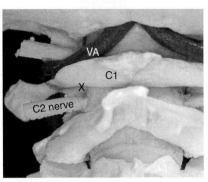

Figure 2 Posterior view photograph of the occipitocervical junction. The entry point for the C1 lateral mass screw is indicated (X). C1 = the posterior arch of C1, VA = the vertebral artery as it runs in the groove of the superior aspect of the C1 posterior arch, C2 nerve = the C2 nerve root. The C1-C2 facet joint lies just anterior to the C2 nerve.

The most challenging aspect of implanting C1 lateral mass screws is the exposure of the C1 lateral mass and C1-C2 joint from a cranial to caudal direction. The key to this exposure is mobilization of the C2 nerve root. Although most spine surgeons are comfortable with exposing the C1-C2 joint from a caudal to cranial fashion, as is routinely performed to insert transarticular C1-C2 screws, the dissection of this joint from a cranial to caudal path with mobilization and retraction of the C2 nerve caudally is not common. There has not been a previous reason to expose the C1 lateral mass because there was no advantage or technique to fixate it before the development of universal screw/rod instrumentation.

Dissection of the posterior arch of C1 lateral to 1.5 cm from the midline is performed with caution because the vertebral artery runs in a groove on the superior surface of the posterior arch. It is usually protected by a thin rim of bone from the superior border of this posterior arch,

but it may be exposed; therefore, lateral exposure is focused from the middle aspect to the inferior part of the posterior arch of C1. The venous plexus around the C2 nerve root is cauterized with a bipolar and the C2 root is mobilized caudally. Subperiosteal dissection is performed from the inferior aspect of the posterior arch of C1 and anteriorly down to the lateral mass of C1. The lateral mass of C1 inferior to the C1 arch is exposed. The medial wall of the lateral mass is identified using a forward angle curet to identify the medial limit of screw placement. The medial aspect of the transverse foramen can also be identified and serves as the lateral limit for screw placement. The entry point for screw placement is identified 3 to 5 mm lateral to the medial wall of the lateral mass, at the junction of the lateral mass and inferior aspect of the C1 arch (Figure 2). A high-speed drill with a 3-mm burr is used to remove a small portion of the inferior aspect of the posterior C1 arch overlying the entry point and to create a recess for the screw head. Removing this lip from the inferior aspect of the C1 posterior arch also assists in accessing the vertical wall, which leads to the lateral mass. If this lip is not removed, it is extremely difficult to subperiosteally dissect the venous plexus surrounding the C2 nerve from a cephalad to caudal direction (Figure 3). An assistant retracts the C2 nerve inferiorly and protects it during drilling and screw placement. A cervical probe with a diameter equal to the inner diameter of the polyaxial screw is used to forage a path into the cancellous bone of the C1 lateral mass with 10° to 15° of medial angulation and 10° to 20° of cephalad angulation. The medial angulation is important because it helps surgeons to stay away from the lateral vertebral artery. The spinal canal is not at risk because the starting point for this screw on the lateral mass is near the anterior aspect of the canal. The slight cephalad angulation is necessary to keep the screw out of the C1-C2 facet joint, but the screw should not be steeply angled to prevent the screw head from impinging on the C2 nerve root. Removing the lip of bone from the inferior aspect of the posterior arch assists in allowing a more horizontal trajectory. If this lip remains, it forces a steeper path through the lateral mass. The screw head should sit on the inferior aspect of the posterior arch of C1 that was previously prepared by the drill. Using lateral fluoroscopic imaging, the probe is directed toward the anterior tubercle of C1 midway between the superior and inferior facets of C1. Because this is usually a strong screw with excellent purchase in the lateral mass and the screw is rigidly attached to the rod, bicortical purchase is not routinely obtained through the anterior cortex of C1. If there is concern about the sturdiness of the screw, then a 2.5-mm drill can perforate the anterior cortex. The internal carotid artery is usually just lateral to the entry point of this screw; thus, the importance of medial angulation is strengthened with bicortical purchase. The hole is tapped, and either a 3.5- or 4.0-mm screw is placed. Approximately half of this screw will be within the bone of the C1 lateral mass and half will be exposed under the posterior arch of C1. If preferred, a special C1 partially threaded screw can be used so that no screw threads abut the C2 nerve root (Vertex, Medtronic, Memphis, TN). Anatomic landmarks are used to guide the placement of C1 lateral mass screws; however, a lateral fluo-

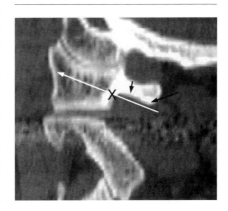

Figure 3 Lateral radiograph of the posterior occipitocervical junction. The entry point for the C1 lateral mass screw is indicated (X). The long arrow shows the trajectory of the screw. The small arrow shows the inferior lip of bone on the posterior arch of C1 that should be removed to allow subperiosteal access to the vertical wall (arrowhead) and provide appropriate trajectory of the screw without excessive cephalad angulation. This also creates a nesting place for the polyaxial screw head on the posterior arch of C1.

roscopic image may be obtained to assure proper sagittal angulation

C2 Pedicle Screws Versus C2 Pars Interarticularis Screws

The pars interarticularis is defined as the portion of the C2 vertebra between the superior and inferior articular surfaces. A screw placed in this portion of C2 has often been called a pedicle screw, but is more appropriately termed a pars interarticularis screw. This screw is placed in a trajectory similar to that of the C1-C2 transarticular screw. The entry point for the C2 pars interarticularis screw is 3 to 4 mm cephalad and 3 to 4 mm lateral to the inferomedial aspect of the inferior articular surface of C2. The screw follows a steep trajectory, paralleling the C2 pars interarticularis. An appropriately steep trajectory ($\geq 40°$) is achieved by aligning the shaft of the drill or screwdriver with the tip of the T1

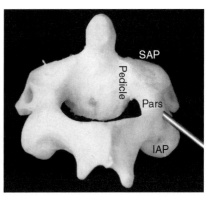

Figure 4 Posterior view photograph of C2. SAP = superior articular process of C2, IAP = inferior articular process of C2.

spinous process. This trajectory may be achieved by using percutaneous stab incisions that are approximately 2 cm lateral to the T1 spinous process. The screws are passed with 10° of medial angulation. Screw length is typically 16 mm, which will stop short of the C1-C2 facet joint. This short screw also usually stops short of the transverse foramen, thereby avoiding injury to the vertebral artery. When possible, a larger (4.0-mm) diameter screw is used to achieve increased pullout resistance because the screw is unicortical.

The C2 pedicle is defined as that portion of the C2 vertebra connecting the dorsal elements with the vertebral body, which is actually a narrow area between the vertebral body and the pars interarticularis (Figure 4). The trajectory of the C2 pedicle screw is different from that of the C2 pars screw, being shallow in relation to the axial plane and more medially angulated.[4] The entry point for C2 pedicle screw fixation is in the pars interarticularis, lateral to the superior margin of the C2 lamina, approximately 2 mm superior and 1 to 2 mm lateral to the entry point for the C2 pars interarticularis screw. The screw is placed with 15° to 25°

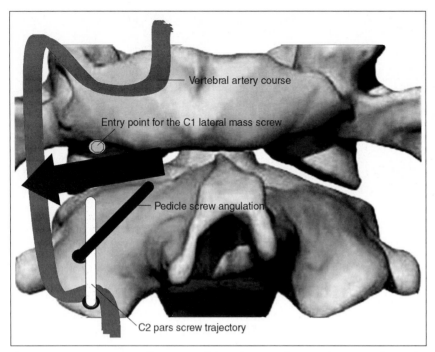

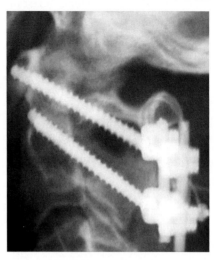

Figure 6 Lateral radiograph of a posterior atlantoaxial fixation construct with C1 lateral mass and C2 pedicle screws. Both screws are 4.0 mm in diameter and 40.0 mm in length.

Figure 5 Posterior view illustration of the atlantoaxial joint. The arrow shows the C2 nerve root course.

of medial angulation, depending on the angulation of the pedicle when palpated by removing a small amount of ligamentum flavum. The thick medial wall of the C2 pedicle will help redirect the screw if necessary and prevent medial wall breakout. The entry point can be adjusted based on the degree of medial angulation of the pedicle as well as the rostrocaudal inclination of the pars interarticularis, which may be determined from the lateral fluoroscopic view. The entry point will generally be 3 to 4 mm lateral to the medial margin of the pars, which may be palpated with a curved spatula. C2 pedicle screws generally should be placed with a slight caudal-to-rostral inclination, which will point toward the ventral C2 body just below the base of the dens. This trajectory (20° up angle) allows safe bicortical purchase if desired and greater resistance to screw pullout. The trajectory of the C2 pedicle screw will be

medial to the C2 transverse foramen (Figure 5).

The fundamental problems with the C2 pars interarticularis screw are that it is short (14 to 18 mm) compared with the C2 pedicle screw (30 to 40 mm) and it carries the same vertebral artery injury risks as the C1-C2 transarticular screw. The C2 pedicle screw, by definition, is positioned into the C2 vertebral body and thus is much longer and biomechanically stronger than the pars interarticularis screw. Also, because it angles medially much more than the pars interarticularis screw, it is less likely to damage the vertebral artery. The pedicle screw also starts more cephalad than the pars interarticularis screw, and this entry point is most often above the vertebral artery as it courses from medial to lateral under the inferior articular process of C2. Because the pars interarticularis screw begins more caudally, its trajectory may take it close to the

underlying vertebral artery in its medial to lateral course. The ability to begin screw placement more cephalad is an advantage because the higher the screw starts, the more likely the vertebral artery has already passed underneath the starting point.

Arthrodesis

Finally, arthrodesis is performed. Posterior arthrodesis with sublaminar cable and interspinous bicortical autograft is preferred if the laminae of C1 and C2 are preserved. Otherwise, lateral arthrodesis is performed by carefully decorticating the exposed surfaces of the C1-C2 joints with a high-speed drill, and then packing cancellous iliac crest autograft into these joints. The rod is then positioned and fixed to the C1 lateral mass and C2 pedicle screws (Figure 6).

Extremely high fusion rates are achieved because of the stability of the segmental C1 and C2 screws, which are rigidly attached to the rods. Postoperative rigid external immobilization is not required. Because pseudarthrosis is rarely needed with this polyaxial screw/rod construct, autogenous iliac crest bone graft harvest is becoming less common. Decortication of the C1-C2 joint surfaces and packing with local bone graft results in a high rate of fusion; the morbidity of the iliac crest bone site is eliminated.

Discussion

This technique can achieve solid fixation of the C1 lateral mass and can be used in a variety of instrumentation constructs for varying indications. The most common indication for the use of C1 lateral mass screws is atlantoaxial instability. Although a variety of techniques exist to treat atlantoaxial instability, certain anatomic factors may preclude their application in specific situations. C1-C2 interspinous fusion techniques using either sublaminar cables or interlaminar clamps in combination with iliac crest autograft require the presence of intact posterior elements.[5,6] These techniques cannot be applied when the C1 arch or C2 laminae have been disrupted by trauma, neoplasm, or other pathologic processes, or when resection of these elements is necessary to achieve neural decompression. Also, rigid postoperative immobilization is required in a halo to achieve satisfactory fusion rates. Even when using the Brooks method of interspinous fusion, which is the most stable of all wire/cable constructs, all patients should be immobilized in a halo vest for 3 months.[7,8]

C1-C2 transarticular screw fixation is likewise precluded by a variety of factors.[2,6,9,10] In up to 20% of patients, a medially located or high-riding vertebral artery will preclude safe passage of C1-C2 transarticular screws unilaterally. In 3% of patients, vertebral artery anatomy will preclude passage of screws bilaterally.[11,12] Irreducible C1-C2 subluxation will likewise preclude placement of C1-C2 transarticular screws. If C1 is displaced anterior to C2, the resulting trajectory of the transarticular screw is flatter (more horizontal), which jeopardizes the vertebral artery (the steeper the trajectory, the safer the vertebral artery).

Cervicothoracic kyphosis may preclude C1-C2 transarticular screw placement by obstructing the trajectory of the instruments used to insert the screws. Destruction or erosion of the osseous substrate for screw fixation by trauma, neoplasm, or other pathologic processes will similarly preclude transarticular screw placement. In these situations, occipitocervical fusion may be considered as an alternative means to treat atlantoaxial instability. Occipitocervical fusion may be avoided by using C1 lateral mass screws to achieve atlantocervical fixation. By avoiding occipitocervical fixation, range of motion at the atlanto-occipital joint is maintained, and potential morbidity from craniocervical malalignment is reduced. Clinical studies also have suggested that avoidance of occipitocervical fusion may decrease the incidence of delayed subaxial subluxation.[13,14] C1 lateral mass screws can achieve atlantocervical fixation in patients who have demonstrated various anatomic characteristics that precluded traditional methods of atlantoaxial fixation. The rigid internal fixation achieved with this technique allows immediate mobilization with a hard cervical collar, avoiding postoperative halo vest immobilization.

C1 lateral mass screws are extremely useful for occipitocervical fixation. C1 lateral mass screws provide additional fixation points for occipitocervical constructs, increasing resistance to construct failure. This additional construct integrity is achieved without fusing additional cervical levels, thus preserving cervical motion segments. As the use of polyaxial screw-rod systems for occipitocervical fixation becomes more widespread, C1 lateral mass screws will be used more frequently because the rods and lateral offset connectors used in these systems will allow C1 screws to be easily incorporated into occipitocervical constructs.

All screw techniques in the posterior cervical spine are used "off label" for Food and Drug Administration purposes. Occipital screws and thoracic pedicle screws are considered class II Food and Drug Administration devices. Despite the off-label status of these screw techniques, many types of posterior cervical screws are routinely used by most spine surgeons and are the standard of care in many indications that require cervical stabilization.

In the future, the decision to use a C1 lateral mass screw construct without interspinous fusion or contralateral transarticular screw fixation should be considered on an individual basis in the context of the pathologic process causing instability, bone quality, and other comorbidities that influence bone fusion, as well as the potential morbidity of the alternative treatment, occipitocervical fusion. Larger studies with long-term follow-up will be necessary to determine the safety and efficacy of C1 lateral mass screw constructs.

Lynch and associates[15] evaluated an atlantoaxial construct with C1 lateral mass screws and C2 pedicle screws with and without supplemental interspinous cable and graft and compared this construct with atlantoaxial transarticular screws.

Melcher and associates[16] also performed a human biomechanical cadaveric study of posterior atlantoaxial fixation techniques in an odontoidectomy model. Screw techniques (transarticular and C1 lateral mass/C2 pedicle screw/rod construct) significantly decreased motion compared with all wire/cable techniques. There were no differences between screw techniques; however, the transarticular screw model was tested with a posterior C1-C2 cable, whereas the screw/rod construct was tested without the posterior cable. These findings suggest that C1 lateral mass screw constructs coupled with C2 pedicle screw/rod constructs provide a reasonable alternative to transarticular screws for achieving atlantoaxial stabilization.

Harms and Melcher[17] used a specially modified screw at C1 with an unthreaded proximal shaft to reduce the risk of greater occipital nerve irritation and screw breakage. Fiore and associates[18,19] used standard screws with threads along the entire shaft and did not observe any instances of occipital neuralgia or screw breakage, indicating that standard screws may be used at C1. The risk of greater occipital nerve irritation is low provided there is adequate space caudal to the C1 screw for passage of the nerve.

The risk of vertebral artery injury must always be assessed when placement of lateral mass screws, C2 pars interarticularis screws, C2 pedicle screws, or transarticular screws is planned. Vertebral artery injury has not been reported during placement of C1 screws. The surgeon must note that the trajectory of the C1 lateral mass screw is different from that of lateral mass screws placed in the subaxial cervical spine. Particularly important is that the C1 screw

is placed with a slight medial angulation to avoid the vertebral artery laterally.

Summary

The placement of C1 lateral mass screws provides a useful alternative method to achieve atlantoaxial fixation when anatomic factors preclude the placement of atlantoaxial transarticular screws. This method achieves immediate rigid stabilization of the atlantoaxial joint and obviates the need for halo vest immobilization. This technique may be used in certain patients as an alternative to occipitocervical fusion and may also be used to increase construct stability when occipitocervical fixation is used. Placement of C1 lateral mass screws is a technically demanding procedure and should only be performed by surgeons who are highly experienced in the treatment of atlantoaxial instability and have an intimate understanding of the anatomy of the region. The uninitiated surgeon can minimize the possibility of complications during C1 lateral mass screw placement by first performing this procedure in a cadaveric setting. Additional biomechanical analysis of this technique should be performed to quantify the strength of constructs using C1 lateral mass screws compared with other fixation methods. Additional clinical studies should also be performed to determine the safety and efficacy of this technique.

References

1. Sasso RC, Jeanneret B, Fischer K, et al: Occipitocervical fusion with posterior plate and screw instrumentation: A long-term follow-up study. *Spine* 1994;19:2364-2368.

2. Reilly TM, Sasso RC, Hall PV: Atlantoaxial stabilization: Clinical comparison of posterior cervical wiring technique with transarticular screw fixation. *J Spinal Disord Tech* 2003;16:248-253.

3. Benzel EC: Anatomic consideration of C2 pedicle screw placement. *Spine* 1996;21:2301-2302.

4. Borne GM, Bedou GL, Pinaudeau M: Treatment of pedicular fractures of the axis: A clinical study and screw fixation technique. *J Neurosurg* 1984;60:88-93.

5. Dickman CA, Sonntag VK, Papadopoulos SM, et al: The interspinous method of posterior atlantoaxial arthrodesis. *J Neurosurg* 1991;74:190-198.

6. Farey ID, Nadkarni S, Smith N: Modified Gallie technique versus transarticular screw fixation in C1-C2 fusion. *Clin Orthop Relat Res* 1999;359:126-135.

7. Boden SD, Dodge LD, Bohlman HH, et al: Rheumatoid arthritis of the cervical spine: A long-term analysis with predictors of paralysis and recovery. *J Bone Joint Surg Am* 1993;75:1282-1297.

8. McCarron RF, Robertson WW: Brooks fusion for atlantoaxial instability in rheumatoid arthritis. *South Med J* 1988;81:474-476.

9. Dickman CA, Sonntag VK: Posterior C1-C2 Transarticular screw fixation for atlantoaxial arthrodesis. *Neurosurgery* 1998;43:275-281.

10. Haid RW, Subach BR, McLaughlin MR, et al: C1-C2 transarticular screw fixation for atlantoaxial instability: A 6-year experience. *Neurosurgery* 2001;49:65-70.

11. Madawi AA, Casey AT, Solanki GA, et al: Radiological and anatomical evaluation of the atlantoaxial transarticular screw fixation technique. *J Neurosurg* 1997;86:961-968.

12. Paramore CG, Dickman CA, Sonntag VK: The anatomical suitability of the C1-2 complex for transarticular screw fixation. *J Neurosurg* 1996;85:221-224.

13. Clark CR, Goetz DD, Menezes AH: Arthrodesis of the cervical spine in rheumatoid arthritis. *J Bone Joint Surg Am* 1989;71:381-392.

14. Kraus DR, Peppelman WC, Agarwal AK, et al: Incidence of subaxial subluxation in patients with generalized rheumatoid arthritis who had previous occipital cervical fusions. *Spine* 1991;16:S486-489.

15. Lynch JJ, Crawford NR, Chamberlain RH, Bartolomei JC, Sonntag VKH: Biomechanics of lateral mass/pedicle screw fixation at C1-2, in *Proceedings of the 2002 Annual Meeting of the American*

Academy of Neurologic Surgeons. Available at: http://www.aans.org/Library/Article.aspx?ArticleId=12334. Accessed July 17, 2006.

16. Melcher RP, Puttlitz CM, Kleinstueck FS, et al: Biomechanical testing of posterior atlantoaxial fixation techniques.

Spine 2002;27:2435-2440.

17. Harms J, Melcher RP: Posterior C1-C2 fusion with polyaxial screw and rod fixation. *Spine* 2001;26:2467-2471.

18. Fiore AJ, Haid RW, Rodts GE, et al: Atlantal lateral mass screws for posterior

spinal reconstruction: Technical note and case series. *Neurosurg Focus* 2002;12:E5.

19. Fiore AJ, Mummaneni PV, Haid RW, Rodts GE, Sasso RC: C1 lateral mass screws: Surgical nuances. *Tech Orthop* 2002;17:272-277.

Contemporary Posterior Occipital Fixation

Gordon H. Stock, MD

Alexander R. Vaccaro, MD

Andrew K. Brown, MD

Paul A. Anderson, MD

Abstract

Occipitocervical fixation is technically demanding but necessary in many clinical scenarios where junctional occiptocervical instability is present. The surgeon must have a thorough knowledge of the associated anatomy, biomechanics of spinal instrumentation, and familiarity with an ever-growing number of stabilization techniques and implants. The nature of the injury, the patient's anatomy, and the quality of the host bone will ultimately determine which form of fixation is optimal. Although the contemporary modular systems, at first glance, appear to add significant surgical complexity, in truth the designs actually simplify the process by allowing the surgeon to place occipital and spinal anchors in optimal anatomic locations.

Instr Course Lect 2007;56:319-328.

Throughout the spine, the vertebral bodies are separated from one another by intervertebral disks. The intervertebral disks provide strength between adjacent segments and limit movement by resisting compressive, rotational, and shear forces placed on the spine. In contrast, the highly mobile occipitocervical (atlanto-occipital and atlantoaxial) joints are synovial joints whose articulations are devoid of an intervertebral disk; instead, they are supported by capsuloligamentous attachments. This region is the most mobile portion of the cervical spine, with nearly one half of cervical flexion-extension and cervical rotation occurring across these cartilaginous articulations. However, the anatomic structures that allow this increased mobility also predispose the joints to instability.

The etiology of occipitocervical instability is vast and includes trauma, rheumatoid arthritis, infection, tumor, congenital deformity, and degenerative processes. Instability in this region may be asymptomatic or may manifest as pain, cranial nerve dysfunction, paresis, paralysis, or even sudden death. It is paramount, therefore, that the surgeon fully understand the complex anatomy of the occipitocervical junction, be aware of the presence of instability and its ramifications, and have a practical understanding of the many

contemporary methods used to stabilize the occipitocervical articulation.

The goals of surgery at this junction are to decompress the neurologic structures if necessary, normalize alignment, and provide immediate stability to promote osseous fusion. Recent anatomic and biomechanical studies have provided data that have led to more efficient and less morbid strategies of fixation, allowing earlier mobilization and more active participation in rehabilitation.

To better understand current implant systems used to stabilize the occipitocervical junction, it helps to review older instrumentation systems and their advantages and shortcomings.

Evolution of Occipitocervical Fixation

Occipitocervical stabilization was described as early as the 1920s by Foerster, who used a fibular strutgraft construct to span the occipitocervical articulation.[1] This was followed by in situ onlay bone grafting with wire fixation and attempts to use methylmethacrylate, with and without internal fixation, to stabilize the occipitocervical junction. Although the constructs provided some support, they were associated with a high failure rate as a result of their inability to maintain occipitocervical alignment until osseous fusion could, if ever, occur. In most instances, extended skeletal traction was required for more than 4 weeks.[2-4] In the presence of posttraumatic ligamentous injury, the distraction and translational forces associated with positional changes during immobilization in a halo vest or orthosis at times proved deleterious.[5]

In 1978, Luque[6] introduced contoured steel rods attached to the lamina with wire fixation for thoracic and lumbar spinal fixation. This concept was later adapted to reinforce fusions in the cervical spine and at the occipitocervical junction.[7] Rods could be contoured to achieve a desired alignment, and they also offered improved stability compared with that provided by previous in situ fusion methods. Unfortunately, cumbersome, prolonged postoperative external immobilization was required to improve the otherwise unacceptably low fusion rates. Furthermore, implants were available only in stainless steel, making postoperative imaging impossible. Apostolides and associates[8] introduced a device that could contour titanium rods, which were then fixed to the occiput and the posterior elements of the cervical spine with cables. Thirty-seven of the 39 patients treated with this method had osseous fusion without requiring halo vest immobilization.

For patients with rheumatoid arthritis, Ransford and associates[9] developed a contoured loop that is fixed to the occiput and cervical spine with wires. The loop compresses around C2 with the goal of maintaining the vertical alignment between the occiput and the cervical spine. Ransford and associates did not routinely attempt fusion with bone graft when they used this device. A review of the long-term results in 150 patients suggested that bone grafting in an attempt to obtain a fusion did not improve the results compared with those following fixation alone.[10]

Pelvic plate-and-screw fixation was subsequently adapted for use as segmental internal fixation of the cervical spine.[11-14] This method provided immediate rigidity to the spinal elements and obviated, in many instances, the need for postoperative halo vest immobilization. It was not necessary to pass sublaminar wires, so the most risky part of the Luque technique of fixation was avoided. However, plate-and-screw fixation still had several limitations: plates have a fixed hole-to-hole distance, which at times prevents optimal screw placement; the completed fixation implant leaves very little space for graft material; and plates provide a limited ability to compress or distract across individual interspaces.

Although the screws provided excellent fixation, the plates were less acceptable. Therefore, the longitudinal components of fixation evolved to rods that allowed unlimited superior and inferior screw placement, greater space caudad to the rod for bone grafting, and the ability to compress or distract between spinal segments as desired.

In 1999, Oda and associates[15] performed a cadaveric biomechanical analysis comparing the stability of five different types of occipitoatlantoaxial fixation systems (Figure 1), and drew several important conclusions. First, they showed that C2 transpedicular and C1- C2 trans-

articular screws significantly increased the stabilizing effect of an occipitocervical implant compared with that provided by rods and sublaminar hooks or wires ($P < 0.05$). Second, the construct with the greatest stability was a combination occipital plate-subaxial rod system with six occipital screws and C2 pedicle screws (Figure 1, E). Their hypothesis that this increased stability would lead to higher fusion rates was supported by an independent clinical study in which all 24 patients treated with rigid internal fixation and bone-grafting obtained an osseous fusion.[16]

An important consideration in the selection of a system is the stiffness of the implants. Anderson and associates[17] recently demonstrated that biomechanical performance correlated with the amount of metallic material and with its distribution as defined by the area moment of inertia. Plates, in general, have a two to three times greater area moment of inertia than do rods. The area moment of inertia correlates directly with biomechanical stiffness. For rods, the area moment of inertia varies to the fourth power of their diameter. Thus, even relatively small increases in rod size can have substantial effects. For example, a change in diameter from 3.2 to 3.5 mm doubles a rod's stiffness. Greater stiffness is believed to be better.

Fixation systems with occipital plates that are not rigidly fixed to the cervical component but can be attached to them with a locking screw mechanism were recently introduced (Figures 2 and 3). This obviates the need for contouring of the longitudinal plate or rod component between the subaxial spine and the occiput and has facilitated implant construction at the time of surgery.

Currently there remains a variety

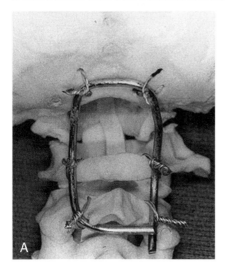

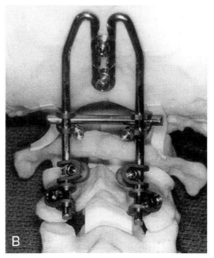

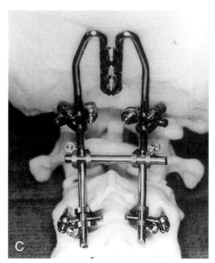

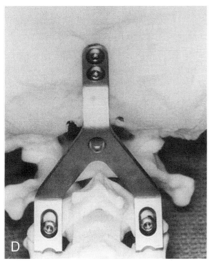

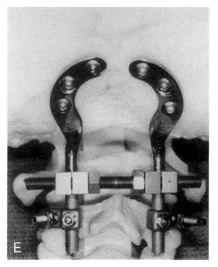

Figure 1 Five different occipitoatlanto-axial fixation devices. **A,** Occipital and sublaminar wiring with a rectangular rod. **B,** Two occipital screws and C2 lamina claw hook/rods. **C,** Two occipital screws, two foramen magnum screws, and C1-C2 transarticular screws/rods. **D,** Two occipital screws and C1- C2 transarticular screws/Y-plate. **E,** Six occipital screws and C2 pedicle screws/rods. (Reproduced with permission from Oda I, Abumi K, Sell LC, Haggerty CJ, Cunningham BW, McAfee PC: Biomechanical evaluation of five different occipito-atlanto-axial fixation techniques. *Spine* 1999;24:2377-2382.)

of fixation methods for stabilization of the occipitocervical junction.[18] There are many factors to consider when choosing which implant to use. The challenge lies in finding a proper balance between the desire for immediate rigid stabilization and the increasing surgical complexity and risk.[19]

In addition to posterior spinal fixation methods, an anterior occipitocervical reconstruction technique with use of screw fixation between the C1 lateral mass and the occipital condyles was recently described by Dvorak and associates.[20,21] Although this method provided stability in axial rotation and lateral bend-

ing, it was inferior to contemporary posterior fixation methods with regard to its ability to resist flexion and extension. Although this anterior method of fixation will have only limited application, it may prove helpful in some unique clinical settings where posterior fixation techniques either are not possible or have previously failed.

Contemporary Universal Occipital-Cervical-Thoracic Systems

Some of the device components discussed in this section have not been approved by the US Food and Drug Administration.

At present, there are two popular occipital-cervical-thoracic spinal fixation methods: dual (subaxial) rod-plate (occiput) systems and subaxial rod-independent occipital plate systems (Figures 2 and 3). Most new designs include variations on these themes with components that are all similarly designed to accomplish the same task. In the subaxial and upper cervical spine it is requisite that the skeletal anchors (screws or hooks) form a rigid connection with the longitudinal components (rods) of the implant system. This connection between the spine anchors and the longitudinal components may be direct, or it may be accomplished with

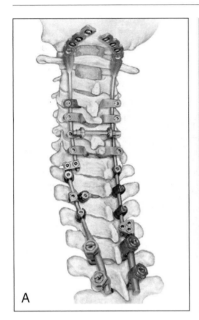

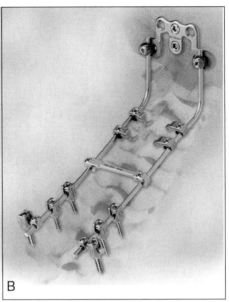

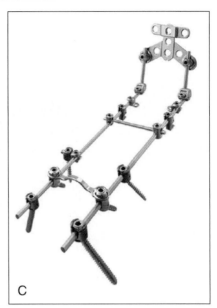

Figure 2 Representative universal posterior fixation systems. **A,** Axon System. (Reproduced with permission from Synthes USA, West Chester, PA.) **B,** Altius M-INI OCT System. (Reproduced with permission from EBI Spine, Parsippany, NJ.) **C,** Mountaineer OCT Spinal System. (Reproduced with permission from DePuy Spine, Raynham, MA.)

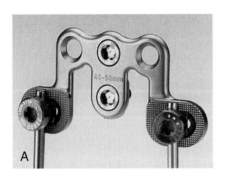

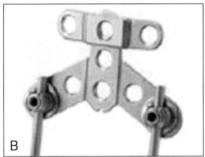

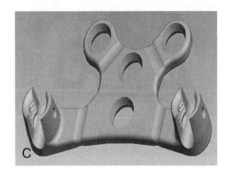

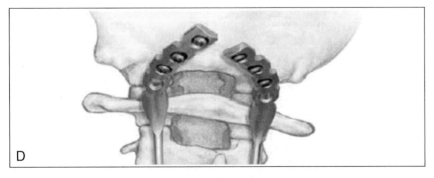

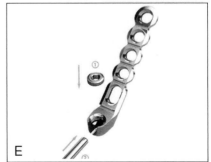

Figure 3 Various independent and bilateral occipitocervical plate designs. **A,** Altius M-INI OCT System. (Reproduced with permission from EBI Spine, Parsippany, NJ.) **B,** Mountaineer OCT Spinal System. The occipital plate is shown with the optional lateral washer. (Reproduced with permission from DePuy Spine, Raynham, MA.) **C,** Vertex Max. (Reproduced with permission from Medtronic Sofamor Danek USA, Memphis, TN.) **D,** Axon System. (Reproduced with permission from Synthes USA, West Chester, PA.) **E,** Oasys. (Reproduced with permission from Stryker, Mahwah, NJ.)

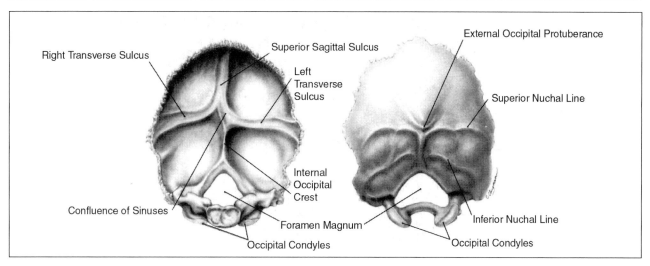

Figure 4   Internal and external osseous anatomy of the posterior aspect of the occiput. (Reproduced with permission from Roberts DA, Doherty BJ, Heggeness MH: Quantitative anatomy of the occiput and the biomechanics of occipital screw fixation. *Spine* 1998;23:1100-1108.)

use of a rod-offset connector or a variable plate-offset connector to allow maximum flexibility in medial-lateral screw or hook location. Additionally, depending on the sagittal contouring of an individual patient's anatomy, the interface between the longitudinal component and the spinal anchors must be able to accommodate substantial screw angulation when needed.

Occipital Fixation

To safely place occipital anchors, it is important to understand the osseous anatomy of the occiput in terms of its thickness in various regions and the location of underlying vascular sinuses[22] (Figure 4). The external occipital protuberance is the most prominent posterior osseous landmark on the occiput. It is located in the midline of the occiput at the confluence of the superior nuchal line and the midoccipital region. From the external occipital protuberance, there are several palpable osseous crests. The superior nuchal line extends laterally from the external occipital protuberance, whereas

the medial nuchal line descends inferiorly along the midline toward the foramen magnum. Finally, the inferior nuchal line extends inferolaterally from the middle of the medial nuchal line bilaterally. On the internal surface of the occiput, there are osseous elevations, or sulci, that contain the large venous sinuses.

In their anatomic study of the occipital bone, Ebraheim and associates[23] projected the course of the large internal venous sinuses onto the external surface of the occiput. The superior nuchal line overlies the transverse sinuses bilaterally whereas the superior sagittal sinus descends from the superior aspect of the cranium inferiorly along the midline to the torcula, or confluence of the sinuses. The torcula lies immediately underneath the external occipital protuberance. These venous structures are at risk for penetrative injury during drilling or screw placement in locations where only the dura mater separates the bone from the lumen of the dural sinuses.

In addition to mapping the large venous sinuses, Ebraheim and asso-

ciates[23] measured the thickness of the occipital bone and used those data to suggest ideal screw-insertion points. They found that the occipital bone is thickest in the midline at the external occipital protuberance. In males it is roughly 11 to 15 mm thick, whereas in females it is 10 to 12 mm thick. Cadaveric sectioning showed that the bone adjacent to the external occipital protuberance was the thickest and densest bone and that the thickness of the bone decreased laterally and inferiorly. Ten- to 12-mm screws can be used close to the external occipital protuberance, and 8-mm screws can be safely inserted lateral and inferior to the external occipital protuberance.

In a separate study on occipital morphology, Zipnick and associates[24] also showed that the occiput was thickest at the external occipital protuberance and that it decreased in thickness in a radial fashion. The outer and middle tables both contributed 45% to the overall bone thickness, whereas the inner table contributed only about 10%. Biomechanical studies have shown that screw pullout strength is related to the thickness of the bone and whether the screw has unicortical or bicortical purchase. Haher and associates[25] found that although unicortical occipital screws had less pullout strength than bicortical screws at the external occipital protuberance, the strength of the unicortical screws was comparable with that of bicortical screws at other locations. Both cortical and cancellous bone-type screws have been tested in occipital bone, but there was no significant biomechanical difference in their pullout strengths.[22]

Fear of venous penetration with bicortical screw fixation limits screw placement to below the superior nuchal line, but the work of Zipnick and associates[24] suggests that unicortical screw purchase both at and above the superior nuchal line is sufficient because the contribution of the inner table to the bone thickness is minimal and that unicortical fixation lowers the risk of intracranial venous penetration.

Because of the thicker bone that descends down the medial nuchal line, midline screws have greater pullout strength than do more laterally placed screws. This finding has been exploited by fixation designs, such as a Y-plate, that involve a single longitudinal series of occipital screw anchors in the midline (Figure 1, D). Although screws placed at the midline had greater pullout strength, this particular design (without lateral support) was found to have much weaker torsional strength than designs that included midline and laterally placed occipital screws.[26] This finding prompted the development of additional designs that either incorporated lateral fixation points in the occiput or even used only lateral fixation, without midline screws.

Anatomic and biomechanical studies have shown that, compared with laterally placed screws, midline screw fixation allows longer screw purchase but decreased torsional resistance.[17] Laterally placed screws theoretically provide better resistance to rotational stresses as a result of the bilateral purchase. In a biomechanical study, Anderson and associates[17] demonstrated that lateral screws had slightly increased stiffness in bending and rotation but not in flexion-extension. This difference was much smaller than that related to changes in rod diameter.[17] A combination of midline and laterally placed screws appears to provide the most optimal screw arrangement to ensure rigid occipital fixation. Most contemporary plates, therefore, have both medial and lateral occipital fixation points incorporated into their design (Figure 3).

To achieve maximum occipital fixation, occipital screws differ from cortical and cancellous bone screws that are used elsewhere; they have a larger diameter and smaller pitch. This design difference is especially important laterally, where the occipital bone is thinner and where shorter screws with a much smaller pitch are necessary for optimal fixation.

An alternative to traditional occipital screw fixation was described by Pait and associates.[27] They described the inside-outside technique, in which a slotted keyhole is first created in the occiput. The head of an occipital screw is then slid down into the created keyhole with the flat head of the screw in the epidural space and with the threads facing out. An occipital bone plate is then secured to the occiput with a nut. Multiple studies[27,28] have shown that this method is also safe and effective for occipital fixation.

A problem with all occipital fixa-

tion devices is implant prominence. Modern occipital plates are designed to be low profile and are precontoured to the approximate shape of the occiput. Bend zones have also been added to some plate designs to facilitate intraoperative manipulation of the plate to achieve an even closer fit between it and the occipital bone. This is shown representatively by the plate in Figure 5, but it can also be seen in Figure 3, C and E. In rod-plate designs, the bilateral occipital plates can be contoured in both the sagittal and the coronal plane for better medial approximation to the occipital bone (Figure 3, D and E).

In designs that use a rod as the longitudinal component connected to an occipital plate, the rod may be a single component that transforms from a rod into a plate in the occipital region (Figure 3, D) or it may be a two-piece design in which the occipital plate and rod are mechanically connected intraoperatively (Figure 3, E). With the latter type of design, the rod is most commonly connected to the plate with use of a slotted connector for flexibility with regard to medial-lateral rod placement. Some of the slotted connections have a fixed orientation (Figure 3, C), whereas others allow one to medialize or lateralize the rod and even rotate the articulation to facilitate plate attachment to the longitudinal rod; this is most clearly seen in Figure 3, A, where up to 5 mm of medial-lateral adjustment and any degree of rotation are possible.

Cervical Spine Fixation
There are multiple techniques for obtaining upper cervical and subaxial spine fixation. A solid upper cervical or subaxial vertebral anchor is the key to a rigid occipitocervical construct. Vertebral anchoring can

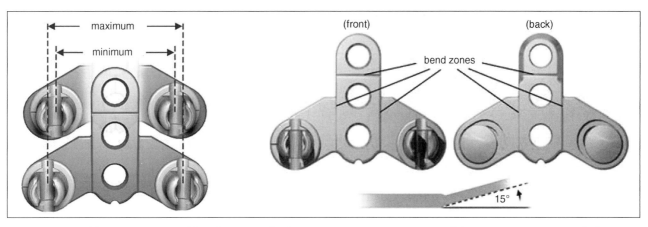

Figure 5 Variable size options and bend zones to facilitate intraoperative contouring of the Mountaineer occipital plate. (Reproduced with permission from DePuy Spine, Raynham, MA.)

be accomplished by using screws (pedicle, lateral mass, or transarticular), laminar hooks, or sublaminar wires. Screws provide the most rigid spinal anchor. Studies have shown that screws can be placed safely in the lateral mass and the cervical pedicles, although the variability in the morphometry and orientation of the pedicles and lateral masses requires very careful preoperative assessment.[29,30] When screws are placed correctly, they avoid the recognized neurologic risks associated with intracanal fixation with laminar hooks, sublaminar wires, or cables.

In addition to the advantage of not violating the canal space, properly placed screws offer several other benefits over laminar hooks that make them preferable for posterior stabilization.

Because hooks engage only the posterior part of the lamina, they can provide only semirigid fixation. On the other hand, a screw in the C1 lateral mass or the C2 pedicle can provide solid three-column fixation. The creation of a stiffer construct often reduces the number of levels that require fusion.

As part of the design versatility of contemporary occipital-cervical-

thoracic systems, the bone anchors in the cervical spine—especially those that are most constrained in their anatomic placement, such as C1 and C2 screws—are typically placed first. Once they are placed, these anchors can be used as a guide for choosing a properly sized occipital plate.

In earlier systems, the screw location was limited and mechanically constrained by the implant system. However, with the newer implants, the large variety of screw and connector designs allows the surgeon to place screws where the patient's anatomy dictates and then take advantage of screw and connector design features to facilitate attachment of the anchors to the rods with minimal rod contouring (Figure 6).

Systems currently feature variable axis or polyaxial screws, meaning that there is a certain degree of freedom between the bone screw and screw head or connecting saddle that attaches to the longitudinal rods. Some screws feature a cone of angulation that allows any position within that cone, whereas other screws are more constrained with lesser degrees of freedom, sometimes allowing movement in just

one plane. The screws depicted in Figure 6 have various degrees of freedom between the screw shaft and head. Additional design features, such as biased-angle screws and modular screw designs with multiple connector options, also facilitate rod-anchor attachment.

Longitudinal Components

There are size and shape differences between the rod-plate systems and the independent occipital plate systems. In a rod-plate system, the longitudinal connector options that are available depend on whether the rod and plate are integrated (Figures 2, A, and 3, D) or are two separate components (Figure 3, E). Integrated rod-plate systems avoid the additional mechanical coupling of the rod and plate intraoperatively, but by design they constrain the surgeon more with regard to the location of the cervical or occipital anchors because of the lack of flexibility between a fixed occipital implant location and the attached longitudinal component.

A modular rod-plate system is a design that is intermediate between a pure rod-plate design and an independent occipital plate design. Such

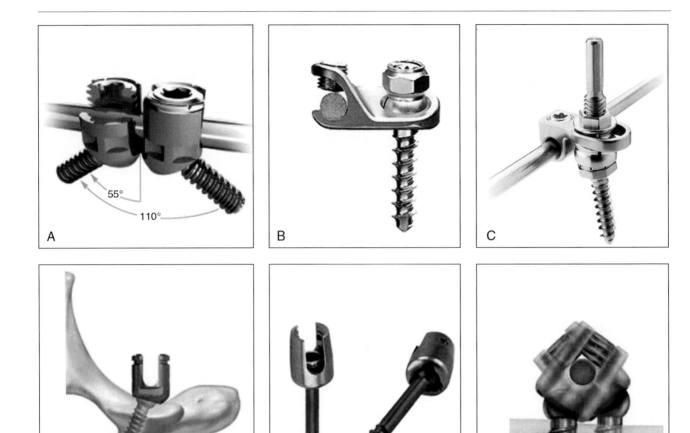

Figure 6 Contemporary screw and connector design features to facilitate attachment of the anchors to the rods with minimal rod contouring. **A,** Oasys biased-angle polyaxial screw. (Reproduced with permission from Stryker, Mahwah, NJ.) **B,** Starlock screw and favored-angle clamp. (Reproduced with permission from Synthes USA, West Chester, PA.) **C,** Altius variable-angle posted screw on lateral connector. (Reproduced with permission from EBI, Parsippany, NJ.) **D,** Mountaineer OCT favored-angle screw. (Reproduced with permission from DePuy Spine, Raynham, MA.) **E,** Vertex multiaxial screw in pivot saddle. (Reproduced with permission from Medtronic Sofamor Danek USA, Memphis, TN.) **F,** Implant detail showing anchor placement versatility. (Reproduced with permission from Medtronic Sofamor Danek USA, Memphis, TN.)

a system gives the surgeon the flexibility of changing the rod during surgery without the need to remove the screws from the occipital plate portion of the rod-plate system. However, the fixed-angle interface between the plate and the rod adds an additional constraint to the implant. For example, the connection between the rod and the occipital plate in one system is fixed at 110°

(Figure 3, *E*). Although additional minor contouring of the rod and plate may take place intraoperatively, this fixed-angle design constraint requires that the patient's anatomy be close to this angle for the device to fit well.

Independent occipital plate systems allow ultimate flexibility in plate placement that is independent of the location of the cervical rod.

This implant design allows interchange or repositioning of the rod without removal of the occipital plate. In the independent occipital plate systems, the rods may come prebent to approximate the anatomy of the occipitocervical junction; minor intraoperative adjustments are then made to further fit the implant to the sagittal plane contouring of the individual patient (Figure 2, *B*).

A recently introduced adjustable rod (Figure 7) features a joint in the rod at the level of the occipitocervical junction. This innovative design feature allows a full range of angulation to be achieved in a single plane within the rod. This has several advantages. First, surgical time is decreased because rod angulation can be fine-tuned during construct development. In addition, as with other rod-plate systems, the rods can be changed intraoperatively without removing the occipital plate. Finally, depending on the biomechanical strength of the design, long-term fatigue failure may be minimized by the lack of a need for rod-bending or stress transfer, which are traditionally required at this interface.

Several other occipitocervical rod designs are available (Figure 8), including a standard rod, a tapered rod, and a transitional rod. Most systems use rods with a constant cross-sectional area that has been precontoured to fit the occipitocervical angle (Figure 8, *A*). Although there is some variation in the diameters of the rods, most of the systems use cervical rods that are 3.5 mm in diameter.

The tapered rod is an alternative design with a different diameter at each end separated by a transition zone (Figure 8, *B*). The increased diameter gives the system added strength, especially at the transition between the occiput and the cervical spine.

A third design is the transitional rod (Figure 8, *C*). This rod is 3 mm in diameter at each end but 4 mm at the apex of the precontoured bend at the level of the occipitocervical junction. This gives the implant added strength at the apex of the curve, where the mechanical stresses are the greatest, while minimizing the size and weight in other locations along the rod.

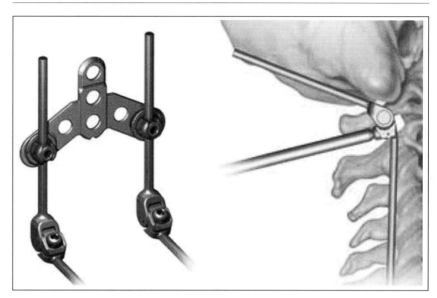

Figure 7 Occipitocervical adjustable rod (Mountaineer OCT Spinal System). The joint allows a full range of angulation in a single plane; angles can be changed intraoperatively without removing the rod. (Reproduced with permission from DePuy Spine, Raynham, MA.)

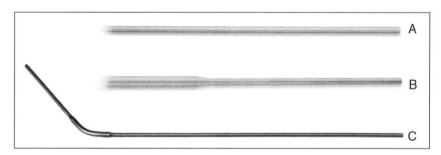

Figure 8 Standard, tapered, and transitional rod designs. **A,** Axon System standard rod. (Reproduced with permission from Synthes USA, West Chester, PA.) **B,** Axon System tapered rod. (Reproduced with permission from Synthes USA, West Chester, PA.) **C,** Summit Spinal System transitional rod. (Reproduced with permission from DePuy Spine, Raynham, MA.)

Other Components of Fixation Systems

To further stabilize the mechanical construct, each system includes cross-connecting bars or transverse connections to stabilize the two rods inferior to the occiput. The cross-connectors attach either directly to the rod or directly onto the heads of the polyaxial screws (head-to-head cross-connectors). The distance between the rods obviously varies with each patient, so each connector has design features that allow it to be easily attached to the rods regardless of the distance between them. Some connectors allow adjustment at the point where the cross-connector connects with the longitudinal rod, whereas others use an adjustable linkage within the connector itself (Figures 1 and 2). The optimal region for attachment of this connector is either right below the occipitocervical bend in the rod or at the cervicothoracic junction for longer constructs to avoid possible contact with the prominent dura in the subaxial spine.

Summary

Occipitocervical fixation is technically very demanding. The surgeon must have a thorough knowledge of the associated anatomy and of the biomechanics of the spinal instrumentation as well as familiarity with an ever-growing number of stabilization techniques and implants. The nature of the injury, the patient's anatomy, and the quality of the host bone ultimately determine which form of fixation is optimal.

Although at first glance the contemporary modular systems appear to add substantial surgical complexity, the designs actually simplify the process by allowing the surgeon to place the spinal anchors in optimal anatomic locations and still easily attach the longitudinal rods with minimal intraoperative contouring of the rods. This flexibility in anchor placement optimizes the chance of obtaining a rigid construct, therefore obviating the need for cumbersome external immobilization. The designs and techniques for obtaining fusion have changed drastically over the past century and will continue to evolve as new design innovations are introduced.

References

1. Foerster O: *Die leitungsbahnen des schmerzgefühls und die chirurgische behandlung der schmerzzustände.* Berlin, Germany, Urban and Schwarzenberg, 1927.

2. Elia M, Mazzara JT, Fielding JW: Onlay technique for occipitocervical fusion. *Clin Orthop Relat Res* 1992;280:170-174.

3. Grantham SA, Dick HM, Thompson RC Jr, Stinchfield FE: Occipitocervical arthrodesis: Indications, technic and results. *Clin Orthop Relat Res* 1969;65:118-129.

4. Hamblen DL: Occipito-cervical fusion: Indications, technique and results. *J Bone Joint Surg Br* 1967;49:33-45.

5. Vaccaro AR, Lim MR, Lee JY: Indications for surgery and stabilization techniques of the occipito-cervical junction. *Injury* 2005;36(suppl 2):B44-B53.

6. Luque ER: The anatomic basis and development of segmental spinal instrumentation. *Spine* 1982;7:256-259.

7. Itoh T, Tsuji H, Katoh Y, Yonezawa T, Kitagawa H: Occipito-cervical fusion reinforced by Luque's segmental spinal instrumentation for rheumatoid diseases. *Spine* 1988;13:1234-1238.

8. Apostolides PJ, Dickman CA, Golfinos JG, Papadopoulos SM, Sonntag VK: Threaded Steinmann pin fusion of the craniovertebral junction. *Spine* 1996;21:1630-1637.

9. Ransford AO, Crockard HA, Pozo JL, Thomas NP, Nelson IW: Craniocervical instability treated by contoured loop fixation. *J Bone Joint Surg Br* 1986;68:173-177.

10. Moskovich R, Crockard HA, Shott S, Ransford AO: Occipitocervical stabilization for myelopathy in patients with rheumatoid arthritis: Implications of not bone-grafting. *J Bone Joint Surg Am* 2000;82:349-365.

11. Grob D, Dvorak J, Panjabi M, Froehlich M, Hayek J: Posterior occipitocervical fusion: A preliminary report of a new technique. *Spine* 1991;16(3 suppl):S17-S24.

12. Lieberman IH, Webb JK: Occipitocervical fusion using posterior titanium plates. *Eur Spine J* 1998;7:308-312.

13. Sasso RC, Jeanneret B, Fischer K, Magerl F: Occipitocervical fusion with posterior plate and screw instrumentation: A long-term follow-up study. *Spine* 1994;19:2364-2368.

14. Smith MD, Anderson P, Grady MS: Occipitocervical arthrodesis using contoured plate fixation: An early report on a versatile fixation technique. *Spine* 1993;18:1984-1990.

15. Oda I, Abumi K, Sell LC, Haggerty CJ, Cunningham BW, McAfee PC: Biomechanical evaluation of five different occipito-atlanto-axial fixation techniques. *Spine* 1999;24:2377-2382.

16. Abumi K, Takada T, Shono Y, Kaneda K, Fujiya M: Posterior occipitocervical reconstruction using cervical pedicle screws and plate-rod systems. *Spine* 1999;24:1425-1434.

17. Anderson PA, Oza AL, Puscak TJ, Sasso R: Biomechanics of occipitocervical fixation. *Spine* 2006;31:755-761.

18. Menezes AH: Complications of surgery at the craniovertebral junction: Avoidance and management. *Pediatr Neurosurg* 1991;17:254-266.

19. Singh SK, Rickards L, Apfelbaum RI, Hurlbert RJ, Maiman D, Fehlings MG: Occipitocervical reconstruction with the Ohio Medical Instruments Loop: Results of a multicenter evaluation in 30 cases. *J Neurosurg* 2003;98(suppl 3):239-246.

20. Dvorak MF, Fisher C, Boyd M, Johnson M, Greenhow R, Oxland TR: Anterior occiput-to-axis screw fixation: Part I. A case report, description of a new technique, and anatomical feasibility analysis. *Spine* 2003;28:E54-E60.

21. Dvorak MF, Sekeramayi F, Zhu Q, et al: Anterior occiput to axis screw fixation: Part II. A biomechanical comparison with posterior fixation techniques. *Spine* 2003;28:239-245.

22. Roberts DA, Doherty BJ, Heggeness MH: Quantitative anatomy of the occiput and the biomechanics of occipital screw fixation. *Spine* 1998;23:1100-1108.

23. Ebraheim NA, Lu J, Biyani A, Brown JA, Yeasting RA: An anatomic study of the thickness of the occipital bone: Implications for occipitocervical instrumentation. *Spine* 1996;21:1725-1730.

24. Zipnick RI, Merola AA, Gorup J, et al: Occipital morphology: An anatomic guide to internal fixation. *Spine* 1996;21:1719-1724.

25. Haher TR, Yeung AW, Caruso SA, et al: Occipital screw pullout strength: A biomechanical investigation of occipital morphology. *Spine* 1999;24:5-9.

26. Sutterlin CE III, Bianchi JR, Kunz DN, Zdeblick TA, Johnson WM, Rapoff AJ: Biomechanical evaluation of occipitocervical fixation devices. *J Spinal Disord* 2001;14:185-192.

27. Pait TG, Al-Mefty O, Boop FA, Arnautovic KI, Rahman S, Ceola W: Inside-outside technique for posterior occipitocervical spine instrumentation and stabilization: Preliminary results. *J Neurosurg* 1999;90(suppl 1):1-7.

28. Sandhu FA, Pait TG, Benzel E, Henderson FC: Occipitocervical fusion for rheumatoid arthritis using the inside-outside stabilization technique. *Spine* 2003;28:414-419.

29. Ebraheim N, Rollins JR Jr, Xu R, Jackson WT: Anatomic consideration of C2 pedicle screw placement. *Spine* 1996;21:691-695.

30. Jones EL, Heller JG, Silcox DH, Hutton WC: Cervical pedicle screws versus lateral mass screws. Anatomic feasibility and biomechanical comparison. *Spine* 1997;22:977-982.

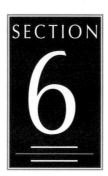

SECTION

6

Trauma

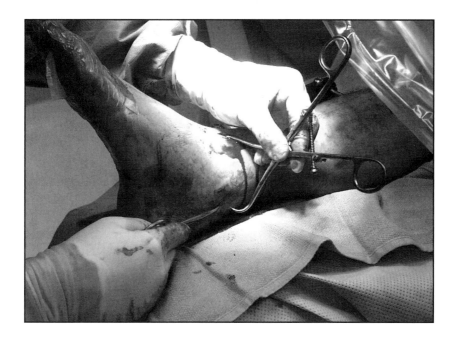

Fractures of the Tibial Plafond

J. Lawrence Marsh, MD
Joseph Borrelli, Jr, MD
Douglas R. Dirschl, MD
Michael S. Sirkin, MD

Abstract

Tibial plafond fractures comprise a diverse group of articular, metaphyseal, and occasionally diaphyseal injuries and have in common injury to the articular surface of the distal tibia and significant associated soft-tissue injury. Injury to the soft tissues combined with the complex fracture patterns has led to high complication rates from surgical attempts to reduce and stabilize these fractures. Currently, there is a wide range of treatment techniques available for a wide spectrum of injury severity, surgeon experience, and surgeon preferences. Patient outcomes vary widely. Because these injuries are relatively uncommon, the amount of clinical data available to guide treatment decisions is limited. Careful classification and assessment of the fracture pattern and associated soft-tissue injury and an understanding of the principles of modern concepts of treatment should allow the surgeon to choose from among several treatment protocols, all of which emphasize minimizing complications to optimize patient outcomes.

Instr Course Lect 2007;56:331-352.

This chapter reviews the latest concepts in assessment, management, and expected outcomes for patients with fractures of the tibial plafond. The ongoing controversy between whether to treat these complex fractures with external fixation or plate fixation will be highlighted, and the factors that relate to outcome will be reviewed.

Classification and Assessment
Fracture Classification
The two most common classification systems used currently to assess fractures of the distal tibia are that of the AO/Orthopaedic Trauma Association (OTA) (Figure 1) and the system described by Ruedi and Allgöwer (Figure 2). Although both of these classification systems are commonly discussed in the literature, recent publications favor the AO/OTA classification.

The AO/OTA classification system is a complex fracture classification that assesses which bone is involved, the part of the bone that is involved, the number of fragments, the complexity of the fracture pattern, and in patients with articular injuries, the amount of joint involvement. For distal tibia fractures, the designation of bone involvement is 43: 43-A fractures are extra-articular, 43-B fractures are partial articular, and 43-C fractures are complete articular. Although further subclassifications are based on these criteria, it has been shown that beyond the most rudimentary divisions of A, B, and C, the classification is not reliable; therefore, any usefulness beyond this level may be limited,[1-3] especially when comparing results of treatment.

The classification system of Ruedi and Allgöwer is based on the amount of comminution of the articular surface[4] (Figure 2). Type I fractures are nondisplaced, type II fractures are displaced but not comminuted, and type III fractures are displaced and comminuted. Although this classification system is simple and easy to remember, it has been shown to have poor observer reliability and may not provide enough detail to meaningfully guide treatment.[2]

Soft-Tissue Assessment and Classification
Understanding the importance of the soft-tissue injury in tibial plafond fractures is paramount to successful treatment. Complications

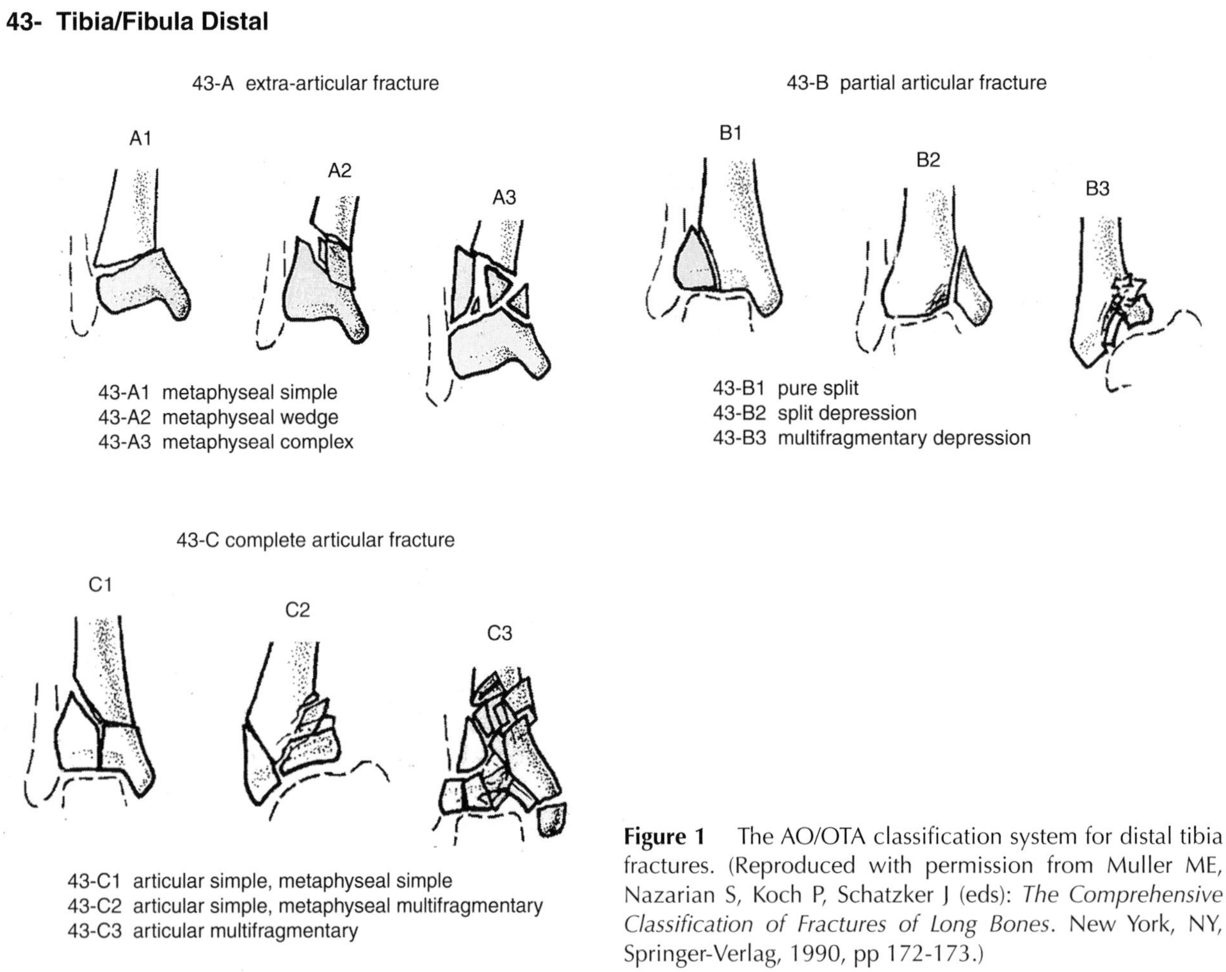

43- Tibia/Fibula Distal

43-A extra-articular fracture

A1

A2

A3

43-A1 metaphyseal simple
43-A2 metaphyseal wedge
43-A3 metaphyseal complex

43-B partial articular fracture

B1

B2

B3

43-B1 pure split
43-B2 split depression
43-B3 multifragmentary depression

43-C complete articular fracture

C1

C2

C3

43-C1 articular simple, metaphyseal simple
43-C2 articular simple, metaphyseal multifragmentary
43-C3 articular multifragmentary

Figure 1 The AO/OTA classification system for distal tibia fractures. (Reproduced with permission from Muller ME, Nazarian S, Koch P, Schatzker J (eds): *The Comprehensive Classification of Fractures of Long Bones.* New York, NY, Springer-Verlag, 1990, pp 172-173.)

related to the surrounding soft-tissue envelope may be the most difficult to treat and are responsible for devastating and long-term problems, such as chronic osteomyelitis or even amputation. The most commonly used system to classify soft-tissue injuries associated with fractures is that described by Tscherne[5] (Table 1).

The degree and amount of soft-tissue injury at times can be difficult to fully appreciate. Surgeons can assess the presence or absence of fracture blisters; if present, it can be determined whether they are clear or hemorrhagic. Blisters are one sign of severe soft-tissue injury. Visible

bruising and contusion over the injured area as described in the Tscherne classification system are other signs of soft-tissue injury (Figure 3). However, even in the absence of blisters or visible bruising and contusion, swelling itself can represent a soft-tissue injury that should preclude aggressive surgery until it resolves. The presence of the wrinkle sign has been described as one measure of resolution of swelling, but to the authors' knowledge, the usefulness of this measure has not been systematically tested. If there is any concern for the status of the soft tissues, definitive treatment should be delayed, especially when

considering formal open reduction of the articular component. Performing surgery through swollen, contused, and damaged tissue is unwise and will typically lead to disastrous complications.

Before surgeons had full understanding of the significance of the associated soft-tissue injury, treating high-energy pilon fractures was fraught with complications.[6-11] To prevent these severe soft-tissue–related problems, several strategies have been developed and tested, including definitive unilateral external fixation,[12-17] hybrid external fixation,[18-25] staged protocols with open reduction,[26-28] and most re-

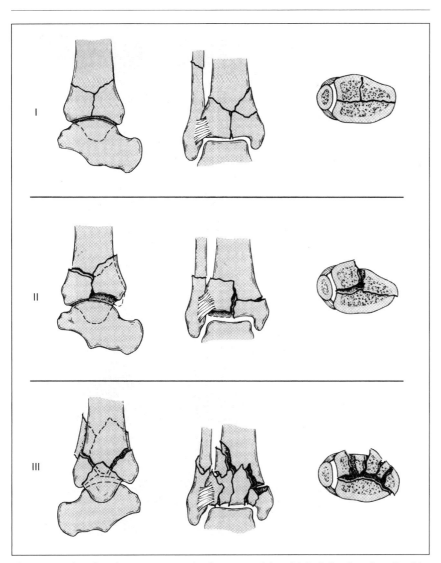

Figure 2 The classification system for fractures of the tibial plafond as described by Ruedi and Allgöwer is based on the amount of comminution of the articular surface. Type I fractures are nondisplaced, type II fractures are displaced but not comminuted, and type III fractures are displaced and comminuted. (Reproduced with permission from Ruedi TP, Allgöwer M: The operative treatment of intra-articular fractures of the lower end of the tibia. *Clin Orthop Relat Res* 1979;138:105-110.)

Table 1
Classification System for Soft-Tissue Injuries Associated With Fractures

Type 0	Minimal soft-tissue injury, torsion fractures
Type I	Superficial abrasion or contusion, mild to moderate fracture configuration
Type II	Deep, contaminated abrasion or muscle contusion, segmental fractures
Type III	Extensive soft-tissue injury, decompressed compartment syndromes

(Adapted with permission from Tscherne H, Oestern HJ: A new classification of soft-tissue damage in open and closed fractures (author's transl). *Unfallheilkunde* 1982;85:111-115.)

cently limited open reduction and percutaneous plating.[26,29-31] Soft-tissue complications from treatment have been reduced to a more acceptable level by using one or more of these techniques.

Temporizing Spanning External Fixation

Most modern treatment protocols recommend delaying definitive surgery to allow soft-tissue recovery. During this time, the use of a temporizing external fixator allows the patient to be mobilized while the length and alignment of the fracture is maintained. Use of these devices has become commonplace in the management of high-energy tibial plafond fractures.

Temporizing spanning external fixation uses the fixator to provide portable traction. Distraction and ligamentotaxis realign the limb; and although the fixator maintains length and rotation, it does not typically restore articular congruity. The ankle spanning external fixator can only facilitate the approximation of the articular fracture fragments (via ligamentotaxis); it cannot accurately reduce articular fragments.

Definitive articular reduction and bony stabilization is performed after swelling and edema have resolved, making surgical incisions safer. The spanning fixator provides some stability to the fractured area that minimizes additional soft-tissue injury and improves patient comfort, while the soft tissues recover. Once the surgeon determines that the soft tissues have recovered sufficiently, the fracture pattern has been thoroughly assessed, and a preoperative plan has been developed, additional surgical stabilization of the distal tibia, such as plate fixation and removal of the external fixator, can safely be performed.[27,28]

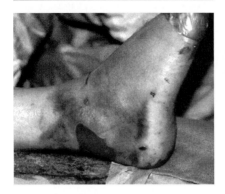

Figure 3 Photograph of a Tscherne type III soft-tissue injury in a patient with a tibial plafond fracture. (Reproduced with permission from Tscherne H, Oestern HJ: A new classification of soft-tissue damage in open and closed fractures (author's transl). *Unfallheilkunde* 1982;85:111-115.)

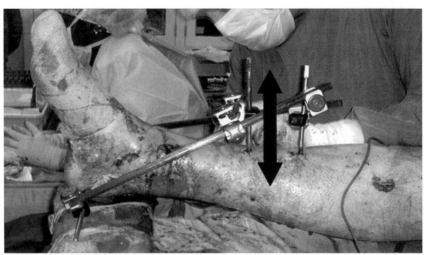

Figure 4 Photograph showing application of the temporizing transarticular fixator. The distal pin in the tibia controls the position of the foot in the sagittal plane. By sliding the frame up or down on this pin (*arrow*), the ankle can be translated anterior or posterior in relation to the tibial shaft. After locking this clamp, the alignment will be maintained even if an anteriorly directed force is placed on the distal segment by resting the foot on the bed.

Temporizing spanning external fixation uses half-pins in the tibia and a calcaneal transfixation pin. Two pins initially are placed into the tibia on the anteromedial portion of the tibial crest in the sagittal plane. These pins should be placed well proximal away from the zone of injury and away from the area where the future plate may be placed. It is best to avoid overlapping the pin sites with definitive implants to avoid contamination. A transcalcaneal pin is then placed. This centrally threaded pin is placed through the posterior calcaneus in the safe zone to avoid injury to the lateral plantar nerve, the most posterior plantar nerve, and the medial calcaneal nerve.[32] This pin should be placed parallel to the distal tibial articular surface and parallel to floor, with the patient's foot pointing straight up. Bars are then connected in a triangle from the most proximal tibial pin to the calcaneal pin, manual traction is applied, and a reduction is obtained. The distal tibial pin is then connected to the construct to maintain rigidity in the sagittal plane and allow for small adjustments to the

ankle reduction (Figure 4). If the foot lies in equinus after the frame is tightened, a supplemental 4-mm pin can be inserted into the base of the first metatarsal and attached to the medial rod of the frame to maintain the foot and ankle in a plantigrade position.

Radiographs should be obtained after reduction and carefully assessed for any residual shortening or ankle subluxation. Guides to correct length include the fibula or the Chaput fragment (anterolateral tibial fragment). Correct length of the tibia must be obtained with this initial fixator to avoid undue tension on the skin at the time of definitive fixation when tibial length must be restored (Figure 5). The talus must be reduced under the tibia, especially on a lateral radiograph; if not, anterior skin necrosis may occur from direct pressure of underlying bone. A poorly applied spanning frame that does not achieve length and overall alignment serves little purpose.

Although a large, multiplanar, one-piece external fixator typically used for definitive treatment can accomplish these same goals, it has two important disadvantages when used as a temporary spanning frame. First, one of the distal pins is placed within the talar neck, which therefore is close to the location of secondary incisions for internal fixation. Second, the cost of these external fixators is considerable compared with the cost of half-pins and bars. Simpler frames with transfixation pins placed through the tibia and the calcaneus can also be applied to accomplish the same goals, but offer no additional benefits and are associated with increased risk of neurovascular injury. The frames previously described are sometimes placed in the emergency department without bringing the patient to the operating room.

Rationale for Plate Fixation
Open reduction and internal fixation of intra-articular distal tibia

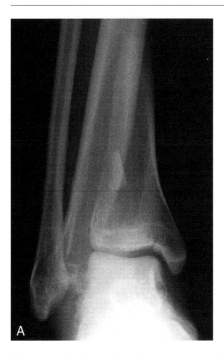
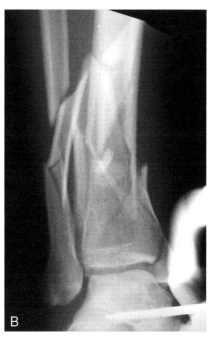

Figure 5   Radiographs of transarticular fixation in which the talus is left shortened and limb length is not realigned. Note the position of the intact fibula and lateral tibia as the guide to length **(A)** and the short fibula **(B)**.

Table 2
Advantages of Open Reduction and Internal Fixation Over External Fixation in the Treatment of Pilon Fractures

Anatomic reduction of moderate to severely displaced articular fracture fragments is only possible with formal open reduction and internal fixation, particularly for fractures with centrally displaced fragments

With newer plating techniques and approaches, reduction and stabilization of the articular block to the tibial diaphysis can be performed with less soft-tissue stripping and smaller incisions; as a result, formal open reduction and internal fixation is safer, more soft-tissue friendly, and results in a considerably lower complication rate when combined with use of an initial spanning external fixator

Locking plate technology has allowed fixation of very distal fractures and in patients with osteoporosis, without having to span the ankle and subtalar joints, making early range of motion possible

Patients treated with open reduction and internal fixation do not require long-term pin site care and are therefore not subject to the morbidity commonly associated with the use of external fixators; additionally, if subsequent surgical procedures are necessary (bone graft of the metaphysis to treat delayed union or nonunion), contaminated pins and pin sites do not have to be prepped into the field

Although an external fixator can be used as effectively as a plate to buttress metaphyseal fractures, the longer the fracture takes to heal, the longer the frame has to remain in place, making pin tract complications even more likely

fractures was originally popularized in the 1970s.[4,33] Unfortunately, because of many unfavorable outcomes, including wound dehiscence, deep infection, and amputation, this technique fell out of favor for the treatment of these challenging injuries. Over the past 30 years, methods and implants have changed to make this technique safer and more beneficial to the patient. One such advance is the temporary ankle spanning external fixator, which helps delay surgery in patients with acute injury. Other advances have been made in the surgical approaches used to treat distal tibia fractures, which are often high-energy injuries.[27-29,34] The decrease in the rate of complications has allowed plate fixation to again be one of the more popular techniques of treatment of articular fractures of the distal tibia. Formal open reduction and internal fixation of pilon fractures also offers certain advantages over the use of external fixation. These advantages are listed in Table 2 .

Treatment of high-energy displaced intra-articular distal tibia fractures is challenging. Although several treatment options are available, many surgeons continue to prefer formal open reduction and internal fixation to maximize the articular reduction and avoid the use of external fixators. The surgical approaches to the distal tibia allow direct visualization of fracture reduction, which optimizes the reconstruction of the damaged articular surface. Conversion of the temporary external fixator to internal fixation frees the ankle, allowing patients to perform range-of-motion exercises without encumbering the external fixation components.

There are several potential surgical approaches to the distal tibia through which plate fixation can be accomplished. Each of these approaches has relative indications and its own sets of advantages and disadvantages. The choice of approach should depend on the extent and location of the soft-tissue damage, the fracture pattern, and the surgeon's familiarity, training, and comfort with the approach.

Approaches and Techniques of Definitive Plate Fixation
Anteromedial Approach
The "workhorse" for the open treatment of distal intra-articular tibia fractures is the anteromedial ap-

proach, which is commonly used to treat fractures with involvement of the anterior, medial, and central plafond and with limited involvement of the lateral aspect. The anteromedial approach should only be undertaken once the soft tissues surrounding the distal leg have recovered from the trauma. Recovery of the skin, including reduction of swelling, is often evident by wrinkling of the skin at the base of the toes and the ankle and reepithelization of the blistered areas.[35] Care should be taken during the anteromedial approach, manipulation of the fracture fragments, and closure to minimize further soft-tissue trauma. Additional trauma to these areas can be avoided by not grasping the skin edges with forceps and by minimizing the use of self-retaining retractors and inattentive assistants.[36,37] If open reduction and internal fixation of the fibula is to be performed, the fibular incision should be placed slightly posterior to the midcoronal plane to ensure that at least a 7-cm skin bridge is present between the fibular and tibial incisions.

The anteromedial approach is started proximally at (or just above) the proximal extent of the fracture, one-half fingerbreadth lateral to the palpable tibial crest. The incision is extended distally, curving gently toward the talonavicular joint, paralleling the path of the anterior tibialis tendon. The incision should not be curved sharply around the medial malleolus because this will limit the exposure of the plafond. The extensor retinaculum is exposed medial to the anterior tibialis tendon and incised, leaving the tendon(s) undisturbed within the paratenon. The periosteum is left attached to the underlying fracture fragments, and the anterior tibialis, extensor hallu-

cis longus, and extensor digitorum communis tendons, along with the dorsalis pedis artery and venae and the superficial peroneal nerve, are retracted laterally. Previously, it was recommended that this approach be performed between the anterior tibialis and extensor hallucis longus tendons by retracting the anterior tibialis tendon medially and the extensor hallucis longus tendon laterally.[38] This technique, however, exposes the nearby neurovascular bundle and theoretically increases the risk of injury. Once the joint capsule is exposed, an arthrotomy is performed, and the articular surface and fragments are exposed. While gently retracting the skin, tendons, and dorsalis pedis arteries, the articular fragments of the distal tibia can be further displaced in a manner comparable to opening the pages of a book. Reconstruction of the joint should generally begin with the largest, least displaced fracture fragments and then proceed to the smaller, more displaced fragments. Occasionally, large articular fragments can first be reduced to the distal tibial diaphysis, and then the rest of the articular fragments reduced next. If this method is chosen, it is imperative that the articular fragments are anatomically reduced to the diaphysis because any malposition of these fragments will result in an even greater displacement at the articular surface. In either instance, image intensification in the AP, lateral, and oblique views will aid in assessing the reduction of the articular surface. If possible, the articular reduction can also be assessed via direct visualization by looking into the joint from below. It is important to keep in mind that if the metaphyseal aspect of the fibula has been plated, then the plate will obscure the articular surface when the

image intensifier is in the true lateral position. If recognized in advance, temporary stabilization of the fibula can be performed with small reduction forceps, and then definitive fixation can be performed after the tibial plafond has been reduced and stabilized. If the fibula has already been reduced and plated, oblique images of the distal tibia can be used to assess the adequacy of the reduction. Temporary stabilization of the reduced articular fragments is obtained with Kirschner wires (1.6 mm or 2.0 mm) and pointed reduction forceps, which are subsequently replaced with interfragmentary small-fragment lag screws or cannulated screws. Once the articular block is reconstructed, it is then reduced to the tibial shaft. It is held reduced with pointed reduction forceps and/or Kirschner wires (1.6 mm or 2.0 mm) while making sure that length, alignment, and rotation are restored. Definitive fixation of the distal tibia is then performed with small, low-profile implants. Generally, plates are placed along the medial aspect of the tibia to secure the articular block while resisting varus drift. Small plates are often needed anteriorly to buttress the anterior articular and metaphyseal fragments. Again, small, low-profile plates are best for this area. If the soft-tissue attachments are maintained during the surgery, these fragments will often heal relatively quickly; large fragment plates are not needed for strength and, because of their size, can become quite bothersome to the overlying soft tissues[29,39,40] (Figure 6).

Anterolateral Approach

An alternative approach to the tibial plafond that is gaining in popularity is the anterolateral approach. The relative indications for this approach

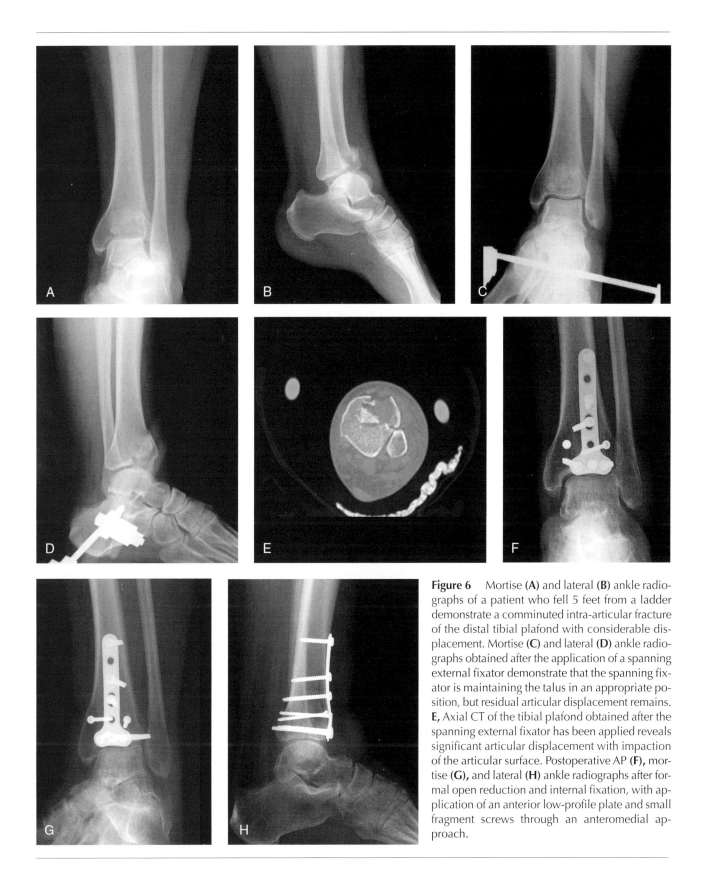

Figure 6 Mortise (**A**) and lateral (**B**) ankle radiographs of a patient who fell 5 feet from a ladder demonstrate a comminuted intra-articular fracture of the distal tibial plafond with considerable displacement. Mortise (**C**) and lateral (**D**) ankle radiographs obtained after the application of a spanning external fixator demonstrate that the spanning fixator is maintaining the talus in an appropriate position, but residual articular displacement remains. **E**, Axial CT of the tibial plafond obtained after the spanning external fixator has been applied reveals significant articular displacement with impaction of the articular surface. Postoperative AP (**F**), mortise (**G**), and lateral (**H**) ankle radiographs after formal open reduction and internal fixation, with application of an anterior low-profile plate and small fragment screws through an anteromedial approach.

over the anteromedial approach are the presence of an open or previously open medial wound, significant medial soft-tissue swelling and contusion, fractures with primarily lateral and anterolateral articular comminution, and fractures with widely displaced Chaput fragments. The primary advantages this approach has over the anteromedial approach are that on closure there is a thicker, more vascular coverage of the implants and fracture and, because the skin and soft tissues in this area are usually less severely injured than they are medially, both the fibula and the tibia can be stabilized through this single approach.[41] Although the dorsalis pedis artery can be injured from below, the superficial peroneal nerve is more at risk during this approach. Specially contoured plates are typically used when this approach is used to repair distal tibial fractures.

The approach is started along the anterolateral aspect of the distal leg parallel to and just anterior to the fibula. The incision is taken down through the skin and subcutaneous tissue, and the superficial peroneal nerve is identified, carefully mobilized, and retracted medially. The superior and inferior retinaculae are exposed and incised longitudinally for later repair. The interval between the extensor digitorum communis and the fibula is developed, the tendons and muscle bellies are elevated off of the interosseous membrane, and the distal tibia and ankle joint are exposed. In this approach, all of the tendons and dorsalis pedis and superficial peroneal nerves are retracted medially. The fibula is exposed and can be stabilized with an anterolateral or laterally placed plate; the articular fragments are reduced, and restoration of limb length, alignment, and rotation are achieved. Stabilization of

the articular fragments is typically performed with small fragment lag screws or cannulated screws, and specially designed distal tibial plates and other low-profile plates are used to restore continuity between the articular block and the diaphysis (Figure 7).

Posterolateral Approach

A posterolateral approach for the treatment of high-energy distal tibia fractures has been described, although the safety and indications for this approach have not been fully developed.[34] The rationale for the posterolateral approach, as with the anterolateral approach, is that the incision is made through skin that is less severely injured than with the anteromedial approach. Because of the robust nature of the posterior soft tissues, the implants and fracture will be well covered. In addition, because these tissues are more robust, they will be less likely to break down postoperatively. The disadvantages of this approach include limited access to the anterior articular fragments, patient positioning (prone), and the risk of injury to the sural nerve.

To perform the posterolateral approach to the distal tibia, the patient is positioned prone. The incision is made just medial, posterior, and parallel to the distal fibula and the peroneal tendons. The incision is carried down through the subcutaneous tissues, and the sural nerve is isolated and protected throughout. The interval between the peroneal brevis or peroneal longus and the flexor hallucis longus tendons is developed. The flexors are elevated off of the interosseous membrane and the posterior aspect of the distal tibia, and the fracture fragments are addressed in the usual manner. Plate fixation of the distal fibula and tibia are per-

formed through the same incision, with either specialty plates or straight plates contoured to the bone.

Medial Approach

A direct medial approach to the distal tibia for the treatment of intra-articular distal tibia fractures should be avoided for two reasons. First, the medial soft tissues are often compromised and cannot tolerate further surgical trauma and therefore are prone to develop wound dehiscence that can lead to deep infections. Second, even if these tissues are capable of tolerating a second insult, often, to close the incision over the implant and tibia, considerable tension of the skin is required. In this instance, wound dehiscence can occur and there is further loss of surrounding soft tissues, requiring a vascularized free-tissue transfer for secondary coverage.[10] If a wound problem occurs when using the other recommended approaches (anteromedial, anterolateral, and posterolateral), the wound, because of its location over muscle, retinaculum, and tendons, can be treated with local wound care and allowed to heal, thereby avoiding major soft-tissue reconstruction.

A medial approach should only be used for true percutaneous plating. With this technique, the articular surface is either not injured (AO/OTA type A fracture) or is reduced and fixed percutaneously. A precontoured plate is then placed medially to stabilize the articular segment to the tibial shaft using small percutaneous incisions.

Rationale for External Fixation for Definitive Treatment

Whether to treat high-energy tibial plafond fractures with open reduction and internal fixation or external fixation is a controversial issue

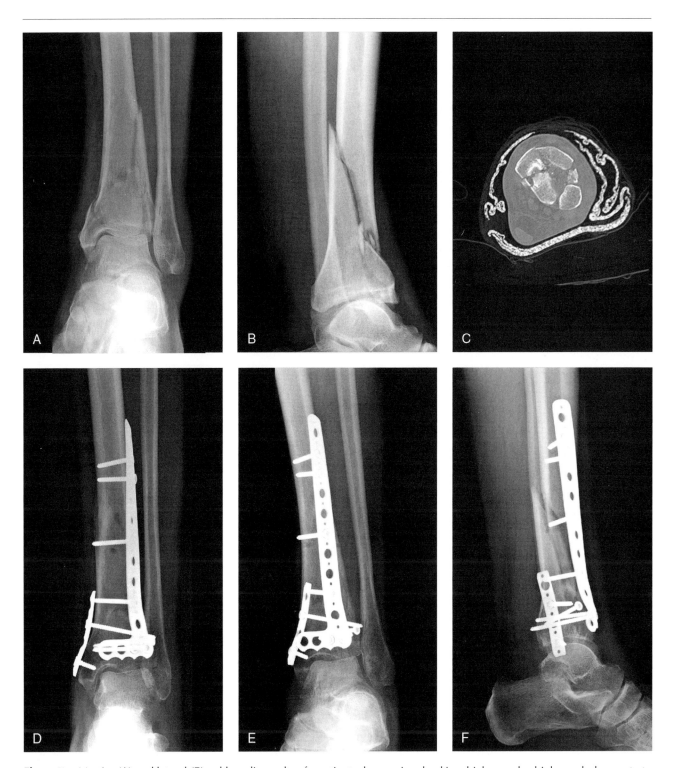

Figure 7 Mortise (**A**) and lateral (**B**) ankle radiographs of a patient who was involved in a high-speed vehicle crash demonstrate a comminuted, intra-articular fracture with shortening and a long posterolateral fragment. **C,** Axial CT scan demonstrates the intra-articular displaced fractures. Postoperative AP (**D**), mortise (**E**), and lateral (**F**) ankle radiographs after open reduction and internal fixation was performed via an anterolateral approach and supplemental stabilization was performed via a percutaneously placed medial plate.

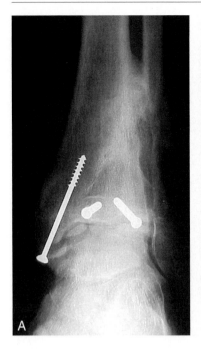 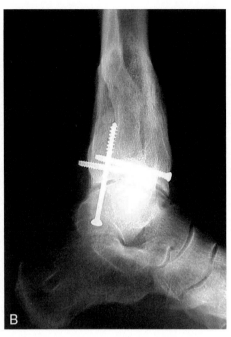 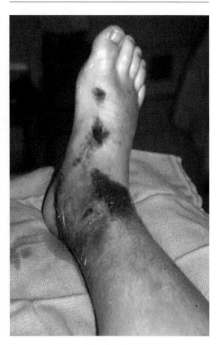

Figure 8 AP (**A**) and lateral (**B**) radiographs obtained 5 years after a highly comminuted tibial plafond fracture reveal nonanatomic reduction and severe osteoarthrosis. The patient had no pain and an excellent ankle score.

Figure 9 Photograph of a patient with a tibial plafond fracture shows massive soft-tissue swelling, fracture blisters, and deep contusion to the skin and muscle. Early open surgical treatment in this situation should be avoided.

among orthopaedic traumatologists. It is not uncommon to hear dogmatic statements about the treatment of these injuries, with dichotomous terms such as "always/never" or "good/evil" used to describe treatment choices and their relative merits. In examining why this controversy exists, five factors come to mind. First, dogma and surgeon biases indicate that intra-articular fractures should undergo anatomic reduction; the literature, however, is divided on the preeminence of articular reduction.[42-48] Second, there is a strong legacy of using open reduction and internal fixation to treat these injuries, beginning in the 1970s with the work of Ruedi and Allgöwer.[33] Third, individual surgeon training and experience provide varying levels of expertise and comfort with the various reduction and stabilization techniques. Fourth, the functional outcomes of these injuries are unpredictable and do

not correlate well at all with the radiograph appearance.[49] Fifth, valid functional outcomes data indicating one technique is superior to another simply do not exist.

Tibial plafond fractures are devastating injuries to both the bone and soft tissues; consequently, the outcomes following treatment of these injuries are unpredictable. A patient with an anatomic reduction with a stable fixation and radiographic evidence of healing often will still have severe pain and a poor functional outcome. Conversely, a patient with a great deal of comminution and a nonanatomic reduction, who, after healing, has radiographic evidence of severe arthrosis, may have no pain and an excellent functional result (Figure 8). In trying to understand why this is so, surgeons must consider whether the extent of the soft-tissue and articular cartilage injury may have as much or more influence on the functional

outcome as the bony injury.[47,48] High-energy tibial plafond fractures are characterized by severe, early, soft-tissue swelling and the frequent occurrence of fracture blisters. These fractures often result in chronic soft-tissue changes such as swelling, extensive scar formation, tendon impingement, or complex regional pain syndrome. The extent and nature of soft-tissue injury are the factors that increase the risk of treatment complications in the management of these injuries.[36,50] The sequelae of such complications can be devastating and include amputation of the limb. Thus, the treatment undertaken for these injuries must ensure that devastating soft-tissue complications can be avoided (Figure 9).

External fixation as definitive treatment of high-energy tibial

Table 3
Advantages of Using External Fixation to Treat High-Energy Tibial Plafond Fractures

External fixation completely spans the zone of injury and requires minimal or no soft-tissue dissection within the zone of injury; furthermore, it burns no bridges—it can always be converted later to internal fixation if the need arises

Surgery for articular reduction and stabilization (usually done on a delayed basis) can be performed with an external fixator in place; the fixator assists in maintaining length and alignment during surgery

External fixation is the easiest of the available techniques to apply and, once the spanning external fixator is in place, it allows a graded approach to the articular surface; fractures with minimal soft-tissue swelling are amenable to open reduction techniques, but those with massive soft-tissue swelling and scarring should have limited approaches to the articular surface

External fixation affords one technique for all fractures (there is no need to worry about whether to do a medial, lateral, or even a posterior approach); the technique for fixator application is the same in all fractures

An external fixator is as good a buttress as is a plate. This is a fact that is often ignored by those who prefer internal fixation; however, an external fixator, if appropriately applied, serves as an effective buttressing device in the same way as does a plate applied inside the body

It is not possible to achieve perfect anatomic reduction in all high-energy tibial plafond fractures because comminution of the central portion of the tibial plafond is present in almost all of these injuries and there is often loss of bone or articular cartilage from this central area of the plafond; therefore, restoration of the cortical rim of the plafond is nearly always possible with any technique, but restoration of the central bone and the lost articular cartilage is almost always impossible in the highest-energy fractures—external fixation acknowledges this fact because the goal of this technique is not to make the articular surface perfect in every patient

External fixation has good long-term (5- to 11-year) outcomes reported in the literature

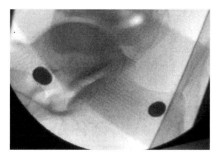

Figure 10 Lateral intraoperative fluoroscopic view of the foot illustrating the appropriate positions for half-pins in the talus and calcaneus. Care should be taken to ensure that the pins are parallel to the talar dome on the AP radiograph and that the subtalar joint is in neutral alignment when the second pin is inserted.

plafond fractures can help avoid complications because it is the safest technique available for the treatment of these fractures.[49] External fixation offers several advantages, which are listed in Table 3.

It is clear that external fixation of high-energy distal tibia fractures began as a reaction to the high complication rates encountered with using open reduction and internal fixation to treat these fractures.[36,50] However, external fixation has now evolved and has been integrated into a philosophy of care for patients with high-energy periarticular fractures, a philosophy that involves spanning the zone of injury with the fixation device and making limited approaches to the fracture fragments with minimal dissection within the zone of injury.[12,49]

To apply the technique of definitive external fixation, the surgeon must understand that soft-tissue injuries are major contributors to poor outcomes. Therefore, further soft-tissue injury—particularly further surgical dissection within the zone of injury—should be limited. The surgeon must understand that reconstruction of a stable and functional ankle mortise is paramount, but that this does not necessarily mean reconstructing the entire tibia and fibula. The surgeon must understand that proper alignment of the mortise—both in an angular and rotational fashion—beneath the tibial shaft is important.

Spanning External Fixation as Definitive Treatment

The application of an external fixator for definitive care is similar to that used for temporary spanning external fixation. There is, however, one key difference: the external fixator used in this technique serves as a buttressing device for at least 12 weeks after injury. Thus, the fixator pins used and the fixator construct attached to those pins must be strong and able to withstand physiologic forces for at least 12 weeks.[51] To achieve these goals, the following key points should be considered.

The pins inserted in the hindfoot should be large in diameter (the authors use 6-mm to 5-mm tapered pins), should be inserted in the coronal plane (directly from the medial side), and should have a cortical thread profile. The cortical thread profile maximizes the core diameter of the pin, which is important because these pins are loaded primarily in bending rather than in pullout.

One pin should be inserted in the talus and one in the calcaneus (Figure 10). The quality of the bone in the talar neck is superior to that in the calcaneus; this is an important factor to consider when using an external fixator frame that is to remain in place for 12 weeks. Because pins in this configuration will immobilize the subtalar joint, the surgeon must be careful to ensure that the joint is in neutral or slight valgus alignment

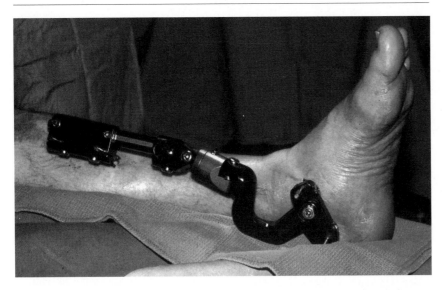

Figure 11 Photograph showing that pins should be inserted in the coronal plane in the tibial shaft to ensure that the tibial pins are in nearly the same plane as the pins in the foot and will allow for more potential for angular adjustment in the frame and a more cosmetic appearance of the device.

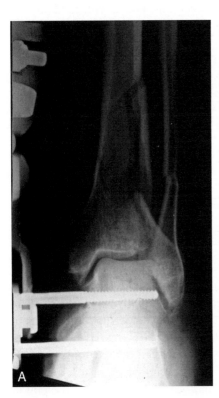 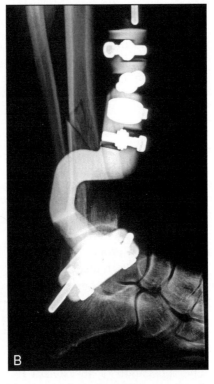

Figure 12 After application of the external fixator, the limb should be out to length and the talus centered under the tibial shaft on both AP **(A)** and lateral **(B)** radiographic views. Anterior translation of the talus relative to the tibial shaft should be avoided.

at the time of fixator application. Varus alignment should be avoided.

Pins inserted into the tibial shaft must be outside (superior to) the zone of injury and in the coronal plane. It is important that the tibial pins remain outside the zone of injury as well as proximal to where any plate would lie on the tibia, should the surgeon choose at a later date to plate the fracture. Putting pins in the coronal plane, rather than perpendicular to the subcutaneous border of the tibia, allows for better alignment of the external fixator frame and easier adjustment of the position of the ankle and the limb within the frame.

The authors use a unified body type of external fixator frame (as opposed to a pin-to-bar construct) for this application (Figure 11). The unified body type of frame has been shown to provide excellent performance in static and fatigue testing,[51] is highly adjustable, and offers a lower profile and more cosmetic appearance than a pin-to-bar construct. Additionally, the unified body type of device is designed for use with the stronger 6-mm to 5-mm tapered external fixator pins.

Once the frame is applied, the limbs should be distracted with a frame to restore the limb to anatomic length and alignment. At the completion of the fixator application, the limb should be out to length and the talus should be centered beneath the tibial shaft on both AP and lateral fluoroscopic views. The surgeon should be particularly aware of (and should not accept) any anterior translation of the talus relative to the tibial shaft, a phenomenon that is common with highly comminuted fractures (Figure 12).

With the spanning fixator properly applied, limited internal fixation is then delayed until soft-tissue swell-

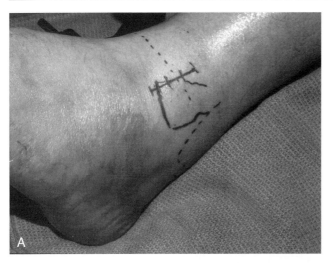
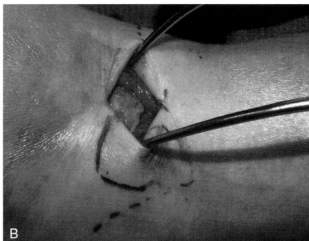

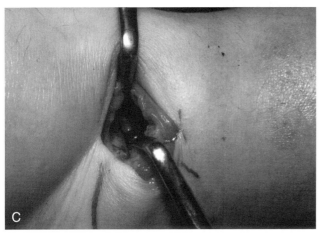

Figure 13   **A,** The incision should be centered on the ankle joint (*dotted line*) and made over the major anterolateral fracture fragment (*marked*). **B,** Dissection proceeds lateral to the peroneus tertius and the fracture fragment is exposed and retracted laterally. **C,** With the anterolateral fragment retracted laterally, the ankle joint is visualized, and the coronal split in the distal tibia can be identified and reduced.

ing has subsided and fracture blisters have epithelialized. In many patients, this delay is 14 to 21 days before performing the secondary procedure. Several principles should be followed in performing limited internal fixation of the articular surface in these injuries.

The external fixator should be prepped into the surgical field—it cannot be removed because it is needed to obtain overall limb alignment. It is the authors' preference to wash the fixator thoroughly with chlorhexidine, cleanse it further with alcohol, and then paint it with povidone-iodine as part of the skin preparation.

The patient should be positioned supine in such a way that allows easy access to the limb for both surgery and obtaining the necessary AP and lateral fluoroscopic views. Using a narrow foot piece for the operating room table, with the opposite leg in a hemilithotomy position, is ideal; however, a regular operating room table with the surgical leg elevated on towels is also acceptable.

The surgeon should ensure that the limb is out to length and the talar dome is centered beneath the tibial shaft in both AP and lateral fluoroscopic views before proceeding with internal fixation. Appropriate length and rotational and angular

alignment in the fixator should be ensured before an incision is made for limited open reduction and internal fixation. The external fixator serves to obtain and maintain length and overall alignment to make reduction and limited internal fixation of the articular fragments easier.

The surgical incisions should be centered on the joint line and positioned so as to use the major fracture lines as windows to see into the ankle joint (Figure 13). To facilitate this positioning, it is helpful to understand that there are some fracture fragments that are consistently present in most tibial plafond fractures. The anterolateral (Tillaux)

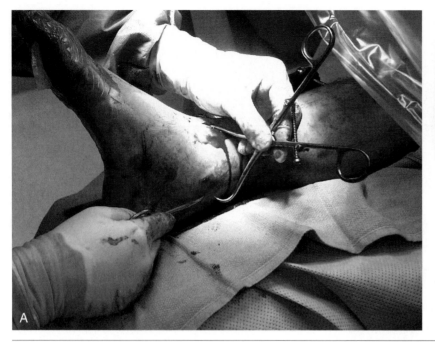

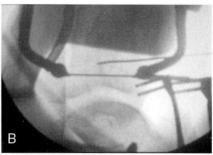

Figure 14 **A,** Intraoperative photograph showing reduction forceps and Kirschner wires used through stab incisions to reduce and stabilize the articular fragments. **B,** The reduction is assessed fluoroscopically.

fracture fragment is the most consistently present fragment in fractures of the distal tibia; as such, the anterolateral fracture line is the most frequent location in which the skin incision is made. A skin incision over this fracture line places the surgical approach lateral to the peroneus tertius tendon in a safe interval. Lateral retraction of this fracture fragment allows viewing of the ankle joint and also allows for visualization of the coronal split, which is also a typical finding in tibial plafond fractures. The comminuted central portion of the articular surface—another consistently present feature of these fractures—also can be visualized through this small window. The medial malleolar articular fragment, yet another consistently present fracture fragment in these injuries, is the only fracture fragment that cannot be visualized well through this small surgical approach centered at the level of the ankle joint.

Probes, dental picks, small elevators, tenacula, and pointed forceps are then used to "tease" the various articular fracture fragments into place. These reduction tools are used through the small surgical incisions or through stab incisions made at various locations about the ankle to enable them to provide a bit of pressure on the articular fragments to gently rotate or translate them into proper position (Figure 14, *A*).

Once fracture fragments have been realigned (alignment is confirmed by visualization through the ankle joint and by fluoroscopy), they can then be stabilized with Kirschner wires or guide pins for cannulated screws. Screws are then inserted to compress the fracture fragments together and complete the reconstruction of the articular surface (Figure 14, *B*).

When using this methodology, care should be taken that surgical dissection does not extend proximally into the area of metaphyseal comminution because any dissection into this area will place it at risk for delayed union or nonunion. It is difficult at times to resist the temptation to expose this area for a lag

screw or a small plate, but this should be avoided. The external fixator will serve as an effective buttressing device such that additional fixation in the metaphysis or diaphysis is not necessary (Figure 15).

Final adjustments to the external fixator are made to ensure that the articular block of the tibial plafond is perfectly aligned beneath the tibial shaft with the appropriate angular and rotational alignment.

When the articular fragments have been stabilized with screws and the limb is aligned and stabilized by the external fixator, which now serves as a buttressing device, the surgical procedure is complete. Although this procedure will adequately stabilize the fracture against physiologic forces, it does not provide rigid stabilization. Rigid stability, however, is not necessary because the fixator will remain as the buttressing device during the entire treatment period. Essentially, the fixator serves as a buttress plate applied outside of the body.

Postoperatively, routine pin care

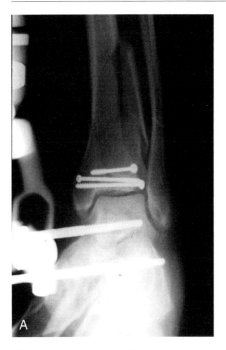 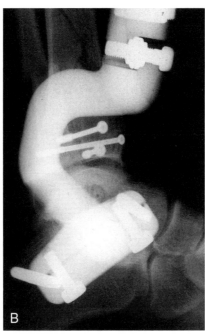

Figure 15 AP (**A**) and lateral (**B**) radiographs showing the articular fragments stabilized with screws. Final adjustments of the external fixator achieve proper alignment. No plate is required because the external fixator serves as a buttressing device. No dissection in the area of the tibial shaft is performed; this fracture will heal well without intervention (dissection in this area may lead to soft-tissue complications and will delay healing).

is begun in 48 hours (at the time of removal of the surgical dressing). Patients are also permitted at this time to bathe and shower the leg and fixator. The limb and fixator may be washed with regular soap and water in either the shower or the bath, but patients are encouraged not to enter swimming pools and/or hot tubs in which chemical additives are in the water. Patients should not bear weight (touch down only) on the limb for approximately 8 weeks after surgery. Following that period, patients are encouraged to bear weight as tolerated on the limb, with the fixator still in place, for 8 to 12 weeks following surgery. During the third postoperative month, the calcaneal pin typically will become inflamed and will be somewhat loose by 12 weeks after surgery. This is of no concern because the fixator will

have done its job and will be removed in the office at 12 weeks, provided the radiographs show healing of the metaphyseal portion of the fracture and the patient can bear weight without pain in the office with the frame removed and the pins still in place. After fixator removal, patients are usually placed in a short leg walking cast or removable orthotic device for an additional 4 weeks. Return to work almost never occurs before 6 months in patients who are laborers.

Hybrid External Fixation

When using hybrid external fixation to treat fractures of the distal tibia, there are no fixator elements distal to the ankle joint. Motion of the ankle joint is allowed and encouraged through most of the treatment course. Fixation is accomplished

with diaphyseal half-pins connected to metaphyseal or epiphyseal multiple thin tensioned wires through the use of rings, bars, and clamps. As this technique has evolved, it has become a staged protocol consisting of initial spanning fixation accompanied by definitive articular reconstruction and conversion to a non-bridging frame.[18,52] The articular reconstruction may occur at the time of initial external fixation or it may occur at conversion to a nonbridging construct. The timing will depend on the amount of articular displacement, the conditions of the soft tissue, and whether an open or a percutaneous technique of reduction will be used.

The technique of hybrid external fixation is initially similar to that of temporizing fixation. After soft-tissue stabilization has occurred, definitive fixation may be safely performed. If articular reduction has not been accomplished, this is performed first. Limited incisions, based on imaging, should be placed directly over articular fragments that need to be reduced. Percutaneously placed clamps and lag screws are then used to gain and hold reductions of the articular surface. Once articular congruity has been established, the reduction must be stabilized by way of the hybrid fixator.

Thin wires (usually 2 mm) are placed in the distal tibia. The first of these wires is typically placed from posterolateral, through the fibula, to anteromedial, and exiting the tibia medial to the tendon of the tibialis anterior. The second wire is placed from posteromedial on the tibia, beginning anterior to the neurovascular bundle and aimed to come out between the anterior and lateral compartments of the leg. The greater the angle that can be obtained between these two key wires, the more

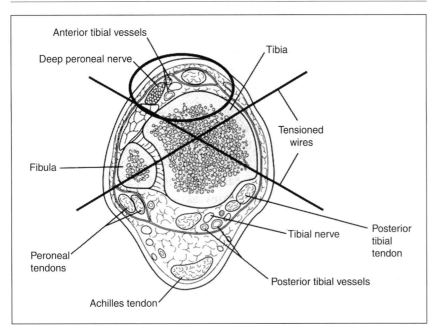

Figure 16   Illustration of the safe zone position for placement of thin wires in distal tibia; anterior compartments are the structures that are at risk (*circle*). (Reproduced with permission from Tornetta P III, Weiner L, Bergman M, et al: Pilon fractures: Treatment with combined internal and external fixation. *J Orthop Trauma* 1993;7:489-496.)

stable the fixation.[53] Even when using these "safe corridors," the thin wires across the distal tibia will impale a tendon in 55% of patients and a neurovascular structure in 38% of patients. Wires within 20 mm of the anterior joint line or 30 mm of the tip of the medial malleolus will be intracapsular and therefore may put patients at risk for septic arthritis[54] (Figure 16).

After these wires have been placed and tensioned to a ring, they are connected to the previously placed half-pins. The limb is manipulated and a reduction is obtained while the frame is tightened to maintain the fracture reduction.

Postoperatively, after the incision has healed, patients are allowed a 5-minute shower and are instructed to wash their legs and frames with soap and water. Weight bearing, except in patients with the most severe articular injuries, is begun quickly,

with progression to full weight bearing at approximately 6 to 8 weeks postoperatively. Frame removal occurs in the operating room after fracture healing has progressed, which is typically at 4 months after injury.

Factors Related to Outcome

To make informed choices on treatment decisions, a surgeon must have an understanding of the factors that affect patient outcome. Patient outcomes vary widely, and often the factors that surgeons believe are most important seem to have little bearing on the eventual function of the ankle and patient pain and impairment. Clinical data are either not available or are not robust enough to answer important questions. For all these reasons, assessing the most important factors for optimal outcome for a given patient is difficult and challenging.

Outcomes after rotational ankle fractures are generally good, and the factors that affect good versus poor outcomes are well known. Patient factors such as advanced age, diabetes, and obesity have been shown to correlate with poor results. Factors associated with the injury are also important, including associated open wounds, osteochondral fractures, and the number of malleoli involved. The type and quality of treatment is clearly important because an accurate reduction of the talus in the mortise is critical to avoid early posttraumatic osteoarthritis. After high-energy axial loading plafond fractures, outcomes are less favorable and the important factors are less well understood. For instance, the relative effect of an anatomic articular reduction and the severity of injury are unknown.

It is important, therefore, that surgeons have an understanding of what can be expected at 1 year, 2 years, and at greater than 5 years after a tibial plafond fracture. To do so, surgeons must be familiar with available data on the interaction between the effect of the severity of injury and the quality of the articular reduction on outcome as well as the effects of other injury and patient demographic factors.

Complications

It is well known that complications during treatment such as infection, wound breakdown, nonunion, and malunion create grave situations that may lead to amputation and other unfortunate outcomes.[55] Data from studies performed in the 1990s indicate that complications during that period were frequent. For instance, Wyrsch and associates[11] reported that three of 18 closed fractures treated with plates resulted in amputation. In one study in which infections occurred in 37% of patients with high-energy fractures, more than 30 additional surgeries were required in 18 of 30 patients with Ruedi and Allgower type III fractures.[50]

Current techniques have substantially reduced but not eliminated complications. Table 4 details complication rates that have been reported in recent publications on the treatment of tibial plafond fractures using three contemporary techniques.

Changes in treatment techniques that have decreased complication rates include a long delay to definitive surgery, temporary spanning fixation, definitive external fixation, low-profile implants, indirect reduction techniques, and percutaneous techniques for reduction and placement of implants. Because complications have not been eliminated to the extent that there is always a risk of serious complications, surgeons must remember that when complications occur, they significantly influence patient outcome—often negatively. If a surgeon can minimize complications, the overall results for the patients will be positively influenced.

Typical Outcomes

Compared with other types of injury, other fracture problems, and specifically other articular fractures, patients with high-energy fractures of the tibial plafond have poorer outcomes and near-normal ankle function is rarely restored. For instance, compared with similar multiply injured patients without foot and ankle trauma, multiply injured patients with foot and ankle trauma have poorer outcomes, which demonstrates the negative effect of severe foot and ankle injuries.[56,58] As an-

Table 4
Complication Rates From Treatment With Current Techniques

Technique	Authors (year of study)	No. of Patients	Complication Rate (%)
Spanning external fixator	Marsh et al[16] (1995)	43	0
	Wyrsch et al[11] (1996)	20	5
	Mitkovic et al[17] (2002)	26	0
External fixation same side	Court-Brown et al[56] (1999)	24	4
	Tornetta et al[25] (1993)	26	7
Delayed plating	Patterson and Cole[27] (1999)	22	5
	Wyrsch et al[11] (1996)	20	5
	Mitkovic et al[17] (2002)	26	0

other example, patients with high-energy tibial plateau fractures have significantly better outcomes for the involved joint and better general health status than patients with tibial plafond fractures.[49,59] This point is illustrated by comparing two series of patients who were treated at the same institution. In a series of patients with high-energy tibial plateau fractures, all of whom were treated with external fixation, Weigel and Marsh[59] found that in the second 5-year period after injury the knee scores averaged 90 on a 100-point scale and that few knees had progressive osteoarthritis. In contrast, at a similar follow-up, patients with tibial plafond fractures had decreased general health status, marked ankle pain and disability, and a high percentage of severe posttraumatic osteoarthritis.[49] These two studies demonstrate that unlike the knee, which seems to tolerate high-energy articular fractures reasonably well, the ankle frequently develops posttraumatic osteoarthritis, secondary pain, and decreased function after high-energy articular fractures.

The measurable effect on the general health status of patients with tibial plafond fractures has been illustrated in studies in which the Medical Outcomes Study 36-Item Short-Form Health Survey (SF-36)

was administered years after injury. This long-lasting negative effect appears to be irrespective of treatment technique because it has been reported in separate series of patients who were treated with plates, external fixators, and both devices.[16,49,60,61] At 2 to 4 years after injury, most patients can expect to still have some pain that prevents full participation in normal recreational activities.[16,60] Most patients, however, will return to work, and arthrodesis is unusual. In the second 5-year period after injury, tibial plafond fractures have been shown to still affect the lives of patients. In one study, SF-36 scores showed that tibial plafond fractures had a significant effect on physical function, the role of physical function, and bodily pain compared with the scores of age-matched control subjects at 5 to 11 years after injury.[49] Not surprisingly, Ankle Osteoarthritis Scale scores were dramatically different in both groups as well; however, most patients were satisfied with the results and most had not required late arthrodesis (arthrodesis rate, 5.4%).

Most data indicate that recovery is slow and prolonged. In the first 2 years after injury, most patients can expect to still be recovering and improving by having gradually less pain and increasing function. In one study, patients reported that maximum medical improvement occurred at an average of 2.4 years after injury; in nine patients from whom sequential ankle scores were obtained (at 2 years and at < 5 years after injury), all reported improvement between these time points.[49] Because these data suggest a high likelihood of continued improvement, surgeons should delay reconstructive procedures in the first 12 to 18 months after injury.

Arthrosis is common and nearly universal after severe fractures. In one study, moderate or severe arthrosis was present in 30% of fractures by 2 to 4 years after injury; in another study, more than 70% of ankles were moderately or severely arthritic in the second 5-year period after injury.[16,49]

Factors Affecting Outcome

It is reasonable to conclude that high-energy, more comminuted fractures have poorer outcomes than low-energy, less comminuted fractures; these outcomes may be modified to a certain extent by the skill of the surgeon and the quality of the surgical repair. However, the limited data available indicate that patient outcome after these fractures is difficult to predict based on any criteria, including severity of injury and quality of articular reduction (Figures 17 and 18). In two studies using the same assessment of reduction, fair reductions were reported in 14% of patients and arthrodesis was required in 9%,[27] whereas another study reported fair or poor reductions in 30% of patients and arthrodesis was required in only 3%.[16] Two other studies that specifically assessed the quality of reduction and severity of injury found these variables were associated with arthrosis but not with clinical outcome.[62,63]

Severe injuries may result in an ankle that is as good as or better (in terms of function and pain) than ankles with less severe injuries because severe fractures develop peripheral buttressing osteophytes that cause ankylosis of the joint, thereby protecting the remaining articular surface from painful and damaging shear stresses. Less severe injuries preserve movement, and the loads on the damaged articular surfaces are not protected, leading to a higher risk of progressive cartilage loss. This concept is illustrated in a rotational ankle fracture in which a slightly wide mortise (a relatively nonsevere injury) left untreated can lead to rapidly progressive posttraumatic osteoarthritis.

Patient demographics have been shown to be an important predictor of outcome after calcaneal fractures to the extent that sex, age, and work status can be used to guide treatment. For fractures of the tibial plafond, the data are less robust; therefore, the effect of patient demographics on patient outcome is uncertain. In one study, females and white-collar workers had better outcomes at 2 to 4 years after injury.[16,62] These results were not seen in another study at 5 to 11 years after injury.[49] The effect of workers' compensation status on patient outcome, which has been shown to have a strong negative effect for other injuries, has not been studied for patients with fractures of the tibial plafond.

Important clinical implications arise from the inability to predict the outcome of a certain patient with a certain fracture pattern. First, based on the lack of a strong correlation of outcome with severity of injury, surgeons should not be quick to recommend arthrodesis for patients with severe injuries or for injuries with poor articular reductions. Most patients improve over time, and most do not require arthrodesis. Because some of the worst fractures can actually have satisfactory outcomes, patience may be rewarded. Another important clinical consideration arises when making treatment decisions during the early treatment phases for patients with tibial plafond fractures. The risk versus benefit ratio of treatment choices must be considered. Complications always lead to bad outcomes, and the extent that outcome is improved with aggressive surgical approaches is at best unclear.

Summary

Tibial plafond fractures have a long-lasting adverse effect on patient general health status and a more significant adverse effect on ankle pain and function. Few patients with tibial plafond fractures experience restoration of normal ankle function. Many patients begin to show radiographic evidence of arthrosis by 2 years after injury, and most have significant posttraumatic arthrosis by the second 5-year period after injury. The effect of radiographic findings on clinical outcome is not clear, however, because most patients improve over time and most do not require arthrodesis. Patients may continue to experience some pain and decreased function, but they typically do not have enough symptoms to warrant reconstructive surgery. Complications must be avoided because they typically lead to repeat surgeries and poor patient outcomes. The factors that affect variations in outcome are uncertain. In particular, the severity of injury and the quality of articular reduction do not have as close an association with subsequent clinical outcome as has generally been believed.

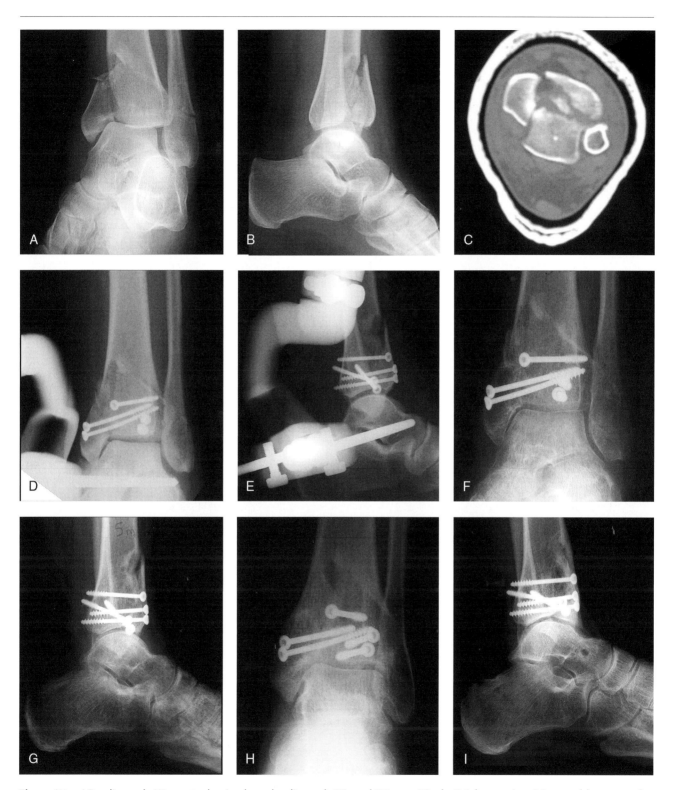

Figure 17   AP radiograph **(A)**, postreduction lateral radiograph **(B)**, and CT scan **(C)** of a B-3 fracture in a 38-year-old woman who fell from a horse show that only mild comminution is present. AP **(D)** and lateral **(E)** radiographs obtained after the application of a spanning fixator and fixation of the articular surface with screws show that articular reduction is excellent. AP **(F)** and lateral **(G)** radiographs obtained 6 months after injury show evidence of healing; however, the patient reported severe pain and inability to walk. At 4 years after injury, AP **(H)** and lateral **(I)** radiographs show an anterior osteophyte and anterior joint narrowing. The patient was fitted with a brace, reported moderate pain, and was able to return to work in a hospital kitchen; her ankle score was 72.

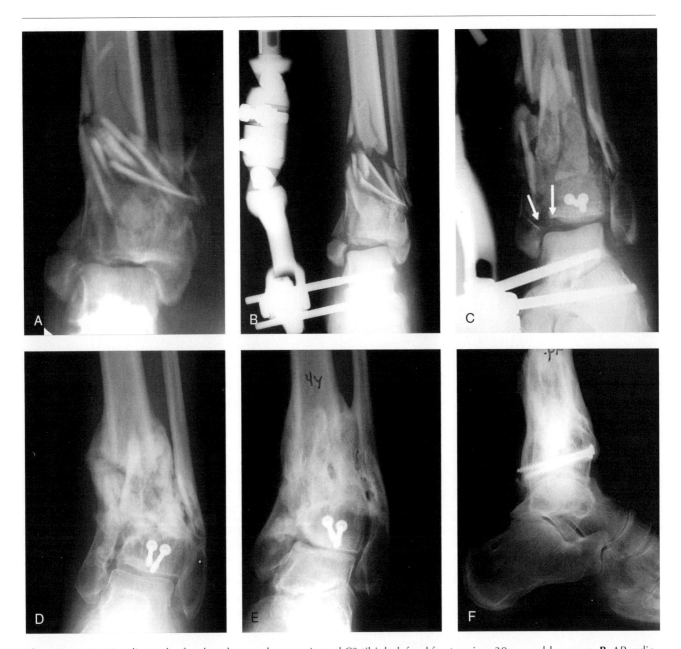

Figure 18 **A,** AP radiograph of a closed, severely comminuted C3 tibial plafond fracture in a 30-year-old woman. **B,** AP radiograph showing alignment in a spanning fixator. **C,** Radiograph of the fracture after fixation of the articular surface demonstrates residual articular incongruity (*arrows*). **D,** Radiograph obtained 1 year after injury shows a varus malunion. AP **(E)** and lateral **(F)** radiographs obtained 4 years after injury show maintained joint space. The patient, a teacher, was able to return to work and return to full participation in recreational activities; her ankle score was 95.

Because of the lack of clear data for preferred treatment techniques based on patient outcome, surgeons should choose treatment based both on characteristics of an injury and their own surgical skill and experience. Satisfactory results have been reported in series using predominantly plate fixation and in series using predominantly external fixation. With either technique, priority must be given to the soft-tissue injury to minimize complications. Techniques discussed in this chapter such as temporary spanning fixation, long delays to definitive surgery, the use of external fixation, low-profile plates, limited approaches, and avoiding the medial tibia have all had a role in decreasing complications and therefore improving outcomes.

References

1. Dirschl DR, Adams GL: A critical assessment of factors influencing reliability in the classification of fractures, using fractures of the tibial plafond as a model. *J Orthop Trauma* 1997;11:471-476.

2. Martin JS, Marsh JL, Bonar SK, DeCoster TA, Found EM, Brandser EA: Assessment of the AO/ASIF fracture classification for the distal tibia. *J Orthop Trauma* 1997;11:477-483.

3. Swiontkowski MF, Sands AK, Agel J, Diab M, Schwappach JR, Kreder HJ: Interobserver variation in the AO/OTA fracture classification system for pilon fractures: Is there a problem? *J Orthop Trauma* 1997;11:467-470.

4. Ruedi T: Fractures of the lower end of the tibia into the ankle joint: Results 9 years after open reduction and internal fixation. *Injury* 1973;5:130-134.

5. Tscherne H, Oestern HJ: [A new classification of soft-tissue damage in open and closed fractures (author's transl)]. *Unfallheilkunde* 1982;85:111-115.

6. Bourne RB, Rorabeck CH, Macnab J: Intra-articular fractures of the distal tibia: The pilon fracture. *J Trauma* 1983;23:591-596.

7. Ovadia DN, Beals RK: Fractures of the tibial plafond. *J Bone Joint Surg Am* 1986;68:543-551.

8. Helfet DL, Koval K, Pappas J, Sanders RW, DiPasquale T: Intraarticular "pilon" fracture of the tibia. *Clin Orthop Relat Res* 1994;298:221-228.

9. Mast JW, Spiegel PG, Pappas JN: Fractures of the tibial pilon. *Clin Orthop Relat Res* 1988;230:68-82.

10. Trumble TE, Benirschke SK, Vedder NB: Use of radial forearm flaps to treat complications of closed pilon fractures. *J Orthop Trauma* 1992;6:358-365.

11. Wyrsch B, McFerran MA, McAndrew M, et al: Operative treatment of fractures of the tibial plafond: A randomized, prospective study. *J Bone Joint Surg Am* 1996;78:1646-1657.

12. Bonar SK, Marsh JL: Unilateral external fixation for severe pilon fractures. *Foot Ankle* 1993;14:57-64.

13. Bonar SK, Marsh JL: Tibial plafond fractures: Changing principles of treatment. *J Am Acad Orthop Surg* 1994;2:297-305.

14. Bone L, Stegemann P, McNamara K, Seibel R: External fixation of severely comminuted and open tibial pilon fractures. *Clin Orthop Relat Res* 1993;292:101-107.

15. Marsh JL: External fixation is the treatment of choice for fractures of the tibial plafond. *J Orthop Trauma* 1999;13:583-585.

16. Marsh JL, Bonar S, Nepola JV, Decoster TA, Hurwitz SR: Use of an articulated external fixator for fractures of the tibial plafond. *J Bone Joint Surg Am* 1995;77:1498-1509.

17. Mitkovic MB, Bumbasirevic MZ, Lesic A, Golubovic Z: Dynamic external fixation of comminuted intra-articular fractures of the distal tibia (type C pilon fractures). *Acta Orthop Belg* 2002;68:508-514.

18. Anglen JO: Early outcome of hybrid external fixation for fracture of the distal tibia. *J Orthop Trauma* 1999;13:92-97.

19. Barbieri R, Schenk R, Koval K, Aurori K, Aurori B: Hybrid external fixation in the treatment of tibial plafond fractures. *Clin Orthop Relat Res* 1996;332:16-22.

20. French B, Tornetta P III: Hybrid external fixation of tibial pilon fractures. *Foot Ankle Clin* 2000;5:853-871.

21. Gaudinez RF, Mallik AR, Szporn M: Hybrid external fixation in tibial plafond fractures. *Clin Orthop Relat Res* 1996;329:223-232.

22. Griffiths GP, Thordarson DB: Tibial plafond fractures: Limited internal fixation and a hybrid external fixator. *Foot Ankle Int* 1996;17:444-448.

23. Manca M, Marchetti S, Restuccia G, Faldini A, Faldini C, Giannini S: Combined percutaneous internal and external fixation of type-C tibial plafond fractures: A review of twenty-two cases. *J Bone Joint Surg Am* 2002;84(Suppl 2):109-115.

24. Pugh KJ, Wolinsky PR, McAndrew MP, Johnson KD: Tibial pilon fractures: A comparison of treatment methods. *J Trauma* 1999;47:937-941.

25. Tornetta P III, Weiner L, Bergman M, et al: Pilon fractures: Treatment with combined internal and external fixation. *J Orthop Trauma* 1993;7:489-496.

26. Blauth M, Bastian L, Krettek C, Knop C, Evans S: Surgical options for the treatment of severe tibial pilon fractures: A study of three techniques. *J Orthop Trauma* 2001;15:153-160.

27. Patterson MJ, Cole JD: Two-staged delayed open reduction and internal fixation of severe pilon fractures. *J Orthop Trauma* 1999;13:85-91.

28. Sirkin M, Sanders R, DiPasquale T, Herscovici D Jr: A staged protocol for soft tissue management in the treatment of complex pilon fractures. *J Orthop Trauma* 1999;13:78-84.

29. Helfet DL, Shonnard PY, Levine D, Borrelli J Jr: Minimally invasive plate osteosynthesis of distal fractures of the tibia. *Injury* 1997;28(Suppl 1):A42-A47.

30. Khoury A, Liebergall M, London E, Mosheiff R: Percutaneous plating of distal tibial fractures. *Foot Ankle Int* 2002;23:818-824.

31. Oh CW, Kyung HS, Park IH, Kim PT, Ihn JC: Distal tibia metaphyseal fractures treated by percutaneous plate osteosynthesis. *Clin Orthop Relat Res* 2003;408:286-291.

32. Casey D, McConnell T, Parekh S, Tornetta P III: Percutaneous pin placement in the medial calcaneus: Is anywhere safe? *J Orthop Trauma* 2002;16:26-29.

33. Ruedi TP, Allgöwer M: The operative treatment of intra-articular fractures of the lower end of the tibia. *Clin Orthop Relat Res* 1979;138:105-110.

34. Gobezie RG, Ponce BA, Vrahas MS: Pilon fractures: Use of the posterolateral approach for ORIF. *Operative Techniques in Orthopaedics* 2003;13:113.

35. Tull F, Borrelli J Jr: Soft-tissue injury associated with closed fractures: Evaluation and management. *J Am Acad Orthop Surg* 2003;11:431-438.

36. McFerran MA, Smith SW, Boulas HJ, Schwartz HS: Complications encountered in the treatment of pilon fractures. *J Orthop Trauma* 1992;6:195-200.

37. Thordarson DB: Complications after treatment of tibial pilon fractures: Prevention and management strategies. *J Am Acad Orthop Surg* 2000;8:253-265.

38. Hoppenfeld DP, Hutton R (eds): *Surgical Exposures in Orthopaedics: The Anatomic Approach.* Philadelphia, PA, Lippincott, 1994.

39. Borrelli J Jr, Catalano L: Open reduction and internal fixation of pilon fractures. *J Orthop Trauma* 1999;13:573-582.

40. Borrelli J Jr, Ellis E: Pilon fractures: Assessment and treatment. *Orthop Clin North Am* 2002;33:231-245.

41. Shantharam SS, Naeni F, Wilson EP: Single-incision technique for internal fixation of distal tibia and fibula fractures. *Orthopedics* 2000;23:429-431.

42. Wright V: Post-traumatic osteoarthritis: A medico-legal minefield. *Br J Rheumatol* 1990;29:474-478.

43. Mitchell N, Shepard N: Healing of articular cartilage in intra-articular fractures in rabbits. *J Bone Joint Surg Am* 1980;62:628-634.

44. Llinas A, McKellop HA, Marshall GJ, Sharpe F, Kirchen M, Sarmiento A: Healing and remodeling of articular incongruities in a rabbit fracture model. *J Bone Joint Surg Am* 1993;75:1508-1523.

45. Matta JM: Fractures of the acetabulum: Accuracy of reduction and clinical results in patients managed operatively within three weeks after the injury. *J Bone Joint Surg Am* 1996;78:1632-1645.

46. Honkonen SE: Degenerative arthritis after tibial plateau fractures. *J Orthop Trauma* 1995;9:273-277.

47. Marsh JL, Buckwalter J, Gelberman R, et al: Articular fractures: Does an anatomic reduction really change the result? *J Bone Joint Surg Am* 2002;84-A:1259-1271.

48. Dirschl DR, Marsh JL, Buckwalter JA, et al: Articular fractures. *J Am Acad Orthop Surg* 2004;12:416-423.

49. Marsh JL, Weigel DP, Dirschl DR: Tibial plafond fractures: How do these ankles function over time? *J Bone Joint Surg Am* 2003;85-A:287-295.

50. Teeny SM, Wiss DA: Open reduction and internal fixation of tibial plafond fractures: Variables contributing to poor results and complications. *Clin Orthop Relat Res* 1993;292:108-117.

51. Dirschl DR, Obremskey WT: Mechanical strength and wear of used EBI external fixators. *Orthopedics* 2002;25:1059-1062.

52. Watson JT, Moed BR, Karges DE, Cramer KE: Pilon fractures: Treatment protocol based on severity of soft tissue injury. *Clin Orthop Relat Res* 2000;375:78-90.

53. Geller J, Tornetta P III, Tiburzi D, Kummer F, Koval K: Tension wire position for hybrid external fixation of the proximal tibia. *J Orthop Trauma* 2000;14:502-504.

54. Vives MJ, Abidi NA, Ishikawa SN, Taliwal RV, Sharkey PF: Soft tissue injuries with the use of safe corridors for transfixion wire placement during external fixation of distal tibia fractures: An anatomic study. *J Orthop Trauma* 2001;15:555-559.

55. Dillin L, Slabaugh P: Delayed wound healing, infection, and nonunion following open reduction and internal fixation of tibial plafond fractures. *J Trauma* 1986;26:1116-1119.

56. Court-Brown CM, Walker C, Garg A, McQueen MM: Half-ring external fixation in the management of tibial plafond fractures. *J Orthop Trauma* 1999;13:200-206.

57. Turchin DC, Schemitsch EH, McKee MD, Waddell JP: Do foot injuries significantly affect the functional outcome of multiply injured patients? *J Orthop Trauma* 1999;13:1-4.

58. Tran T, Thordarson D: Functional outcome of multiply injured patients with associated foot injury. *Foot Ankle Int* 2002;23:340-343.

59. Weigel DP, Marsh JL: High-energy fractures of the tibial plateau: Knee function after longer follow-up. *J Bone Joint Surg Am* 2002;84-A:1541-1551.

60. Sands A, Grujic L, Byck DC, Agel J, Benirschke S, Swiontkowski MF: Clinical and functional outcomes of internal fixation of displaced pilon fractures. *Clin Orthop Relat Res* 1998;347:131-137.

61. Pollak AN, McCarthy ML, Bess RS, Agel J, Swiontkowski MF: Outcomes after treatment of high-energy tibial plafond fractures. *J Bone Joint Surg Am* 2003;85:1893-1900.

62. Williams TM, Nepola JV, DeCoster TA, Hurwitz SR, Dirschl DR, Marsh JL: Factors affecting outcome in tibial plafond fractures. *Clin Orthop Relat Res* 2004;423:93-98.

63. DeCoster TA, Willis MC, Marsh JL, et al: Rank order analysis of tibial plafond fractures: Does injury or reduction predict outcome? *Foot Ankle Int* 1999;20:44-49.

Locked and Minimally Invasive Plating

Judith Siegel, MD
Paul Tornetta III, MD
Joseph Borrelli, Jr, MD
Philip Kregor, MD
William M. Ricci, MD

Abstract

Plate fixation of fractures began before the start of the 20th century. Initially, plates and screws were used to decrease deformity. There was minimal interest in the biology of fracture union. As knowledge increased in regard to the science of bone healing, fixation techniques and implants also evolved, from the development of rudimentary rigid constructs to stable locked plating.

Instr Course Lect 2007;56:353-368.

Plate fixation of fractures continues to evolve. Although surgical technique and plate and screw design are distinct, they are intimately related and each drives the evolution of the other. Recent advances in plating techniques aim to maximize the biologic potential of fractures to heal. Some of these techniques are surgeon-controlled and are related to the degree of iatrogenic injury and disruption of the soft tissues induced during plate fixation. Implant design has also evolved toward the goals of minimizing injury to bone and maximizing the surgeon's ability to implant plates with minimal soft-tissue injury. Implant design characteristics, most recently locked plate-screw devices, have also evolved to improve plate fixation in bone and hence minimize implant-related failures before fracture union. This chapter details the evolution of the latest advances in plate technology and locked plate devices; discusses the advantages, disadvantages, and potential pitfalls of the use of locked plates; compares current methods of implanting plates (nonlocked, locked, and hybrid fixation methods); and summarizes how locked plates are naturally compatible with minimally invasive plating techniques.

History of Locked Plating
Early Plating
Before the science of bone healing was understood, internal fixation was introduced as a method to decrease deformity associated with a healed fracture[1-5] (Table 1). The mechanical aspects of plating fractures were developed without any regard to biology. At the start of the 20th century, two surgeons, Lambotte and Lane, first advocated for the internal fixation of fractures. Lambotte, a Belgian surgeon who has been credited with coining the term "osteosynthesis," is universally regarded as the father of modern internal fixation. He created numerous different plates and screws and the instruments needed to use them for fracture fixation.[1,6] Ultimately, Lambotte's goal was rigid fixation so no external splinting was necessary. At approximately the same time, Lane, an English surgeon and prolific writer, began performing open reduction and internal fixation of fractures. He published drawings, photographs, and radiographs demonstrating his internal fixation devices in 1905. In 1907, he introduced the Lane plate, a narrow, flat plate that acted to splint long bone fractures but offered no rotational control. Despite his enthusiasm for internal fixation of fractures, these

One or more of the authors or the departments with which they are affiliated have received something of value from a commercial or other party related directly or indirectly to the subject of this chapter.

Table 1
Timeline of Plate Fixation of Fractures

1890-1910	Lane (open fracture treatment)[1]
	Lane plate[2]
	Lambotte's series[1]
	W. Sherman (metal alloys)[1]
	Hey-Groves (locking screw)[1]
1920-1930	American Surgical Association
	Radiographs for fracture treatment
	Rush rods
1940-1950	Kirschner (intramedullary nails)
1950-1960	Danis (osteosynthesis)[2]
	Compression plating
	Müller (AO founded)[1]
1970-1980	Anatomic open reduction and internal fixation
1980-1990	Indirect reduction
1990-2000	Blatter and Weber (waveplate)[3]
	Minimally invasive percutaneous osteosynthesis
	Schuhli nut[4]
	Locking plates[5]
2000-2010	Locking and minimally invasive percutaneous osteosynthesis hybrid

methods were not well received by his colleagues at the time.[1,6]

Others who reported on early techniques of internal fixation include Sherman and Tait, who both used screws to stabilize articular fractures in dogs. They advanced this concept to periarticular fractures in humans with good results.[1] Sherman popularized the use of steel plates and screws in the United States. Because of his frustration with frequent postoperative hardware failure, he incorporated engineering principles in the creation of new plates and self-tapping screws from vanadium steel alloy—a major

advance.[1] The English successor of Lane was Hey-Groves. His experimental studies in fracture healing led to many improvements in internal fixation devices. Intramedullary fixation, interfragmentary compression screws with neutralization plates, and double-onlay plates with bolts fixing the plates together were developed from his ideas.[1,6] He also introduced curved plates for better apposition to the diaphysis of long bones and continued to endorse rigid fixation for anatomic healing.

In the 1930s and 1940s, Danis, a surgeon in Brussels, began reporting his observations on the use of rigid fixation devices in the treatment of fractured bones. His philosophy of fracture surgery included firm stabilization to allow for soft-tissue healing, joint mobility, and muscle function. To achieve these goals, he devised a compression plate (coapteur) that would be applied after anatomic reduction of individual fracture fragments. He also noted that this fixation resulted in bony healing that he called "soudure autogène" or welding.[1,2] Today, this process is referred to as direct or primary bone healing and represents haversian remodeling rather than endochondral bone formation.

The 1950s and 1960s brought about the birth of the Arbeitsgemeinschaft für Osteosynthesefragen (AO) philosophies. A Swiss surgeon, Müller, read the work of Danis and was immediately drawn to his philosophy of fracture fixation and his observations on bone healing. In 1958 in Chur, Switzerland, a study group formed to investigate the internal fixation of bone.[1]

The principles of the AO group became the standard for the management of fractures in the 1970s. The original management concepts included recreating normal anat-

omy, providing stability, preserving blood supply, and starting early motion.[7] The group was dedicated to the basic science and biomechanical research of osteosynthesis and to the design of necessary instrumentation and implants to achieve these goals.

Neutralization and Compression Plating

Absolute stability and precise surgical reduction to allow immediate function was the goal of the compression technique of fracture treatment. Restoring smooth congruent articular surfaces to avoid the concentration of stresses on the articular cartilage was believed to prevent posttraumatic arthrosis. This concept of exact reduction was also applied to diaphyseal and metaphyseal long bone fractures to improve stability.

The use of interfragmentary lag screws grew from this concept. Applying local compression at the bony ends with a screw perpendicular to either the fracture line or to the long axis of the bone, depending on the fracture pattern, would aid in avoiding displacement.[2] Neutralization plates were added in these circumstances to protect the lag screw fixation from various external forces. Primary fracture healing occurred without external callus.

Compression plating subsequently arose as another method to achieve anatomic reduction, rigid stability, and direct bone healing. Several methods of creating static compression of the fracture ends developed. Articulated tensioning devices were originally used by Danis. The technique of overbending a plate before application provided compression to the far cortex of the fracture. Dynamic compression was accomplished using compression plates with oblong holes and inclined shoulders in association with eccentrically placed screws with chamfered heads. The fracture ends are drawn together as the screws engage the plate, applying compression at the fracture site.[8] All of these concepts use extensive fracture site exposure and soft-tissue stripping.

Locked Plating Designs

The continued evolution of plating techniques led to further attempts to provide better angular stability of articular end segments. The current fixed-angle plates use threaded screw heads that lock into the threaded holes of these locking plates. Although the use of locking screws is increasing dramatically, the concept used is not new. In 1916, Hey-Groves described converging screws placed through a plate and threading screws placed into the socket of a plate as two ways of maintaining firm fixation in which the grip of the metal screw to the metal plate secures the fixation to prevent loosening. With these ideas, Hey-Groves designed his own locking plates.[1,6] Soft-tissue preservation was not a consideration in fracture care at this time.

The Schuhli nut, Swiss-German for "little shoe," is a device that created an early version of the locked plate. It allows a cortical screw placed through a standard dynamic compression plate to achieve a fixed angle. The Schuhli nut sits between the bone and the plate within the oval compression hole, contacting the bone through its three sharp projections and thereby elevating the plate from the bone. It engages the screw, and locks the construct at 90°, creating a low-profile internal fixator. Schuhli nuts have been effective in acting as a substitute cortex when a defect is present and markedly improve stability over a

standard plate in this situation.[4] These devices have also proved beneficial in osteopenic bone.[4,9-11] They prevent stripping of the screw threads in weak bone and require failure of the entire construct before fracture stability is lost. The locking mechanism inhibits screw toggle, which prevents the screw from loosening and backing out of the plate. Another advantage is the protection of the biology of the cortex of the bone because the plate is elevated from the surface. This augmented construct shows higher load to failure than standard constructs.[12]

Another plate design that uses a locked screw mechanism is the point contact fixator device. It also minimizes the contact between the undersurface of a plate and a bone while using unicortical screws that locked into the plate. A Morse cone mismatch between the screw hole in the plate and the screw head prevents toggle.[13,14] Despite the theoretic advantage of preserved blood supply with this "splint" elevated off of the bone, recent studies have shown no advantage to the point-contact fixator over conventional bicortical plates.[14,15] Conversely, several clinical studies have documented high union rates and low complication rates with its use in the treatment of long bone fractures.[14,16] Success with such devices led to the creation of precontoured locking plates to treat periarticular fractures, which often require a fixed-angle device to achieve adequate metaphyseal stability.

Koval and associates[5] described a locking plate prototype to improve stability in the treatment of elderly patients who had distal femur fractures with loss of the medial buttress. Traditionally, fixed-angle devices such as blade plates or dynamic condylar screws were used; how-

ever, when significant intra-articular comminution is present, these devices are less than ideal. Condylar buttress plates better serve the articular fracture, but when the medial metaphyseal buttress is compromised, the fracture may collapse into varus. Sanders and associates[17] recommended double plating to treat these fractures, but this technique would involve stripping the soft tissues on both the medial and lateral condyles. The plate studied by Koval and associates[5] consisted of threaded nuts welded to lateral condylar buttress plates. This plate was compared with a standard lateral condylar buttress plate and a standard 95° blade plate in cadavers. Results revealed greater fixation stability with the locked plate than either the standard buttress plate or the blade plate.

Another technique, intramedullary plating, uses similar biologically friendly, cortical-substituting fixation.[18] Standard dynamic compression plates are placed in the intramedullary canal, spanning the fracture site in seven recalcitrant femoral nonunions, to substitute for the deficient medial cortex. A standard lateral plate is also used, and screws are threaded through both plates to lock both plates and the bone together as a composite. The soft-tissue sleeve is preserved, and autologous bone graft is used in all patients. In the study by Matelic and associates,[10] all fractures achieved union (average time to union, 19.2 weeks).

The less invasive stabilization system was introduced in the 1990s as a method to combine minimally invasive, biologically friendly, fixed-angle concepts in stabilization of Orthopaedic Trauma Association (OTA) type A and type C periarticular fractures.[19] This system made it easier to place a fixed-angle device than previously available dynamic compression screws or blade plates.[20] Thus, stability is provided to fractures with metaphyseal comminution that were often subjected to hardware failure and varus collapse secondary to the loss of a medial buttress.[21]

Locking plate design and fixation concepts are in constant evolution. Surgeon-friendly designs allow more freedom in avoiding the lag screws initially placed to reconstruct the joint surface. Hybrid fixation, which is the ability to use standard bicortical screws in addition to locking screws within a locking plate, allows for a more anatomic indirect reduction because the plate, with initially placed nonlocking screws, can assist with the reduction. As biomechanical and clinical data are collected on these plates, the technology will likely expand to include other locations and uses in the body. As with all other implants and techniques introduced throughout history, caution should be exercised until the science meets the innovation.

For more than a century, fracture management with internal fixation has advanced as the science of bony union was elucidated. Although eliminating deformity was the original driving force of internal fixation, functional recovery soon became an additional goal and benefit. As the pioneers of plate fixation introduced new ideas, more questions arose. Initially, a rigid implant was thought to be ideal, and concepts developed to create the most stable bone-plate construct possible. There was little early consideration given to the biology of the fracture. Callus was unwanted. As respect for the blood supply and the soft tissues grew, more biologically friendly tech-

niques for fracture reduction and implant placement were explored. Primary fracture healing and rigid fixation were sacrificed, and a new wave of implants was introduced. Indirect reduction and soft-tissue preservation have become the standard treatment for most periarticular fractures, and with the introduction of locking plates, an instrument became available that would provide angularly stable fixation. Additionally, these implants provide better fixation for osteopenic bone, aiding in the treatment of fractures in the elderly and in nonunions.

Advantages, Disadvantages, and Potential Pitfalls of Locked Plating

As with any new technology, surgeons must be aware of the advantages, disadvantages, and potential pitfalls of locked plating and decide on its use based on an evaluation of the fracture configuration, bone quality, and location of the fracture (diaphyseal versus metaphyseal).

Advantages of Locked Plating
The advantages of locked plating include improved fixation in metaphyseal bone, prevention of coronal plane collapse (varus/valgus) for end-segment fractures, and ease of percutaneous screw placement.

Improved Fixation in Metaphyseal Bone Especially in osteoporotic bone, the ability to place locked screws seems biomechanically helpful, particularly in the distal tibia, proximal humerus, and about the knee. It should be recognized, however, that there are no randomized prospective studies demonstrating the superiority of locked plating in these areas.

Prevention of Varus Collapse Prior to the advent of locked plating, varus collapse in distal femoral and proxi-

mal tibial fractures was problematic, especially in the setting of osteoporotic bone.[22-24] In the distal femur, multiple methods to prevent this complication were suggested, including double plating of the distal femur,[17] placement of a diagonal screw into the medial femoral condyle,[25] and placement of a medial external fixator. Similarly, both dual plating (medial and lateral)[26] or placement of a medial external fixator have been used for the treatment of bicondylar tibial plateau fractures.

Biomechanically, a locked plate design for the distal femur has been shown to have significantly improved fixation in an osteoporotic supracondylar femoral fracture model when compared with a blade plate or intramedullary nail.[27] Clinically, a fixed-angle locked internal fixator will maintain the reduction that is obtained intraoperatively, even in the setting of a short distal segment and/or osteoporosis. In a series of 103 distal femur fractures, no loss of varus/valgus angulation was reported.[28]

Similarly, fixed-angled screws have increased biomechanical stability for fixation of bicondylar tibial plateau fractures and unstable proximal metaphyseal fractures[29,30] (Figure 1). Fixed-angle plates prevent varus collapse in the treatment of proximal tibial fractures.[31] This allows surgeons to use a laterally based plate to prevent collapse of the medial column and obviates the requirement for a separate medial incision. One caveat is that the reliability of such lateral fixed-angle plates to adequately stabilize posterior medial coronal fracture fragments remains suspect. In such instances, the use of separate posterior medial buttress plates may be prudent.

Lack of Need for Precise Plate Contouring When using a locked

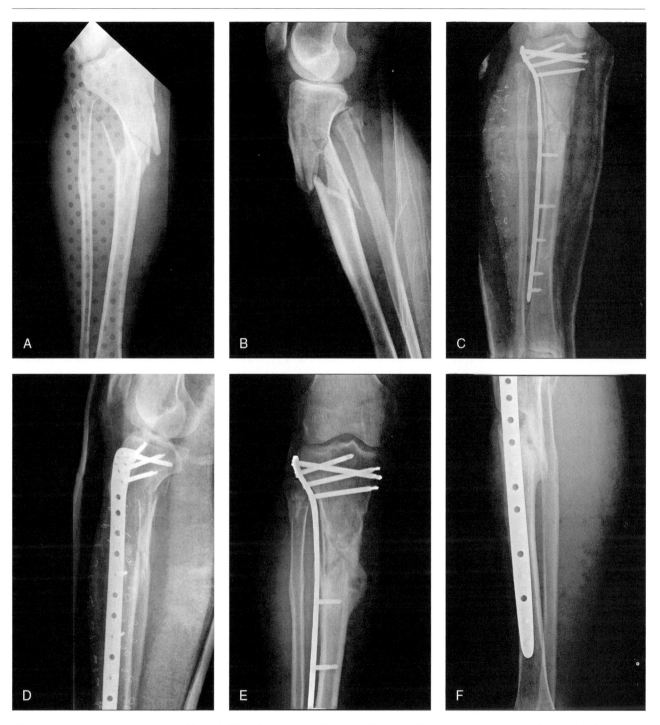

Figure 1   Preoperative AP (**A**) and lateral (**B**) radiographs of the right tibia of a 48-year-old man who had a crush injury to his right leg and sustained a proximal tibial fracture. Initially, the patient had significant soft-tissue swelling with potential impending compartment syndrome; therefore, he had a four-compartment fasciotomy of his lower extremity and a spanning external fixator placement. Postoperative AP (**C**) and lateral (**D**) radiographs of the right tibia after removal of the external fixator, fixation of the tibial fracture, and closure of the fasciotomy wound. Multiple fixed-angle locked screws give appropriate fixation of the relatively short proximal tibial block. Unicortical distal locked screws are used. One-year postoperative AP (**E**) and lateral (**F**) radiographs show complete consolidation of the fracture. The patient was able to bear full weight at 8 weeks. Note the exuberant secondary bone healing, which is characteristic of the bridge plating often used with locked fixators.

plate without conventional screws, placement of locked screws will not alter the reduction that has been obtained. This is a key concept. When considering, for example, medial plate fixation for a distal tibial fracture, surgeons should place concave and internal rotation contouring on the distal aspect of the plate (Figure 2). If this plate is placed in a subcutaneous manner, however, precise contouring of the plate may be difficult. Thus, appropriate reduction of the distal tibial region can be obtained indirectly independently of the plate (by use of a femoral distractor or by plating of the fibula). The use of a locked plate in this instance will be helpful because of improved metaphyseal fixation that will be obtained by locked screws, and even if a precise anatomic contouring of the locked plate is not obtained, the fracture will not be malreduced with the placement of the locked screws (as the plate will not approximate the bone to the slightly malcontoured plate.)

Easier Screw Placement Because of the improved fixation of locked screws, the number of screws necessary in a specific segment of bone may be less than with conventional screws. In addition, the ease of placement of locked screws in a percutaneous manner may be easier because the screws may be placed in a unicortical manner, and thus precise measurement of screw length is not necessary.

Lower Infection Risk The exclusive use of locked screws makes it unnecessary for the plate to be compressed to the bone. Therefore, the periosteal blood supply remains relatively intact as has been demonstrated in several cadaveric studies.[31-33] The use of an insertion guide additionally minimizes muscular devitalization. There is some clinical evidence that the minimized devitalization leads to a decreased infection risk in distal femur fractures.[34]

Disadvantages/Potential Pitfalls of Locked Plating

Lack of Compression at the Articular Surface For locked screws placed across periarticular fracture lines, it is recognized that if the locked screws are placed first through the plate, there will be no compression across the articular fracture line. If the articular surface has already been compressed by some other means, then this may not be a disadvantage. If locked plates are used to treat an articular fracture, the reduction and fixation of the articular surface should be performed first, after which the articular block may be connected to the diaphysis by means of a locked plate. Alternatively, newer plate designs have the ability to accept both locked and nonlocked screws. Thus, nonlocked screws may be used to compress the articular surface through the plate first, and then locked screws may be placed.

Locked plates may often be misused in the setting of tibial plateau fractures, particularly with simple split or split-depression tibial plateau fractures (Schatzker type I through IV injuries). With the exception of patients with severe osteoporosis, the use of pure locked plates (without nonlocked screws) in the treatment of these fractures is disadvantageous because it does not allow the plate to slowly compress the split component of the fracture by conventional lag screws. Surgeons must compare the advantage of increased biomechanical stability provided by locked plating with the lack of compression of the articular surface.

Lack of Compression of the Diaphyseal Simple Fracture Biologic plating is the concept of plating fractures in which the emphasis is placed on obtaining the length, rotation, and angulation of the limb[18] without an anatomic reduction of all fragments and without disturbing the soft-tissue attachments to the fragments. In this situation, locked plating works well; however, with a simple, diaphyseal, transverse fracture, the fracture should undergo traditional compression plating. Thus, the only way locked plating should be used in this instance is if locked screws are used in osteoporotic bone in which conventional screws are first used to compress the fracture, and then locked screws are used secondary to the osteoporotic bone.

Cost As with most new technology, locked plating is associated with increased cost. For example, the cost of a locked straight eight-hole narrow 4.5-mm plate may be as much as five times greater than a similar nonlocked plate. Similar trends are seen for periarticular plates, for which a locked plate can cost twice as much as a nonlocked plate.

Comparison of Plating Methods: Nonlocked, Locked, and Hybrid Plating

Available options for plate implantation have increased in complexity. Techniques including open, submuscular, subcutaneous, and percutaneous plating each have a role. Regardless of the chosen insertion technique, the fixation method can vary. Each of the three methods, nonlocked, locked, and hybrid plating, are discussed separately, along with their biomechanical principles, failure modes, and ability to be used as reduction tools.

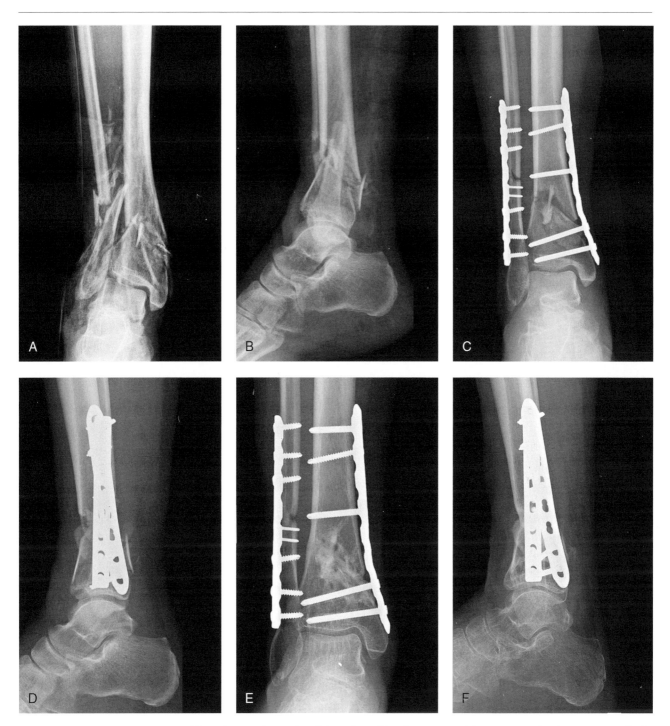

Figure 2   Preoperative AP (**A**) and lateral (**B**) radiographs of the right ankle of a 48-year-old woman involved in a motor vehicle collision and who sustained a right type IIIA open distal tibial fracture with an associated fibular fracture. Postoperative AP (**C**) and lateral (**D**) radiographs after fixation. The fibula was plated using traditional plating techniques providing an indirect reduction of the distal tibial fracture. A locked plate was slid along the distal medial tibia in a subcutaneous manner through the open transverse medial wound. The use of locked screws distally allowed for improved fixation of the short distal tibial block and for an imprecise contouring of the distal aspect to the plate. Even if the plate was not perfectly contoured, the locked distal screws would maintain the reduction that has been obtained via the indirect reduction of the fibula. Postoperative AP (**E**) and lateral (**F**) radiographs at 4 months show evidence of healing. The patient was able to bear weight at 10 weeks postoperatively.

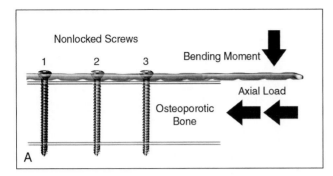
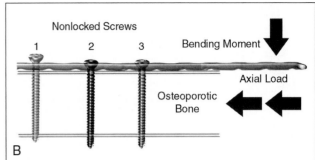
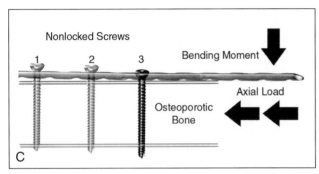
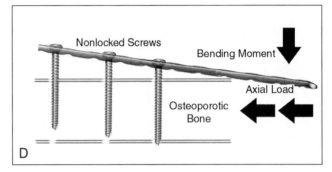

Figure 3 Illustration of the "sequential" screw failure mode of a nonlocked screw construct in osteoporotic bone subject to axial load with a bending moment. **A,** Screw 1 has the greatest insertion torque and bears the greatest load. **B,** As screw 1 loosens, screw 2 (now with the greatest insertion torque) bears the greatest load. **C,** As screw 2 loosens, screw 3 (now with the greatest insertion torque) bears the greatest load. **D,** Once all screws have sequentially loosened, construct stability is completely lost.

Nonlocked Plating

Traditional nonlocked plating methods essentially lag or compress the plate to bone. The force of friction is essential to construct stability. The frictional force between the plate and bone is proportional to the construct's coefficient of friction multiplied by the normal force between plate and bone. The normal force is proportional to the screw insertion torque. The more a screw is tightened, the more frictional force is generated between plate and bone, and the more stability is imparted to the construct. The magnitude of screw insertion torque required to eliminate motion between plate and bone is approximately 3 Nm.[35-37] Such a force is easily generated in healthy bone with thick cortices; however, in osteoporotic bone, screws can be stripped before this amount of torque is generated, leav-

ing the construct with marginal or insufficient stability.[35-37]

In nonlocked constructs, the screw with the greatest torque bears the greatest load. When these constructs are subjected to repetitive stress, the nonlocked screws can fail by fatigue fracture, loosen from bone, or pull out. As the frictional force between plate and bone are overcome during loading, the fixation strength becomes dependent on a single screw. As one screw loosens, force is transmitted to another single screw, and this process repeats, such that the construct fails by sequential screw failure (Figure 3). The weakest link in a nonlocked construct is the shear interface between screw and bone.[36] The force required to move a screw through bone is the resistance of bone to such shear stress multiplied by the contact area between screw and bone. This

mechanism of failure is different than the failure mode of locked plate constructs.

Because nonlocked screws lag bone to plate, fracture reduction in the plane of the screws is largely determined by the contour of the plate. In this way, the plate can be used as a reduction aid (Figure 4, *A* and *D*). Also, by beading the plate, the reduction can be adjusted.

Locked Plating

Pure locked plating methods use all locked screws, and these constructs are often described as internal fixators. A critical distinction between nonlocked and locked plating methods is that locked screws, by definition, lock into the plate and therefore do not lag bone to plate. The heads of the screws are threaded to match threads in plate screw holes. The axial orientation of these locked

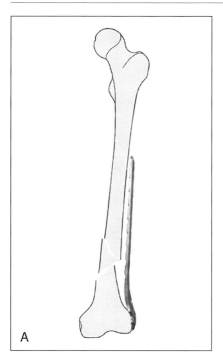

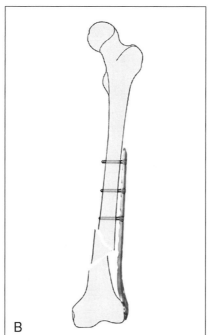

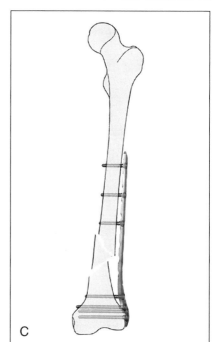

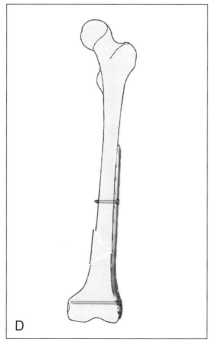

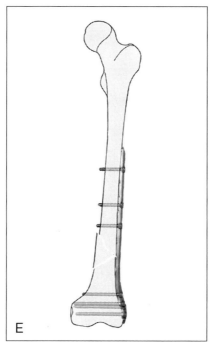

Figure 4 Illustration of the reduction and fixation of a comminuted supracondylar femur fracture with the locked and hybrid plating methods. **A,** Comminuted distal femur fracture. **B,** The plate is secured to the proximal fragment with locking screws. Bone is not reduced to the plate. **C,** Locking screws are added to the distal fragment. The fracture reduction is not affected by the addition of locking screws. The plate is an internal fixator, not a reduction aid. **D,** With the hybrid plating technique, the plate is secured to the proximal fragment with a nonlocking screw and then to the distal fragment with a nonlocking screw to obtain satisfactory fracture reduction. **E,** Locking screws are then added to create a fixed-angle device distally and to add additional fixation stability in the osteoporotic proximal fragment.

screws is therefore controlled and enhances the screw-plate construct by creating a single-beam construct. The single beam is defined by absence of motion between all components of the beam. Single-beam constructs are four times stronger than similar constructs in which motion can occur between individual components.[38] Nonlocked constructs can only function as single-beam constructs under ideal conditions when the insertion torque and the coefficient of friction between plate and bone are sufficient to eliminate motion between plate and screw under physiologic loads (Figure 5, *A*). When insertion torque is insufficient to resist motion between plate and bone, axial loads produce shear stress (Figure 5, *B*). In contrast, when locked plate constructs are exposed to axial load, potential shear stress between plate

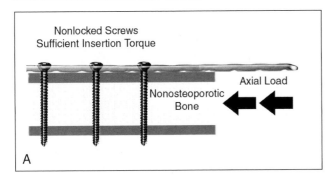

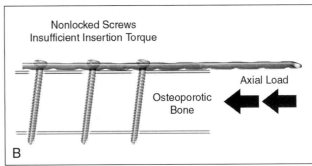

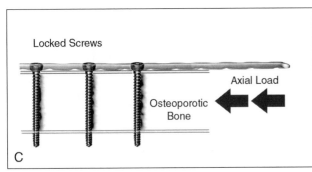

Figure 5 Illustration of the failure modes of single-beam versus load-sharing beam constructs. **A,** With a nonlocked screw construct in nonosteoporotic bone, sufficient insertion torque to eliminate motion between plate and bone creates a stable single-beam construct. **B,** With a nonlocked screw construct in osteoporotic bone, insufficient insertion torque to eliminate motion between plate and bone during axial loading results in an unstable load-sharing beam construct that fails under shear stress. **C,** With a locked screw construct in osteoporotic bone, fixed-angle screws create a stable single-beam construct in which axial load results in compression at the screw-bone interface.

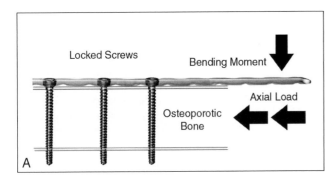

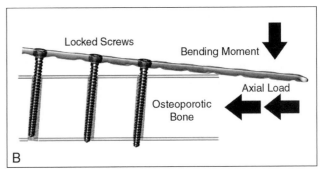

Figure 6 Illustration of simultaneous screw failure mode of locked screw construct. **A,** A locked screw construct in osteoporotic bone is subject to axial load with a bending moment. **B,** The locked screws must simultaneously cut through the entire shaded area of bone simultaneously to fail.

and bone (as seen with nonlocked constructs) are converted to compressive stress at the bone-screw interface (Figure 5, C). This mode of loading offers improved stability compared with nonlocked constructs because of bone's greater resistance to compression than shear, and because with locked plates the strength of fixation is the sum of each screw bone interface rather than dependent on a single screw. Furthermore, under axial load combined with bending, in contrast to the sequential screw failure that can occur with nonlocked screw constructs (Figure 3), and because locked screws remain at a fixed angle to the plate, all screws must simultaneously cut through bone for pullout to occur (Figure 6).

The insertion trajectory of locked screws must be colinear with the axis of the threads in the plate to properly lock into the plate and to avoid cross-threading. Locked plate systems, therefore, provide instrumentation to ensure that the pilot hole for a locked screw is colinear with the plate-hole thread axis. Most commonly, this consists of a drill guide that threads into the screw hole. A drill hole made through this guide is therefore aligned properly with the plate hole. Assuming the screw follows the pilot hole, the screw will be on axis and securely lock into the plate without cross-threading. Based on clinical practice, this is a reasonable assumption when placing screws through diaphyseal bone of good quality. When placing screws through osteoporotic or relatively soft metaphyseal bone, other methods should be considered to ensure that the screw will follow the pilot hole. Cannulated screws provide on-axis assurance when placed over a guidewire that is inserted through a guide that is screwed into the plate. Nested guides provide both an on-axis pilot hole and engage the head of the screw to ensure on-axis screw insertion (Figure 7). Outrigger systems similarly guide both pilot holes and screw insertion, and additionally enable easy percutaneous insertion. The outrigger is secured to the plate, and holes in the outrigger are designed to be aligned with the screw holes in the plate and accommodate sleeves for drill and screw insertion. In such circumstances, the plate should not be bent, otherwise the on-axis relationship between outrigger and plate will be violated and cross-threading of the screw head could occur.

The clinical consequence of off-axis screw insertion remains largely unknown. In a single biomechanical study that compared off-axis with on-axis screw insertion, an off-axis insertion angle of 5° resulted in up to a 43% reduction in bending strength, and an off-axis insertion angle of 10° resulted in up to a 68% reduction in bending strength.[39] These tests were performed using 4.5-mm locked screws inserted into plates with combination holes. The open section of these holes accounts for directional variation in the testing results. Screw insertion in the direction opposite of the dynamic compression portion of the combination hole yielded poorer strength than insertion toward the dynamic

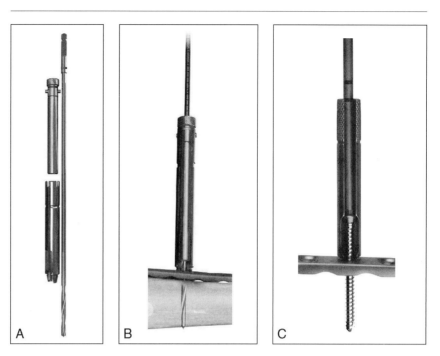

Figure 7 Illustration of how nested guides ensure on-axis screw insertion. **A,** The components of nested screw guide include the outer sleeve, the inner sleeve, and the drill bit. **B,** The outer sleeve threads into the plate, and the inner sleeve guides the drill. **C,** The inner sleeve is removed, and the outer sleeve guides screw insertion.

compression portion of the hole. Other locked plate designs with closed locking holes provide circumferential contact with the screw head and are likely to yield better bending strength when cross-threaded. Although a minimum screw insertion torque of locked screws is not required to compress plate to bone, adequate insertion torque is required for the threaded screw head to lock into the plate. Overtightening of small screws in thin plates can lead to stripping of the threads. Larger screws in thick plates are not likely to be stripped under loads generated by hand tightening. The phenomenon of cold welding can occur after overtightening of titanium implants. However, stainless steel implants are less likely to cold weld because of the harder material properties of stainless steel compared with titanium.

Fracture reduction is substantially different when using pure locked plate constructs compared with nonlocked constructs. Because locked screws do not lag bone to plate, such plate-screw constructs cannot be used as a reduction tool. Fracture reduction and plate contour are completely independent (Figure 4); therefore, fracture reduction should be obtained before locked screw placement. Once a satisfactory reduction is obtained, definitive locked screw fixation is performed on both sides of the fracture. Accordingly, the plate does not necessarily have to have the same contour as the bone nor does it have to be in contact with the bone. Not compressing plate to bone avoids crushing of the periosteum, an advantage of locked plating for which the clinical benefit remains unknown. Because most current locked plates are precontoured to match the anatomic area for which they are designed, reduction tools have been devised to be used in conjunction with locked plate internal fixators to allow the plate to be used as a reduction aid as with hybrid plating methods.

Hybrid Plating

Hybrid plating uses both nonlocked and locked screws within the same plate-screw construct and has become the most common method of plating with locked screws. Using nonlocked screws, the plate can be used as a reduction aid, and fracture fragments can be lagged and/or dynamically compressed. Locked screws added secondarily improve fixation by creating a fixed-angle device during treatment of end-segment metaphyseal fractures and improving fixation in osteoporotic bone. There are some guidelines that should be followed when using the hybrid plating method. In any given fracture fragment, if nonlocked screws are used, they should be placed before any locked screws in that fragment. This is because nonlocked screws require friction between plate and bone for construct stability. If a locked screw were inserted first, subsequent insertion of a nonlocked screw would not further compress plate to bone (without bending the plate). A locked screw inserted first can hold the plate completely off of the bone. Subsequent insertion of a nonlocked screw would not be able to generate any friction between plate and bone; therefore, the nonlocked screw would not impart significant additional stability to the construct. Another guideline for hybrid plating is based on similar reasoning. Dynamic compression of the fracture, if used, should be obtained with nonlocked screws before insertion

of locked screws in the fragment that is moving relative to the plate. It should, therefore, be clear that locked screws can certainly be inserted in one fragment before insertion of nonlocked screws in a separate fragment. This technical variation is preferable in certain situations, especially when compression or the push-pull technique is used in association with osteoporotic bone. For example, treatment of a shortened lateral malleolus fracture is associated with osteoporotic bone, where restoration of fibular length is obtained with the push technique by fixing the plate to the distal fragment and then translating the plate (and distal fragment) distally by pushing against a screw affixed outside and proximal to the plate. Nonlocked screws in the distal fragment, especially unicortical screws in osteoporotic bone, are less likely to resist this axial shear stress than fixed-angle locked screws.

The biomechanically ideal hybrid construct remains uncertain. However, two distinct goals, fracture site stability and bone/plate fixation, must be differentiated when considering the biomechanics of any plate-screw construct. Fracture site strain is critical to fracture healing. The stress/strain properties of plate constructs are most significantly affected by the working distance across the fracture site (the distance between the most proximal screw in the distal fragment and the most distal screw in the proximal fragment), the stability imparted by direct contact and compression of the fracture fragments, the physical dimensions of the plate, and the plate material. The type of screw fixation, whether nonlocked, locked, hybrid, unicortical, or bicortical, is a secondary factor affecting fracture site stability, assuming that plate fixation to bone is

secure. This assumption becomes potentially invalid after a construct is loaded to near its ultimate failure or, as more commonly occurs in clinical practice, is fatigued through cyclic stress with noncritical (physiologic) loads. There is some evidence to suggest that locked screws should be placed at both ends of the fracture to maximally resist axial load and bending. To resist torsion, the position of a locked screw relative to the fracture has less effect on stability.[40]

Another advantage of the hybrid plating technique is that the plate can easily be used as a reduction tool as with nonlocked plating. Because most periarticular locked plates are manufactured with anatomic contour, little if any plate bending is required for the plate to be effectively used as a reduction tool. When locked plates are bent, the threaded holes are potentially damaged. The consequences of such deformations on locked screw stability remain unknown.

Minimally Invasive Plating Techniques

Open reduction and internal fixation of fractures dates back more than 80 years. With the development of improved anesthetic techniques and surgical implants and the availability of antibiotics, surgical treatment of fractures gained popularity in the 1950s. As a result, previously unrealized complications began to occur, including wound dehiscence and infections, often resulting in less than optimal outcomes and amputation in some patients. In an effort to avoid these complications, minimize soft-tissue scarring and patient discomfort, and improve patient outcomes, early plating techniques have undergone considerable refinement.

Conventional rigid plating techniques required anatomic reduction of individual fracture fragments to accomplish compression. This necessitated large skin incisions, significant soft-tissue dissection, and periosteal stripping and created a biologically unfriendly environment for fracture healing. Intramedullary fixation techniques for long bone fractures described by Kuntscher[41] provided adequate, but not rigid, fracture stability such that secondary bone healing occurred with callus formation. Kuntscher's success generated interest in preserving the biologic environment at the fracture site during plate fixation. Thus, alternatives to rigid fixation were sought.

Initial modifications of the traditional open methods of fracture fixation focused on decreased soft-tissue stripping from about the fractured bone fragments while still providing restoration of limb length, alignment, and rotation. Blatter and Weber[3] introduced the wave plate, which spans the fracture site and is situated away from the fracture ends, leaving the blood supply to the fracture site undisturbed. The wave plate also allows bone graft to be packed beneath it. Kinast and associates[42] were among the first to evaluate clinical results of indirect reduction techniques. Subtrochanteric femur fractures were internally stabilized with 95° condylar blade plates by one of two different reduction techniques. The first technique used direct anatomic reduction with a traditional degree of soft-tissue stripping; the second technique used an indirect anatomic reduction with care taken to minimize soft-tissue stripping from about the fracture, without anatomic reduction of individual fracture fragments, but with restoration of overall limb alignment. The average time to union for the direct anatomic reduction group was 5.4 months, with 17% of the fractures going on to delayed union or nonunion. The indirect anatomic reduction group achieved union in 4.2 months, and there were no nonunions. Kinast and associates concluded that anatomic reduction of fracture fragments is not necessary for union. These findings paved the way for the concept of indirect reduction: obtaining length, alignment, and rotation of long bones while bypassing the area of comminution.

Further advances with indirect reduction techniques continued to develop. Mast and associates[18] described using ligamentotaxis and the plate as reduction tools to reestablish fracture alignment while maintaining a biologically friendly environment. Although this technique still used large incisions, the soft-tissue envelope around the fracture site remained intact because traditional plates were slid submuscularly. The plate simply bridged the fracture site. This fixation technique, because of a lack of anatomic fracture fragment reduction and therefore a lack of fracture compression, provided relative but not rigid stability, and fractures united by secondary bone healing with visible fracture callus. The technique was most helpful in treating fractures with areas of comminution.

Bolhofner and associates[43] evaluated these soft-tissue sparing, indirect reduction techniques with standard plates. They treated 57 AO type A or C supracondylar femur fractures with a condylar blade or buttress plate, using biologic reduction techniques, without any need for bone graft, and with immediate postoperative continuous passive motion. The average time to union for the fractures was 10.7 weeks, and there were no reported nonunions. They found that this reduction technique yielded satisfactory union results with minimal hardware failure.

The next step in the evolution of biologic plating techniques was to extend the soft-tissue preservation to the more superficial tissues. In two studies, Krettek and associates[44,45] further advanced biologically friendly fixation techniques. Using small incisions and conventional plates, implants were placed submuscularly through tunnels created in the soft tissues. The fracture site was left undisturbed. Screws were then placed percutaneously through the plate. Longer plates were used to ensure adequate stability, whereas fewer holes were filled to decrease damage to the bone and provide the correct amount of flexibility.[41] This concept, known as minimally invasive percutaneous osteosynthesis, resulted in fracture union with abundant fracture callus formation. The use of these smaller incisions results in a decrease in the amount of soft-tissue disruption, and therefore decreased muscle scarring, contracture, and weakness, and potentially an increase in functional recovery compared with more invasive techniques. Indirect reduction techniques, including manual traction, use of the femoral distractor, and strategically placed pointed reduction forceps, continue to be required. Fixation constructs are created with implants that are carefully passed along the bone, beneath the musculature, and fixed with screws at either end to bridge the fracture, much like an intramedullary nail placed in the treatment of a diaphyseal fracture.

Multiple clinical and basic science studies have since been published reporting the advantages of

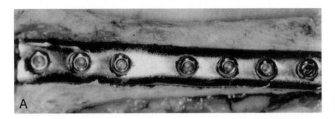 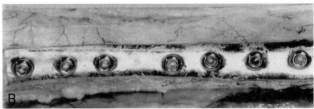

Figure 8 Specimen photographs show the medial aspect of a distal tibia plated via an open technique (**A**) and a percutaneous technique (**B**). Note the reduced extraosseous vessels anterior to the plate of the open specimen relative to the percutaneously plated specimen.

minimally invasive techniques. Baumgaertel and associates[46] used three groups of sheep in which a closed subtrochanteric femur fracture was created. Group A underwent formal open reduction and internal fixation, group B underwent open and indirect reduction and internal fixation, and group C underwent indirect reduction and fixation with point contact fixation plates and unicortical screws. Groups B and C had superior healing (evident by earlier and increased bone formation) and better blood supply compared with group A. Farouk and associates[33] investigated the effect of minimally invasive percutaneous osteosynthesis and traditional techniques on femoral blood supply in a human cadaveric injection study. Group I specimens underwent standard open reduction and internal fixation of the intact distal femur, and group II underwent a minimally invasive application of a similar plate on the distal femur. After injection with India ink and latex, all of the minimally invasive percutaneous osteosynthesis specimens showed that each of the perforating and nutrient arteries remained intact, whereas traditional plating had caused considerable disruption of these vessels.

Helfet and associates[47] published one of the first clinical series describing the use of minimally invasive plating techniques for the treatment of fractures of the distal tibia. In this series of lower-energy distal tibia fractures, a flattened one-half tubular plate was passed percutaneously along the medial tibia, the fracture was indirectly reduced, and screw fixation was applied through individual stab incisions. All fractures healed with good alignment, none required secondary procedures, and only one patient had a complication (cellulitis), which resolved with antibiotics.

Borrelli and associates[48] demonstrated the effects on the distal tibia periosteal blood supply relative to different plating techniques. In this matched cadaveric injection study, the medial distal tibia was plated either via a traditional open procedure or a minimally invasive percutaneous osteosynthesis procedure. The specimens were then doubly injected with India ink and latex. The minimally invasive percutaneous osteosynthesis specimens were found to have a statistically significant greater number of intact periosteal arteries compared with the openly plated specimens (Figure 8). These data support the contention that minimally invasive percutaneous osteosynthesis techniques are more likely to preserve bone blood supply than traditional open techniques.

Although minimally invasive percutaneous osteosynthesis techniques are gaining in popularity and have been shown to preserve more of the local blood supply than open techniques, there are some disadvantages. These techniques are more technically demanding than traditional formal open reduction and internal fixation and require an increased utilization of fluoroscopy. More user-friendly jigs and implants are becoming available, but further modifications are necessary for these procedures to gain universal acceptance. Also, because these newer implants are often made of titanium and frequently not every hole in the plate is being filled, minimally invasive means of hardware removal must also be developed. Despite these limitations, minimally invasive percutaneous osteosynthesis techniques offer real advances and advantages over more traditional open plating techniques.

The results of this evolving method of fracture care are encouraging. Acceptably lower complication rates and higher fracture union rates have been reported for some of the most challenging injuries.[28,49] It is not yet known, however, whether minimally invasive percutaneous osteosynthesis methods lead to faster fracture healing or earlier return of function than open indirect techniques. Unresolved issues, including the realization that this technique is more demanding than formal open reduction and internal fixation and requires increased use of image intensification, have spurred the development of newer implants and insertion instruments. As this technique for fracture fixation has gained in popularity, implant removal has also been identified as a potential problem.

Summary

Locked and minimally invasive plating are two of the most recent advances in plate fixation of long bone fractures. Locked plating technology provides for fixed angle support of end segment fractures and improved construct stability in osteoporotic bone. Minimally invasive plating techniques preserve the soft-tissue envelope surrounding the fracture to maximize the potential for fracture healing. These two advances, locked and minimally invasive plating, are not synonymous, but work well together toward providing improved stability and a more optimal biologic environment for fracture healing compared to traditional plating techniques. Although these advances represent improvements, the optimal biomechanical construct to maximize fracture healing potential remains unknown and represents the next frontier for plate and screw fixation of fractures.

References

1. Peltier L: The internal fixation of fractures, in *Fractures: A History and Iconography of Their Treatment*. San Francisco, CA, Norman Publishing, 1990, pp 114-167.

2. Danis MR: The operative treatment of fractures: 1947. *Clin Orthop Relat Res* 1993;292:10-12.

3. Blatter G, Weber BG: Wave plate osteosynthesis as a salvage procedure. *Arch Orthop Trauma Surg* 1990;109: 330-333.

4. Kolodziej P, Lee FS, Patel A, et al: Biomechanical evaluation of the Schuhli nut. *Clin Orthop Relat Res* 1998;347:79-85.

5. Koval KJ, Kummer FJ, Bharam S, Chen D, Halder S: Distal femoral fixation: A laboratory comparison of the 95 degrees plate, antegrade and retrograde inserted reamed intramedullary nails. *J Orthop Trauma* 1996;10:378-382.

6. The operative treatment of fractures: General considerations of indications and technique, in *On Modern Methods of Treating Fractures*. Bristol, England, John Wright & Sons, 1916, pp 176-208.

7. Schatzker J: AO philosophy and principles, in Reudi T, Murphy W (eds): *AO Principles of Fracture Management*. New York, NY, Thieme, 2000, pp 1-4.

8. Bagby GW: Compression bone-plating: historical considerations. *J Bone Joint Surg Am* 1977;59:625-631.

9. Kassab SS, Mast JW, Mayo KA: Patients treated for nonunions with plate and screw fixation and adjunctive locking nuts. *Clin Orthop Relat Res* 1998;347: 86-92.

10. Matelic TM, Monroe MT, Mast JW: The use of endosteal substitution in the treatment of recalcitrant nonunions of the femur: Report of seven cases. *J Orthop Trauma* 1996;10:1-6.

11. Ring D, Perey BH, Jupiter JB: The functional outcome of operative treatment of ununited fractures of the humeral diaphysis in older patients. *J Bone Joint Surg Am* 1999;81:177-190.

12. Simon JA, Dennis MG, Kummer FJ, Koval KJ: Schuhli augmentation of plate and screw fixation for humeral shaft fractures: A laboratory study. *J Orthop Trauma* 1999;13:196-199.

13. Perren SM, Buchanan J: Basic concepts relevant to the design and development of the Point Contact Fixator (PC-Fix). *Injury* 1995;26(suppl 2):SB1-SB41.

14. Tepic S, Perren SM: The biomechanics of the PC-Fix internal fixator. *Injury* 1995; 26(suppl 2):SB5-SB10.

15. Leung F, Shew-Ping C: A prospective, randomized trial comparing the limited contact dynamic compression plate with the point contact fixator for forearm fractures. *J Bone Joint Surg Am* 2003; 85:2343-2348.

16. Haas N, Hauke C, Schutz M, Kaab M, Perren SM: Treatment of diaphyseal fractures of the forearm using the Point Contact Fixator (PC-Fix): Results of 387 fractures of a prospective multicentric study (PC-Fix II). *Injury* 2001;32(suppl 2):B51-B62.

17. Sanders R, Swiontkowski M, Rosen H, Helfet D: Double-plating of comminuted unstable fractures of the distal part of the femur. *J Bone Joint Surg Am* 1991;73: 341-346.

18. Mast J, Jakob R, Ganz R: *Planning and Reduction Technique in Fracture Surgery*. Berlin, Germany, Springer-Verlag, 1989.

19. Frigg R, Appenzeller A, Christensen R, Frenk A, Gilbert S, Schavan R: The development of the distal femur Less Invasive Stabilization System (LISS). *Injury* 2001;32(suppl 3):SC24-SC31.

20. Schandelmaier P, Partenheimer A, Koenemann B, Grun OA, Krettek C: Distal femoral fractures and LISS stabilization. *Injury* 2001;32(suppl 3):SC55-SC63.

21. Mize RD, Bucholz RW, Grogan DP: Surgical treatment of displaced, comminuted fractures of the distal end of the femur. *J Bone Joint Surg Am* 1982; 64:871-879.

22. Benum P: The use of bone cement as an adjunct to internal fixation of supracondylar fractures of osteoporotic femurs. *Acta Orthop Scand* 1977;48:52-56.

23. Schatzker J, Home G, Waddell J: The Toronto experience with the supracondylar fracture of the femur: 1966-72. *Injury* 1974;6:113-128.

24. Struhl S, Szporn MN, Cobelli NJ, Sadler AH: Cemented internal fixation for supracondylar femur fractures in osteoporotic patients. *J Orthop Trauma* 1990;4:151-157.

25. Simonian PT, Thompson GJ, Emley W, Harrington RM, Benirschke SK, Swiontkowski MF: Angulated screw placement in the lateral condylar buttress plate for supracondylar femoral fractures. *Injury* 1998;29:101-104.

26. Barei DP, Nork SE, Mills WJ, Henley MB, Benirschke SK: Complications associated with internal fixation of high-energy bicondylar tibial plateau fractures utilizing a two-incision technique. *J Orthop Trauma* 2004; 18:649-657.

27. Zlowodzki M, Williamson S, Cole PA, Zardiackas LD, Kregor PJ: Biomechanical evaluation of the less invasive stabilization system, angled blade plate, and retrograde intramedullary nail for the internal fixation of distal femur fractures. *J Orthop Trauma* 2004;18:494-502.

28. Kregor PJ, Stannard JA, Zlowodzki M, Cole PA: Treatment of distal femur fractures using the less invasive stabilization system: Surgical experience

and early clinical results in 103 fractures. *J Orthop Trauma* 2004;18:509-520.

29. Cole PA, Zlowodzki M, Kregor PJ: Treatment of proximal tibia fractures using the less invasive stabilization system: Surgical experience and early clinical results in 77 fractures. *J Orthop Trauma* 2004;18:528-535.

30. Ricci WM, O'Boyle M, Borrelli J, Bellabarba C, Sanders R: Fractures of the proximal third of the tibial shaft treated with intramedullary nails and blocking screws. *J Orthop Trauma* 2001;15:264-270.

31. Farouk O, Krettek C, Miclau T, Schandelmaier P, Guy P, Tscherne H: Minimally invasive plate osteosynthesis and vascularity: Preliminary results of a cadaver injection study. *Injury* 1997; 28(suppl 1):A7-12.

32. Farouk O, Krettek C, Miclau T, Schandelmaier P, Guy P, Tscherne H: Minimally invasive plate osteosynthesis: Does percutaneous plating disrupt femoral blood supply less than the traditional technique? *J Orthop Trauma* 1999;13:401-406.

33. Farouk O, Krettek C, Miclau T, Schandelmaier P, Tscherne H: Effects of percutaneous and conventional plating techniques on the blood supply to the femur. *Arch Orthop Trauma Surg* 1998; 117:438-441.

34. Zlowodzki M, Bhandari M, Marek DJ, Cole PA, Kregor PJ: Operative treatment of acute distal femur fractures: Systematic review of two comparative studies and 45 case series (1989 to 2005). *J Orthop Trauma* 2006;20:366-371.

35. Borgeaud M, Cordey J, Leyvraz PE, Perren SM: Mechanical analysis of the bone to plate interface of the LC-DCP and of the PC-FIX on human femora. *Injury* 2000;31(suppl 3):C29-C36.

36. Egol KA, Kubiak EN, Fulkerson E, Kummer FJ, Koval KJ: Biomechanics of locked plates and screws. *J Orthop Trauma* 2004;18:488-493.

37. Hofer HP, Wildburger R, Szyszkowitz R: Observations concerning different patterns of bone healing using the Point Contact Fixator (PC-Fix) as a new technique for fracture fixation. *Injury* 2001;32(suppl 2):B15-B25.

38. Gautier E, Perren SM, Cordey J: Effect of plate position relative to bending direction on the rigidity of a plate osteosynthesis: A theoretical analysis. *Injury* 2000;31(suppl 3):C14-C20.

39. Kaab MJ, Frenk A, Schmeling A, Schaser K, Schutz M, Haas NP: Locked internal fixator: sensitivity of screw/plate stability to the correct insertion angle of the screw. *J Orthop Trauma* 2004;18:483-487.

40. Stoffel K, Dieter U, Stachowiak G, Gachter A, Kuster MS: Biomechanical testing of the LCP: How can stability in locked internal fixators be controlled? *Injury* 2003;34(suppl 2):B11-B19.

41. Kuntscher G: Intramedullary surgical technique and its place in orthopaedic surgery. *J Bone Joint Surg Am* 1965;47: 809-818.

42. Kinast C, Bolhofner BR, Mast JW, Ganz R: Subtrochanteric fractures of the femur: Results of treatment with the 95 degrees condylar blade-plate. *Clin Orthop Relat Res* 1989;238:122-130.

43. Bolhofner BR, Carmen B, Clifford P: The results of open reduction and internal fixation of distal femur fractures using a biologic (indirect) reduction technique. *J Orthop Trauma* 1996;10: 372-377.

44. Krettek C, Schandelmaier P, Miclau T, Bertram R, Holmes W, Tscherne H: Transarticular joint reconstruction and indirect plate osteosynthesis for complex distal supracondylar femoral fractures. *Injury* 1997;28(suppl 1):A31-A41.

45. Krettek C, Schandelmaier P, Miclau T, Tscherne H: Minimally invasive percutaneous plate osteosynthesis (MIPPO) using the DCS in proximal and distal femoral fractures. *Injury* 1997; 28(suppl 1):A20-A30.

46. Baumgaertel F, Buhl M, Rahn BA: Fracture healing in biological plate osteosynthesis. *Injury* 1998;29(suppl 3):C3-C6.

47. Helfet DL, Shonnard PY, Levine D, Borrelli JJ: Minimally invasive plate osteosynthesis of distal fractures of the tibia. *Injury* 1997;28(suppl 1):A42-A47.

48. Borrelli J Jr, Prickett W, Song E, Becker D, Ricci W: Extraosseous blood supply of the tibia and the effects of different plating techniques: A human cadaveric study. *J Orthop Trauma* 2002;16:691-695.

49. Stannard JP, Wilson TC, Volgas DA, Alonso JE: The less invasive stabilization system in the treatment of complex fractures of the tibial plateau: Short-term results. *J Orthop Trauma* 2004;18:552-558.

Unstable Fracture-Dislocations of the Elbow

Dean G. Sotereanos, MD

Nickolaos A. Darlis, MD

Thomas W. Wright, MD

Robert J. Goitz, MD

Graham J. King, MD

Abstract

Fracture-dislocations of the elbow are devastating injuries. The surgeon must maintain a high index of suspicion when evaluating an elbow dislocation to avoid missing critical associated injuries. Patterns of unstable fracture-dislocations include the "terrible triad" injury of the elbow (elbow dislocation, radial head fracture, and coronoid fracture), transolecranon fracture-dislocations, and the posterior Monteggia lesion. Complex fracture-dislocations of the elbow are treated surgically and are challenging injuries to manage. Elbow stability must be restored by addressing the specific components of the injury. The proximal ulna must be anatomically reduced and internally fixed, the radial head must be repaired or replaced, and substantial coronoid fractures must be repaired or reconstructed. Soft-tissue injuries must also be treated. The lateral ulnar collateral ligament and extensor origin reattachment can be easily performed. The next critical step is to intraoperatively assess the stability of the elbow with a range-of-motion assessment with the forearm in pronation. If the elbow remains unstable, application of a hinged elbow external fixator or repair of the medial collateral ligament must be considered. The goal of reconstruction is early mobilization within a stable arc of motion. This treatment protocol has the potential to improve the suboptimal outcomes reported in the literature for such injuries.

Instr Course Lect 2007;56:369-376.

The elbow is an inherently stable joint. Its stability is maintained by osseous, ligamentous, capsular, and musculotendinous restraints.[1,2] When more than one of those restraints fail as a result of an injury, the potential of complex elbow instability exists. A simple elbow dislocation is characterized by posterior displacement of the ulna relative to the humerus, without a significant associated fracture. In a patient with a simple elbow dislocation, the joint will be stable and will not redislocate after it is reduced unless placed in a position of near full extension and supination. In contrast, a complex elbow dislocation is either irreducible or after reduction it is inherently and immediately unstable unless surgical repair is performed.

Elbow Stability

The main osteoarticular components of elbow stability are the ulnohumeral and radiocapitellar articulations. In the ulnohumeral articulation, integrity of both the proximal ulna and distal humerus is necessary to maintain stability. The trochlear notch of the ulna forms a 180° arc around the trochlea of the humerus. The olecranon sits in the olecranon fossa and the coronoid process provides an anterior buttress to posterior elbow dislocation. The medial aspect of the coronoid is also the insertion site of the important anterior bundle of the medial collateral ligament (MCL). The spool-shaped trochlea of the distal humerus conforms to the proximal ulna and has a 30° anterior tilt of the articular surface that is important in maintaining stability. Studies have shown that the integrity of the olecranon is crucial to maintaining stability. Elbow stability increases linearly with larger amounts of olecranon excision.[3]

The second osteoarticular component contributing to elbow stability is the radiocapitellar articulation. The radial head provides approximately 30% of the resistance to valgus stress when all other ligamentous structures are intact. The radial head also provides an anterior buttress to posterior elbow dislocation. The radial head is oval and its axis of rotation is offset laterally approximately 15°. The contribution of the radial head to stabilizing the elbow against valgus stress increases dramatically when the MCL is injured.[4]

Capsular and ligamentous components of elbow stability include the MCL, lateral collateral ligament (LCL), and (to a lesser degree) the joint capsule. The MCL consists of an anterior bundle that is a distinct structure and the posterior transverse bundles, which could be considered more as thickenings of the capsule. The anterior bundle of the MCL extends from the inferior surface of the medial epicondyle to the sublime tubercle of the ulna and is biomechanically the most important structure. It is a nearly isometric structure; parts of the anterior bundle remain tight both in flexion and extension of the elbow.[5-7] It is the primary stabilizer of the elbow to valgus stress, providing 30% to 50% of the resistance to valgus stress (depending on the amount of flexion).[4,8] Fractures of the base of the coronoid distal to the insertion of the anterior bundle spare the ligament from anatomic injury, but are biomechanically equivalent to a complete rupture. In recent years, the importance of fractures of the medial facet of the coronoid have been increasingly recognized and specialized plates for internal fixation have been developed.[9-11] When the MCL is damaged, the radial head, which under normal circumstances is a secondary constraint to valgus stress, becomes essential for elbow stability.

In recent years, the contribution of the LCL to elbow stability has been increasingly recognized. The LCL inserts into the lateral epicondyle of the humerus at the axis of ulnohumeral rotation. The part of the LCL that inserts into the crista supinatoris of the ulna is called the lateral ulnar collateral ligament (LUCL). Fibers of the LCL also insert into the annular ligament. The LCL maintains apposition of the radial head to the capitellum and it prevents posterolateral rotatory instability.[12] Although the LCL is the primary restraint to posterolateral instability, it has been shown that other lateral musculotendinous structures (the extensor muscles, the fascial bands of the extensor carpi ulnaris, and intermuscular septa) provide secondary restraints.[13] The anterior capsule also provides a secondary restraint both in valgus and varus stress.[14]

Elbow stability is closely related to forearm stability. The forearm can be considered an osteoligamentous ring. Double or multiple injuries to that ring are common and elbow and forearm instability can coexist. Three structures play a key role in forearm stability: the radial head, the interosseous membrane of the forearm, and the triangular fibrocartilage complex. The forearm interosseous membrane contributes 70% to forearm stability and may be injured in association with elbow fractures.[15,16] In such instances, the resultant longitudinal instability of the forearm and disruption of the distal radioulnar joint is called the Essex-Lopresti injury.

Pathophysiology
Elbow dislocations represent a wide spectrum of instability ranging from isolated ligamentous injury to complete osteoligamentous disruption.

The most common mechanism of injury is a fall at ground level that produces axial compression to the elbow, forces the forearm into supination, and forces the elbow into valgus. The combination of these three forces (axial compression, supination, valgus vector) creates a posterolateral rotatory stress. Approximately 90% of all dislocations of the elbow are associated with posterolateral displacement of the olecranon, which follows a predictable pattern (Figure 1). Ligamentous injuries caused by dislocation follow a predictable lateral to medial path that is known as the Horii circle.[12] The LUCL is injured first, followed by the capsule, the posterior aspect of the MCL, and the anterior bundle of the MCL.

Simple elbow dislocations with no associated fractures have a favorable prognosis; early closed reduction and early mobilization usually achieve excellent results.[17] Patients with complex elbow fracture-dislocations have an increased risk of recurrent or chronic instability and arthrosis. In general, whenever instability remains after closed reduction of a complex fracture-dislocation, surgical treatment is needed to restore stability for an optimal outcome.

Injury patterns that are often associated with significant elbow instability include the "terrible triad" of the elbow (Figure 2), transolecranon fracture-dislocations (Figure 3), and the posterior Monteggia lesion[18-22] (Figure 4). The Essex-Lopresti injury must be treated using the same principles used to treat complex elbow fracture-dislocations. The terrible triad of the elbow consists of an elbow dislocation, radial head fracture, and coronoid fracture. It is a terrible injury because it results in severe instability, is

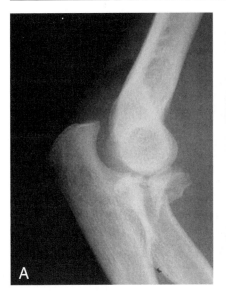
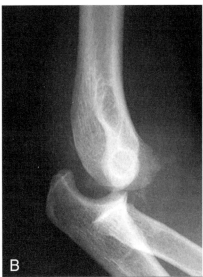
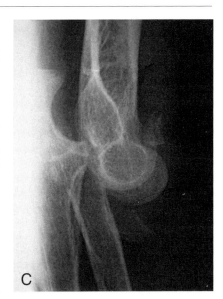

Figure 1   The stages of posterolateral rotatory instability of the elbow. **A,** Subluxated. **B,** Perched. **C,** Dislocated. Each stage is associated with increasing degrees of soft-tissue disruption from lateral to medial.

difficult to manage, and has a poor prognosis. The significance of this injury pattern can be easily missed; treatment with simple closed reduction will result in recurrent instability (Figure 2). The radiographs of patients with elbow dislocations must be carefully evaluated to diagnose a terrible triad injury. A consistent treatment protocol for this injury pattern can improve the suboptimal results that have been reported in the literature.[23,24]

Evaluation
Fracture-dislocations of the elbow are characterized by notable pain, swelling, and deformity. A concomitant injury of the wrist and shoulder occurs in 10% to 20% of patients. All injuries should be assessed before a closed reduction is attempted. A detailed neurovascular evaluation is performed before and after reduction. The ulnar nerve is the most vulnerable structure because of its position directly medial to the joint. Median and radial nerve injuries have been reported and the median

nerve has occasionally been found trapped in the joint. Radiographs of the distal radioulnar joint are needed to rule out Essex-Lopresti injury. The muscles of the forearm should be monitored for compartment syndrome.

Plain radiographs of the elbow are helpful to assess the extent and severity of concomitant fractures. Because of the overlap of structures, plain tomograms and CT (especially with three-dimensional reconstruction) also are useful in appreciating the size and the displacement of the fracture fragments.

Treatment
Surgical treatment is imperative for patients with complex elbow instability. Nonsurgical treatment is not an option. Although treatment must be individualized based on the osseous or ligamentous structures that have been disrupted, some general principles can be described for all injuries (Figure 5).

Many of these injuries can be treated with a lateral approach to the

elbow. A posterolateral (Kocher) skin incision can be used. If a concomitant proximal ulnar fracture exists or if a medial approach to the elbow is contemplated, a posterior midline skin incision can be used. The lateral approach is performed through the Kocher interval between the anconeus and extensor carpi ulnaris. This interval can be identified from the rim of adipose tissue between those two muscles or by the presence of small vessels perforating the fascia. A more simple approach uses an incision line that extends from the tip of the lateral epicondyle to a point bisecting the width of the radial head. If necessary, this approach is extended proximally by detaching the extensor muscles from the distal humerus. By staying anterior to the lateral epicondyle, further injury to the LCL can be avoided. Injuries to the radial nerve can be avoided by keeping the forearm in full pronation or by exposing the nerve proximally. In some instances, soft-tissue injuries are extensive and the fractures can

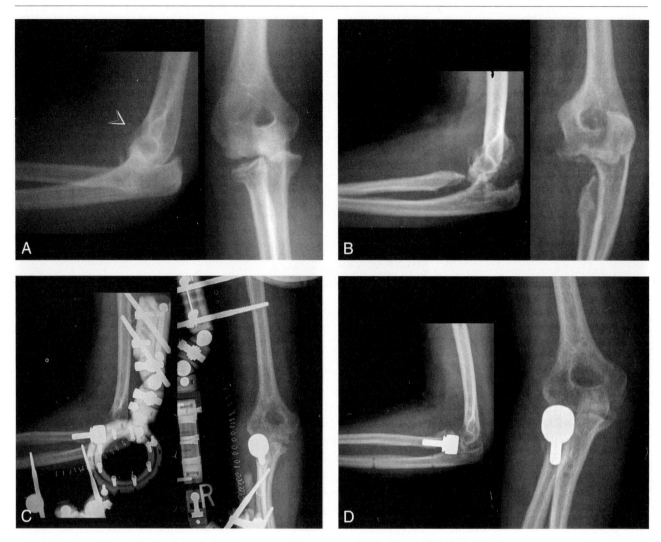

Figure 2 **A,** Lateral (left) and AP (right) views of a terrible triad injury of the elbow consisting of elbow dislocation, radial head fracture, and coronoid fracture (*arrow*). Note the posteromedial direction of the dislocation. **B,** The nature of the injury was missed by the treating surgeon and a radial head excision was undertaken, resulting in recurrent elbow dislocation. Lateral view (left) and AP view (right) show recurrent elbow dislocation and the development of ectopic bone around the elbow. **C,** Final treatment included radial head replacement, LCL reattachment to the lateral epicondyle using two bioabsorbable suture anchors, and application of a hinged external elbow fixator. Lateral view (left) and AP view (right). **D,** After removal of the external fixator, concentric reduction of the elbow was maintained. Lateral view (left) and AP view (right).

be safely accessed through the path of soft-tissue injury, thus eliminating the need for a formal approach.

When a concomitant proximal ulna fracture coexists, anatomic reduction and internal fixation is essential. In those instances, reconstruction is usually initiated with fixation of the proximal ulna through a posterior approach. Shortening of the ulna can be detrimental to elbow stability and can lead to arthrosis. In some instances, the anterior fragment of the proximal ulna includes the coronoid process. Fixation of this fragment with lag screws to the shaft restores the anterior buttress of the coronoid. Dual plating may also be used, especially in patients with a large anteromedial facet coronoid fracture (Figure 3). Tension band fixation of the proximal ulna should be reserved only for simple transverse fracture patterns. Specialized anatomic proximal ulnar plates and locking plates are now available and are useful when treating comminuted proximal ulnar fractures that are commonly associated with complex elbow instability.

In patients without a concomitant proximal ulna fracture, reconstruction is initiated by assessing the radi-

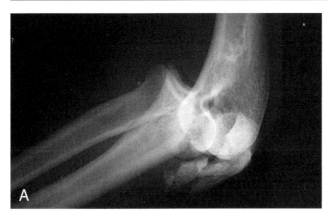
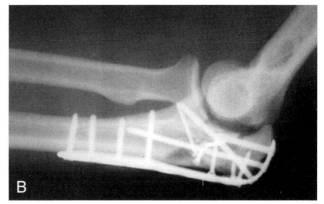

Figure 3   **A,** Transolecranon fracture-dislocation of the elbow. **B,** Open reduction and internal fixation using a precontoured proximal ulna plate was used to restore congruence of the ulnohumeral articulation. (Courtesy of C.G. Zalavras, MD, University of Southern California.)

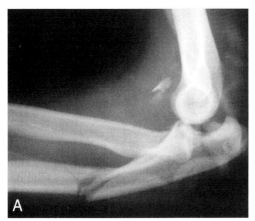
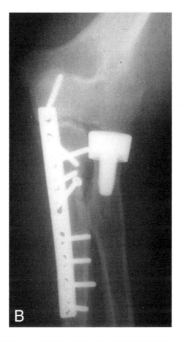
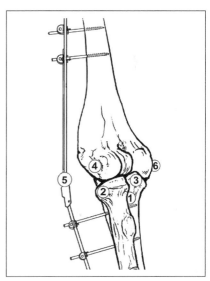

Figure 4 The posterior Monteggia lesion. **A,** Note the avulsion of the tip of the coronoid process. **B,** Treatment with anatomic reduction and internal fixation of the ulna, radial head replacement, and LCL reattachment using transosseous sutures. The coronoid was not repaired in this patient.

Figure 5 Schematic drawing showing the usual order of surgical steps taken to treat an unstable elbow fracture-dislocation. Concomitant proximal ulna fractures are (1) anatomically reduced and fixed first, followed by (2) radial head reconstruction or replacement, (3) coronoid fixation or reconstruction, and (4) LCL reattachment to the lateral epicondyle. If the elbow remains unstable after these steps, consideration must be given to (5) hinged external elbow application or (6) MCL repair or reconstruction. Not all steps are necessary for every patient. Stability of the elbow is reassessed after each step. The order of surgical steps may be altered depending on the patient's fracture pattern (for example, large coronoid fragments can be often fixed in conjunction with proximal ulna fixation).

al head. Radial head excision without prosthetic replacement is not recommended in patients with complex elbow instability.[1,19,25-27] The radial head buttress is essential if the MCL is injured. Options for treating the radial head include open reduction and internal fixation or prosthetic replacement. Radial head fractures with fragments of substantial size are amenable to internal fixation. Fixation can be achieved with small fragment screws, headless compression screws (such as the Herbert screw), Kirschner wires, and low-profile plates. A combination of these fixation devices may be needed; however, it is important to adhere to the safe zone of hardware replacement to avoid restrictions in pronosupination. The safe zone is a 110° arc of the radial head facing laterally with the forearm in neutral rotation.[28] It is important to avoid overretraction of the soft tissues anterior to the radial head to prevent posterior interosseous nerve injuries. Fixation of radial neck fractures can be challenging; specialized plates have recently become available for use in such fixation.

In comminuted radial head fractures, side-table reassembly of the radial head and reattachment to the radial shaft is no longer a favored treatment method. Comminuted radial head fractures associated with elbow dislocations are better treated by prosthetic replacement. If prosthetic replacement is elected, the radial head fragments are removed and a neck osteotomy is performed. The radial head fragments are reassembled at the side table and the head diameter is measured. In recent years, a metallic prosthesis has become the implant of choice in radial head replacement.[29] Silicone implants are not currently favored. When a concomitant coronoid fracture exists, the space provided by radial head resection can be used to access the coronoid and stabilize the fragments before the radial head implant is inserted. Proper sizing of the radial head is necessary. Overstuffing the joint with a large radial head implant should be avoided. A radial head implant with the smallest diameter that corresponds to the size of the native radial head should be used. In patients with severe comminution, the height of the radial head can be difficult to assess. Visual inspection of the proximal radioulnar joint can be helpful in determining the appropriate radial head height, which should not extend more proximal than the proximal radioulnar joint. Most contemporary radial head implant designs do not require press-fit fixation of the implant stem to the radial shaft. A loose fit that permits rotation of the implant relative to the radius is preferred.

Coronoid fractures are assessed next. The Regan-Morrey classification is useful in managing those fractures. Fractures involving more than 50% of the coronoid should be fixed.[30] Fixation of smaller fragments also is desirable if technically feasible. Fixation of larger coronoid fractures can be achieved with a retrograde screw through the dorsal ulna. Suture fixation with drill holes placed retrograde through the ulna and suture passage through the anterior capsule is also an option; however, the efficacy of this technique is questionable for small fragments. Specialized plates for fixation of medial facet fractures of the coronoid are now available, but require a separate medial incision and approach. Fixation of a large fragment of the medial facet of the coronoid is important because it is the insertion site for the anterior bundle of the MCL.[10] The fracture can be approached either by transposing the ulnar nerve anteriorly and then splitting the flexor carpi ulnaris where the nerve used to lie, or by a more anterior flexor-pronator mass-splitting approach, or by a more posterior elevation of the entire flexor-pronator mass.[11]

Radial head repair or replacement alone may be insufficient for the treatment of complex fracture-dislocations of the elbow;[31] the LCL must be addressed next. In most complex elbow fracture-dislocations, the LCL is usually avulsed from its origin from the lateral epicondyle and should be repaired with either suture anchors or drill holes through the lateral epicondyle. Dissection of the LCL is not necessary for this repair. The whole extensor origin sleeve (including the LCL) can be reattached to the lateral epicondyle.

MCL repair has become less popular in recent years. Stability of the

elbow can be satisfactorily maintained by addressing all associated fractures and repairing the LCL. With the elbow accurately reduced, isometric healing of the medial structures is expected. If a medial approach to the elbow is necessary for fracture fixation (for example, displaced medial epicondyle or medial facet of a coronoid fracture) or a nerve lesion, the medial ligamentous structures must be assessed and repaired if possible.

Intraoperative assessment of longitudinal stability is imperative, especially in patients with derangement of the distal radioulnar joint. Intraoperative assessment for an interosseous membrane injury is performed with direct longitudinal traction applied to the radius and assessment of forearm stability. If an Essex-Lopresti injury coexists, principles of treatment include radial head reconstruction or replacement, reduction of the distal radioulnar joint, and pinning in supination. The role of interosseous membrane repair or reconstruction or the repair of the triangular fibrocartilage complex in patients with acute injuries is not clearly defined.

After all osseous and ligamentous injuries have been treated, intraoperative assessment of elbow stability is necessary. This assessment is performed both clinically and radiographically under fluoroscopy. The forearm is kept in pronation as the elbow is brought through a range-of-motion evaluation. Elbow flexion and forearm pronation increases elbow stability, whereas elbow extension and forearm supination do not increase stability. As the elbow is tested for range of motion with the forearm in pronation, stability is assessed under fluoroscopy and the stable arc of motion is noted. If the elbow is stable between full flexion and 50° of flexion, the patient can be treated with immobilization in pronation. Early range of motion in a hinged brace, within the range of stability that was noted intraoperatively, is permitted. Hinged brace designs are available that maintain the forearm in pronation while permitting flexion and extension. In these braces, a limit can be set in extension to maintain the range of motion within the safe zone for the first 2 postoperative weeks; extension is gradually added thereafter.

If the elbow is completely unstable after completion of ligamentous and osseous repair, or if the elbow is stable only in a narrow range of motion, MCL repair or the application of an elbow fixator should be considered. Hinged, external elbow fixators allow joint range of motion while maintaining a concentric reduction and protecting any repair or fixation[32-34] (Figure 2). The soft tissues heal in an isometric position when a hinged elbow fixator has been accurately applied. Precise placement of the guide pin and open placement of the humeral half-pins (to avoid injury to the radial nerve) are essential for the successful application of a hinged elbow fixator.

Early range of motion within a safe arc is imperative for maintaining a functional elbow. Intraoperative stability must be adequate to permit early active, active-assisted, and gentle passive ranges of motion. If fracture stability is still questionable after all reasonable treatments have been performed, fracture healing takes precedence over early mobilization.

The protocol described allows most of the elements of these devastating elbow injuries to be comprehensively addressed. Consistent treatment protocols for these injuries rarely appear in the literature. In a re-cent study of patients with terrible triad injuries of the elbow, 77% of those treated with a similar protocol had good or excellent results at a mean follow-up of 3 years.[35] The long-term risk for degenerative joint disease is still unknown. Factors that adversely affect patient outcome are delayed treatment, previously unsuccessful surgery, comminution of the coronoid and proximal ulna, and severe soft-tissue injury. The age of the patient also can affect the outcome. In selected older patients, total elbow replacement can be considered as an alternative treatment to achieve improved function and pain relief.

Complications

Complications of complex fracture-dislocations include neurovascular injury, compartment syndrome, and infection. Recurrent instability can also occur. In those instances, LUCL reconstruction with a tendon graft or reconstruction of the coronoid with a bone block can be considered. Elbow stiffness can be avoided by early immobilization; however, fracture healing takes precedence over early mobilization. Mobilizing a fracture with questionable stability has no merit. Elbow stiffness can be treated with soft-tissue releases. The development of heterotopic ossification can impair the final outcome. The use of nonsteroidal anti-inflammatory drugs to prevent heterotopic ossification is unproven for patients with traumatic elbow injuries and may impair fracture healing. In recent years, early excision (6 to 12 months) of post-traumatic elbow heterotopic ossification has produced satisfactory results.[36-38] The assessment of the maturity of the heterotopic bone using bone scans or alkaline phosphatase levels has not been proved necessary. The development of de-generative arthritis can be addressed with a total elbow arthroplasty in older patients or a fascial interposition arthroplasty in younger patients.

Summary

Fracture-dislocations of the elbow are destructive and are challenging injuries to treat. A high index of suspicion is needed when evaluating apparently routine elbow dislocations. Complex fracture-dislocations of the elbow are treated surgically. Elbow stability must be restored by treating the specific components of the injury. Fracture repair is an essential element of treatment. The proximal ulna must be anatomically reduced and fixed, the radial head must be repaired or replaced, substantial coronoid fractures must be repaired or reconstructed, and soft-tissue injuries should be treated. LUCL and extensor origin reattachment are easily performed; however, repair of the MCL is rare unless a medial approach to the elbow is necessary for another reason. The stability of the elbow must be assessed intraoperatively by testing range of motion with the forearm in pronation. A hinged, elbow external fixator or repair of the MCL should be considered if the elbow remains unstable. Early mobilization within a stable arc of motion is the goal of elbow reconstruction.

References

1. Ring D, Jupiter JB: Fracture-dislocation of the elbow. *J Bone Joint Surg Am* 1998;80:566-580.

2. Ring D, Jupiter JB: Fracture-dislocation of the elbow. *Hand Clin* 2002;18:55-63.

3. An KN, Morrey BF, Chao EY: The effect of partial removal of proximal ulna on elbow constraint. *Clin Orthop Relat Res* 1986;209:270-279.

4. Morrey BF, Tanaka S, An KN: Valgus stability of the elbow: A definition of

primary and secondary constraints. *Clin Orthop Relat Res* 1991;265:187-195.

5. Callaway GH, Field LD, Deng XH, et al: Biomechanical evaluation of the medial collateral ligament of the elbow. *J Bone Joint Surg Am* 1997;79:1223-1231.

6. Zimmerman NB: Clinical application of advances in elbow and forearm anatomy and biomechanics. *Hand Clin* 2002;18:1-19.

7. Armstrong AD, Ferreira LM, Dunning CE, Johnson JA, King GJ: The medial collateral ligament of the elbow is not isometric: An in vitro biomechanical study. *Am J Sports Med* 2004;32:85-90.

8. Hotchkiss RN, Weiland AJ: Valgus stability of the elbow. *J Orthop Res* 1987;5:372-377.

9. Cohen MS: Fractures of the coronoid process. *Hand Clin* 2004;20:443-453.

10. Sanchez-Sotelo J, O'Driscoll SW, Morrey BF: Medial oblique compression fracture of the coronoid process of the ulna. *J Shoulder Elbow Surg* 2005;14:60-64.

11. Doornberg JN, Ring DC: Fracture of the anteromedial facet of the coronoid process. *J Bone Joint Surg Am* 2006;88:2216-2224.

12. O'Driscoll SW, Morrey BF, Korinek S, An KN: Elbow subluxation and dislocation: A spectrum of instability. *Clin Orthop Relat Res* 1992;280:186-197.

13. Cohen MS, Hastings H II: Rotatory instability of the elbow: The anatomy and role of the lateral stabilizers. *J Bone Joint Surg Am* 1997;79:225-233.

14. Morrey BF, An KN: Articular and ligamentous contributions to the stability of the elbow joint. *Am J Sports Med* 1983;11:315-319.

15. Hotchkiss RN, An KN, Sowa DT, Basta S, Weiland AJ: An anatomic and mechanical study of the interosseous membrane of the forearm: Pathomechanics of proximal migration of the radius. *J Hand Surg [Am]* 1989;14:256-261.

16. Skahen JR III, Palmer AK, Werner FW, Fortino MD: The interosseous membrane of the forearm: Anatomy and function. *J Hand Surg [Am]* 1997;22:981-985.

17. Mehlhoff TL, Noble PC, Bennett JB, Tullos HS: Simple dislocation of the elbow in the adult: Results after closed treatment. *J Bone Joint Surg Am* 1988;70:244-249.

18. Morrey BF (ed): *The Elbow and its Disorders*, ed 2. Philadelphia, PA, WB Saunders, 1993.

19. Sotereanos DG, Hotchkiss RN: Complex traumatic elbow dislocation, in Green DP, Hotchkiss RN, Pederson WC (eds): *Green's Operative Hand Surgery*, ed 5. Philadelphia, PA, Churchill Livingstone, 2005, pp 907-918.

20. Ring D, Jupiter JB, Simpson NS: Monteggia fractures in adults. *J Bone Joint Surg Am* 1998;80:1733-1744.

21. Ring D, Jupiter JB, Sanders RW, Mast J, Simpson NS: Transolecranon fracture-dislocation of the elbow. *J Orthop Trauma* 1997;11:545-550.

22. McKee MD, Pugh DM, Wild LM, Schemitsch EH, King GJ: Standard surgical protocol to treat elbow dislocations with radial head and coronoid fractures: Surgical technique. *J Bone Joint Surg Am* 2005;87(suppl 1):22-32.

23. Josefsson PO, Gentz CF, Johnell O, Wendeberg B: Dislocations of the elbow and intraarticular fractures. *Clin Orthop Relat Res* 1989;246:126-130.

24. Ring D, Jupiter JB, Zilberfarb J: Posterior dislocation of the elbow with fractures of the radial head and coronoid. *J Bone Joint Surg Am* 2002;84:547-551.

25. O'Driscoll SW: Classification and evaluation of recurrent instability of the elbow. *Clin Orthop Relat Res* 2000;370:34-43.

26. O'Driscoll SW, Jupiter JB, King GJ, Hotchkiss RN, Morrey BF: The unstable elbow. *Instr Course Lect* 2001;50:89-102.

27. Ball CM, Galatz LM, Yamaguchi K: Elbow instability: Treatment strategies and emerging concepts. *Instr Course Lect* 2002;51:53-61.

28. Smith GR, Hotchkiss RN: Radial head and neck fractures: Anatomic guidelines for proper placement of internal fixation. *J Shoulder Elbow Surg* 1996;5:113-117.

29. King GJ: Management of comminuted radial head fractures with replacement arthroplasty. *Hand Clin* 2004;20:429-441.

30. Morrey BF: Complex instability of the elbow. *Instr Course Lect* 1998;47:157-164.

31. Beingessner DM, Dunning CE, Gordon KD, Johnson JA, King GJ: The effect of radial head excision and arthroplasty on elbow kinematics and stability. *J Bone Joint Surg Am* 2004;86:1730-1739.

32. Fox RJ, Varitimidis SE, Plakseychuk A, Vardakas DG, Tomaino MM, Sotereanos DG: The Compass Elbow Hinge: Indications and initial results. *J Hand Surg [Br]* 2000;25:568-572.

33. Jupiter JB, Ring D: Treatment of unreduced elbow dislocations with hinged external fixation. *J Bone Joint Surg Am* 2002;84:1630-1635.

34. Ring D, Hannouche D, Jupiter JB: Surgical treatment of persistent dislocation or subluxation of the ulnohumeral joint after fracture-dislocation of the elbow. *J Hand Surg [Am]* 2004;29:470-480.

35. Pugh DM, Wild LM, Schemitsch EH, King GJ, McKee MD: Standard surgical protocol to treat elbow dislocations with radial head and coronoid fractures. *J Bone Joint Surg Am* 2004;86:1122-1130.

36. McAuliffe JA, Wolfson AH: Early excision of heterotopic ossification about the elbow followed by radiation therapy. *J Bone Joint Surg Am* 1997;79:749-755.

37. Viola RW, Hanel DP: Early "simple" release of posttraumatic elbow contracture associated with heterotopic ossification. *J Hand Surg [Am]* 1999;24:370-380.

38. Moritomo H, Tada K, Yoshida T: Early, wide excision of heterotopic ossification in the medial elbow. *J Shoulder Elbow Surg* 2001;10:164-168.

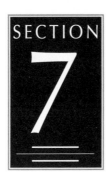

SECTION 7

Sports Medicine

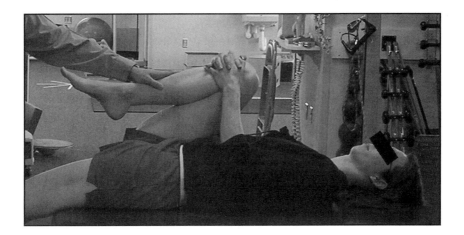

Core Strengthening

Elizabeth A. Arendt, MD

Abstract

Several recent studies have evaluated interventional techniques designed to reduce the risk of serious knee injuries, particularly noncontact anterior cruciate ligament injuries in female athletes. Maintenance of rotational control of the limb underneath the pelvis, especially in response to cutting and jumping activities, is a common goal in many training programs. Rotational control of the limb underneath the pelvis is mediated by a complex set of factors including the strength of the trunk muscles and the relationship between the core muscles. It is important to examine the interrelationship between lower extremity function and core stability.

Instr Course Lect 2007;56:379-384.

The effect of core stability on the spinal column has often been discussed in orthopaedic literature. Core stability has been defined as the ability of the lumbopelvic hip complex to prevent buckling of the vertebral column and return it to a condition of equilibrium following perturbation.[1] Several recent studies have evaluated core stability as a component in training programs aimed at preventing injuries to female athletes.[2] A definition that is more relevant to athletic activities would describe core stability as a base or platform of musculoskeletal strength that results in control of the trunk (axial skeleton) and allows optimal performance of limb activity.

Core Stability

Core stability, as it relates to the lower extremity, involves the lumbar vertebral column, the pelvis, and the lower extremity appendages (especially the hip articulation that connects the femur to the pelvis). This view of core stability designates a stable platform or core (proximal control) as the primary factor for controlling limb rotation. Adequate strength and neuromuscular feedback are also needed from other elements in the limb to maintain a stable limb position. Although rotational limb control in landing and cutting activities have elements of distal feedback (foot and ankle kinematics that relate to ultimate position), this distal control plays a secondary role in limb stability. In this view of core stability, rotational limb control is achieved through interplay of a complex set of factors including balance, rotation, and body awareness.

In addition to local control of the limb, the contribution of central control is acknowledged, but less well understood. A review of current neuromuscular programs indicates that feedback appears to be a necessary element of a successful program.[3] The type of feedback and its timing and duration are not yet determined. Does central control change the timing and sequence of muscle firing? Does training improve anticipatory reactions at the central level, improving local control? Is the improvement in limb control a consequence of increased strength at a local level, adjustments in the timing and firing of muscles regulated more centrally, or both? Despite the unanswered questions, mounting evidence supports the concept that core stability plays a key role in limb function and is therefore an important factor in injury prevention.

Core Stability and Lower Extremity Function

The relationship between core stability and lower extremity function was presented by Bouisset[4] when he proposed that "postural support" must occur before the initiation of voluntary extremity movements. Other studies acknowledge the roles of both the lumbar spine and hip/gluteal musculatures in extremity function.[5,6]

Many studies have correlated the relationship between core strength and athletic performance. Hewett and associates[7] studied musculoskeletal knee performance by evaluating jumping and landing kinematics in 11 female high school volleyball players. The athletes then participated in a neuromuscular program that included plyometrics and strength training. Pretesting and posttesting results showed an improvement in neuromuscular control as evidenced by a reduction in knee adduction and abduction moments during landing from a jump, and an increase in the height of the vertical jump.

Evidence supporting a relationship between core muscle strength and lower extremity musculoskeletal injury is more difficult to establish. However, a small but emerging body of data shows a correlation between core weakness and lower extremity injuries. The absence of low back extensor endurance is associated with low back pain in adults in occupations requiring physical labor.[8,9] A study of injuries in rugby players acknowledged that abdominal muscle fatigue is a contributing factor in hamstring injuries.[10] A review of patients with previous severe ankle sprains showed a delay in the onset of firing patterns in their gluteal muscles.[11] In another study, young female patients with patellofemoral pain exhibited weakness in hip abduction and external rotation.[12]

Few evidence-based studies show a correlation between core weakness and acute lower extremity injury; however, this finding can be inferred from the positive results of current interventional studies in decreasing the rate of noncontact anterior cruciate ligament injuries.[1] In these interventional studies, athletes were trained using programs that emphasized core principles, awareness or body sense in athletic movements, and plyometric strengthening. To date, no population-based interventional studies have been done that include pretraining and posttraining data that identify the elements of movement and function that were changed by the training regimens. The outcome variable in these studies was injury. The explanation of why the training programs are beneficial was inferred from observing the movement patterns of athletes rather than from an analysis of quantifiable data. Despite the fact that the evidence supporting the link between core stability and orthopaedic injury is largely theoretic, promoting the acquisition and maintenance of core stability seems justifiable for a variety of orthopaedic injuries, especially noncontact anterior cruciate ligament injuries.

Core Stability and Clinical Tests

Tests to assess an individual's core stability can be discussed, with the acknowledgment that no single test can completely measure this complex skill. In a research setting, core stability is usually measured using sophisticated electromyographic techniques, which evaluate the timing patterns of muscle activation during the performance of various tasks. This data also can be used to model movement patterns.

A patient with core weakness has clinical characteristics that include weak abdominal muscles (these muscles help to control the position of the pelvis), weak gluteal muscles (these muscles help to control femoral rotation), and weak hamstrings (these muscles help to control pelvic position primarily through its proximal insertions).

In a clinical setting, several tests are currently used by physical therapists and athletic trainers. These tests are easy to administer, provide feedback to the patient and the clinician, and can be followed up over time. Timed tests of isometric muscle function have been a mainstay of testing for patients with conditions of the lower back. Using these tests, McGill and associates[13] compiled a table of normative scores for healthy young adults.

In preseason screening and conditioning evaluations, many athletes, particularly female athletes, have shown poor control of limb rotation in functional activities such as partial squatting and landing techniques. They also have poor weightlifting techniques that are believed to result from two sources. Athletes may have trained muscles (for example, strength in individual muscle groups) but do not have trained movements, which must be learned. In addition, athletes often lack core or trunk stability and/or strength.

In 1995, the University of Minnesota began a screening program to assess core strength. Although the program has evolved, certain elements are still used in the preliminary phase of assessing core strength in athletes and patients. These screening techniques, which can be readily used in the clinic or training room setting, include the ability to perform a pelvic bridge using a single leg (Figure 1); the ability to hold a plank or arrow position (Figure 2); the ability to hold a supine hollow body position (reverse arrow position) (Figure 3); the ability to hold a side bridge (Figure 4); and the ability to perform a partial squat without having a functional valgus knee position (Figure 5). The first four tests can be performed using time as a variable. Alternatively, the athlete

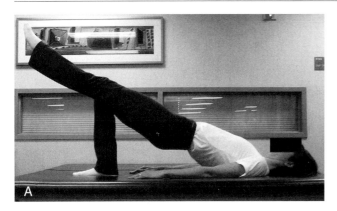
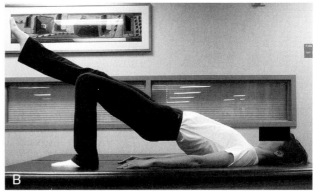

Figure 1   An athlete performing a double-leg pelvic bridge with right leg (**A**) and left leg (**B**).

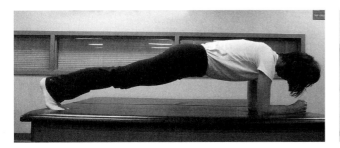
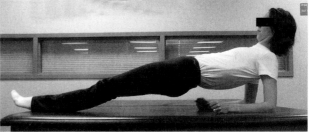

Figure 2   An athlete demonstrates the plank or arrow position.

Figure 3   An athlete demonstrates the supine hollow body position (reverse arrow).

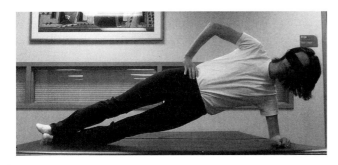
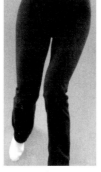

Figure 4   An athlete demonstrates a side bridge.

Figure 5   An athlete demonstrating a single-leg partial squat with left knee collapsing into a valgus position during dynamic testing.

can be asked hold these positions for a set time, usually 30 seconds. The results are recorded in a binary fashion: yes, can perform the exercise; or no, cannot perform the exercise for the set time.

The interventional strategies that are used to train patients with core weakness are beyond the scope of

this chapter; however, a brief outline of approaches includes the following elements. If an athlete cannot perform the core tests, movement training begins with identifying individual muscle weakness and strengthening isolated muscle groups. Conditioning is then expanded to encompass tasks that in-

volve other muscles that are integrated with the weaker muscle group. Movement training usually begins with tasks using single plane directions and advances to tasks that use multiplane directions. The use of core muscles is integrated into performing the tasks of daily living, with advancement to use in sport-

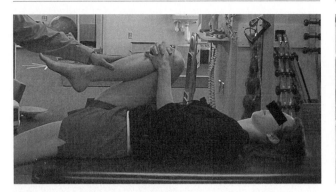

Figure 6   An athlete demonstrates a positive Thomas test on physical examination.

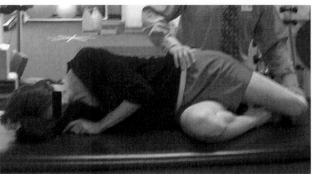

Figure 7   An athlete demonstrates a positive Ober test on physical examination.

specific activities. Patients are encouraged to adopt limb positions that are favorable for knee kinematics (balanced body with knee over toe, flexion of knee and hip in landing) by first training using controlled motions such as stepping down and partial squats and then advancing to faster and more integrated movements such as jump landing and cutting.

Pelvic position, a secondary issue related to core stability and pelvifemoral weakness, is often overlooked during the patient's physical examination. Malalignment includes the familiar clinical presentations of femoral anteversion, genu valgum, squinting patella, tibial vara, external tibial torsion, and foot pronation. The position of the pelvis also can be malaligned and relates specifically to anterior pelvic tilt. Anterior pelvic tilt creates relative femoral internal rotation; this is a coupled motion of lower extremity kinematics.[14] This coupled motion can result in aggravation or predisposition to use the functional valgus knee position in squatting or loading motions. Anterior tilt can occur on both sides of the pelvis, or the pelvis may be hemirotated with just one side tilted anteriorly.

Pelvifemoral malposition is most readily diagnosed by physical examination. The patient has an anteriorly tilted pelvis, which is flexible. When resting supine, the position of the femur is internally rotated. This relationship of the femur to the pelvis is relative, creates relative capsular tightness, and results in a positive Thomas test[15] (Figure 6). This condition is not associated with fixed hip flexor tightness because the pelvis can be reduced and the hip flexion contracture can be eliminated. The patient with an anterior pelvic tilt, while resting in the supine position, will display hamstring tightness on physical examination (90° hip flexion, knee extension) as measured by the popliteal angle. This "tightness" is eliminated with reduction of the pelvic tilt.

Femoral internal rotation malpositions the iliotibial band to the position of a hip flexor and a hip abductor, which results in a positive Ober test on physical examination[15] (Figure 7). The positive Ober test is not absolute tightness of the iliotibial band because the pelvis can be repositioned; retesting eliminates the positive Ober test.

The training goal for a patient with pelvifemoral malpositioning is to reposition the pelvis from an anterior tilt to a neutral position. The patient can learn the physical therapy technique needed to achieve this goal. This technique involves recruitment of proximal hamstrings and gluteal and abdominal muscles to maintain appropriate pelvic and body positioning.[14,16]

At the University of Minnesota, the performances on core strength tests of 10 athletes with overuse-type injuries (including low back pain, patellofemoral pain, and iliotibial band tendinitis) were evaluated (Table 1). Eight of the 10 athletes showed weakness on two or more core strength tests; most showed weakness on four or more tests. At the same university, 20 uninjured athletes (from different sports) were evaluated using the same core strength tests (Table 2). The heptathletes (those participating in the heptathlon) had positive results on all the core strength tests and better results in core strength tests than the athletes participating in a single sport.

Summary

Pelvifemoral and core strength is a cornerstone of trunk and limb stability. Proper pelvic stability and position allows for optimal femoral po-

Table 1
University of Minnesota Review of Injury Types and Core Strength Results for 10 Athletes With Overuse Injuries

Athlete's Sport	Injury	Negative Results (Indicating Weakness) on Six Core Strength Tests*
Gymnastics	LBP	4 of 6
Ice hockey	LBP	4 of 6
Ice hockey	PF	0 of 6
Cross-country running	ITB	4 of 6
Cross country running	LBP	6 of 6
Basketball	PF	4 of 6
Diver	PF	4 of 6
Swimmer	PF	2 of 6
Thrower	LBP/PF	2 of 6
Thrower	PF	4 of 6

LBP = low back pain; PF = patellofemoral pain; ITB = iliotibial band tendinitis
*6/6 = normal strength in all tests

Table 2
University of Minnesota Core Strength Test Results for 20 Athletes Without Overuse Conditions

Athlete's Sport	Positive Results (Indicating Successful Performance) on Six Core Strength Tests
Heptathlon	6 of 6
Heptathlon	6 of 6
Sprinting	6 of 6
Sprinting	3 of 6
Sprinting	3 of 6
Cross-country running	3 of 6
Cross-country running	3 of 6
Cross-country running	1 of 6
Cross-country running	1 of 6
Cross-country running	0 of 6
Volleyball	5 of 6
Volleyball	5 of 6
Volleyball	4 of 6
Volleyball	4 of 6
Volleyball	4 of 6
Volleyball	4 of 6
Volleyball	3 of 6
Volleyball	3 of 6
Volleyball	3 of 6
Volleyball	3 of 6

sition and improved lower limb muscle mechanics. Data suggest that core stability is related to enhanced performance and that core weakness is related to an increased risk of lower limb injury.

References

1. Pope MH, Panjabi M: Biomechanical definitions of spinal instability. *Spine* 1985;10:255-256.

2. Hewett TE, Myer GD, Ford KR: Reducing knee and anterior cruciate ligament injuries among female athletes: A systematic review of neuromuscular training interventions. *J Knee Surg* 2005;18:82-88.

3. Griffin LY, Albohm MJ, Arendt EA, et al: Understanding and preventing noncontact anterior cruciate ligament injuries: A review of the Hunt Valley II meeting, January 2005. *Am J Sports Med* 2006;34:1512-1532.

4. Bouisset S: Relationship between postural support and intentional movement: Biomechanical approach. *Arch Int Physiol Biochim Biophys* 1991;99:A77-A92.

5. Hodges PW, Richardson CA: Contraction of abdominal muscles associated with movements of the lower limb. *Phys Ther* 1997;77:132-144.

6. Bobbert MF, van Zandwijk JP: Dynamics of force and muscle stimulation in human vertical jumping. *Med Sci Sports Exerc* 1999;31:303-310.

7. Hewett TE, Stroupe AL, Nance TA, Noyes FR: Plyometric training in female athletes: Decreased impact forces and increased hamstring torques. *Am J Sports Med* 1996;24:765-773.

8. Biering-Sorensen F: Physical measurements as risk indicators for low-back trouble over a one-year period. *Spine* 1984;9:106-119.

9. Luoto S, Heliovaara M, Hurri H, Alaranta H: Static back endurance and the risk of low-back pain. *Clin Biomech (Bristol, Avon)* 1995;10:323-324.

10. Devlin L: Recurrent posterior thigh symptoms detrimental to performance in rugby union: Predisposing factors. *Sports Med* 2000;29:273-287.

11. Bullock-Saxton JE, Janda V, Bullock M: The influence of ankle sprain injury on muscle activation during hip extension. *Int J Sports Med* 1994;15:330-334.

12. Ireland ML, Willson JD, Ballantyne BT, David IM: Hip strength in females with and without patellofemoral pain. *J Orthop Sports Phys Ther* 2003;33:671-676.

13. McGill SM, Childs A, Liebenson C: Endurance times for low back stabilization exercises: Clinical targets for testing and training from a normal database. *Arch Phys Med Rehabil* 1999;80:941-944.

14. Willson JD, Dougherty CP, Ireland ML, Davis IM: Core stability and its relationship to lower extremity function and injury. *J Am Acad Orthop Surg* 2005;13:316-325.

15. Physical examination of the hip and pelvis, in Hoppenfeld S (ed): *Physical Examination of the Spine and Extremities.* New York, NY, Appleton-Century-Crofts, Prentice Hall, 1976, pp 143-169.

16. McGill S (ed): *Low Back Disorders: Evidence-Based Prevention and Rehabilitation*. Champaign, IL, Human Kinetics, 2002.

Prevention of Catastrophic Injuries in Sports

Barry P. Boden, MD

Abstract

Catastrophic sports injuries are rare but severely debilitating events. Catastrophic injuries are divided into two etiologic categories: direct and indirect. Direct injuries are those resulting directly from participation in a sport, such as a collision in football. Football is associated with the greatest number of direct catastrophic injuries for all major team sports in the United States, whereas ice hockey, pole vaulting, gymnastics, and football have the highest incidence of direct catastrophic injuries per 100,000 male participants. Cheerleading is associated with the highest number of direct catastrophic injuries for all sports in which females participate. Indirect or nontraumatic injuries are caused by systemic failure resulting from exertion while participating in a sport and include cardiovascular conditions, heat illness, exertional hyponatremia, and dehydration. Indirect deaths in athletes are predominantly caused by cardiovascular conditions such as hypertrophic cardiomyopathy and coronary artery disease.

Instr Course Lect 2007;56:385-393.

Information on catastrophic injuries in athletes is collected by the National Center for Catastrophic Sports Injury Research (NCCSIR), the US Consumer Product Safety Commission (CPSC), and other organizations (Table 1). For all sports followed by the NCCSIR, the total incidence of direct and indirect catastrophic injuries[1] is 1 per 100,000 high school athletes and 4 per 100,000 college athletes.[2] The National Collegiate Athletic Association (NCAA) and the National Federation of State High School Associations (NFSH) review injury epidemiology annually and publish a rules book for each sport with the intent of promoting safe play.

Direct Injuries
Football
Head Injury

Football is associated with the highest number of severe head and neck injuries per year for all high school and college sports.[2] Head injuries are the most common direct cause of death among football players, accounting for 497 of 714 football fatalities from 1945 through 1999.[3] Most head-related fatalities are associated with subdural hematomas (86%) and occur during game situations.[3] Unlike most direct catastrophic injuries, which have a higher incidence in college athletes, the incidence of subdural hematomas is three times more common in high school athletes.[4] Most subdural hematomas occur as a result of head trauma, either from tackling or being tackled. In the author's experience, more than 50% of athletes who sustained a subdural hematoma were found to have suffered a minor head injury earlier in the season. There has been a dramatic decrease in brain injury–related fatalities since the late 1960s. A major factor in the decline of head injuries is improvement in helmet design and the establishment of safety standards by the National Operating Committee on Standards for Athletic Equipment. Improved medical care and technology are also likely responsible for the decline in fatalities. New data indicate that athletes need to be monitored closely for concussions and should never return to play until full neurologic recovery has been achieved.[4]

Ice Hockey

The incidence of catastrophic injuries in ice hockey is high compared with other sports.[2] Most catastrophic injuries are reported to occur to the cervical spine as a result of checking from behind and being hurled horizontally into the boards[5] (Figure 1). Contact with the boards typically occurs to the crown of the player's head, subjecting the neck to

Table 1
Sources of Information on Sport Safety

Acronym	Organization	Web Site
AACCA	American Association of Cheerleading Coaches and Advisors	http://www.aacca.org
CPSC	Consumer Product Safety Commission	http://www.cpsc.gov
NCAA	The National Collegiate Athletic Association	http://www.ncaa.org
NCCSIR	National Catastrophic Center for Sports Injury Research	http://www.unc.edu/dept/nccsi/
NCIPC	National Center of Injury Prevention and Control at the US Centers for Disease Control and Prevention	http://www.cdc.gov/ncipc
NFHS	National Federation of State High School Associations	http://www.nfhs.org
NOCSAE	National Operating Committee on Standards for Athletic Equipment	http://www.nocsae.org
PVSCB	Pole Vault Safety Certification Board	http://www.skyjumpers.com.
USAB	USA Baseball	www.usabaseball.com

(Reproduced from Boden BP: Direct catastrophic injury in sports. *J Am Acad Orthop Surg* 2005;13:445-454.)

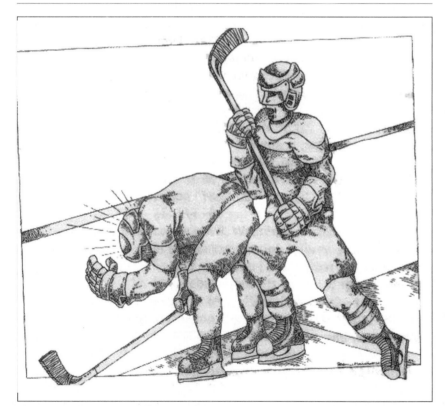

Figure 1   Illustration of body checking from behind in ice hockey, which can lead to axial injury to the cervical spine and quadriplegia. (Reproduced with permission from Molsa JJ, Tegner Y, Alaranta H, et al: Spinal cord injuries in ice hockey in Finland and Sweden from 1980 to 1996. *Int J Sports Med* 1999;20:64-67.)

an axial load.[5] Preventive strategies include the "heads-up, don't duck" program, which teaches ice hockey players to avoid contact with the top of the head when taking a check, giving a check, or sliding on the ice. The Safety Toward Other Players Program involves placing a patch on the back of the jersey of amateur athletes as a visual reminder not to hit an opponent from behind.

Head and facial injuries are also common in ice hockey, resulting from collisions, fighting, or being hit by the puck or stick. The frequency and severity of head and neck injuries may be reduced by enforcing current rules against pushing or checking from behind, padding the boards, and encouraging the use of helmets and face masks. In a prospective analysis of facial protection in elite amateur ice hockey players, it was documented that players wearing no protection were injured twice as often as players wearing partial protection and nearly seven times more often than those wearing full protection.[6]

Pole Vaulting

Pole vaulting is a technically demanding sport in which athletes often land from heights ranging from 15 to 20 feet. Pole vaulting has one of the highest rates of direct catastrophic injuries per 100,000 participants for all sports monitored by the NCCSIR.[7] Most catastrophic injuries caused by pole vaulting are head injuries in high school male athletes.[7] The overall incidence of catastrophic injuries from pole vaulting is 2.0 per year, whereas the incidence of fatalities is 1.0 per year.[7] Although the number of fatalities in pole vaulting seems small, it is a significant concern because there are only approximately 25,000 to 50,000 high school athletes participating in pole vaulting each year.

Because most catastrophic injuries from pole vaulting occur as a result of athletes missing the landing pad, both the NCAA and NFHS have increased the minimum pole vaulting landing pad area from 16 feet × 12 feet to 19 feet 8 inches × 16 feet 5 inches as of January 2003 (Figure 2). These organizations also proposed enforcing a rule that any hard or unyielding surfaces such as concrete or asphalt around the landing pad must be padded or cushioned. A new rule has also been adopted for placing the crossbar farther back over the landing pad to reduce the risk of an athlete landing in the vaulting or planting box. The use of a coaching box (a painted square in the middle of the landing pad) is also being promoted and should help train athletes to instinctively land near the center of the landing pad. The value of using helmets in reducing head injuries in high school pole vaulting is controversial. Without conclusive data as to the protective effect of helmets in pole vaulting, helmet use is optional at the time of this writing.

Cheerleading

Over the past 20 years, cheerleading has evolved from cheering on the sidelines to a competitive sport demanding high levels of skill, athleticism, and complex gymnastics maneuvers. Although cheerleading is associated with a low overall incidence of injuries, it has a high risk of catastrophic injuries. The NCCSIR reports approximately two direct catastrophic injuries in cheerleaders per year or 0.6 per 100,000 cheerleaders.[8] In 2000, the CPSC estimated that a total of 1,258 head injuries and 1,814 neck injuries occurred in cheerleaders of all ages that year.

The cheerleading maneuvers that most commonly result in cata-

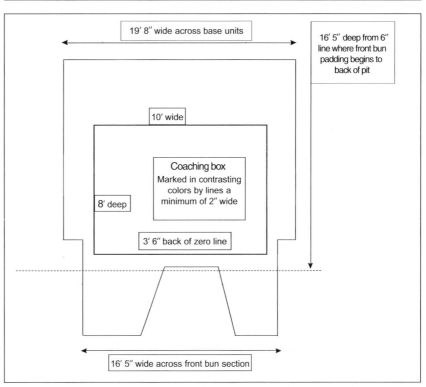

Figure 2 Illustration of the footprint of the high school landing pad for pole vaulters before and after the rule change requiring a larger landing pad area. The illustration also shows the recommended dimension of the coaching box. (Reproduced with permission from Boden BP, Mueller FO: Catastrophic injuries in pole-vaulters. *Sports Med Update* 2003;Jan-Feb:4-7.)

strophic injury are the pyramid (with the cheerleader at the top of the pyramid most frequently injured) and the basket toss.[8] The NFHS and NCAA have attempted to reduce pyramid injuries by limiting the height and complexity of a pyramid and specifying a required number of spotters. Height restrictions on pyramids are limited to two levels in high school and 2.5 body lengths in college. The cheerleaders at the top of the pyramid are required to be supported by one or more individuals (the base) who are in direct weight-bearing contact with the performing surface. Spotters must be present for each person extended above shoulder level. The cheerleader at the top of the pyramid is not allowed to be inverted (head

below horizontal) or to rotate on the dismount.

A basket toss is a maneuver in which a cheerleader is thrown into the air, often between 6 and 20 feet, by either three or four throwers (Figure 3). Safety measures have also been developed for the basket toss, such as limiting the basket toss to four throwers, starting the throw from the ground level (no flips), and having one of the throwers positioned behind the top person (flyer) during the throw. The flyer is trained to maintain a vertical position and not allow the head to drop backward out of alignment with the torso or below a horizontal plane with the body.

Cheerleading coaches must place as much time and attention on the

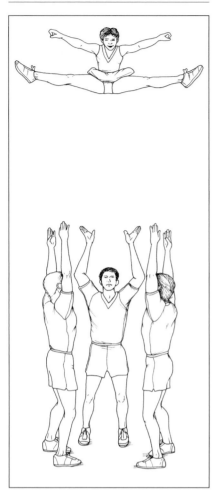

Figure 3 Illustration of a basket toss in cheerleading. (Reproduced with permission from Boden BP, Tacchetti R, Mueller FO: Catastrophic cheerleading injuries. *Am J Sports Med* 2003;31:881-888.)

technique and attentiveness of spotters in practice as with the performance of the maneuvers. Cheerleading coaches are encouraged to complete a safety certification, especially for any teams that perform the pyramid or basket toss maneuvers. Participation in pyramid and basket toss maneuvers should be limited to experienced cheerleaders who have mastered all other skills and should not be performed without qualified spotters or landing mats.

Baseball

Baseball is associated with a low rate of noncatastrophic injuries, but a relatively high incidence of catastrophic injuries. Head injuries constitute most catastrophic injuries in baseball. There are approximately two direct catastrophic injuries reported to the NCCSIR per year or 0.5 injuries per 100,000 participants.[2,9] The most common mechanism of catastrophic injury in baseball is a collision between fielders or between a base runner and a fielder.[9] Proper training is the best way to prevent collisions between fielders. When two infielders are running for a pop-up, the pitcher should determine who catches the ball. In circumstances in which an outfielder and infielder are racing for a ball, the outfielder should determine who catches the ball. These drills should be reinforced in practice sessions so they become instinctual in game situations.

Collisions between base runners and the catcher can result in an axial compression cervical injury when the base runner dives headfirst into a catcher.[9] Baseball rules state that the runner should avoid the fielder who has the right to the base path. Unfortunately, this rule is not always enforced at home plate. Because the speed of headfirst sliding has been shown not to be statistically different from feetfirst sliding, the headfirst slide needs to be reassessed at the high school and college levels.[10] In Little League baseball, headfirst sliding is not allowed at any base.

After collisions, a pitcher hit by a batted ball is the next most common catastrophic injury mechanism in high school and college baseball players. In major and minor league baseball, only wood bats are allowed; however, at the high school and college levels, bats made of aluminum and metal alloys are used almost exclusively. Because of their lighter weights, aluminum bats can be swung faster than wood bats, resulting in a higher baseball exit velocity.[11] In response to the potential risk of injury, the NCAA and the NFHS now require all high school and college baseball bats to be labeled with a permanent certification mark indicating that the baseball exit speed ratio cannot exceed 97 miles per hour as set by the Baum Hitting Machine (Baum Research and Development, Traverse City, MI). New rules also regulate the diameter and weight of the bat as well as the hardness of the baseball. Protective screens (L-screens) for pitchers are recommended at all times during practice sessions. Pitchers also have the option of wearing protective headgear.

Another area of concern in baseball is commotio cordis, arrhythmia often associated with sudden death from low-impact blunt trauma to the chest.[12] The condition occurs most commonly when a batter is struck by a pitched baseball, but it has also been reported in hockey, softball, lacrosse, and other sports.[2] The proposed mechanism of injury is impact just before the peak of the T wave on an echocardiogram, which induces ventricular fibrillation. Cardiac arrest may occur immediately or on a delayed basis. Although the rate of rescue from commotio cordis was initially documented to be extremely low, more recent reports indicate that survival is possible with immediate resuscitative measures such as a precordial thump or with the use of automatic external defibrillators.[13,14] The pediatric population may be more susceptible to commotio cordis because of increased compliance of the immature rib cage, less chest musculature, and slower protective reflexes.

Unfortunately, neither chest protectors nor softer-core baseballs have been shown to eliminate the risk of commotio cordis and may exacerbate the force to the chest.[15,16] Preventive strategies are currently limited to teaching youth baseball players to turn their chest away from a wild pitch, a batted baseball, or a thrown baseball. Analysis of the etiology of commotio cordis and the effectiveness of resuscitative measures, especially with automatic external defibrillators, require further study.

Soccer

Fatalities in soccer are usually associated with either movable goalposts falling on a victim or player impact with the goalpost.[17] The CPSC identified 21 deaths over a 16-year period associated with movable goalposts. Goalpost injuries in soccer can be prevented by never allowing children to climb on the net or goalpost framework (Figure 4). Soccer goalposts should be secured at all times. During the off-season, goalposts should be placed in a safe storage area or disassembled. Goalposts should be moved only by trained personnel and used only on flat fields. The use of padded goalposts may also reduce the incidence of impact injuries with the goalposts.[17]

Swimming

Most catastrophic swimming injuries are caused by diving into the shallow end of a pool.[2] The NFHS and NCAA have implemented rules to prevent injuries during the racing dive. At the high school level, swimmers must start the race in the water if the water depth at the starting end is less than 3.5 feet. If the water depth is 3.5 feet to less than 4 feet at the starting end, the swimmer may start in the water or from the deck. If the water depth at the starting end is

4 feet or more, the swimmer may start from a platform up to 30 inches above the water surface. The NCAA requires a minimum water depth of 4 feet at the starting end of the pool. During practice sessions in which platforms may not be available, swimmers are advised to only dive into the deep end of the pool or to jump into the water feet first.

Indirect Injuries

Indirect or nontraumatic catastrophic injuries and deaths in athletes have been identified to be predominantly caused by cardiovascular conditions such as hypertrophic cardiomyopathy, coronary artery anomalies, arrhythmogenic right ventricular dysplasia, myocarditis, and dysrhythmias.[18] Noncardiac conditions that cause catastrophic indirect injuries are heat illness, dehydration, exercise-associated hyponatremia, shallow water blackout, rhabdomyolysis, status asthmaticus, and electrocution caused by lightning.

Cardiac Conditions

The most common etiology of sudden cardiac death in athletes younger than 35 years is hypertrophic cardiomyopathy and coronary artery disease for those older than 35 years.[18] Athletes with hypertrophic cardiomyopathy are typically asymptomatic before sudden cardiac death, but they may have prodromal symptoms such as chest pain or syncope with or without exercise. Half of all athletes who experience hypertrophic cardiomyopathy have specific genetic mutations. A systolic murmur may be appreciated on auscultation and usually increases in the standing position or with a Valsalva maneuver. Athletes with murmurs that are grade III or greater in intensity, continuous, holosystolic, dia-

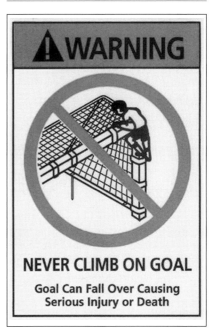

Figure 4 Warning sticker developed by the US Consumer Product Safety Commission to prevent children from climbing on goalposts. (Reproduced with permission from the US Consumer Product Safety Commission.)

stolic, or unclear should be referred to a cardiologist for an echocardiogram. The preparticipation physical examination is the recommended method for detecting cardiac conditions that may be life-threatening. However, there is controversy whether widescale screening is necessary because there is no cost-effective test that is 100% sensitive and specific. A test with 99% specificity will lead to numerous false-positive results, often forcing healthy individuals to limit sports activities. In general, any athlete with a personal history of chest pain, exertional syncope, exercise intolerance, palpitations, or a family history of sudden death identified during the preparticipation physical examination should be referred for further evaluation. A summary of the contraindications to vigorous exercise are listed in Table 2.

Table 2
Guidelines on Restriction of Exercise for Cardiovascular Disease: Contradictions to Vigorous Exercise

Hypertrophic cardiomyopathy

Idiopathic concentric left ventricular hypertrophy

Marfan syndrome

Coronary heart disease

Uncontrolled ventricular arrhythmias

Severe valvular heart disease (especially aortic stenosis and pulmonic stenosis)

Coarctation of the aorta

Acute myocarditis

Dilated cardiomyopathy

Congestive heart failure

Congenital anomalies of the coronary arteries

Cyanotic congenital heart disease

Pulmonary hypertension

Right ventricular cardiomyopathy

Ebstein's anomaly of the tricuspid valve

Idiopathic long Q-T syndrome

Require close monitoring and possible restriction

Uncontrolled hypertension

Uncontrolled atrial arrhythmias

Hemodynamic significant valvular heart disease (aortic insufficiency, mitral stenosis, and mitral regurgitation)

(Reproduced from Boden BP: Direct catastrophic injury in sports. *J Am Acad Orthop Surg* 2005;13:445-454.)

Heat Illness

Heat illness or dehydration is a common cause of death in athletes.[2] Risk factors for heat illness include obesity, fever, recent respiratory or gastrointestinal viral illness, sickle cell trait, use of stimulants, illicit drug use, alcohol use, sleep deprivation, sunburn, unfit athletes, and use of supplements such as ephedrine.[19] Heat illness usually occurs during unseasonably hot conditions at times of extreme exertion. A typical scenario in which heat illness occurs is an obese football lineman wearing a football uniform and playing two practices a day during late summer tryouts in the southeastern United States.

There are various forms of heat illness based on the core body temperature.[19] Heat syncope is associated with an abrupt loss of consciousness in a heat-exposed athlete whose core temperature is normal or mildly elevated. The condition often occurs toward the completion of exercise because of reduced cardiac return and postural hypotension. Heat exhaustion occurs at core temperatures between 100.4°F and 104.0°F and is defined as the inability to continue to exercise in the heat because the cardiovascular system fails to respond to the workload. Symptoms of heat exhaustion can include muscle cramping, mild confusion, headache, dizziness, chills, nausea, and often collapse. Heatstroke is the most dangerous type of heat illness and carries a significant risk of mortality if treatment is delayed. Heatstroke begins at temperatures in excess of 104°F and is associated with central nervous system dysfunction and can manifest as mental status changes. The athlete may or may not be sweating. The condition can result in a variety of life-threatening problems such as rhabdomyolysis, renal failure, disseminated intravascular coagulopathy, liver failure, and brain injury.

Diagnosis of heat illness is based on the history, physical examination, core body temperature, and differentials, including exercise-associated hyponatremia and cardiac conditions. Rectal temperature is the optimal method for detecting core body temperature. Treatment involves rapid cooling techniques such as moving to a cooler environment, removing clothing, tepid water spray, fans, and the application of ice to the neck, groin, and axillae. Hydration should include both oral intake and intravenous fluids. Rehydration with sports drinks containing electrolytes is preferred over water. Athletes with core temperatures greater than 104°F should be considered for cold water immersion. Cooling efforts should be discontinued when the rectal temperature reaches 101°F to 102°F to prevent overcorrection with resultant hypothermia. Emergency medical services should be contacted for athletes with heat exhaustion and heatstroke.

Preventive strategies for heat-related illness include educating athletes, parents, and coaches about the potential hazards of high intensity exercise in hot, humid climates as well as the importance of acclimatization (the body's physiologic adaptation to heat stress) and proper hydration. Acclimatization typically takes 7 to 10 days.[20] The NCAA mandates a 5-day acclimatization period during which players may participate in no more than one practice session at the beginning of the season for no longer than 3 hours.[21] The equipment worn by players is also restricted with helmet only for the first and second days, helmet and shoulder pads only for the third and fourth days, and full equipment on the fifth day. After the fifth day, multiple sessions with a maximum of 5 hours practice per day are allowed on an alternating day basis with single sessions.

Maintaining adequate hydration is also of paramount importance. Hydration should begin before the exercise period. For events longer than 1 hour, the replacement fluid should contain electrolytes, which are standard components of commercial sports drinks. The incidence of heat illness can also be significantly reduced by monitoring daily weights, medication use, and status of recent illnesses, as well as identifying at-risk athletes. Prompt, effective treatment can significantly lower the mortality rate of heat stroke.

Dehydration-related deaths and medical complications have been a problem in wrestlers as a result of unhealthy weight-reduction methods.[22] Great strides have been made in reducing the incidence of these injuries through rules restricting rapid weight loss. A minimum body fat of 7% for high school and 5% for college male wrestlers has been established by the NFHS and the NCAA to reduce weight-loss injuries. The NFHS also instituted a rule that competitors cannot lose more than 1.5% of body weight per week. Both groups have banned the use of laxatives, diuretics, and other rapid weight-loss techniques such as exercising in rubber suits. They have also discouraged excessive weight-reduction measures by mandating that weigh-ins occur within 1

or 2 hours of meets and tournaments.

Exercise-Associated Hyponatremia

Exercise-associated hyponatremia is caused by the inappropriate, excessive intake of water before, during, and after endurance events, often in combination with the inappropriate secretion of vasopressin (an antidiuretic hormone).[23-25] As distance athletes have become more educated about preventing dehydration, many athletes overhydrate, which can be more dangerous than underhydration. Marathon runners often drink several liters of water before running, a small cup of water every mile, and continue drinking after the race. Replacing sweat with excessive water can lead to dilution of sodium or hyponatremia. Risk factors for exercise-associated hyponatremia are low body weight, female sex, slow performance, high availability of fluids, and hotter than anticipated conditions.[23] Early signs of exercise-associated hyponatremia typically develop when sodium levels fall below 130 mmol/L and include nausea, vomiting, headache, and dizziness, symptoms that are similar to those for and often mistaken for dehydration.[23] When the sodium level drops below 120 mmol/L, cerebral edema develops, often causing mental status changes, seizures, coma, and even death.

Exercise-associated hyponatremia is distinguished from heat illness by a normal core body temperature. The definitive diagnosis of exercise-associated hyponatremia is made by measurement of serum sodium. Because many long-distance events do not have machines available to measure sodium, the diagnosis is often delayed until the athlete reaches the hospital. Treatment of

exercise-associated hyponatremia begins with intravenous access, avoiding the administration of isotonic or hypotonic fluids that may worsen the condition. Oxygen should be administered, and patients should be emergently transferred to a hospital. Patients with cerebral edema should be treated with 100 mL of 3% sodium over 10 minutes before transfer to an emergency department.[23] Emergency department treatment should entail administration of hypertonic solutions of sodium or mannitol until the patient regains consciousness. Consultation with a nephrologist and/or endocrinologist is recommended.

The best treatment of exercise-associated hyponatremia is prevention. Coaches, trainers, athletes, and parents need to be educated on the dangers of drinking large amounts of regular water during endurance events. The primary means of preventing exercise-associated hyponatremia is to drink fluid only when thirsty instead of automatically reaching for water at every water station. Although sports drinks are recommended over water, the sodium concentration of sports drinks is far lower than that of blood and will not prevent exercise-associated hyponatremia in athletes who overconsume fluids.[23] There is no available evidence to support the suggestion that consuming extra sodium prevents the development of exercise-associated hyponatremia.[23] Many marathon events are also reducing the number of water stations and being less aggressive about promoting water intake. Runners can test their hydration needs during training by weighing themselves before and after a distance run. If the athlete has gained weight, less fluid should be ingested; however, if more than 3% of body weight has

Table 3
Summary of Safety Measures for Sports

Direct Injuries

Football
    Never return to play with any neurologic symptoms following a head injury
    Helmet improvements (NOCSAE standards)
    Banning spear tackling
    Assess spinal stenosis before return to play after cervical cord neurapraxia episode

Pole Vaulting
    Larger landing pad
    Soft surrounding surfaces adjacent to landing pad
    Moving crossbar closer to landing pad

Cheerleading
    Limit height and complexity of pyramids
    Maintain vertical position for flyer
    Improving the skills of spotters

Baseball
    Proper training to prevent collisions
    Avoiding head-first sliding
    Protecting pitchers (L-screens, bat and ball regulations)
    External defibrillators for commotio cordis

Soccer
    Goalpost safety (anchor properly, no climbing)
    Proper heading technique
    Smaller ball at youth level

Ice Hockey
    Avoid checking from behind
    Helmet and face masks

Swimming
    Adhere to rules on racing dive

Indirect Injuries

Cardiac
    Preparticipation physical

Heat Illness
    Acclimatization
    Proper hydration
    Identifying at-risk athletes

Exercise-Associated Hyponatremia
    Avoid overhydration prior to race
    Weighing athlete before and after exercise

Shallow Water Blackout
    Avoid hyperventilation
    Break surface of water to breathe before 15 meters

been lost, then the athlete requires more hydration. On-site sodium analysis screening should also be available to determine when treatment is necessary.

Shallow Water Blackout

Hyperventilating just before swimming is a technique that is often used by elite swimmers during practice sessions to enhance performance.[26] Hyperventilating lowers the carbon dioxide level in the bloodstream, which is the body's primary signal to breathe. This fools the brain into thinking it does not need to breathe, even when its oxygen stores are dangerously low. Early symptoms include muscle cramps, tingling, dizziness, and eventually loss of consciousness and drowning. The NFHS mandates that swimmers break the surface of water to breathe at or before 15 meters to prevent shallow water blackout.

Summary

It has been clearly documented that physical activity has many health-related benefits. Nonetheless, there is a low risk of catastrophic injuries in certain organized sports, especially football, pole vaulting, ice hockey, and cheerleading. The cost of catastrophic injures can be tremendous to the injured athlete and to society. In addition to the decreased quality of life for the athlete, the lifetime cost to treat a quadriplegic individual can easily surpass $2 million.[27] It has been estimated that the annual aggregate cost of treatment for sport-related spinal cord injuries in the United States in 1995 was approximately $700 million.[27] Prevention is the most effective means of reducing the incidence and costs associated with catastrophic head and neck sports injuries (Table 3). Continued research of the epidemiology and mechanisms of catastrophic injuries is critical to prevent these injuries.

References

1. Mueller FO: Introduction, in Mueller FO, Cantu RC, VanCamp SP (eds): *Catastrophic Injuries in High School and College Sports.* Champaign, IL, HK Sport Science Monograph Series, 1996, pp 1-4.

2. Mueller FO, Cantu RC: *Twentieth Annual Report, Fall 1982-Spring 2002.* Chapel Hill, NC, National Center for Sports Injury Research, 2002, pp 1-25.

3. Cantu RC, Mueller FO: Brain injury-related fatalities in American football, 1945-1999. *Neurosurgery* 2003;52:846-853.

4. Boden BP, Tacchetti R. Cantu R, Knowles SB, Mueller FO: Catastrophic head injuries in high school and college football players. *Am J Sports Med* 2006; submitted for publication.

5. Molsa JJ, Tegner Y, Alaranta H, Myllynen P, Kujala UM: Spinal cord injuries in ice hockey in Finland and Sweden from 1980 to 1996. *Int J Sports Med* 1999;20:64-67.

6. Stuart MJ, Smith AM, Malo-Ortiguera SA, Fischer TL, Larson DR: A comparison of facial protection and the incidence of head, neck, and facial injuries in junior A hockey players: A function of individual playing time. *Am J Sports Med* 2002;30:39-44.

7. Boden BP, Pasquina P, Johnson J, Mueller FO: Catastrophic injuries in pole-vaulters. *Am J Sports Med* 2001;29:50-54.

8. Boden BP, Tacchetti R, Mueller FO: Catastrophic cheerleading injuries. *Am J Sports Med* 2003;31:881-888.

9. Boden BP, Tacchetti R, Mueller FO: Catastrophic injuries in baseball. *Am J Sports Med* 2004;32:1189-1196.

10. Kane SM, House HO, Overgaard KA: Head-first versus feet-first sliding: A comparison of speed from base to base. *Am J Sports Med* 2002;30:834-836.

11. Crisco JJ, Greenwald RM, Blume JD, Penna LH: Batting performance of wood and metal baseball bats. *Med Sci Sports Exerc* 2002;34:1675-1684.

12. Maron BJ, Poliac LC, Kaplan JA, Mueller FO: Blunt impact to the chest leading to sudden death from cardiac arrest during sports activities. *N Engl J Med* 1995;333:337-342.

13. Strasburger JF, Maron BJ: Images in clinical medicine. *N Engl J Med* 2002;347:1248.

14. Viano DC, Andrzejak DV, King AI: Fatal chest injury by baseball impact in children: A brief review. *Clin J Sport Med* 1992;2:161-165.

15. Janda DH, Viano DC, Andrzejak DV, Hensinger RN: An analysis of preventive methods for baseball-induced chest impact injuries. *Clin J Sport Med* 1992;2:172-179.

16. Janda DH, Bir CA, Viano DC, Cassatta SJ: Blunt chest impacts: Assessing the relative risk of fatal cardiac injury from various baseballs. *J Trauma* 1998;44:298-303.

17. Janda DH, Bir C, Wild B, Olson S, Hensinger RN: Goal post injuries in soccer: A laboratory and field testing analysis of a preventive intervention. *Am J Sports Med* 1995;23:340-344.

18. Maron BJ: Sudden death in young athletes. *N Engl J Med* 2003;349:1064-1075.

19. Coyle JF: Thermoregulation, in Sullivan, JA, Anderson, SJ (eds): *Care of the Young Athlete*. Rosemont, IL, American Academy of Orthopaedic Surgeons, 2000, pp 65-80.

20. American Academy of Pediatrics, Committee on Sports Medicine and Fitness: Climatic heat stress and the exercising child and adolescent. *Pediatrics* 2000;106:158-159.

21. Schluep C (ed): *NCAA Sports Medicine Handbook, 2002-2003*. Indianapolis, IN, National Collegiate Athletic Association, 2003.

22. Kiningham RB, Gorenflo DW: Weight loss methods of high school wrestlers. *Med Sci Sports Exerc* 2001;33:810-813.

23. Hew-Butler T, Almond C, Ayus JC, et al: Consensus statement of the 1st International Exercise-Associated Hyponatremia Consensus Development Conference, Cape Town, South Africa. *Clin J Sport Med* 2005;15:208-213.

24. Noakes T, IMMDA: Fluid replacement during marathon running. *Clin J Sport Med* 2003;13:309-318.

25. Gardner JW: Death by water intoxication. *Mil Med* 2002;167:432-434.

26. Craig AB Jr: Summary of 58 cases of loss of consciousness during underwater swimming and diving. *Med Sci Sports* 1976;8:171-175.

27. DeVivo MJ: Causes and costs of spinal cord injury in the United States. *Spinal Cord* 1997;35:809-813.

Overview of Anterior Cruciate Ligament Injury Prevention

Barry P. Boden, MD

The anterior cruciate ligament (ACL) is one of the most commonly disrupted ligaments in the knee. Each year in the United States there are approximately 150,000 ACL injuries or 1 in 3,000 in the general population. It has been demonstrated that female athletes have a twofold to eightfold higher incidence of ACL rupture than their male counterparts in soccer and basketball.[1] Hewett and associates[2] have shown that landing patterns in girls are similar to those in boys before puberty. However, after puberty females tend to land with their knees in a more precarious valgus position, which is a risk factor for ACL rupture.[2] Therefore, a critical time to implement prevention programs in females is during or shortly after puberty.

Hormonal, anatomic, environmental, and neuromuscular theories have been proposed to explain the etiology of noncontact ACL disruptions. The focus of preventive strategies is typically on neuromuscular control of the knee, more specifically training athletes to avoid vulnerable leg positions. It has been demonstrated through videotape analysis of athletes while sustaining an ACL injury that approximately 70% of these injuries occurred via a noncontact mechanism or only minimal contact.[3,4] The two most common actions at the time of injury were landing or an abrupt deceleration. It was demonstrated that the athletes usually contacted the ground on a flat foot with the knee close to extension and often in a valgus position.[3,4] Therefore, prevention programs usually emphasize teaching athletes to reverse this technique by landing on the balls of the feet with the knees flexed, and avoiding valgus collapse at the knee.

In a comprehensive neuromuscular training study, Hewett and associates[5] analyzed the effect of a 6-week plyometric, stretching, and weight-training program in female athletes. Athletes were trained to land on the balls of the feet with the knees flexed and the chest over the knees, avoiding inward buckling of the knee (Figure 1). Soft, silent landings with toe-to-heel rocking of the foot were recommended to decrease ground reaction forces. A variety of different jumps (wall tucks, broad jump, squat jump, and cone jumps) were performed on soft mats in progressively increasing repetitions and time intervals. Verbal cues that assisted in teaching proper tech-

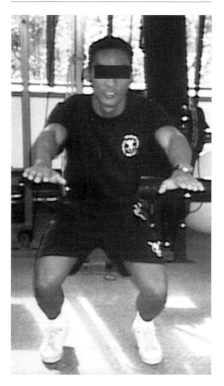

Figure 1 Photograph of an athlete demonstrating proper landing technique.

nique included "light as a feather", "recoil like a spring", "be a shock absorber", and "land on your toes."[6] At the completion of the training period, the authors found a decrease in landing forces as well as adduction and abduction knee moments.[6] In addition, the training program resulted in an increase in jump height and hamstring-to-quadriceps ratios. The authors then prospectively evaluated the effect of the program and found a decrease in the incidence of ACL injuries.[7]

In addition to the previously described technique to prevent ACL injuries that are caused by improper landing, a strategy to lower the incidence of ACL injury from an abrupt deceleration (the three-step stop-deceleration pattern) was introduced by Henning and Griffis.[8] By training athletes to decelerate over a series of three steps, as opposed to one step, the ground reaction forces that are transmitted to the knee can be reduced, potentially lowering the risk of ACL injury.

The current trend in ACL prevention is to incorporate neuromuscular training drills on the practice field. On-field ACL prevention programs stress the same principles of proper landing, plyometrics, and balance training as the original preventive studies. Although there are minor differences in the programs, they all emphasize proper landing and deceleration techniques, with ground contact occurring with the foot in plantar flexion, the knee in flexion, and avoiding excessive valgus at the knee. An example in soccer is a drill where athletes jump over a soccer ball and are trained to land on the balls of their feet with the knees flexed and the chest over the knees. Feedback on proper knee positioning to prevent inward buckling is critical to the success of the program. On-field balance exercises may include throwing a ball with a partner while balancing on one leg. Alternatively, single-leg core stability may be enhanced by training athletes to jump and land on the leg with the knee flexed and then momentarily holding the position. Although ACL injury prevention programs have not been found to be universally effective, most programs have demonstrated a reduction in ACL injury incidence by 35% to 90%.[9-11] Effective programs have shown that training sessions are necessary more than once per week, and the duration of the training program must be a minimum of 6 weeks in length.[12] It is difficult to determine if the use of ACL prevention programs is widespread, but their popularity appears to be growing. Future research should be directed at identifying the exact mechanism of ACL injury, risk factors for injury, and the most effective intervention program. Several research programs currently underway include analysis of injury mechanism based on injury videotapes, assessment of risk factors for ACL injury at military academies, and assessing the effect of several variables on ACL injury prevention programs.

References

1. Arendt E, Dick R: Knee injury patterns among men and women in collegiate basketball and soccer: NCAA data and review of literature. *Am J Sports Med* 1995;23:694-701.

2. Hewett TE, Myer GD, Ford KF: Decrease in neuromuscular control about the knee with maturation in female athletes. *J Bone Joint Surg Am* 2004;86:1601-1608.

3. Boden BP, Dean GS, Feagin JA Jr, Garrett WE Jr: Mechanisms of anterior cruciate ligament injury. *Orthopedics* 2000;23:573-578.

4. Olsen O, Myklebust G, Engebretsen L, Bahr R: Injury mechanisms of anterior cruciate ligament injuries in team handball: A systematic video analysis. *Am J Sports Med* 2004;32:1002-1012.

5. Hewett TE, Stroupe AL, Nance TA, et al: Plyometric training in female athletes: Decreased impact forces and increased hamstring torques. *Am J Sports Med* 1996;24:765-773.

6. Hewett, TE, Noyes, F: Cincinnati Sportsmetrics: A jump training program proven to prevent knee injury, videotape. Cincinnati, OH, Cincinnati Sportsmedicine Research 6 Education Foundation, 1998.

7. Hewett TE, Lindenfeld TN, Riccobene JV, Noyes FR: The effect of neuromuscular training on the incidence of knee injury in female athletes: A prospective study. *Am J Sports Med* 1999;27:699-706.

8. Henning CE, Griffis ND: Injury prevention of the anterior cruciate ligament (videotape). Wichita, KS, Mid-America Center for Sports Medicine, 1990.

9. Caraffa A, Cerulli G, Projetti M, Aisa G, Rizzo A: Prevention of anterior cruciate ligament injuries in soccer: A prospective controlled study of proprioceptive training. *Knee Surg Sports Traumatol Arthrosc* 1996;4:19-21.

10. Myklebust G, Engebretsen L, Braekken IH, Skjolberg A, Olsen OE, Bahr R: Prevention of anterior cruciate ligament injuries in female team handball players: A prospective intervention study over three seasons. *Clin J Sport Med* 2003;13:71-78.

11. Mandelbaum BR, Silvers JH, Watanabe DS, Knarr JF, Garrett W Jr: Effectiveness of a neuromuscular and proprioceptive training program in prevention anterior cruciate ligament injuries in female athletes: 2-year follow-up. *Am J Sports Med* 2005;33:1003-1010.

12. 12.Hewett TE, Ford KR, Myer GD: Anterior cruciate ligament injuries in female athletes: Part 2. A meta-analysis of neuromuscular interventions aimed at injury prevention. *Am J Sports Med* 2006;34:490-498.

Dynamic Neuromuscular Analysis Training for Preventing Anterior Cruciate Ligament Injury in Female Athletes

Timothy E. Hewett, PhD
Gregory D. Myer, MS, CSCS
Kevin R. Ford, MS
James R. Slauterbeck, MD

Abstract

Female athletes are four to six times more likely to sustain an anterior cruciate ligament (ACL) injury than male athletes. Since the enactment of Title IX, male athletic participation at the high school level has remained steady (3.8 million), whereas female athletic participation has increased tenfold (from 0.3 to 3.0 million). Geometric growth in athletic participation and the higher injury rate in female athletes have led to gender inequity in ACL injury rates. Most ACL injuries occur as a result of noncontact mechanisms such as during landing from a jump or while making a lateral pivot. Dynamic knee instability, caused by ligament dominance (decreased dynamic neuromuscular control of the joint), quadriceps dominance (decreased hamstring strength and recruitment), and leg dominance (side-to-side differences in strength and coordination) may be responsible for gender inequity in ACL injury rates.

Instr Course Lect 2007;56:397-406.

The National Collegiate Athletic Association (NCAA) reports that approximately 150,000 women participate in varsity sports each year.[1] In the NCAA 1990 to 1993 injury survey of approximately 15% of member institutions, an average knee injury rate of approximately one injury for every 10 female athletic participants was reported.[1-10] Based on these figures, more than 15,000 debilitating knee injuries are expected to occur in female athletes at the var-

sity intercollegiate level alone during any given year. The total number of knee injuries is at least four times as high at the high school level.[2,10] The 2002 high school athletic participation survey conducted by the National Federation of State High School Associations reported approximately 3 million female participants in high school sports programs.[10] Approximately one in 70 female athletes at the high school level sustains an anterior cruciate lig-

ament (ACL) injury during any given year of varsity sports.[2,11] High school athletics contributes to greater than 40,000 serious knee injuries in female athletes annually (more than 50,000 serious knee injuries if collegiate athletes are included). The cost of reconstructing and rehabilitating the ACL in these athletes, at a conservative cost of $17,000[11] per athlete, would exceed $680 million annually. This cost is in addition to the traumatic effect of potentially losing an entire season of sports participation, the possible loss of scholarship funding, and significantly lowered academic performance.[12]

Posttraumatic osteoarthritis after ACL injury may occur from 5 to 14 years after the index injury,[13,14] with 50% of patients developing osteoarthritis after 10 years.[14] If ACL injury occurs in the second decade of life, osteoarthritis could become a painful problem in these patients in the fourth decade of life, which is nearly 20 years earlier than other studied populations. In another study, patients with radiographic signs of posttraumatic osteoarthritis following ACL injury are on average 15 to 20 years younger than patients with primary osteoarthritis when they seek medical help for their symptoms.[15]

Dynamic Neuromuscular Analysis Training

ACL injury prevention training should be dynamic, neuromuscularly targeted, and analysis based (threefold neuromuscular imbalance in the female athlete is discussed later in this chapter). As evidenced in videotaped athletics, the training should be fast-paced, sport-specific, and based on sound biomechanics.[6,16] As demonstrated in soccer studies conducted by Caraffa and associates,[17] neuromuscular control of the center of mass should be targeted with the training, and the training should incorporate sport-specific balance drills. Because dynamic neuromuscular analysis training is primarily neural in nature, significant changes in technique and landing force can be achieved in relatively short periods, often in a matter of weeks. Constant and consistent trainer analysis and feedback should be incorporated into the training program, the goal of which should be technique perfection using sound biomechanical principles.[18]

Dynamic neuromuscular analysis training includes several components that have been validated in different studies.[16] Optimal biomechanics using safe and effective technique is of the utmost importance; and biofeedback, primarily via verbal and visual cues, is an effective tool to help achieve safe and effective technique. Plyometrics, which uses the muscle stretch response to achieve greater power, can help achieve rapid neuromuscular adaptation and, perhaps most importantly, deceleration of the body's center of mass in an optimal and efficient manner. Core strength and stability are emphasized in a dynamic neuromuscular analysis training program through kinetic chain control, balance drills, and perturbation control exercises. Strength is also developed, primarily through functional speed and multidirectional power drills, but traditional weight-training exercises also may be used.

Technique Perfection

It is critical for athletes in training to perform each exercise with near-perfect technique. To accomplish this, technique should be critically evaluated by the trainer or coach, and constant feedback should be provided. The analysis component helps correct poor technique and potentially harmful body alignment. Strong athletic positioning should be taught to young female athletes from the outset of training. The stance of a boxer, football linebacker, or hockey goalie can be used to help athletes visualize and enforce proper athletic positioning. Good body control and high efficiency of movement should also be emphasized and drilled; supervision and analysis will help achieve this as well. Progression, which is a crucial element of training, should also incorporate proper technique, safety guidelines, and trained feedback. Exercise drills should be progressively more difficult, which will expand the athlete's "envelope of experience" in stable, controlled positions.

Biomechanics and technique can be taught and drilled with many variable parameters. For example, exercise selection and progression can be selected and performed at different intensities, rates of progression can be modified, and the intensity of a particular exercise can be modified by altering the arm position, closing the eyes, increasing or decreasing speed of movement, adding unanticipated movements or perturbations, or adding sport-specific skills.

Plyometrics

Plyometric training involves the use of neuromuscular adaptation to stretch, which significantly enhances force and power of muscle contraction and may be accomplished in accordance with three potential force-enhancing mechanisms: the series elastic mechanism (rubber band theory), muscle spindle mechanism (thermostat theory), and the actin-myosin cross-bridge mechanism (gear theory). Whether one or all of these three mechanisms in combination produce a greater contraction force, plyometric training requires a combination of both stretch and speed of movement. As a result, plyometrics can enhance core strength and control. This is accomplished via the decrease of the amortization phase or the deceleration (deadening) phase of the movement and involves a rapid deceleration of body mass followed by almost immediate rapid acceleration of the mass in the opposite direction. Plyometric training should include sport-specific exercises, and allows safe adaptation to the rigors of explosive sports. Plyometric training should focus on proper technique and body mechanics and has been shown to be effective in reducing serious ligamentous injuries.[6,19,20] Plyometric training should not include high-impact or dangerous exercises (depth jumping or hurdle jumping), and it has been shown to be no more harmful than other established forms of sports training.[6]

In addition to strong athletic positioning, plyometric training tech-

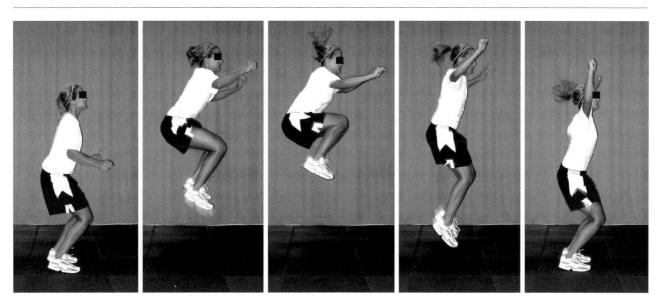

Figure 1   Photographs of the tuck jump exercise in progression.

niques include emphasizing an erect athletic position with the knees over the balls of feet and the chest over the knees. Excellent body control is also important. During vertical jumping there should be no side-to-side or forward-backward motion. The athlete should be ready to react in all planes of motion. The athlete must also learn to use the feet to dissipate impact force and should be taught to use a toe-to-midfoot rocker on vertical landings and a heel to ball of the foot rocker during horizontal landings. Soft, quiet impacts should be emphasized.

Visualization cues, such as hit like a feather, roll the feet, flex the body and get deep with gluteus instant recoil for next jump, drop like a shock absorber, and take off like a spring should be used. The goal of the functional core strength training is to provide the athlete with a dynamically stable core that is prepared to respond to the extreme forces generated at distal body parts during athletic competition, thereby reducing the risk of injury and preparing the athlete to achieve optimal per-

formance levels. The program design or exercises can be circuit-based or linear in nature, consistent versus pyramid-structured, or periodized versus noncyclical. Whichever program design and exercises are selected, intensity versus volume and anaerobic versus aerobic workouts should be emphasized.

Correcting Neuromuscular Imbalances in Female Athletes
Promoting Muscle Dominance
To correct ligament dominance in female athletes, a neuromuscular training program must be designed to teach the athlete to control dynamic knee motion in the coronal (valgus) plane. The first concept that the athlete and coach are taught is that the knee is a single-plane hinge, not a ball-and-socket joint. Reeducation of the female neuromuscular system away from multiplanar motion of the knee to dynamic control of knee motion in the sagittal plane can be achieved only through a progression of single and then multiplanar exercises.

The wall jump exercise is useful for two reasons. First, it provides an athlete with a moderate to low intensity exercise to warm up the joints and muscles. Second, beginning with low to moderate intensity exercise allows athletes to relax and gain confidence that they can succeed through the remainder of the training.

The tuck jump exercise requires a significantly increased level of intensity compared with the wall jump as well as a high level of effort from the athlete (Figure 1). When first performing the tuck jump, the athlete simply focuses on the performance of this difficult exercise. Because the athlete usually devotes minimal attention to technique during the first few repetitions, the athletic trainer assesses the athlete for abnormal coronal plane knee displacement during jumping and landing.

The broad jump allows the therapist or athletic trainer to assess the athlete's knee motion while progressing forward in the sagittal plane. This is important because the

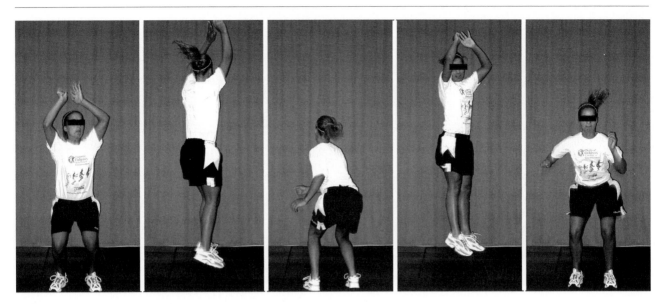

Figure 2   Photographs of the 180° jump exercise in progression.

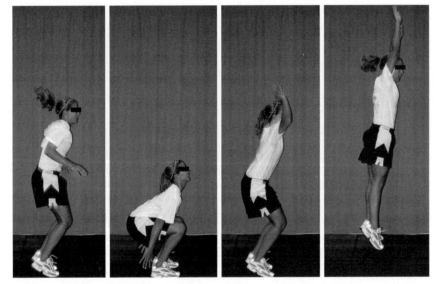

Figure 3   Photographs of the squat jump exercise in progression.

active knee control gained through training must closely match the multiplanar movements required during sports participation. When performing the broad jump, the ligament-dominant athlete will often display a lack of knee control during takeoff.

The 180° jump is an exercise that teaches dynamic body and knee control in the transverse plane (Fig-

ure 2). The 180° jump creates rotational force in the transverse plane that must be decelerated and immediately redirected in the opposite direction. This movement helps teach the athlete to recognize and control rotational forces.

Barrier jumps from side to side are used as part of a progression program that directly creates and targets the dynamic control of potentially

dangerous valgus and varus moments at the knee. The shifting of the athlete's body from side to side along the coronal plane creates significant valgus and varus torques on the knee during landing. This training conditions the athlete to quickly dampen, decelerate, and redirect these forces while gaining proper neuromuscular control of the knee.

Increasing Knee Flexor Recruitment

Exercises that emphasize cocontraction of the knee flexor and extensor muscles can decrease quadriceps dominance by increasing recruitment of the knee flexors while strongly activating the knee extensors.[21] At angles greater than 45°, the quadriceps is an antagonist to the ACL.[22,23] Therefore, it is important to use deep knee flexion angles to put the quadriceps into an ACL-agonist position. By training athletes with deep knee flexion jumps, they learn to increase the amount of knee flexion and decrease the amount of time being in the more

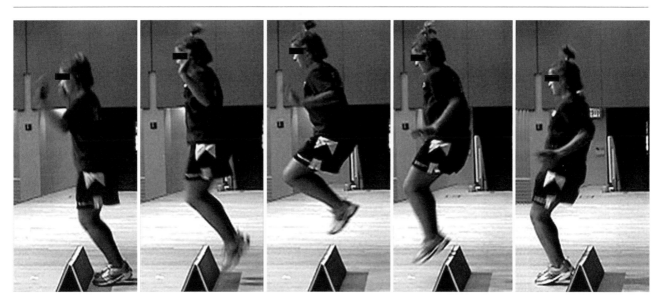

Figure 4   Photographs of the front-to-back barrier jump exercise in progression.

dangerous straight-legged position. At the same time, athletes reprogram peak flexor/extensor firing patterns, thereby increasing cofiring and quadriceps firing in deep flexion for greater protection of the ACL.

Squat jumps specifically help increase control of sagittal plane moments (Figure 3). Squat jumps require athletes to go into deep knee flexion angles greater than 90°. Deep knee flexion angle jumps recruit the hamstrings muscles, which when fired, prevent anterior tibial motion and decrease shearing forces on the ACL. Knee flexion angles greater than 45° allow the quadriceps to be an ACL agonist (decrease strain on the ACL with activation) rather than an ACL antagonist. Deep knee flexion training and the requirement to hold deep knee flexion positions for long periods can help correct quadriceps dominance.

Front-to-back barrier jumps recruit the knee flexor musculature (Figure 4). This movement requires the repetitive recruitment and co-contraction of the knee flexors and extensors, which forces loading of the weaker and less mechanically advantaged hamstring and gastrocnemius muscles, providing the mechanism for greater strength adaptations. In addition, the low external knee flexor moment that occurs during front to back barrier jumps, as a result of low knee range of motion and high ankle range of motion, limits quadriceps activity while maximizing the gastrocnemius contribution. Front-to-back barrier jumps also allow for training of the biarticular gastrocnemius muscle, which is a knee flexor, even though the primary motion is plantar flexion. The cumulative effects of front-to-back barrier jumps provide an increased knee flexor to knee extensor work ratio.

Balancing the Lower Extremities
The correction of dynamic contralateral imbalances can be addressed throughout the entire training protocol. Equal leg-to-leg strength and balance and foot placement should be stressed throughout the training program. To correct for leg dominance, the training program should progressively emphasize double and then single movements throughout the three training phases.

Lunges and scissors jumps are a bridge for the athlete to progress from double leg jumps to the single leg hops (Figure 5). Scissors jumps are performed with the front leg serving as the support leg that maintains most of the upper extremity's balance and weight (with the body's center of gravity leaning forward). The back leg provides secondary support and balance during the jump while maintaining a ballast position that is comparable to the position used in the single-leg hop-and-hold exercise.

The single-leg hop-and-hold exercise is incorporated into the training program only after the athlete has mastered the less difficult broad jump with a 5-second hold (Figure 6). It is important to maintain this progression because most noncontact ACL injuries occur when landing or decelerating on a single limb.

Bounding exercises should be incorporated into the training pro-

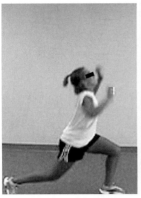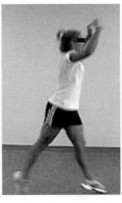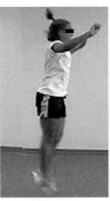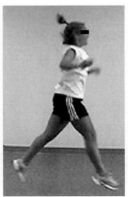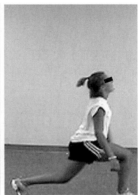

Figure 5   Photographs of the scissors jump exercise in progression.

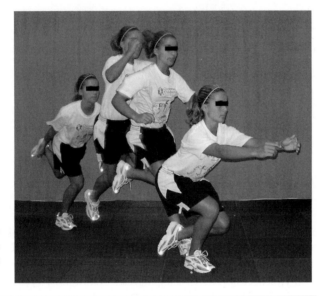

Figure 6 Photograph of the hop and hold exercise in progression.

gram to aid in the correction of lower extremity imbalances and coordinate multiplanar movements (Figure 7). Bounding exercises require that athletes jump with maximum distance in both the vertical and horizontal planes and incorporate high-intensity jumps and landings on a single limb.

Correction of leg dominance also requires that athletes learn to coordinate multiple joint actions and multiplanar movements into power-skill movements that can be used during competitive play. One exercise that helps accomplish this goal is the jump-jump-jump vertical jump exercise, which requires that athletes transfer horizontal momentum into vertical movement.

The box drop 180°-maximum vertical exercise can be incorporated into the training program to focus on lower extremity balance and side-to-side control. The execution of this complex jump requires the coordination of both limbs to maintain body alignment and control during a multiplanar jump. Improper or unbalanced limb contribution to any step of the sequence makes the jump difficult to execute. As athletes eventually learn to perform this jump, they will also learn bilateral limb control.

Progression from double-leg to single-leg power maneuvers is a requirement for correcting dominant leg imbalances. In addition, the incorporation of multiplanar movements that equally recruit both lower extremities for optimal performance is necessary. More complex movement patterns require greater synchronization and coordination in side-to-side performance, which leads to greater balance in side-to-side muscle recruitment and equalization of leg-to-leg coordination and power. Training can be team oriented or trainer intensive. Feedback is critical. Care should be taken not to allow athletes to perfect improper or dangerous techniques.

Dynamic Neuromuscular Training Decreases the Incidence of ACL Injury

Hewett and associates[11] conducted an epidemiologic study to prospectively evaluate the effect of neuromuscular training on ACL injury rates in female athletes and reported that trained female athletes had a 72% lower incidence of ACL injury than untrained female athletes. Trained female athletes demonstrated an incidence of ACL inju-

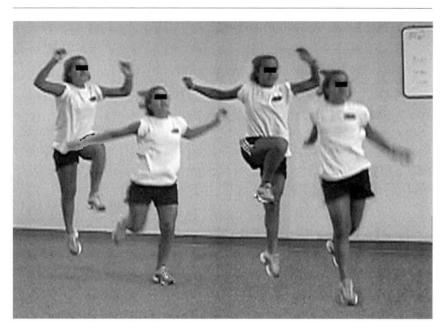

Figure 7   Photograph of the bounding in place exercise in progression.

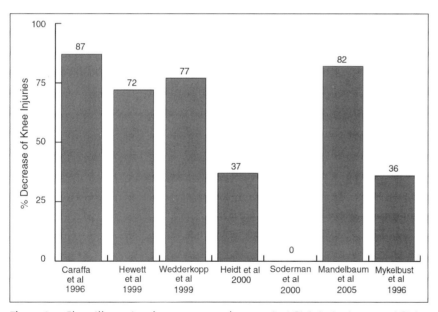

Figure 8   Chart illustrating the percentage decrease in ACL injuries in seven ACL injury prevention-training studies.

the relative decreases in knee injury rates as a result of various training programs.[11,16-20]

A Review of Neuromuscular Training Programs

Several studies have been published that examined the effects of neuromuscular training programs on ACL injury.[6,19,20,24,26-29] Some of the training programs described in these studies have shown a decrease in the rate of ACL injury, a decrease in the rate of knee injury, or no effect. The studies showing no effect did not achieve the power necessary to make the conclusion of no effect.

Hewett and associates[6] used a prospective cohort designed study that monitored high school soccer, volleyball, and basketball athletes. Eight hundred ninety-seven athletes were studied (463 of whom received intervention and 434 served as control subjects). The intervention group received a 6-week plyometric, strength training, and flexibility training program. Trained female athletes had significantly fewer non-contact ACL injuries and fewer knee injuries than the untrained females.

Wedderkopp and associates[26] used a randomized controlled trial that monitored European handball athletes. Eleven teams with 111 players were randomized to an intervention group and 11 teams with 126 players were randomized to a control group. The intervention group received ankle disk training and participated in a warm-up program. The overall injury rates were less than those in the intervention groups. Although eight ACL injures occurred in the control group and two occurred in the intervention group, statistical significance was not achieved. Sufficient power was not achieved to show no effect by the training program.

ry similar to that of untrained male athletes. Neuromuscular training resulted in even greater differences in noncontact ACL injuries between the female athlete groups. These results indicate that neuromuscular training decreases injury risk in female athletes. Although this was the first study to demonstrate significant decreases in ACL injury rates with neuromuscular training, specifically in female athletes, other studies have demonstrated similar significant decreases or trends toward significant changes in female, male, and mixed gender populations. Figure 8 shows

Heidt and associates[24] used a prospective study that monitored high school soccer athletes. Three hundred athletes were studied (42 of whom received intervention 258 served as control subjects). The intervention group received speed, agility, and jump training over a 7-week preseason program. Overall, the intervention group had fewer injures, but there was no difference in ACL injury rates between the two groups. Sufficient power was not achieved to show no significance between the intervention group and control subjects.

Soderman and associates[29] used a prospective randomized controlled trial that monitored professional soccer athletes in Sweden. One hundred forty athletes were studied (62 of whom received intervention and 78 served as control subjects). The intervention group performed an at-home, self-monitored balance board training program in preseason and during the season. No difference in the rates of ACL or serious knee injuries was identified between the groups; however, the study lacked power to show no significant difference between the two groups.

Myklebust and associates[20,28] used a prospective cohort study that monitored elite-level team handball athletes. Over three seasons, 2,647 athletes were monitored. The first season was a control season and injuries were assessed. The second and third seasons included interventions. The intervention groups received floor, wobble board, and balance training. In the most elite athletes, there was a significant drop in the rate of ACL injuries.

Mandelbaum and associates[19] used a prospective cohort study that monitored 14- to 18-year-old soccer athletes over a 2-year period. In the first year, 2,946 athletes were studied

(1,041 of whom received intervention and 1,905 served as control subjects); 2,757 athletes were studied in the second year (844 of whom received intervention, and 1,913 served as control subjects). The intervention group followed a 20-minute warm-up plan consisting of stretching, strengthening, plyometrics, and soccer and agility drills. A significant reduction in the rate of ACL injuries occurred over the two seasons in the intervention group.

Olsen and associates[27] used a cluster randomized controlled trial to monitor youth team handball. A total of 1,837 athletes were studied (958 of whom receive intervention and 879 served as control subjects). The intervention group received a warm-up program to improve running, cutting, and landing techniques as well as balance and strength training. Significantly fewer injuries were observed in the intervention group.

Most of these studies report success in decreasing either knee injury or ACL injury rates. The studies that reported no success in decreasing injury rates lacked sufficient power to statistically make the statement that no effect was observed by the intervention. Overall, plyometric, strength, technique, balance, and stability training all appear to induce some neuromuscular change that is associated with decreased knee and or ACL injury rates in trained individuals. However, the exact mechanism and/or the precise exercise(s) that result in this benefit are unknown.

Dynamic Neuromuscular Imbalances
One theory to account for higher knee injury incidence in female athletes is that neuromuscular imbalances resulting from training deficiencies, developmental differences,

or perhaps hormonal influences lead to higher rates of injury. This review focuses on the neuromuscular theory because intervention and prevention are likely to have the greatest impact at the neuromuscular level where adaptation readily occurs.

The primary goal of the applied research into decreasing ACL ligament injury rates in female athletes must be to determine the factors that make women more susceptible than men to knee ligament injury. Once these factors are determined, treatment modalities should be developed to aid in the prevention of these injuries. If preventive modalities such as dynamic neuromuscular training can decrease the incidence of female athlete knee injury from five times that of male athletes to a rate that is equal to that of males, 40,000 knee injuries could be prevented in high school and collegiate women's sports annually. In addition, with the increasing popularity of high-risk jumping and pivoting sports such as soccer, volleyball, and basketball and the rapidly growing number of participants each year, a higher number of future injuries could be avoided.

Neuromuscular training alters active knee joint stabilization and aids in decreasing ACL injury rates in female athletes. Hewett and associates[11] reported the first prospective study of the effects of a neuromuscular training program on knee injury in the high-risk female athlete population. The rate of serious knee injury was decreased 72% in the trained group relative to the untrained group. This prospective study was the first published in the literature to demonstrate that neuromuscular training can reduce ACL injury risk in the high-risk female athlete population. These findings have been subsequently con-

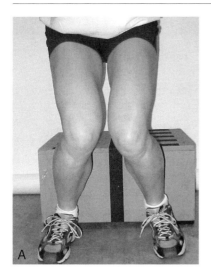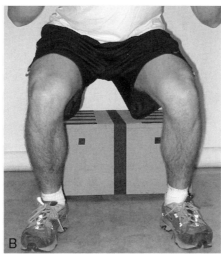

Figure 9   Photographs showing the differences in valgus knee motion between a female (**A**) and male (**B**) athlete when jumping off of a box and progressing into a maximum vertical jump.

firmed by follow-up studies that used similar neuromuscular training protocols in young female athletes.[24,25] These studies provide strong evidence that neuromuscular training is likely to be an effective solution to gender inequity in ACL injury rates.

The Female Athlete: Threefold Neuromuscular Imbalance

Three neuromuscular imbalances (ligament dominance, quadriceps dominance, and leg dominance) are often encountered in female athletes. Andrews[30] first recognized the presence of ligament dominance in female athletes and reported that female athletes allow stress on ligaments before muscle activation to absorb ground reaction forces. During single-leg landing, pivoting, or deceleration, as often occurs during knee ligament injury, the female athlete typically allows the ground reaction force to control the direction of motion of the lower extremity joints, especially the knee joint. The lack of dynamic muscular control of the joint leads to increased valgus motion, increased force, and high torque at the knee. Figure 9 shows the differences in valgus knee motion between a female and a male athlete when jumping off of a box and progressing into a maximum vertical jump.

With quadriceps dominance, female athletes activate their knee extensors preferentially over their knee flexors during athletic movements to stabilize the knee joint, which accentuates and perpetuates strength and coordination imbalances between these muscles.[6,7] At low knee flexion angles, such as those that occur during ACL injury, the quadriceps increases strain on the ACL, while the hamstrings likely decrease ACL strain. Hewett and associates[6] have demonstrated that quadriceps dominance can be addressed and overcome with dynamic neuromuscular training.

Leg dominance is the imbalance between muscular strength and coordination on opposite limbs, with the dominant limb often demonstrating greater strength and coordination. Limb dominance may place the weaker, less-coordinated limb and the stronger limb at increased risk of ACL injury. The weaker limb is compromised in its ability to manage average forces and torques, whereas the stronger limb may experience exceptionally high forces and torques because of increased dependence and increased loading on that side in high-force situations. Female athletes have been reported to generate lower hamstrings torques on the nondominant rather than the dominant leg.[6] Side-to-side imbalances in neuromuscular strength, flexibility, and coordination have been shown to be important predictors of increased injury risk.[6,11,31] Knapik and associates[31] demonstrated that side-to-side balance in strength and flexibility is important for the prevention of injuries; they also demonstrated that when imbalances are present, the athlete is more prone to injury. Baumhauer and associates[32] found that individuals with muscle strength imbalances exhibited a higher incidence of ankle injury.

Summary

Correction of neuromuscular imbalances in all three planes of movement (the sagittal, coronal, and transverse planes) is critical for improving the biomechanics of athletic movements and reducing knee injury incidence. Widespread use of neuromuscular training for ACL injury prevention and enhanced biomechanical performance promises to advance the field of injury prevention in women's athletics. Intervention programs should focus on plyometric, strength, technique, balance, and stability training in those who are identified as being at high risk for ACL injury.

References

1. Hutchinson MR, Ireland ML: Knee injuries in female athletes. *Sports Med* 1995;19:288-302.

2. Chandy TA, Grana WA: Secondary school athletic injury in boys and girls: A three-year comparison. *Phys Sportsmed* 1985;13:106-111.

3. Ferretti A, Papandrea P, Conteduca F, Mariani PP: Knee ligament injuries in volleyball players. *Am J Sports Med* 1992;20:203-207.

4. Gerberich SG, Luhmann S, Finke C, Priest JD, Beard BJ: Analysis of severe injuries associated with volleyball activities. *Phys Sportsmed* 1987;15:75-79.

5. Gray J, Taunton JE, McKenzie DC, Clement DB, McConkey JP, Davidson RG: A survey of injuries to the anterior cruciate ligament of the knee in female basketball players. *Int J Sports Med* 1985;6:314-316.

6. Hewett TE, Stroupe AL, Nance TA, Noyes FR: Plyometric training in female athletes: Decreased impact forces and increased hamstring torques. *Am J Sports Med* 1996;24:765-773.

7. Huston LJ, Wojtys EM: Neuromuscular performance characteristics in elite female athletes. *Am J Sports Med* 1996;24:427-436.

8. Whiteside PA: Men's and women's injuries in comparable sports. *Phys Sportsmed* 1980;8:130-140.

9. Zelisko JA, Noble HB, Porter M: A comparison of men's and women's professional basketball injuries. *Am J Sports Med* 1982;10:297-299.

10. *National Federation of State High School Associations: 2002 High School Participation Survey.* Indianapolis, IN, National Federation of State High School Associations, 2002.

11. Hewett TE, Lindenfeld TN, Riccobene JV, Noyes FR: The effect of neuromuscular training on the incidence of knee injury in female athletes: A prospective study. *Am J Sports Med* 1999;27:699-706.

12. Freedman KB, Glasgow MT, Glasgow SG, Bernstein J: Anterior cruciate ligament injury and reconstruction among university students. *Clin Orthop Relat Res* 1998;356:208-212.

13. Gillquist J, Messner K: Anterior cruciate ligament reconstruction and the long-term incidence of gonarthrosis. *Sports Med* 1999;27:143-156.

14. Myklebust G, Bahr R: Return to play guidelines after anterior cruciate ligament surgery. *Br J Sports Med* 2005;39:127-131.

15. Sharma L, Song J, Felson DT, Cahue S, Shamiyeh E, Dunlop DD: The role of knee alignment in disease progression and functional decline in knee osteoarthritis. *JAMA* 2001;286:188-195.

16. Hewett TE, Myer GD, Ford KR: Reducing knee and anterior cruciate ligament injuries among female athletes: a systematic review of neuromuscular training interventions. *J Knee Surg* 2005;18:82-88.

17. Caraffa A, Cerulli G, Projetti M, Aisa G, Rizzo A: Prevention of anterior cruciate ligament injuries in soccer: A prospective controlled study of proprioceptive training. *Knee Surg Sports Traumatol Arthrosc* 1996;4:19-21.

18. Ettlinger CF, Johnson RJ, Shealy JE: A method to help reduce the risk of serious knee sprains incurred in alpine skiing. *Am J Sports Med* 1995;23:531-537.

19. Mandelbaum BR, Silvers HJ, Watanabe D, et al: Effectiveness of a neuromuscular and proprioceptive training program in preventing the incidence of ACL injuries in female athletes: Two-year follow up. *Am J Sports Med* 2005;33:1003-1010.

20. Myklebust G, Engebretsen L, Braekken IH, Skjolberg A, Olsen OE, Bahr R: Prevention of anterior cruciate ligament injuries in female team handball players: A prospective intervention study over three seasons. *Clin J Sport Med* 2003;13:71-78.

21. Fitzgerald G, Axe M, Snyder-Mackler L: Proposed practice guidelines for nonoperative anterior cruciate ligament rehabilitation of physically active individuals. *J Orthop Sports Phys Ther* 2000;30:194-203.

22. Andriacchi TP, Andersson GBJ, Fermier RW, Stern D, Galante JO: Study of lower-limb mechanics during stair-climbing. *J Bone Joint Surg Am* 1980;62:749-757.

23. Daniel DM, Malcom LL, Losse G, Stone ML, Sachs R, Burks R: Instrumented measurement of anterior laxity of the knee. *J Bone Joint Surg Am* 1985;67:720-726.

24. Heidt RS, Sweeterman LM, Carlonas RL, Traub JA, Tekulve FX: Avoidance of soccer injuries with preseason conditioning. *Am J Sports Med* 2000;28:659-662.

25. Mandelbaum B: ACL prevention strategies in the female athlete and soccer: Implementation of a neuromuscular training program to determine its efficacy on the incidence of ACL injury, in *AAOSM 2002 Specialty Day.* Dallas, TX, AAOSM, 2002.

26. Wedderkopp N, Kaltoft M, Lundgaard B, Rosendahl M, Froberg K: Prevention of injuries in young female players in European team handball: A prospective intervention study. *Scand J Med Sci Sports* 1999;9:41-47.

27. Olsen OE, Myklebust G, Engebretsen L, Holme I, Bahr R: Exercises to prevent lower limb injuries in youth sports: Cluster randomised controlled trial. *BMJ* 2005;330(7489):449.

28. Myklebust G, Maehlum S, Holm I, Bahr R: A prospective cohort study of anterior cruciate ligament injuries in elite Norwegian team handball. *Scand J Med Sci Sports* 1998;8:149-153.

29. Soderman K, Werner S, Pietila T, Engstrom B, Alfredson H: Balance board training: Prevention of traumatic injuries of the lower extremities in female soccer players? A prospective randomized intervention study. *Knee Surg Sports Traumatol Arthrosc* 2000;8:356-363.

30. Andrews J: Overuse syndromes of the lower extremity. *Clin Sports Med* 1983;2:137-148.

31. Knapik JJ, Bauman CL, Jones BH, Harris JM, Vaughan L: Preseason strength and flexibility imbalances associated with athletic injuries in female collegiate athletes. *Am J Sports Med* 1991;19:76-81.

32. Baumhauer J, Alosa D, Renstrom A, Trevino S, Beynnon B: A prospective study of ankle injury risk factors. *Am J Sports Med* 1995;23:564-570.

Prevention of Noncontact Anterior Cruciate Ligament Injuries in Elite and Adolescent Female Team Handball Athletes

Grethe Myklebust, PT, PhD
Lars Engebretsen, MD, PhD
Ingeborg Hoff Brækken, Msci, PT
Arnhilo Skjølberg, PT
Odd-Egil Olsen, PT, PhD
Roald Bahr, MD, PhD

Abstract

To assess the effect of a neuromuscular training program on the incidence of anterior cruciate ligament (ACL) injuries in female team handball athletes, a prospective intervention study of female team handball athletes from divisions I, II, and III in Norway was conducted. The control season (1998-1999) included 60 teams (942 athletes), the first intervention season (1999-2000) included 58 teams (855 athletes), and the second intervention season (2000-2001) included 52 teams (850 athletes). For the intervention teams, a five-phase program (duration, 15 minutes) with three different balance exercises focusing on neuromuscular control and planting and landing skills was developed and introduced to the athletes in the autumn of 1999 and revised before the start of the season in 2000. Each intervention team was instructed in the program and supplied with an instructional video, poster, six balance mats, and six wobble boards. Additionally, a physical therapist was assigned to each team for follow-up during the second intervention season. The number of ACL injuries during the three seasons and compliance with the program were assessed. Twenty-nine ACL injuries occurred during the control season, 23 during the first intervention season (odds ratio [OR], 0.87 [0.50-1.52]; P = 0.62), and 17 during the second intervention season (OR, 0.64 [0.35-1.18]; P = 0.15). In the elite division, 13 injuries occurred during the control season, 6 during the first intervention season (OR, 0.51 [0.19-1.35]; P = 0.17), and 5 during the second intervention season (OR, 0.37 [0.13-1.05]; P = 0.06). For the entire cohort, no difference in injury rates was noted during the second intervention season between compliers and noncompliers (OR, 0.52 [0.15-1.82], P = 0.31). In the elite division, the risk of injury was reduced among athletes who completed the ACL injury prevention program (OR, 0.06 [0.01-0.54], P = 0.01) compared with those who did not. The results demonstrate that it is possible to prevent ACL injuries with specific neuromuscular training.

Instr Course Lect 2007;56: 407-418.

Anterior cruciate ligament (ACL) injuries occur in many athletic activities, particularly among women.[1-3] The risk of ACL rupture is five times higher among female than male athletes, and the gender difference is even higher at the elite athletic level.[4,5] Some studies indicate that it may be possible to reduce the incidence of knee and ankle injuries among adults and adolescents; however, these studies are small and mainly nonrandomized, with important methodologic limitations.

A reported incidence as high as 1.6 injuries per 1,000 hours of athletic activity has been reported for elite female athletes during team handball matches,[5] and this incidence is at least as high as that reported for other team sports.[1-3,6] Thus far, few studies have examined the short-term and long-term consequences of ACL injury in elite athletes. The return rate to athletic participation has been reported to range between 30% and 50%.[7,8] In a recent study of Norwegian team handball athletes, a return rate of 58% after surgery and 82% in non-surgically treated patients was reported.[9] However, the same study showed that as many as half of the injured athletes reported significant problems with instability, pain, and loss of range of motion when examined 8 to 10 years after the injury.

One potential long-term problem after an ACL injury, whether treated surgically or nonsurgically, is osteoarthritis of the knee. Gillquist and Messner[10] concluded that the prevalence of radiographic gonarthrosis is increased after all types of knee injuries compared with the uninjured joint of the same patient. A total rupture of the ACL seems to increase the risk tenfold compared with an age-matched uninjured population,[10] and gonarthrosis seems to occur despite the ability to rectify the instability surgically. There is no evidence to suggest that ACL reconstruction decreases the rate of posttraumatic osteoarthritis in the knee.[11] In fact, it may even be hypothesized that an effective ACL reconstruction increases the risk of future osteoarthritis (because of re-injury or the high demands placed on the knee) by enabling the athlete to return to participation in high-performance pivoting sports. In a follow-up study on team handball athletes, approximately 50% of the injured athletes had radiologic signs of osteoarthritis 8 to 10 years postinjury.[9]

Because most ACL injuries are noncontact injuries (approximately 80% of the injuries occur in a plant-and-cut situation or when landing after a jump shot),[4,5] it was hypothesized that improving awareness of the knee position as well as improving balance, cutting, and landing techniques could reduce the fre-

quency of ACL injuries. Balance board training has been used as an injury prevention model in several studies of injuries to the lower extremity, and some of these studies have reported good results.[12-15] Caraffa and associates[12] recently demonstrated a remarkable reduction of the ACL injury rate in Italian male soccer athletes after introducing a proprioceptive training program using exercises on wobble boards. Conversely, Soderman and associates[16] reported no significant effect of a balance board training program on the incidence of injuries to the lower extremity in a randomized study of female soccer athletes. In two separate studies, Hewett and associates[17,18] observed a reduced incidence of severe knee injuries in female volleyball athletes using a 6-week jump training program in which the athletes focused on changing landing technique to decrease forces by learning neuromuscular control of the lower extremity during landing.

Because the long-term consequences of an ACL injury are serious, and team handball is a high-risk sport for these injuries, there is an urgent need to develop effective ACL injury prevention strategies for this population. Thus, the aim was to assess the effectiveness of a neuromuscular training program on the incidence of ACL injuries in female team handball athletes. The program was designed to improve awareness and knee control during standing, cutting, jumping, and landing. A randomized controlled trial was conducted to investigate the effect of a structured program of warm-up exercises used to prevent acute injuries of the lower limb in young athletes. To minimize overlap within clubs, a cluster design was used.

Materials and Methods
Study I
This intervention study covered three consecutive seasons of the three top divisions in the Norwegian Handball Federation. During the first season (control season, 1998-1999), baseline data were collected on the incidence of ACL injuries. Then an ACL injury prevention program was introduced before the start of each of the following two seasons (first intervention season, 1999-2000; second intervention season, 2000-2001). Injury registration was continued throughout the intervention seasons to assess the effectiveness of the ACL injury prevention program. The Data Inspectorate and the Regional Ethics Committee for Medical Research approved the study, and the injured athletes gave their written consent to provide medical information from hospital records.

Participants The Norwegian Handball Federation league system ranks the participating teams according to skill level into four division levels. Normally, 12 teams play in the elite division, 12 teams play in the second division conference, and 12 teams play in each of the four third division conferences. All the teams in the three top divisions were asked to participate in the study, except for teams from northern Norway that were excluded for practical reasons. Each conference plays using a double round-robin competition format during the season from mid-September to mid-April, and two teams advance and two teams are relegated between divisions according to final league standing at the end of each season. In addition, most teams also participate in a single-elimination cup tournament for the Norwegian Cup Championship, and the teams can play in sev-

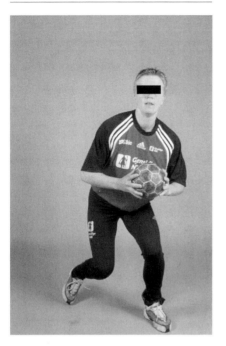

Figure 1 Photograph of a female athlete performing a floor exercise. (Reproduced with permission from Myklebust G, Engebretsen L, Braekken IH, Skjølberg A, Olsen OE, Bahr R: Prevention of ACL injuries in female team handball players: A prospective intervention study over three seasons. *Clin J Sport Med* 2003;13:71-78.)

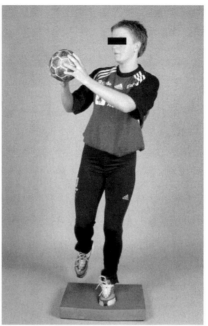

Figure 2 Photograph of a female athlete performing a mat exercise. (Reproduced with permission from Myklebust G, Engebretsen L, Braekken IH, Skjølberg A, Olsen OE, Bahr R: Prevention of ACL injuries in female team handball players: A prospective intervention study over three seasons. *Clin J Sport Med* 2003;13:71-78.)

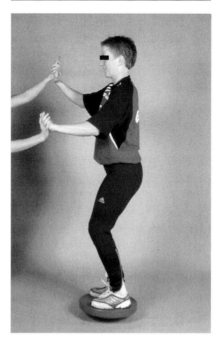

Figure 3 Photograph of a female athlete performing a wobble board exercise. (Reproduced with permission from Myklebust G, Engebretsen L, Braekken IH, Skjølberg A, Olsen OE, Bahr R: Prevention of ACL injuries in female team handball players: A prospective intervention study over three seasons. *Clin J Sport Med* 2003;13:71-78.)

eral national and international tournaments throughout the season.

During the control season, 60 teams (942 athletes) took part in the injury registration, 12 of which were in the elite division, 12 in the second division, and 36 in the third division. During the first intervention season, 58 teams (855 athletes) participated, 12 of which were in the elite division, 13 in the second division, and 33 in the third division (2 teams withdrew, and 1 declined to participate in the study). During the second intervention season, 52 teams (850 athletes) participated, 12 of which were in the elite division, 11 in the second division, and 29 in the third division (4 teams withdrew, and 4 teams declined). A total of six teams declined to participate

in the study during the two intervention seasons, which is 5% of the potential participating teams and unlikely to have introduced any selection bias.

ACL Injury Intervention Program An ACL injury prevention program with three different sets of exercises (Figures 1 through 3) was developed, each with a five-step progression from easy to more difficult (Table 1). Before the first intervention season, the teams were visited once in the preparatory period. They were supplied with an instructional video, posters, six balance mats, and six wobble boards. The teams were instructed to use the program three times weekly during a 5- to 7-week training period, and then once weekly during the season. The

coaches were responsible for carrying out the program and were also asked to record the total number of ACL injury prevention training sessions that the team completed.

After the results of the first intervention season were evaluated, it was decided to continue the intervention, but now with improved control over the quantity and quality of the ACL prevention program. The teams in the elite division all had physical therapists working closely with the teams, but few teams in the lower divisions had established a relationship with a physical therapist. Therefore, physical therapists were recruited to supervise each of the teams. All the physical therapists participated in an 8-hour seminar in which they were

Table 1
Final ACL Injury Prevention Program

	Floor Exercises	Mat Exercises	Wobble Board Exercises
Week 1	Running and planting, partner running backward and giving feedback on the quality of the movement, change position after 20 seconds	Two players standing on one leg on the mat throwing to each other	Two players two-legged on the board throwing to each other
Week 2	Jumping exercise—right leg–right leg over to left leg–left leg and finishing with a two-foot landing with flexion in both hips and knees	Jump shot from a box (30 to 40 cm high) with a two-foot landing with flexion in hip and knees	Squats on two legs, then on one leg
Week 3	Running and planting (as in week 1), now doing a full plant and cut movement with the ball, focusing on knee position	"Step" down from box with one-leg landing with flexion in hip and knee	Two players throwing to each other, one foot on the board
Week 4	Two and two players together two-leg jump forward and backward, 180° turn, and the same movement backward; partner tries to push the player out of control, but still focusing on landing technique	Two players both standing on balance mats trying to push partner out of balance, first on two legs, then on one leg	Two players with one foot on the board, bouncing the ball with their eyes shut
Week 5	Expanding the movement from week 3 to a full plant and cut, then a jump shot with two-legged landing	The players jump on a mat catching the ball, then make a 180° turn on the mat	Two players, both standing on balance boards trying to push partner out of balance, first on two legs, then on one leg

(Adapted with permission from Myklebust G, Engebretsen L, Braekken IH, Skjølberg A, Olsen OE, Bahr R: Prevention of ACL injuries in female team handball players: A prospective intervention study over three seasons. *Clin J Sport Med 2003*;13:71-78.)

given theoretic and practical training on how to conduct the ACL injury prevention program as well as on the procedures of data collection. The physical therapists were asked to attend team training sessions three times weekly for a 5- to 7-week period, and then once weekly during the season to supervise the training program. They were also asked to record individual attendance during each of the ACL injury prevention sessions. Videos and posters were given to all the teams. New teams were supplied with balance mats and wobble boards.

During the training sessions, the teams were divided into three groups: one doing the floor exercises, one using wobble boards (disk diameter, 38 cm; Norpro A/S, Notodden, Norway), and one using balance mats (40 × 50 cm, 7-cm thick; Alusuisse Airex AG, Sins, Switzerland). The athletes changed positions every 5 minutes, for a pro-gram duration of approximately 15 minutes. When performing one-leg exercises, the athletes were told to use the alternate leg after approximately 15 seconds.

Modifications were made to some of the training exercises before the second intervention season based on feedback from athletes and coaches after the first season. The changes aimed to make the exercises more specific to team handball as well as more challenging. However, the focus of the exercises—to improve awareness and knee control during standing, cutting, jumping, and landing—did not change. The athletes were encouraged to be focused and conscious of the quality of their movements and to give emphasis to core stability and hip and knee position in relation to the foot—the "knee over toe" position. The athletes were also asked to watch their partner closely and give feedback to each other during training.

Injury and Exposure Registration

During all three seasons, the coaches and/or the team physical therapists were asked to report all ACL injuries, and they were contacted by telephone every 1 to 2 months to ensure that no knee injuries were missed. Athletes with suspected ACL injuries (knee injuries that caused more than 1 week of missed participation in training or matches) were interviewed by trained physical therapists, either in person or by telephone, using a standard questionnaire. The information requested in each case included personal data, menstrual history, and mechanism of injury. The menstrual cycle date was adjusted to an average cycle length of 28 days, with day 1 of the cycle designated as that day on which bleeding began. Injuries were classified as occurring in four different menstrual phases (day 1 through 7: menstrual phase; day 8 through 14: follicular phase; day 15 through

21: early luteal phase; day 22 through 28: late luteal phase).

Each instance of a suspected ACL injury was either self-referred or referred for examination by an orthopaedic surgeon. Most patients underwent an arthroscopic examination and MRI, and their medical records were obtained to confirm the diagnosis.

The coaches supplied information on the training schedule and attendance as well as the number of official training games, tournament games, and cup and league games during each of the seasons. Competition exposure for each team was calculated as the number of games multiplied by the duration of each game (some tournament games lasted less than the regulation time of 2 × 30 minutes) multiplied by seven athletes. Training exposure was calculated based on the average weekly number of training hours multiplied by the average attendance for training sessions reported by the coaches.

In the second intervention season, the physical therapists registered every training session in which the athletes performed the ACL injury prevention program.

Injuries reported from August 15 to May 31 (the ACL injury prevention program did not start until early August) were included to compare the injury incidence among the three seasons. Injury incidence was calculated as the number of ACL injuries reported per 1,000 hours of athletic activity (competition and/or training, as appropriate).

Statistical Methods To fulfill the compliance requirement, the teams had to have conducted a minimum of 15 ACL injury prevention sessions during the 5- to 7-week period with more than 75% athlete participation. For nominal categorical data, a χ^2 test or Fisher's exact test was used to determine whether there were significant differences among groups. Comparisons of rates were done using Wald's test. An α level of 0.05 was considered as statistically significant.

Study II

All 145 teams in the 16-year-old and 17-year-old divisions from central and eastern Norway as organized by the Norwegian Handball Federation received an invitation to participate in the study during one 8-month season (September 2002 to April 2003). Of these teams, 123 agreed to participate, and were block randomized into an intervention or control group. To reduce potential confounding, the teams were matched by region, playing level, gender, and number of athletes. Teams allocated to the intervention group received a program of warm-up exercises. Teams in the control group were asked to train as usual during the season and would receive the intervention program at the start of the subsequent season.

Intervention The warm-up program was developed by medical staff from the Oslo Sports Trauma Research Center and coaching staff from the Norwegian Handball Federation. Its feasibility had been tested in four teams during the previous season. The program included four different sets of exercises, each of increasing difficulty.

At the start of the league season (September), teams in the intervention group received one visit from an instructor from the handball federation, with a follow-up visit midway through the season (January). The instructors had been familiarized with the program during a 2-hour seminar. The teams received an exercise book, five wobble boards, and five balance mats. The coaches were asked to use the program at the beginning of every training session for 15 consecutive sessions and then once a week during the remainder of the season.

The main focus of the exercises was to improve awareness and control of knees and ankles during standing, running, cutting, jumping, and landing. The program consisted of exercises with the ball, including the use of the wobble board and balance mat during warm-up exercises and for technique, balance, and strength.

The athletes were encouraged to be focused and conscious of the quality of their movements and give emphasis to core stability and position of the hip and knee in relation to the foot (the "knee over toe" position). They were also asked to watch each other closely and give each other feedback during the training. They were instructed to spend 4 to 5 minutes on each exercise group for a total duration of 15 to 20 minutes.

Data on injury and exposure were anonymous and reported by the physiotherapists and confirmed by the coaches.[19]

Outcome Measures The primary outcome was defined as an acute injury to the knee or ankle. A secondary outcome was defined as any injury to the lower limbs. Secondary analyses of injuries overall (including all injuries) and injuries to the upper limb were also included. All injuries reported after an intervention team had completed the first session of the training aiming to prevent injuries (and from the same date in the control teams randomized in the same block) were included to compare the number of injured athletes and the incidence of injury of the intervention and control groups.

Ten research physiotherapists who were blinded to group alloca-

Table 2
Intention to Treat Analysis*

Season	Match						Training					
	Match exposure (hours)		No. of ACL Injuries		Incidence		Training exposure (hours)		No. of ACL Injuries		Incidence	
	All	Elite	All	Elite	All	Elite	All	Elite	All	Elite	All	Elite
Control (1998-1999)	15,547	3,941	23	11	1.48	2.79	193,389	64,491	6	2	0.03	0.03
First Intervention (1999-2000)	14,854	3,822	17	4	1.14	1.05	157,838	48,830	6	2	0.04	0.04
Second Intervention (2000-2001)	12,865	3,822	14	5	1.09	1.31	173,940	67,499	3	0	0.02	0.00

*Total exposure, number of ACL injuries, and injury incidence during matches (including official and unofficial matches) for all divisions (All) and the elite division (Elite) for the control season (1998-1999), the first intervention season (1999-2000), and the second intervention season (2000-2001). Match exposure has been calculated as the number of matches multiplied by the duration of each match multiplied by seven players on each team. The incidence is reported as the number of injuries per 1000 playing hours.
(Adapted with permission from Myklebust G, Engebretsen L, Braekken IH, Skjølberg A, Olsen OE, Bahr R. Prevention of ACL injuries in female team handball players: A prospective intervention study over three seasons. *Clin J Sport Med* 2003;13:71-78.)

tion recorded injuries in both groups, using definitions and a standardized injury questionnaire.[20]

The physiotherapists were in contact with the coaches at least once a month to record injured athletes and exposure data. They interviewed injured athletes, most often within 4 weeks (range, 1 day to 4 months) of injury. The physiotherapists were responsible for approximately the same number of teams from each of the groups (11 to 13 teams each).

The team coaches receiving the intervention recorded compliance on a designated form as the number of injury prevention sessions, the duration of each session in minutes, and the average attendance of the athletes (in percentages). At the end of the season, information was also obtained on prevention training conducted by the control teams, including the types and volume of exercises used.

Statistical Methods The relative risk of the number of injured athletes was used, according to the intention to treat principle, to compare the risk of an injury in the intervention and control groups.

Cox regression analysis was used for the primary and secondary outcomes, taking into account the cluster randomization. The number needed to treat to save one injury was calculated as well as exposures to training and matches and the incidence of injury.

The rate ratio of the two groups (intervention versus control), gender (female versus male), severity of injury (slight, minor, moderate, major), and club activities (match, training) were compared.[19]

Results
Study I
ACL injuries During the control season, there were 29 ACL injuries, whereas 23 injuries occurred during the first intervention season (odds ratio [OR], 0.87 [0.50-1.52]; $P = 0.62$ versus the control season, Wald's test), and 17 injuries occurred during the second intervention season (OR, 0.64 [0.35-1.18]; $P = 0.15$ versus the control season) (Table 2). The corresponding total injury incidence was 0.14 ± 0.05 per 1,000 athlete hours (control season), 0.13 ± 0.06 per 1,000 athlete hours (first intervention season), and 0.09

± 0.06 per 1,000 athlete hours (second intervention season). In the elite division, there were 13 injuries during the control season, 6 injuries during the first intervention season (OR, 0.51 [0.19-1.35]; $P = 0.17$ versus the control season), and 5 injuries in the second intervention season (OR, 0.37 [0.13-1.05]; $P = 0.06$ versus the control season).

Five (7.2%) of the athletes injured the ACL for the second time, and 11 (16%) had injured the ACL in the other knee previously—all while playing team handball. The average age of the injured athletes was 22 years (standard deviation, $\pm$ 4 years).

Compliance With ACL Injury Prevention Program In the 1999-2000 season, 26% of the teams fulfilled the compliance criteria and completed more than 15 ACL injury prevention program sessions with 75% athlete participation. In the elite division, 42% of the teams fulfilled the compliance criteria. In the 2000-2001 season, the overall team compliance for the three divisions was 29%, and 50% in the elite division.

Of the 23 athletes injured during the first intervention season, 11 had

Table 3
Per-Protocol Analysis*

Season	All Divisions					Elite Division				
	No Training		Completed ACL Injury Prevention Program		No. of Injuries	No Training		Completed ACL Injury Prevention Program		No. of Injuries
	Noninjured	Injured	Noninjured	Injured		Noninjured	Injured	Noninjured	Injured	
1998-1999	913	29 (3.1%)			29 (3.1%)	212	13 (6.1%)			13 (6.1%)
2000-2001	631	14 (2.2%)	260	3 (1.1%)†	17 (1.9%)	41	4 (8.9%)	175	1 (0.6%)‡	5 (2.3%)

*The number of ACL injuries for players who did or did not complete the ACL injury prevention program are presented for the entire cohort as well as the elite division separately during for the control season and intervention season II. Compliance during the second intervention season (2000-2001) was determined based on individual weekly reports from the physical therapists. Data on individual compliance were not collected during the first intervention season I (1999-2000).
† Not significant
‡ $P = 0.0134$ (Fisher exact test)
(Adapted with permission from Myklebust G, Engebretsen L, Braekken IH, Skjølberg A, Olsen OE, Bahr R: Prevention of ACL injuries in female team handball players: A prospective intervention study over three seasons. *Clin J Sport Med* 2003;13:71-78.)

performed the program as prescribed, whereas 3 of 17 injured athletes in the second intervention season had followed the program as prescribed. When comparing the risk of injury during the second intervention season (at which time individual training records were collected by the physical therapists) between athletes who did or did not complete the ACL injury prevention program for the entire cohort, there was no difference between compliers and noncompliers (OR, 0.52 [0.15-1.82], $P = 0.31$, Fisher exact test) (Table 3). However, in the elite division, the risk of injury was reduced among those who completed the ACL injury prevention program (OR, 0.06 [0.01-0.54], $P = 0.01$).

Injury Mechanisms Fifty-eight (84%) of the injuries occurred during the attacking phase, and 10 (16%) occurred when performing defensive actions. Fifty-one (74%) of the athletes were handling the ball at the time of injury. Of the injured athletes, 39 (57%) were back players, 19 (28%) were wing players, four (6%) were line players, and five (7%) were goalkeepers.

Thirty-three (48%) of the injuries were reported as contact injuries, and 35 (51%) were reported as noncontact injuries. A reduction in the total number of noncontact injuries was observed from 18 injuries in the control season to 7 injuries in the second intervention season ($P = 0.04$, χ^2 test).

Menstrual History A reliable menstrual history was obtained from 46 of 69 injured athletes; of these, 28 used oral contraception. Of the 46 injured athletes from whom a reliable menstrual history was obtained, 23 (50%) were injured in the menstrual phase, 12 (26%) were injured in the follicular phase, 5 (11%) were injured in the early luteal phase, and 6 (13%) were injured in the late luteal phase ($\chi^2_3 = 17.3$; $P < 0.0001$). Among the 18 injured athletes who did not use oral contraception, 9 (50%) were injured in the menstrual phase, 4 (22%) were injured in the follicular phase, 1 (6%) was injured in the early luteal phase, and 4 (22%) were injured in the late luteal phase ($\chi^2_3 = 7.3$; $P = 0.06$). Of the 28 injured athletes who used oral contraception, 14 (50%) were injured in the menstrual phase, 8 (29%) were injured in the

follicular phase, 4 (14%) were injured in the early luteal phase, and 2 (7%) were injured in the late luteal phase ($\chi^2_3 = 12.0$; $P = 0.018$).

Study II
After exclusions, 61 teams (958 athletes) were included in the intervention group and 59 teams (879 athletes) were included in the control group. Athletes in the two groups were similar in gender distribution, age, and dropout rates.[19] All but eight (13%) of the teams in the intervention group used the program of warm-up exercises to prevent injuries during the study period. Additionally, 13 (22%) of the teams in the control group used specific exercises intended to prevent injuries (including training on the balance mat and wobble board) as a part of training.

Injury Characteristics During the 8-month season, 262 (14%) of the 1,837 athletes who were included in the study had 298 injuries. Of these, 241 (81%) were acute injuries and 57 (19%) were overuse injuries.[19]

Effect of Prevention Significantly fewer injured athletes were in the intervention group than in the control group for injuries overall, lower limb injuries, acute knee or ankle injuries, and acute knee and upper limb injuries, whereas a 37% reduction in acute ankle injuries did not reach significance (Table 1). The degrees of clustering at the team level (intracluster correlation coefficient) were estimated to be 0.043 to 0.071. The number needed to treat to prevent one injury varied from 11 to 59 athletes.

The exposure in hours for the intervention group was 93 to 812 (11 to 210 hours spent in matches, 82 to 602 hours in training); the exposure in hours for the control group was 87 to 483 hours (10 to 783 hours in matches, 76 to 700 hours in training). The incidence of injuries overall, acute injuries, and acute knee or ankle injuries differed significantly when the intervention and control groups were compared. The overall difference in the incidence of match and training injuries was also statistically significant, whereas acute injuries and acute knee or ankle injuries differed only for matches (Table 2). The 13 teams in the control group using training exercises to prevent injuries had a significantly lower incidence of injuries than the teams in the control group that were doing no prevention training (rate ratio: all injuries = 0.48; 95% confidence interval [CI], 0.31 to 0.73; $P < 0.001$) (rate ratio: lower-limb injuries = 0.35; 95% CI, 0.19 to 0.63; $P = 0.001$) (rate ratio: acute injuries = 0.47; 95% CI, 0.29 to 0.76; $P = 0.002$) (rate ratio: acute knee or ankle injuries = 0.22, 95% CI, 0.09 to 0.55; $P = 0.001$). No category of injury differed by gender.

Discussion
Study 1
The main finding of this study was that there was a reduction in the incidence of ACL injuries from the control season to the second intervention season among the elite athletes who completed the training program. A significant reduction in the risk of noncontact ACL injuries was also demonstrated.

Methodologic   Considerations
There are several factors that must be considered when interpreting the results from an intervention study such as this. It was not possible to plan this investigation as a randomized study because the power calculations showed that approximately 2,000 athletes would have been needed to detect a 50% reduction in ACL injuries. Even using a pre-intervention-postintervention comparison, almost every team in the three upper divisions in Norway would have had to be included to achieve adequate statistical power. Teams in the fourth division, the only other group available for inclusion, do not practice sufficiently and play too few matches to have been used.

It could be claimed that the high number of ACL injuries in the control season or the reduction after intervention is a coincidental result of natural variation and that a reduction in the following season could be expected independent of the intervention. Although data were not systematically collected on potential confounding variables such as floor type, shoe type, previous knee injuries, age, or coaching style during the study period, it is unlikely that there were substantial changes that can explain these findings. Prospective studies in Norwegian team handball have showed an increase in the number of ACL injuries from the late 1980s up to the late 1990s, which supports the fact that the intervention was effective among those who performed the intervention exercises. In addition, the study shows a downward trend in the number of injuries during the study period, as compliance seemed to improve.[4,5] In fact, the injury rate observed in the control season, 0.14 ACL injuries per 1,000 hours, is lower than that observed in an earlier study, 0.31 ACL injuries per 1,000 hours.[5]

In any epidemiologic study the reliability of the injury and exposure registration are critical. The present study was performed using a prospective study design, and the teams were requested to report any knee injury as soon as it occurred. In addition, the investigators remained in close contact with the team coaches and physical therapists throughout the study period. Also, the athletes were covered by the compulsory injury insurance policy of the Norges Håndballforbund, and all insurance claims were examined to identify additional ACL injuries. Nonetheless, there is always a possibility that an injury may have been overlooked; however, an ACL injury usually causes pain, swelling, and disability, and it is unlikely that an athlete may have had an injury and was able to continue playing without the need for medical treatment. Moreover, all of the reported ACL injuries were later verified arthroscopically, and reconstructive surgery was performed. It is therefore highly unlikely that false-positive ACL injuries have been recorded during the study period.

With respect to exposure registration, it was not possible to base this on individual attendance records for all practices and matches during the study period. Data on the number of matches were obtained from the coaches and included out-of-season tournaments and training matches, which should ensure good reliability. The training data are based on the average number of training hours per week reported by the coaches. Athlete lists were received from each team, and the exposure registration was adjusted for training attendance.

Effect of the Training Program Although there was a trend toward a reduction in the number of ACL injuries during the three seasons, it was not statistically significant ($P = 0.15$ for all division and $P = 0.06$ for the elite division). However, a statistically significant difference in injury rates in the elite division was observed when data for athletes who completed the program were compared with data for those who did not. It could be argued that there was a selection bias because the teams who completed the program were more conscious of the risk of ACL injuries and therefore behaved differently in other ways as well. However, it is more likely that the teams that completed the program were those that had experienced significant problems with ACL injuries in the past. An ACL injury in team handball typically occurs in a noncontact situation in which the athlete performs a plant-and-cut movement or lands after a jump shot.[21,22] That a decrease in the number of noncontact injuries was demonstrated is promising because the ACL injury prevention program was designed to prevent noncontact injuries.

One explanation for the better results among the elite athletes could be the fact that these athletes have 5 to 10 practice sessions per week and therefore have the opportunity to achieve "enough" ACL injury prevention training to have protective effect. The low compliance in the study was surprising in light of the attention ACL injuries have received from the media and within the handball community.[4,5] Despite the high incidence of ACL injury, the dire future consequences to knee function in injured athletes,[9] and close follow-up of the teams by physical therapists, acceptable compliance was achieved in less than half of the athletes. Athletes may perceive ACL injuries to be less serious than they may be in the long term because they believe (and as is often portrayed in the media) that the only consequence is to undergo surgery and 6 to 9 months of missed participation. Compliance may be improved by communicating more clearly that although the ensuing instability after an ACL injury can be rectified surgically, future normal knee biomechanics and function usually cannot be ensured. The results also demonstrate the importance of recording individual compliance with the training program in a study of this nature.

The findings of this study show that a preventive neuromuscular program works on most elite and perhaps more motivated athletes and that a more intense follow-up is necessary to motivate athletes in the lower divisions to focus on preventive training. Conversely, if the goal is to develop more "ACL-friendly" movements, it may be more effective to educate younger athletes who have not yet established their motion patterns.

Injury Prevention Program The ACL injury prevention program exercises were developed based on the exercises used by Caraffa and associates[12] on different wobble boards. Exercises on a balance mat were also included to further challenge neuromuscular control. In addition, floor exercises were included because they were thought to be applicable to team handball. The focus on the knee position ("knee over toe") was supported by data from Ebstrup and Bojsen-Moller[21] and Olsen and associates.[22] Their video analyses of ACL injuries in team handball athletes indicated that athletes could derive benefit from not letting their knees sag medially or laterally during plant-and-cut movements or when suddenly changing speed. The ACL injury prevention program also emphasizes two-feet landing after jump shots and hip and knee flexion based on volleyball data reported by Hewett and associates.[17] The ACL injury prevention program also aims to influence the athlete's way of performing the two-feet plant-and-cut movement toward a narrower stance as well as the knee-over-toe position. No data have been obtained to detect any changes in technique after the intervention, and such data may be difficult to obtain from mature athletes. In fact, the ACL injury prevention program that was tested is multifaceted and addresses many aspects of risk for injury (agility, balance, awareness of vulnerable knee positions, and playing technique), and it is not possible to determine exactly which part of the program that may be effective in preventing ACL injury. However, educating coaches to teach young athletes a more "ACL-friendly" way of doing the plant-and-cut movement by not allowing their knees to sag medially when cutting and landing may prove beneficial. Further studies are necessary to determine the effects of each program component on injury risk as well as on the potential physiologic risk factors for injury (balance, joint position sense, strength, and muscle recruitment patterns).

When compared with the findings of Caraffa and associates,[12] the results are not impressive, but this difference may be because of differences in gender, sport, level of play, surface, or the use of a different exercise program. It should be noted, however, that no other studies have thus far been able to repeat the results of Caraffa and associates. Soderman and associates[16] showed no effect of wobble board exercises on the incidence of lower extremity injuries in female soccer players. Actually, the intervention group in this study had more ACL injuries than the control group.

Menstrual History The observation of an apparent relationship between menstrual phase and ACL injury risk must be interpreted with caution because it is based on a small number of observations, and hormonal data to confirm menstrual status were not available. Also, the athletes were not followed with a continuous record of menstrual status throughout the study period, and a reliable menstrual history could not be obtained from some athletes. Nonetheless, these results are similar to the results reported in a previous study,[5] and they are in contrast to the results from Wojtys and associates[23] who reported an increased risk of ACL injury during the ovulatory phase. All of these studies should be interpreted with caution, however, because they are small and the menstrual status of the study participants is uncertain. Based on data reported in the study conducted by Wojtys and associates, the authors suggested that the use of oral contraception increases dynamic stability and may reduce the risk of serious knee injury in high-risk athletes.[23] Karageanes and associates[24] found no significant change in ACL laxity during the menstrual cycle and concluded that the menstrual cycle did not affect ACL laxity in adolescent female athletes. Additional studies are therefore necessary to examine this relationship, and although it is conceivable that hor-

monal fluctuations may have effects on ligamentous tissue, convincing evidence to support this hypothesis is not available.

Study II

The rate of injuries in adolescent athletes using a structured warm-up program as a part of a training was shown to have improved clinically and statistically, especially the rate of severe injuries to the knee and ankle. The reduction in the relative risk is highly significant and has been adjusted for the cluster sampling. To our knowledge, our study is the first randomized controlled trial of adolescents athletes with a sufficient sample size to show that acute knee or ankle injuries can be reduced by 50% and severe injuries even more.

Data Validation The randomized controlled trial had good external and internal validity, and the method of injury and exposure registration should ensure good reliability and validity of these data as well as good reliability for comparing the data for the intervention and control groups.

Compliance A considerably higher rate of compliance (87%) occurred among the youth teams compared with the rate of compliance reported in a similar nonrandomized study of adult athletes (29%).[25] The intervention study may have motivated some of the youth teams to include exercises to prevent injuries as part of their training program, as evidenced by the cross-over observed in 22% of the control teams; these teams also had a significantly lower incidence of injuries than the other control teams.

Not all teams continued to use the program of warm-up exercises after the initial intensive introduction period. Because an intention to treat analysis was used in the study,

the effect of the program may therefore be even higher.

Structured Program of Warm-up Exercises to Prevent ACL Injuries The exercises used in the program were developed on the basis of previous intervention studies in team handball[25,26] and other sports,[27-29] and were feasibility tested and modified to be suitable for team handball. The focus on alignment of the hip, knee, and ankle—especially the knee over toe position—was supported by data from Ebstrup and Bojden-Moller[30] and Olsen and associates.[31] The program focused on the proper technique for planting and cutting movements, aiming at a narrower stance as well as a knee-over-toe position. A study that assessed another program of balance and cutting exercises focusing on knee control found that dynamic balance was improved and maintained for at least 12 months.[32] A static balance training program using a balance board has also shown to result in a substantial decrease in the rate of injuries to the ACL.[27]

The prevention program that was tested is multifaceted, and it is not possible to determine exactly which part of the program may be effective. The program also emphasized landing on both legs after jumps rather than just one leg as well as increased hip and knee flexion. The program also included a strength exercise, the "Nordic hamstring lower" exercise. Because the hamstrings can act as agonists to the ACL during stop and jump tasks, it is possible that stronger hamstring muscles can prevent injuries to the ligament; however, this theory has never been tested.

Generalizability Results indicate that youth elite athletes as well as intermediate and recreational athletes would benefit from using the warm-up program to prevent injuries. It is not known whether these results can be generalized to other age groups or to other youth sports such as football, basketball, or volleyball. However, these sports have a high incidence and similar pattern of knee and ankle injuries, and the injury mechanisms are also comparable (most injuries resulting from pivoting and landing movements). It seems reasonable to assume that the prevention program also could be modified for these sports. It is also recommended that programs focusing on technique (cutting and landing movements) and balance training (on wobble boards, mats, or similar equipment) should be implemented in athletes as young as 10 to 12 years (before the athletes have established motion patterns).

Summary

Prevention of ACL injuries is possible with the use of neuromuscular training in female elite team handball athletes, but successful prevention depends on good compliance from the team athletes. Additional research is needed to determine the effect of each component of the training program on neuromuscular function and injury risk. A structured warm-up program designed to improve awareness and knee and ankle control during landing and pivoting movements can help prevent knee and ankle injuries among young athletes. Such programs have been shown to reduce the incidence of knee and ankle injuries by at least 50%.

Acknowledgments

The Oslo Sports Trauma Research Center has been established at the Norwegian University of Sport and Physical Education through generous grants from the Royal Norwegian Ministry of Culture, the Norwegian Olympic Committee and Confederation of Sport, Norwegian Lottery AS, and Pfizer AS. We thank the physical therapists and the athletes who participated in this study. We are grateful for the statistical advice of Ingar Holme, PhD.

References

1. Engstrom B, Johansson C, Tornkvist H: Soccer injuries among elite female players. *Am J Sports Med* 1991;19:372-375.

2. Lindenfeld TN, Schmitt DJ, Hendy MP, Mangine RE, Noyes FR: Incidence of injury in indoor soccer. *Am J Sports Med* 1994;22:364-371.

3. Hippe M, Flint A, Lee R: University basketball injuries: A five-year study of women's and men's varsity teams. *Scand J Med Sci Sports* 1993;3:117-121.

4. Myklebust G, Maehlum S, Engebretsen L, Strand T, Solheim E: Registration of cruciate ligament injuries in Norwegian top level team handball: A prospective study covering two seasons. *Scand J Med Sci Sports* 1997;7:289-292.

5. Myklebust G, Maehlum S, Holm I, Bahr R: A prospective cohort study of anterior cruciate ligament injuries in elite Norwegian team handball. *Scand J Med Sci Sports* 1998;8:149-153.

6. Arendt E, Dick R: Knee injury patterns among men and women in collegiate basketball and soccer: NCAA data and review of literature. *Am J Sports Med* 1995;23:694-701.

7. Roos H, Ornell M, Gardsell P, Lohmander LS, Lindstrand A: Soccer after anterior cruciate ligament injury–an incompatible combination? A national survey of incidence and risk factors and a 7-year follow-up of 310 players. *Acta Orthop Scand* 1995;66:107-112.

8. Daniel DM, Stone ML, Dobson BE, Fithian DC, Rossman DJ, Kaufman KR: Fate of the ACL-injured patient: A prospective outcome study. *Am J Sports Med* 1994;22:632-644.

9. Myklebust G, Bahr R, Engebretsen L, Holm I, Maehlum S: Clinical, functional and radiological outcome 6-11 years after ACL injuries in team handball players: A follow-up study. *Am J Sports Med* 2003;31:981-989.

10. Gillquist J, Messner K: Anterior cruciate ligament reconstruction and the long-term incidence of gonarthrosis. *Sports Med* 1999;27:143-156.

11. Jomha NM, Borton DC, Clingeleffer AJ, Pinczewski LA: Long-term osteoarthritic changes in anterior cruciate ligament reconstructed knees. *Clin Orthop Relat Res* 1999;358:188-193.

12. Caraffa A, Cerulli G, Projetti M, Aisa G, Rizzo A: Prevention of anterior cruciate ligament injuries in soccer: A prospective controlled study of proprioceptive training. *Knee Surg Sports Traumatol Arthrosc* 1996;4:19-21.

13. Bahr R, Bahr IA: Incidence of acute volleyball injuries: a prospective cohort study of injury mechanisms and risk factors. *Scand J Med Sci Sports* 1997;7:166-171.

14. Wedderkopp N, Kaltoft M, Lundgaard B, Rosendahl M, Froberg K: Prevention of injuries in young female players in European team handball: A prospective intervention study. *Scand J Med Sci Sports* 1999;9:41-47.

15. Tropp H, Askling C, Gillquist J: Prevention of ankle sprains. *Am J Sports Med* 1985;13:259-262.

16. Soderman K, Werner S, Pietila T, Engstrom B, Alfredson H: Balance board training: Prevention of traumatic injuries of the lower extremities in female soccer players? A prospective randomized intervention study. *Knee Surg Sports Traumatol Arthrosc* 2000;8:356-363.

17. Hewett TE, Stroupe AL, Nance TA, Noyes FR: Plyometric training in female athletes: Decreased impact forces and increased hamstring torques. *Am J Sports Med* 1996;24:765-773.

18. Hewett TE, Lindenfeld TN, Riccobene JV, Noyes FR: The effect of neuromuscular training on the incidence of knee injury in female athletes: A prospective study. *Am J Sports Med* 1999;27:699-706.

19. Olsen OE, Myklebust G, Engebretsen L, Holme I, Bahr R: Exercises to prevent lower limb injuries in youth sports: A cluster randomized controlled trial. *BMJ* 2005;330:449-452.

20. Olsen OE, Myklebust G, Engebretsen L, Bahr R: Injury pattern in youth team handball: A comparison of two prospective registration methods. *Scand J Med Sci Sports*. in press.

21. Ebstrup JF, Bojsen-Moller F: Anterior cruciate ligament injury in indoor ball games. *Scand J Med Sci Sports* 2000;10:114-116.

22. Olsen OE, Myklebust G, Engebretsen L, Bahr R: Injury mechanisms for anterior cruciate ligament injuries in team handball: A systematic video analysis. *Am J Sports Med* 2004;32:1002-12.

23. Wojtys EM, Huston LJ, Lindenfeld TN, Hewett TE, Greenfield ML: Association between the menstrual cycle and anterior cruciate ligament injuries in female athletes. *Am J Sports Med* 1998;26:614-619.

24. Karageanes SJ, Blackburn K, Vangelos ZA: The association of the menstrual cycle with the laxity of the anterior cruciate ligament in adolescent female athletes. *Clin J Sport Med* 2000;10:162-168.

25. Myklebust G, Engebretsen L, Braekken IH, Skjolberg A, Olsen OE, Bahr R: Prevention of ACL injuries in female team handball players: A prospective intervention study over three seasons.

26. Wedderkopp N, Kaltoft M, Lundgaard B, Rosendahl M, Froberg K: Prevention of injuries in young female players in European team handball: A prospective intervention study. *Scand J Med Sci Sports* 1999;9:41-47.

27. Caraffa A, Cerulli G, Projetti M, Aisa G: Prevention of anterior cruciate ligament injuries in soccer: A prospective controlled study of proprioceptive training. *Knee Surg Sports Traumatol Arthrosc* 1996;4:19-21.

28. Bahr R, Lian O, Bahr IA: A twofold reduction in the incidence of acute ankle sprains in volleyball after the introduction of an injury prevention program: A prospective cohort study. *Scand J Med Sci Sports* 1997;7:172-177.

29. Hewett TE, Lindenfeld TN, Riccobene JV, Noyes FR: The effect of

Clin J Sport Med 2003;13:71-78.

neuromuscular training on the incidence of knee injury in female athletes: A prospective study. *Am J Sports Med* 1999;27:699-706.

30. Ebstrup JF, Bojsen-Moller F: Anterior cruciate ligament injury in indoor ball games. *Scand J Med Sci Sports* 2000;10:114-116.

31. Olsen OE, Myklebust G, Engebretsen L, Bahr R: Injury mechanisms for anterior cruciate ligament injuries in team handball: A systematic video analysis. *Am J Sports Med* 2004;32:1002-1012.

32. Holm I, Fosdahl MA, Friis A, Risberg MA, Myklebust G, Steen H: Effect of neuromuscular training on proprioception, balance, muscle strength, and lower limb function in female team handball players. *Clin J Sport Med* 2004;14:88-94.

Microfracture: Indications, Technique, and Results

Riley J. Williams III, MD

Heather W. Harnly, MD

Abstract

The so-called "marrow stimulating" technique of microfracture uses an awl to penetrate the subchondral bone in cartilage defects. Disruption of the subchondral bone induces fibrin clot formation in the area of the chondral defect. This clot contains pluripotent, marrow-derived mesenchymal stem cells, which are able to differentiate into fibrochondrocytes, resulting in a fibrocartilage repair with varying amounts of type I, II, and III collagen content. Microfracture is a single-stage procedure that is ideally suited for small, well-contained, Outerbridge grade 3 to 4 cartilage lesions. Most clinical studies of the outcomes after microfracture in the knee show improvement in knee function in 70% to 90% of patients. The long-term results vary. Almost all studies report significant improvement in the first year after surgery; some report a decline in activity levels after 1 year, especially in elite athletes. Other studies have shown a continuation of good results for up to 7 years. Recent studies have shown that a body mass index greater than 30 kg/m^2 and incomplete fibrocartilage fill of a lesion as observed on MRI correlate with a poor outcome. The technical simplicity of the procedure, cost-effectiveness, and relatively low patient morbidity make microfracture an invaluable tool for the treatment of small full-thickness cartilage lesions. Microfracture is a good first-line procedure because it does not prevent the application of other cartilage repair procedures that may be needed in the future.

Instr Course Lect 2007;56: 419-428.

Full-thickness chondral defects of the knee, which rarely heal spontaneously, can be devastating injuries, leading to pain, dysfunction, and arthritis.[1] The search for a treatment for these lesions has spurred great surgical innovations over the past few decades. Although several cartilage-restoring procedures such as mosaicplasty, autologous chondrocyte implantation, and synthetic osteochondral plugs have been developed, microfracture remains a first-line technique for the treatment of posttraumatic femoral cartilage defects.

Microfracture is a commonly accepted procedure that is currently in widespread use for the treatment of articular cartilage lesions in the knee. Originally developed in the 1980s, this procedure has also been used to treat articular cartilage lesions in the talus, hip, and shoulder. Despite its widespread use, much is yet to be learned about the best indi-cations, technique, rehabilitation, and basic science behind this procedure.

History

Attempts to "regenerate" cartilage have met with frustration for centuries. In 1743, Hunter stated "ulcerated cartilage is a troublesome thing and that when destroyed, it is not recovered."[2] However, the surgical treatment of osteoarthritis in the 20th century led to some potential solutions. In the 1940s, it was recognized that chondral lesions that involved the subchondral bone filled in with fibrocartilage. Fibrocartilage fill of cartilage defects does provide some symptomatic relief.[3] Haggart[4] and Magnuson[5] described open chondral abrasion procedures for the treatment of degenerative chondral defects. In 1959, Pridie[6] first described the use of subchondral drilling through eburnated bone to stimulate reparative cartilage formation in osteoarthritic knees. These authors reported mixed long-term clinical results.

In 1976, Mitchell and Shepard[7] demonstrated that drilling of osteochondral lesions in adult rabbits resulted in repair tissue, although the early repair tissue deteriorated after 1 year. In the early 1980s, with the advent of arthroscopic techniques, Johnson[8] introduced arthroscopic abrasion arthroplasty, using a burr to remove 1 to 3 mm of subchondral bone. Rodrigo and associates[9] introduced the microfracture technique by combining this use of arthroscopy and selective subchondral bone penetration, which allowed for clot formation and pluripotent stem cell recruitment without destruction of the bony architecture. An awl was used instead of a drill to avoid thermal necrosis of bone. This so-called marrow-stimulating technique was used for the treatment of acute articular cartilage defects in younger patients. The term *microfracture* was coined to describe this technique, and since the description of this method in the 1990s, it has gained widespread clinical use throughout the world.

Incidence of Chondral Lesions

The incidence of symptomatic chondral lesions is not clear. Most studies estimate that approximately 5% to 10% of all patients who present with knee symptoms have a full-thickness cartilage lesion. Curl and associates[10] retrospectively reviewed 31,516 knee arthroscopies of patients in all age groups and reported chondral lesions in 19,827 patients (63%). The incidence of grade IV lesions in patients younger than 40 years, however, was only 5%. Hjelle and associates[11] reviewed 1,000 arthroscopies and reported a similar incidence of grade III and grade IV chondral lesions in patients younger than 40 years (5.3%). Another recent review of 993 knee arthroscopies found an 11% incidence of localized grade III or grade IV cartilage lesions.[12] Of the localized full-thickness lesions, 55% (6% of all knee arthroscopies) were larger than

2 cm^2, warranting treatment in the authors' opinion because of the large size of the observed lesions. All of these studies were retrospective and included symptomatic patients. There are no current data that directly measure the incidence of articular cartilage defects in the asymptomatic population. However, it is clear that full-thickness cartilage defects are a serious clinical problem for the practicing knee surgeon.

Natural History of Chondral Lesions

The natural history of cartilage lesions in the knee is still unknown. It is widely held that such lesions lead to degenerative arthritis of the knee over time. Some of these lesions can be temporarily asymptomatic. However, long-term studies have shown a definitive link between articular cartilage damage and osteoarthritis. Linden[13] followed patients with the diagnosis of osteochondritis dissecans for an average of 33 years and found an accumulative risk with time, as none of the patients had arthritis at age 40 years, but 70% developed arthritis by age 48 years, and 80% by age 60 years. Messner and Maletius[14] reported on 28 young athletes with severe chondral damage, and approximately 50% of the patients had radiographic joint space reduction at 14-year follow-up. In a series published in 2003, Shelbourne and associates[15] reviewed 123 patients with incidental chondral lesions that were discovered at the time of an anterior cruciate ligament reconstruction and were left untreated at the time of surgery. After a mean of 8.7 years, those patients with chondral lesions reported lower subjective scores than those patients who had no such lesions at the time of ACL reconstruction. This finding suggests that even

initially asymptomatic chondral lesions cause symptoms over time. Lateral chondral lesions resulted in worse subjective scores than medial chondral lesions.

Basic Science

Articular (hyaline) cartilage consists of collagen fibrils, proteoglycan aggregates, and interstitial fluid. The matrix is principally made up of type II collagen, but collagen types V, VI, IX, X, XI, XII, and XIV are also present in smaller amounts. Articular cartilage plays an important role in minimizing the magnitude of contact stress on the joint surface and protects the underlying bone structure by permitting smooth, frictionless movement of diarthrodial joints. Chondrocytes are spread throughout the cartilage matrix. These cells are of mesenchymal origin and are responsible for producing and maintaining the matrix.

The response of articular cartilage to injury depends on the severity and depth of the injury. Superficial damage will injure chondrocytes and lead to decreased proteoglycan concentration, increased matrix hydration, and altered fibrillar organization of collagen. Because articular cartilage is avascular, superficial cartilage injuries do not cause hemorrhage or an inflammatory response. Although chondrocytes respond by proliferating and increasing the synthesis of matrix molecules near the injury site, they cannot restore the surface architecture. Thus, superficial cartilage lesions that do not penetrate bone do not heal.

A full-thickness injury, which penetrates the subchondral bone, however, has some healing potential. Disruption of the subchondral bone induces a fibrin clot formation in the area of the chondral defect. This clot contains pluripotent, marrow-derived mesenchymal stem cells. These cells are able to differentiate into fibrochondrocytes and chondrocytes, resulting in fibrocartilage repair with varying amounts of type I, II, and III collagen content.

Fibrocartilage differs from hyaline cartilage in several key ways. Fibrocartilage contains a higher percentage of collagen, but a lower percentage of proteoglycan molecules. Fibrocartilage contains a high proportion of type I collagen, which transforms into coarse fibers. Collagen of this type has a lower compressive stiffness under normal load, inferior resilience, and poorer wear characteristics compared with type II collagen. Over time, the loading of fibrocartilage results in structural disruption and fissure of the repair tissue.

In an adult rabbit model, Mitchell and Shepard[16] showed that drilling initially resulted in a hyaline-like tissue. This reparative tissue lost its hyaline appearance after 8 months, and at 1 year resembled fibrocartilage with apparent surface fibrillation. Another rabbit study helped define the timing of the sequence of events involved in the healing response. Furukawa and associates[17] showed that deep chondral lesions filled with granulation tissue and that the fibroblasts differentiated into chondrocytes by 7 to 10 days after injury. After 3 weeks, type I collagen comprised most of the repair tissue. By 6 to 8 weeks, radiochemical analysis revealed that type II collagen was predominant. In this study, the quality of the cartilage continued to improve up to 1 year; however, because type I collagen persisted, the repair tissue never fully resembled normal articular cartilage.

Many other animal model studies have shown that type II collagen is present in repair tissue after subchondral cartilage injury. Frisbie and associates[18] reported an increase in type II collagen mRNA expression 6 weeks after microfracture of a cartilage defect compared with control defects without microfracture in equine knees. No significant difference in the expression of other matrix mRNA or protein levels, including type II collagen protein, was noted in the first 8 weeks after microfracture.

Frisbie and associates[19] also used an equine model to study the healing response in articular cartilage after microfracture over a longer period. Chondral defects were created and half were treated with microfracture and half were untreated controls. These samples were examined at 4 and 12 months postoperatively. On gross examination, a greater volume of repair tissue filled the defects after microfracture (74% fill versus 45% fill). Histologically, no difference in relative amounts of different tissue types was observed; all of the samples consisted of a combination of fibrous tissue, fibrocartilage, and small amounts of hyaline cartilage. More type II collagen was found in the 12-month samples compared to the 4-month samples (56% versus 21%).

Gill and associates[20] examined the extent and time course of chondral defect healing after microfracture in a primate model. Full-thickness defects were created in the knees of macaque monkeys and treated with microfracture. The limbs were cast in flexion for 2 weeks postoperatively. After removal of the casts, the animals were allowed to bear weight as tolerated. Evaluation of the defects at 6 and 12 weeks with gross and microscopic examination revealed poor repair at 6 weeks, but marked improvement

at 12 weeks postoperatively. At 6 weeks, the defects had only a thin layer of fibroblastic repair tissue at the base. By 12 weeks, the condylar defects showed 100% filling with hyaline-like tissue. The authors concluded that the repair after microfracture takes longer than 6 weeks and postoperative weight-bearing in the clinical setting may need to be delayed longer than 6 weeks.

In a clinical study on second-look arthroscopies, Gobbi and associates[21] took tissue samples from 10 patients. Histologically, the samples revealed areas of fibromyxoid tissue with differentiation, a transition zone with some cartilage tissue, and areas with initial hyaline transformation, which were described as fibrocartilaginous hybrid tissue. This was supported by a recent clinical study by Knutsen and associates,[22] who performed arthroscopy with biopsy 2 years after microfracture and found that 39% of the biopsy specimens had at least some hyaline cartilage present, whereas 43% had fibrocartilage throughout most of the depth.

Animal and clinical studies have shown that microfracture produces fibrocartilage repair with varying amounts of type I and type II collagen with greater fill than in controls. This process takes at least 6 weeks to 4 months to mature. Because the repair tissue does not fully resemble normal hyaline cartilage, it is prone to fibrillation and breakdown after 1 year or longer.

Indications

Microfracture is a single-stage procedure that is ideally suited for the treatment of small, well-contained, Outerbridge grade 3 to 4 cartilage lesions. The technical simplicity of the procedure, cost-effectiveness,

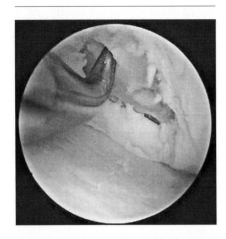

Figure 1 Intraoperative photograph of a full-thickness chondral lesion immediately before penetration of the subchondral bone during a microfracture procedure. Penetrating awls are used to create vascular access channels.

and relatively low patient morbidity make microfracture an invaluable tool for the treatment of small full-thickness cartilage lesions. It is an excellent first-line procedure because it does not prevent the application of other cartilage repair procedures that may be needed in the future.

The size of the cartilage lesion that is best treated with microfracture is controversial. There are few comparison studies in the literature to help provide the appropriate guidelines. Animal and cadaver studies have helped determine a minimum lesion size for treatment. Guettler and associates[23] reported a critical lesion size of 10 mm diameter (0.79 cm^2) over which defect rim stresses increase significantly. They postulated that size of the femoral condyle and shear stress may also play a significant role in lesion progression. Jackson and associates[24] found progressive deterioration of osteochondral defects in a goat model, with defects measuring 6 mm in diameter and depth. These investigators described a zone of in-fluence surrounding the lesion, with collapse of the surrounding area of articular cartilage and subchondral bone. These studies demonstrate that lesions smaller than 6 to 10 mm may be stable, whereas larger lesions are at risk of progression.

Clinical studies have shown poorer outcomes in patients with lesions larger than 2 cm^2 (400 mm^2), suggesting an upper limit of size for treatment with microfracture.[22,25] Most surgeons are willing to attempt using microfracture to treat larger lesions, especially in lower-demand patients, but with expectations of the possibility of poorer outcomes. Microfracture, however, is not recommended for lesions larger than 10 cm^2.

Recently published data also demonstrated the clinical importance of body mass index on functional outcome. In particular, a high body mass index (> 30 kg/m^2) was associated with a significantly poor functional outcome after microfracture, which suggests that high body mass index may be a relative contraindication for microfracture repair in the knee.[3]

Technique

The microfracture technique developed by Steadman and associates[26] is recommended. A well-padded pneumatic tourniquet is applied to the patient's upper thigh, but it is not typically inflated. A comprehensive diagnostic arthroscopic examination of the knee is performed. Other intra-articular procedures should be performed before the microfracture, such as meniscal débridement, meniscal repair, or anterior cruciate ligament reconstruction. Once the microfracture holes are created, blood and fat emanating from them may obscure arthroscopic visualization.

The initial step consists of a thorough débridement of the cartilage lesion back to stable margins and a careful removal of the calcified layer of cartilage. It is important to avoid violation of the subchondral plate when completing any deep débridement. Débridement typically is performed with an arthroscopic shaver and handheld curet. The aggressive use of a motorized burr is not recommended because of the risk of removing excessive amounts of bone.

An arthroscopic awl is then used to make multiple holes in the defect 3 to 4 mm apart to a maximal depth of 5 mm (Figure 1). Care is taken to appropriately position and space the holes to maintain a subchondral bone bridge between them, ensuring subchondral plate integrity. Various angled awls can be used to assist in ensuring that the holes are perpendicular to the joint surface. Once the holes are made, the arthroscopic pump pressure is decreased to visualize the blood and fat droplets emanating from the holes (Figure 2). The tourniquet, if used, is deflated, and suction is applied at this time. A drain should not be used because the success of the procedure relies on the formation of a clot in the defect. A routine second-look arthroscopy is not necessary because postoperative MRI with cartilage sequencing provides an excellent evaluation of the percentage of lesion fill and has the added advantage of evaluating the underlying subchondral plate with respect to integrity and overgrowth (Figure 3).

Rehabilitation

Chondrocytes are sensitive to pressure and deformation. Continuous passive motion (CPM) may help stimulate chondrocyte matrix production. Motion likely has a molding effect, shaping the newly formed

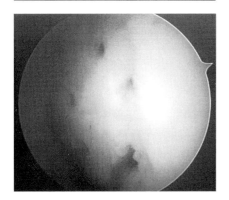

Figure 2 Intraoperative photograph of a full-thickness chondral lesion that has been treated using the microfracture technique. The vascular access channels are created around the lesion's periphery initially. Note the confirmation of bleeding through the channels that is observed following a decrease in the intra-articular pressure.

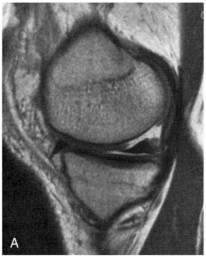 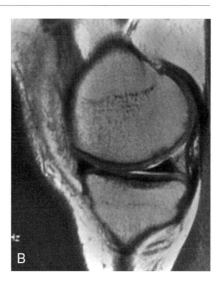

Figure 3 Sagittal fast spin-echo MRI scans of the knee of a 30-year-old patient with a full-thickness lesion of the medial femoral condyle obtained before microfracture (**A**) and 4 months after microfracture (**B**), demonstrating moderate fill of the defect with hyperintense repair tissue signal and smooth peripheral integration. (Reproduced with permission from Mithoefer K, Williams RJ, Warren RF, et al: The microfracture technique for the treatment of articular cartilage lesions in the knee. *J Bone Joint Surg Am* 2005;87:1911-1920.)

repair tissue to conform to the remaining articular surface. Weight bearing, especially in the first 6 weeks after surgery, can cause potential propagation of the microfractures or collapse of the subchondral plate. Shear forces or excessive pressure in this early phase can flatten the repair cartilage or displace the mesenchymal cells and clot from the defect.

A postoperative regimen that includes no weight bearing with crutches for 6 to 8 weeks is recommended. Partial weight bearing may be implemented over a 2-week period and full weight bearing allowed subsequently. CPM should be initiated in the recovery room and continue for 6 to 8 hours a day for 6 weeks. Range-of-motion exercise should be started at 0° to 60° and increased approximately 10° per day until full range of motion is achieved. Cryotherapy (using ice packs or the Cryo Cuff [Aircast, Boca Raton, FL]) should be initiated in the recovery room. A femoral nerve block, although not always necessary, can be helpful for relieving excessive postoperative pain.

The use of CPM postoperatively is largely based on the rabbit model findings of Salter[27] that showed more rapid and complete metaplasia of healing tissue within articular cartilage defects when CPM was used. Rodrigo and associates[9] retrospectively compared a group of patients who used postoperative CPM for 6 to 8 hours a day for approximately 8 weeks after microfracture and a group of patients who were not able to comply with the CPM recommendations. Seventy-seven patients comprised the cohort for this study. Of this cohort, 46 patients were able to comply with CPM recommendations and 31 were not. At second-look arthroscopy, the cartilage repair was visually graded from 1 to 5. The authors found a mean improvement in grade of 2.67 for patients in the CPM group versus 1.67 in the non-CPM group.[9] It should be noted that the arthroscopic assessments of the cartilage repair tissue were performed by the authors of the study, and were not blinded. Forty-five percent of the patients in the non-CPM group had no improvement in grade after microfracture. There was no change in improvement based on the age of the patient, lesion size, or location. The authors did not assess functional outcome in this study.

Although most surgeons use the postoperative regimen originally described by Steadman, at least one study suggests that no weight bearing and CPM may not affect outcome. Marder and associates[28] retrospectively reviewed the outcomes of 50 patients who were treated with microfracture for isolated chondral defects. Twenty-five patients underwent microfracture performed by a senior surgeon who used CPM and touchdown weight bearing for 6 weeks postoperatively. The other 25 patients underwent microfracture performed by another surgeon who did not use CPM and allowed full weight bearing as tolerated postoperatively. Among the 43 patients who were available for 2-year follow-up, no significant differences in pain scores, radiographs, Lysholm scores, or Tegner scores were noted between the two groups. Although this study was limited by the small number of patients and short follow-up, these findings suggest that the postoperative course may not affect outcome as much as other factors.

Isometric exercises and dynamic quadriceps training should start in supervised physical therapy during the first postoperative week. Water-based exercises should be started at 2 weeks postoperatively; patients should be allowed to begin riding a stationary bicycle as soon as range of motion permits. Resistance exercises should be started at 6 weeks postoperatively. Linear running and jumping should be restricted until at least 4 months postoperatively. Quadriceps and core strength must be adequate before running is resumed. Pivoting and sports-related activities, including contact sports, can usually be allowed between 6 and 8 months postoperatively.

Results

Most clinical studies of the outcomes after microfracture in the knee show improvement in knee function in 70% to 90% of patients[3,21,22,25-31] (Table 1). Long-term results vary. Almost all studies report significant clinical improvement in the first year after surgery. Some studies report a decline in activity levels after 1 to 2 years, especially in elite athletes.[21,32] Other studies have shown good results at up to 7-year follow-up.

Steadman and associates[29] reviewed the long-term results (average follow-up, 11 years) after microfracture. The cohort of 71 knees was limited to patients age 45 years and younger with isolated traumatic chondral defects. The average Lysholm score improved from 59 before surgery to 89 at final follow-up. The average Tegner activity level improved from 3 before surgery to 6 at final follow-up. Age older than 35 years was a negative predictor. Statistically, the lesion size did not affect outcome. Using Western Ontario and McMaster Universities Osteoarthritis Index pain scores, 23 knees were pain free, 38 had mild pain, and 10 had moderate pain at final follow-up. Overall, the most improvement occurred during the first year after surgery, but improvement continued for 2 to 3 years postoperatively. Little change was reported from postoperative years 2 to 7 with regard to a patient's ability to perform activities of daily living, sports, and strenuous work.

Gobbi and associates[21] also reported long-term results (mean follow-up, 6 years). They found improvement in the athletes who were treated, but a decline in sports participation over time. They used microfracture to treat chondral lesions in 53 athletes (26 professional athletes and 27 recreational athletes) with an average age of 38 years. Lysholm scores improved from 57 preoperatively to 87 postoperatively. Subjective ratings (maximum score, 100) were 40 before surgery and 70 at final follow-up. Seventy percent of the patients had improvement in knee pain and swelling, normal functional testing, and normal or near-normal International Knee Documentation Committee form scores. The average Tegner activity level in all patients was 3.2 before

surgery, peaked at 6.0 at 2 years after surgery, and declined to 5.0 at final follow-up. Participation in strenuous sports activities increased after surgery in 80% of patients at 2 years, but gradually decreased to 55% of patients at final follow-up.

Blevins and associates assessed functional and arthroscopic improvement in a group of young athletes (48 highly competitive athletes and 188 recreational athletes).[30] The greatest improvement in functional scores occurred in the first postoperative year in both groups. The scores did not continue to increase over the next 4 to 5 years, but no deterioration was seen. Seventy-seven percent of the highly competitive athletes returned to competition. Two thirds of these athletes reported that they were able to perform at a level equal or superior to their preinjury level. Half of the professional athletes were still competing 3 years after undergoing microfracture. Steadman and associates[31] reported results using microfracture to treat chondral injuries in 25 National Football League players, 19 of whom returned to play the season after the surgery. At an average 4.5-year follow-up, the average Lysholm score improved from 52 before surgery to 90 postoperatively. Pain, swelling, and functional level also improved significantly.

Miller and associates[25] also reviewed the outcomes of microfracture for isolated degenerative chondral lesions in patients who were 40 to 70 years of age. At an average 2.6-year follow-up, the average Lysholm score improved from 54 preoperatively to 83, and the average Tegner activity score improved from 2.9 preoperatively to 4.5. There was, however, a higher complication rate in this group; 13 (15.5%) of the 81 patients in this cohort required a

Table 1 Summary of Microfracture Clinical Outcome Studies

Author(s)/Year	Patient Population	No of Patients	Mean Patient Age (years)	Average Follow-Up (years)	Results
Blevins et al[30] (1998)	Group A (professional athletes) Group B (recreational athletes)	Group A: 48 Group B: 188	Group A: 26 (range, 13-58) Group B: 38 (range, 15-68)	Group A: 3.7 (range, 1-7) Group B: 4.0 (range, 1-7)	77% of group A returned to competition Pain scores improved in both groups, with greatest improvement in first postoperative year and then plateaued for the next 4 to 5 years
Steadman et al[31] (2003)	National Football League players	25	29 (range, 22-36)	4.5 (range, 2-13)	76% returned to football the next season Those who returned completed an average of 4.6 seasons (range, 1 to 13 seasons) Average Lysholm score increased from 52 to 90
Steadman et al[29] (2003)	Patients with traumatic chondral defects	71	30.4 (range, 13-45)	11.3 (range, 7-17)	Average Lysholm score was 88.9 Average Tegner score was 5.8 Most increases in scores were seen in first year postoperatively No decline occurred with time
Miller et al[25] (2004)	Patients with degenerative lesions	81	49 (range, 40-70)	2.6 (range, 2-5)	Average Lysholm score increased from 53.8 to 83.1 Average Tegner score increased from 2.9 to 4.5 15.5% of patients required surgery for lysis of adhesions 5.9% required revision microfracture or total knee arthroplasty
Knutsen et al[22] (2004)	Patients with a single symptomatic cartilage defect	80 (40 underwent ACI and 40 underwent microfracture)	ACI group: 33.3 Microfracture group: 31.1	2	Prospective, randomized study comparing ACI to microfracture No significant difference in Lysholm scores between the two groups 78% of patients who underwent ACI had less pain at 2-year follow-up, whereas 75% of patients who underwent microfracture had less pain at 2-year follow-up Patients younger than 30 years in both groups had significantly better clinical outcomes
Gobbi et al[21] (2005)	Athletes	53	38 (range, 19-55)	6 (range, 3-10)	Average Lysholm score increased from 56.8 to 87.2 Average Tegner score improved from 3.2 to 6 At final follow-up, 80% of patients showed decline in sports activity level to Tegner score of 5
Mithoefer et al[3] (2005)	Patients with isolated traumatic chondral defects	48	41 (range, 16-60)	3.4 (range, 2-4.5)	67% good/excellent, 25% fair, and 8% poor results 69% had decline in scores after 2 years MRI fill percentage correlated to outcome Body mass index > 30 kg/m^2 correlated to worse fill and worse outcome

ACI = autologous chondrocyte implantation

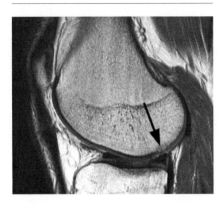

Figure 4 Sagittal fast spin-echo MRI scan obtained 12 months after microfracture treatment of a cartilage defect of the lateral femoral condyle, demonstrating prominent osseous overgrowth of the subchondral bone (*arrow*) with resultant relative thinning of the overlying repair cartilage. (Reproduced with permission from Mithoefer K, Williams RJ, Warren RF, et al: The microfracture technique for the treatment of articular cartilage lesions in the knee. *J Bone Joint Surg Am* 2005;87:1911-1920.)

manipulation after the microfracture procedure. The failure rate, defined as subsequent procedures, was also higher; five patients (5.9%) had either revision microfracture or total knee arthroplasty within 3 years of the index microfracture. There was a trend toward lower Lysholm scores in patients with lesions larger than 400 mm^2 and in patients with lesions on adjacent articular surfaces.

Mithoefer and associates[3] reported on 48 symptomatic patients with isolated full-thickness articular cartilage defects of the femur that were treated with the microfracture technique. At a minimum 24-month follow-up, knee function was rated good to excellent in 32 patients (67%), fair in 12 (25%), and poor in 4 (8%). A lower body mass index correlated with higher scores for the activities of daily living and the physical component of the Med-

ical Outcomes Study 36-Item Short-Form Health Survey (SF-36), whereas the poorest results occurred in patients with a body mass index greater than 30 kg/m^2.

This study also demonstrated a correlation between outcome and percentage fill of the defect as determined by MRI. MRI in 24 knees demonstrated good repair tissue fill in the defect in 13 patients (54%), moderate fill in 7 (29%), and poor fill in 4 (17%). The fill grade correlated with the knee function scores. All knees with good fill demonstrated improved knee function, whereas poor fill grade was associated with limited improvement and decreasing functional scores at 24-month follow-up. However, despite incomplete filling, all patients with a fill volume of more than two thirds of the defect demonstrated significant improvement in knee function after microfracture. This finding suggests that complete filling of the lesion may not be necessary, at least for short-term functional improvement, but more complete fill of the lesion increases the likelihood of clinical improvement. In a second study, these same authors analyzed outcomes of the microfracture technique in a group of high-impact athletes.[32] At a mean follow-up of 41 months, only 66% of athletes reported good or excellent results. Furthermore, only 44% of these patients could ultimately participate in high-impact sports. The authors found that age younger than 40 years, symptom duration less than 12 months, and lesion size less than 200 m^2 correlated with higher clinical outcomes.[32]

Osseous overgrowth following microfracture has not been well described in other studies. This phenomenon was observed in 25% of the patients who underwent MRI in

this study[3] (Figure 4). This overgrowth is believed to result from metaplasia of the deep layer of the repair cartilage after microfracture stimulation. MRI studies in this series demonstrated that osseous overgrowth results in a relative thinning of the overlying repair cartilage, which may have negative biomechanical implications for the repair cartilage and its function and durability.

Only a handful of randomized prospective studies comparing the outcome of microfracture with other techniques have been completed to date. Knutsen and associates[22] compared autologous chondrocyte implantation with microfracture in a prospective randomized study of 80 patients. This well-designed study used a blinded, independent observer and included arthroscopic and histologic outcomes in addition to Lysholm, Tegner, and SF-36 subjective scores. They found that at 2 years postoperatively, the SF-36 physical component scores were significantly better in the microfracture group than in the autologous chondrocyte implantation group. Pain was significantly reduced in both groups, with 78% of the patients treated with autologous chondrocyte implantation and 75% of those treated with microfracture reporting less pain at 2 years follow-up. Younger and more active patients had better outcomes in both groups. With regard to arthroscopic and histologic findings at follow-up, there was no statistically significant difference between the groups, although there was a tendency for autologous chondrocyte implantation to result in more hyaline repair cartilage as assessed by histologic analysis. Conversely, Mosely and associates[33] demonstrated that patients who underwent autologous chondrocyte implantation had greater improvements in their clinical outcome scores in comparison with the patients who underwent microfracture.

Some early research in the use of specific scaffolds and growth factors for stimulating stem cells to improve the natural repair response has been promising, but the results of clinical studies are still pending. It is not yet known whether better quality of repair tissue will make a significant difference in clinical outcomes. To date, no single technique for treating isolated chondral lesions stands out as better than another. No long-term randomized findings have been published to confirm the benefit of replacing articular cartilage with hyaline cartilage rather than fibrocartilage. Although many studies focus on repair methods for symptomatic cartilage defects, interpretation of these results are difficult, because many of these studies include patients who have also undergone other procedures (osteotomy, ligament reconstruction). Prospective randomized studies in this area are needed in order to develop a better understanding of the correct approach to cartilage restoration.

Summary

Microfracture remains an important first-line technique for treating chondral lesions in the knee. The simplicity and low cost of the procedure in comparison with osteoarticular allograft/autograft transplants and autologous chondrocyte implantation, along with reports of good outcomes in 70% to 85% of patients in clinical studies, support the continued use of microfracture as a first-line cartilage repair procedure. However, surgeons must consider certain parameters such as lesion size, body mass index, and rehabili-

tation compliance as indications for surgery. Surgeons also have new tools, such as MRI criteria of lesion fill, to aid in critically analyzing the outcomes of the microfracture technique. Lesion fill correlates with good outcome; as such, MRI can be used to assess this repair method and help the orthopaedic surgeon to make clinical decisions based on this valuable information.[3]

References

1. 1.Hunziker E: Articular cartilage repair: Basic science and clinical progress. A review of the current status and prospects. *Osteoarthritis Cartilage* 2002;10:432-463.

2. Hunter W: Of the structure and disease of articulating cartilages. *Clin Orthop Relat Res* 1995;317:3-6.

3. Mithoefer K, Williams RJ, Warren RF, et al: The microfracture technique for treatment of articular cartilage lesions of the knee: A prospective cohort study. *J Bone Joint Surg Am* 2005;87:1911-1920.

4. Haggart GE: The surgical treatment of degenerative arthritis of the knee joint. *J Bone Joint Surg Am* 1940;22:717-729.

5. Magnuson PB: Joint debridement surgical treatment of degenerative arthritis. *Surg Gyn Obstet* 1941;73:1-9.

6. Pridie KH: A method of resurfacing osteoarthritic knee joints. *J Bone Joint Surg Br* 1959;41:618-619.

7. Mitchell N, Shepard N: The resurfacing of adult rabbit articular cartilage by multiple perforations through the subchondral bone. *J Bone Joint Surg Am* 1976;58:230-233.

8. Johnson LL: Arthroscopic abrasion arthroplasty historical and pathologic perspective: Present status. *Arthroscopy* 1986;2:54-69.

9. Rodrigo JJ, Steadman JR, Silliman JF, Fulston HA: Improvement of full-thickness chondral defect healing in the human knee after debridement and microfracture using continuous passive motion. *Am J Knee Surg* 1994;7:109-116.

10. Curl WW, Krome J, Gordon ES, Rushing J, Smith BP, Poehling GG: Cartilage injuries: A review of 31,516 knee arthroscopies. *Arthroscopy* 1997;13:456-460.

11. Hjelle K, Solheim E, Strand T, Muri R, Brittberg M: Articular cartilage defects in 1000 knee arthroscopies. *Arthroscopy* 2002;18:730-734.

12. Aroen A, Loken S, Heir S, et al: Articular cartilage lesions in 993 consecutive knee arthroscopies. *Am J Sports Med* 2004;32:211-215.

13. Linden B: Osteochondritis dissecans of the femoral condyles. *J Bone Joint Surg Am* 1977;59:769-776.

14. Messner K, Maletius W: The long-term prognosis for severe damage to weight-bearing cartilage in the knee. *Acta Orthop Scand* 1996;67:165-168.

15. Shelbourne KD, Jari S, Gray T: Outcome of untreated traumatic articular cartilage defects of the knee: A natural history study. *J Bone Joint Surg Am* 2003;85(suppl 2):8-16.

16. Mitchell N, Shepard N: The resurfacing of adult rabbit articular cartilage by multiple perforations through the subchondral bone. *J Bone Joint Surg Am* 1976;58:230-233.

17. Furukawa T, Eyre DR, Koide S, Glimcher MJ: Biomechanical studies on repair cartilage resurfacing experimental defects in the rabbit knee. *J Bone Joint Surg Am* 1980;62:79-89.

18. Frisbie DD, Oxford J, Southwood L, et al: Early events in cartilage repair after subchondral bone microfracture. *Clin Orthop Relat Res* 2003;407:215-227.

19. Frisbie DD, Trotter G, Powers BE, et al: Arthroscopic subchondral bone plate microfracture technique augments healing of large chondral defects in the radial carpal bone and medial femoral condyle of horses. *Vet Surg* 1999;28:242-255.

20. Gill TJ, McCulloch PC, Glasson SS, Blanchet T, Morris EA: Chondral defect repair after the microfracture procedure. *Am J Sports Med* 2005;33:680-685.

21. Gobbi A, Nunag P, Malinowski K: Treatment of full thickness chondral lesions of the knees with microfracture in a group of athletes. *Knee Surg Sports Traumatol Arthrosc* 2005;13:213-221.

22. Knutsen G, Engebretsen L, Ludvigsen T, et al: Autologous chondrocyte implantation compared with microfracture in the knee: A randomized trial. *J Bone Joint Surg Am* 2004;86:455-464.

23. Guettler JH, Demetropoulos CK, Yang KH, Jurist KA: Osteochondral defects in the human knee: Influence of defect size on cartilage rim stress and load

redistribution to surrounding cartilage. *Am J Sports Med* 2004;32:1451-1458.

24. Jackson DW, Lalor PA, Aberman HM, Simon TM: Spontaneous repair of full thickness defects of articular cartilage in a goal model. *J Bone Joint Surg Am* 2001;83:53-64.

25. Miller BS, Steadman JR, Briggs KK, Rodrigo JJ, Rodkey WG: Patient satisfaction and outcome after microfracture of the degenerative knee. *J Knee Surg* 2004;17:13-17.

26. Steadman JR, Rodkey WG, Singleton SB, Briggs KK: Microfracture technique for full-thickness chondral defects: Technique and clinical results. *Oper Tech Orthop* 1997;7:300-304.

27. Salter RB: The biologic concept of continuous passive motion of synovial joints: The first 18 years of basic research and its clinical application. *Clin Orthop Relat Res* 1989;242:12-25.

28. Marder RA, Hopkins G, Timmerman LA: Arthroscopic microfracture of chondral defects of the knee: A comparison of two postoperative treatments. *Arthroscopy* 2005;21:152-158.

29. Steadman JR, Briggs KK, Rodrigo JJ, Kocher MS, Gill TJ, Rodkey WG: Outcomes of microfracture for traumatic chondral defects of the knee: Average 11-year follow-up. *Arthroscopy* 2003;19:477-484.

30. Blevins FT, Steadman JR, Rodrigo JJ, Silliman J: Treatment of articular cartilage defects in athletes: An analysis of functional outcome and lesion appearance. *Orthopedics* 1998;21:761-768.

31. Steadman JR, Miller BS, Karas SG, Schlegel TF, Briggs KK, Hawkins RJ: The microfracture technique in the treatment of full-thickness chondral lesions of the knee in National Football League players. *J Knee Surg* 2003;16:83-86.

32. Mithoefer K, Williams RJ 3rd, Warren RF, Wickiewicz TL, Marx RG: High-impact athletics after knee articular cartilage repair: A prospective evaluation of the microfracture technique. *Am J Sports Med* 2006;34:1413-1418.

33. Mosely JB, Anderson A, Browne JE: A controlled study of autologous chondrocyte implantation versus microfracture for articular cartilage lesions of the femur, in *Proceedings from the Annual Meeting of the Arthroscopy Association of North America*, 2003.

Autologous Chondrocyte Implantation

Deryk G. Jones, MD

Lars Peterson, MD, PhD

Abstract

Injuries to joint surfaces can result from acute high-impact or repetitive shear and torsional loads to the superficial zone of the articular cartilage architecture. The use of autologous chondrocyte implantation is promising and is associated with several potential long-term benefits. Proper patient selection and education are important factors for success.

Instr Course Lect 2007;56:429-445.

Direct arthroscopic visualization has suggested that the prevalence of isolated, focal articular cartilage defects is approximately 5%.[1,2] In a retrospective review of more than 31,000 arthroscopic procedures, Curl and associates[1] found a 63% prevalence of chondral lesions with an average of 2.7 lesions per knee. Older patients had more lesions. Curl and associates found grade IV lesions (according to a modification of the Outerbridge classification system[3]) in 20% of the patients, but only 5% of the individuals who had such a lesion were younger than 40 years. Three of four of the patients had a solitary lesion. A prospective study demonstrated chondral or osteochondral lesions in 61% of the patients, whereas focal defects were found in 19%;[2] these percentages are similar to those found in the retrospective analysis.[1] In the prospective assessment, the mean defect size was 2.1 cm^2. A single, well-defined International Cartilage Repair Society (ICRS) grade III or IV defect[4] (at least 1 cm^2) accounted for 5.3%, 6.1%, and 7.1% of the arthroscopic procedures in patients younger than 40, 45, and 50 years old, respectively.[2] The prevalence of articular lesions secondary to work-related and sports activities has been reported to be as high as 22% to 50% in other studies.[5,6] Such injuries alone or in combination with ligamentous instability, meniscal lesions, or mechanical malalignment can be debilitating.

Articular cartilage is an avascular, aneural tissue that has limited repair capabilities compared with other mesenchymal tissues. Chondrocytes also have limited migratory ability and, as a result, the surrounding normal cartilage cells do not fill the defect. Chondrocytes have a transient but insufficient response to injury.[7] They increase their mitotic activity as well as their production of glycosaminoglycan and collagen but only for a short period of time and to a limited degree. Normal articular cartilage has only a few cells, which exist in isolated cell lacunae within the extracellular matrix, further decreasing the healing potential of articular cartilage. These factors in combination with the continued use of the extremity by the individual, producing repetitive compressive and shear forces, create an extremely poor environment for spontaneous repair.

When the injury extends through the subchondral bone and causes bleeding, multipotential mesenchymal stem cells are allowed to fill the articular cartilage defect. Fibrocartilage is produced, but this tissue lacks the biomechanical properties required to protect the underlying subchondral bone, especially in a high-demand patient.[8,9] When the defect is large, the normal articular cartilage no longer protects the subchondral bone at the base of the lesion from direct injury (Figure 1). Exposure of the subchondral bone to repetitive axial and shear forces leads to progressive pain and disability, especially in a high-demand patient.

Several techniques have been used to improve the repair potential of articular cartilage by implanting other cell or tissue phenotypes that have chondrogenic potential.[10-14]

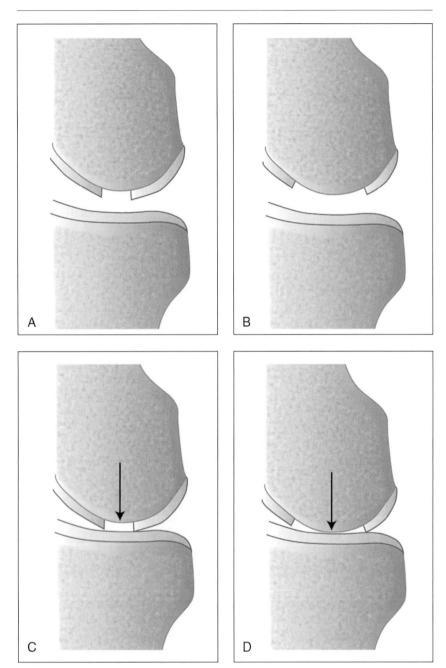

Figure 1   Schematic representation of the loading of focal femoral condyle defects. Small lesions (**A** and **C**) are well contained and protect the tibial surface during activity and movement of the joint. Larger lesions (**B** and **D**) expose the subchondral bone and the margins of the lesion to the tibial articular surface, with a resulting increase in rates of cartilage wear as well as mechanical symptoms and pain.

dure is called autologous chondrocyte implantation.

Indications

Autologous chondrocyte implantation is ideally suited for symptomatic ICRS grade III and IV lesions along the femoral condyle or trochlear regions.[16,17] High-demand patients between 15 and 55 years of age with excellent motivation and potential for compliance are the best candidates. Studies[18,19] have shown a mosaicplasty or microfracture to be an acceptable initial procedure for a lesion of <2 cm². However, autologous chondrocyte implantation is a viable option for a symptomatic patient with a lesion of >2 cm² but ≤12 cm² and for a patient who continues to have pain after a mosaicplasty or microfracture procedure. Bone involvement is not a contraindication, but staged or concomitant autologous bone grafting should be undertaken when the bone involvement is deeper than 6 to 8 mm.[20]

Although the senior author (L.P.) has had experience, and some success, with autologous chondrocyte implantation in some high-demand patients with reciprocal or "kissing" lesions, such lesions are currently considered a contraindication for the technique.[21,22] Surgeons are increasingly using autologous chondrocyte implantation to repair patellar lesions. Although the initial results were not as successful in this region, the concomitant use of tibial tubercle osteotomy and anteromedialization has improved patient outcomes.[23,24]

Preoperative Assessment

To identify appropriate candidates for autologous chondrocyte implantation, all factors that could compromise successful healing of the im-

Grande and associates[15] reported the successful repair of full-thickness cartilage defects following implantation of cultured articular chondrocytes in a rabbit model. On the basis of these promising results, the technique was first used on humans in 1987 and was termed autologous chondrocyte transplantation. In the United States and most of Europe, implantation has been substituted for transplantation and the proce-

plant should be recognized and corrected in a staged or concomitant manner. Key factors to consider while evaluating patients are physiologic age, desired postoperative activity level, etiology, potential for postoperative compliance, and social factors that can delay treatment and complicate postoperative physical therapy regimens such as strenuous postoperative work conditions and limitation of the time that the patient will be allowed off from work. Physical examination should focus on gait status, knee alignment, and body mass index. Weight reduction should be an integral component of the preoperative program. A lower body mass index has been correlated with higher scores for activities of daily living as well as better Short Form-36 Physical Component Summary scores following cartilage repair procedures.[25] No body mass index represents an absolute contraindication to the performance of autologous chondrocyte implantation; however, the goal should be a body mass index of <30 kg/m^2 before surgical intervention to ensure optimal results. The medial and lateral femoral condyles, trochlear groove, and patellar facets are palpated. Tender areas should be correlated with the symptoms. During chondrocyte implantation, it is not uncommon to find isolated regions of ICRS grade II change along the articular surface; if these areas are not tender on examination they should be ignored. Patellofemoral crepitus should be assessed for location and quality (for example, coarse or fine); furthermore, provocative maneuvers such as the patellar grind test should be performed and correlated with symptoms. Associated cruciate ligament insufficiencies should be recognized and further evaluated with MRI. Clinically rele-

vant complete or partial tears should be treated with staged or concomitant reconstruction.[26] Meniscal lesions have a well-defined association with chondromalacia and osteoarthritis.[27] Patients who have undergone a previous meniscectomy may require concomitant or staged meniscal transplantation.

Radiographic Assessment
The initial radiographic assessment should include a posteroanterior weight-bearing view as described by Rosenberg to assess for medial and/or lateral compartment narrowing and bilateral Merchant views to assess for patellar facet wear, subluxation, and tilt.[28-31] Finally, bilateral long-limb standing radiographs (hip to ankle) should be made to determine the mechanical axis and potential sites of increased load to the repair site.[32] A direct side-to-side comparison should be performed on all views to delineate subtle narrowing in comparison with the contralateral side. Asymmetries should not be ignored but should be addressed to unload the involved compartment in preparation for the sensitive chondrocytes that will be implanted.

Magnetic Resonance Imaging
Controversy remains regarding the sensitivity and specificity of MRI in detecting isolated chondral injuries, but it is becoming a reliable, noninvasive method of diagnosing osteochondral injuries. In 1998, Potter and associates[33] used cartilage-sensitive pulse sequencing to detect defects in the articular surface and reported high sensitivity and specificity for chondral lesions with minimal interobserver variability. They concluded that MRI was an accurate and reproducible imaging modality for the diagnosis of chondral lesions in the

knee. Friemert and associates[34] reported that MRI had a sensitivity of 33% to 53% and a specificity of 98% to 99% for detecting advanced articular cartilage lesions when compared directly with diagnostic arthroscopy. Palosaari and associates[35] found an even higher sensitivity (80% to 96%) when diagnosing cartilaginous lesions with MRI. As is the case with cartilage defects detected with direct observation, lesions detected with MRI should be correlated with clinical symptoms and treated only if they produce pain.

Arthroscopic Assessment and Biopsy
Arthroscopic assessment is done after a careful physical examination and the radiographic studies just discussed. Areas of ICRS grade III or IV change are noted and measured, and the reciprocal surface is evaluated for the degree of damage as well. If the patient is deemed an appropriate candidate for chondrocyte implantation, a biopsy is done. The biopsy specimen is best taken from the superomedial edge of the femoral trochlea, but if pathological involvement extends into this region or if there is concern about the patellofemoral articulation, the superolateral trochlear edge can be used. An additional site for biopsy is the lateral aspect of the intercondylar notch, the area typically used for notchplasty during anterior cruciate ligament surgery (Figure 2). The total weight of the biopsy specimen should be 200 to 300 mg, and the specimen should include the entire cartilage surface along with a small portion of the underlying subchondral bone. This tissue should contain between 200,000 and 300,000 cells. Even though cartilage from femoral osteophytes and débrided cartilage have type II collagen and molecular activity consis-

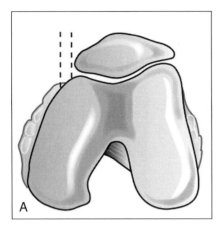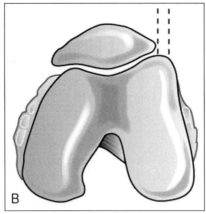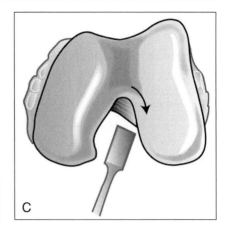

Figure 2 Appropriate cartilage biopsy sites include the superomedial trochlear ridge (**A**), uncovered superolateral trochlear ridge (**B**), and lateral aspect of the intercondylar notch (**C**). All sites should be sharply incised before harvest to avoid gouge slippage. (Reprinted with permission from Minas T, Peterson L: Advanced techniques in autologous chondrocyte transplantation. *Clin Sports Med* 1999;18:13-44.)

tent with that of normal articular chondrocytes, the cells needed for implantation should not be obtained from these "abnormal" sources of cartilage.[36,37] The surgeon should also resist the temptation to use cartilage from a discarded osteochondritis dissecans fragment.

The harvested cells are maintained at 4°C until processing (Figure 3). Isolated defects of up to 6 cm² can be treated with one vial. Each vial typically contains a cell pellet (approximately 12 million cells per vial) and 0.3 to 0.4 mL of Ham F-12 medium with serum supplementation. The number of cells in a vial should allow full coverage of the defect base with a confluent cell population. If there are multiple lesions and areas of >6 cm², more than one vial will be required; lesion size should be taken into account when ordering cells before implantation.

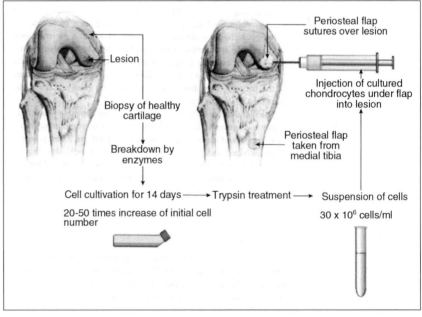

Figure 3 Schematic drawing showing the cartilage biopsy preparation and autologous chondrocyte implantation. (Courtesy of Lars Peterson, MD and Per Renström, MD, PhD)

Surgical Technique
Exposure
A midline skin incision is used. Implantation can be done through a medially or laterally based mini-arthrotomy, to avoid the creation of quadriceps weakness and intra-articular adhesions postoperatively. Alternatively, a subvastus approach can be used, particularly for lesions of the medial femoral condyle. Damage to the anterior horns and central bodies of the menisci should be avoided when dissection is performed along the anterior tibial surface. When a lesion of the tibial plateau is treated, the meniscus should be reflected by releasing the intermeniscal ligament and the anterior meniscal horn of the involved compartment as described previously.[38]

When a concomitant tibial tubercle osteotomy is done, slight lateral placement of the incision avoids injury to the infrapatellar branch of the lesser saphenous nerve.

Preparation of the Defect

The articular defect should be débrided back to normal vertical articular cartilage margins (Figure 4). All fibrillated and partially delaminated cartilage should be removed. The margins of the lesion are first demarcated with a number-15 blade, and the damaged cartilage is then removed, typically with a ring-shaped curet. One should avoid breaking through the subchondral bone plate to prevent bleeding into the defect.

Minimally chondromalacic (grade I and early grade II) areas along the border of the lesion are left alone when appropriate suture fixation is possible. When débridement necessitates extension into poorly contained regions, the bone edge should be prepared for later suture fixation of the periosteal graft. This can be performed with the use of a number-5 Keith needle acting as a drill bit, creating a bone tunnel for later suture placement (Figure 5, *A*). Small suture anchors are commercially available (Microfix; Mitek, Raynham, Massachusetts) and can be used. Prior to placement, the anchors must be reloaded with a 5-0 or 6-0 Vicryl (polyglactin) suture. These anchors are ideal for poorly contained regions such as the intercondylar notch or the peripheral aspect of the femoral condyle or areas such as the posterior edge of a lesion located in the 70° to 90° flexion zone, where it is difficult to place sutures appropriately (Figure 5, *B* through *D*). With extension into the intercondylar notch, interrupted and running suture techniques can be used to supplement graft fixation. Strong fixation of the periosteal graft

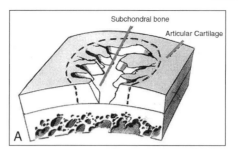
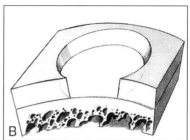
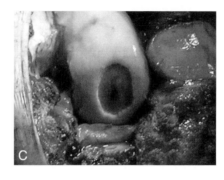

Figure 4   Preparation of the defect. **A,** A fibrillated cartilage lesion. **B,** Débridement to healthy cartilage margins, with smooth vertical borders created on completion. **C,** Isolated cartilage lesion following débridement.

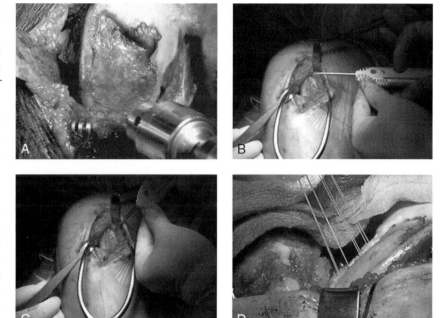

Figure 5   **A,** A number-5 Keith needle used as a drill bit in a poorly contained lesion, creating an osseous tunnel for later suture placement. **B,** Microfix anchor (Mitek, Raynham, Massachusetts). **C,** Following use of the Microfix drill bit and replacement of the nonabsorbable suture with 5-0 Vicryl suture, the anchor is implanted. **D,** Application of several anchors along the poorly contained border of the lesion.

to the defect is critical to prevent future delamination of the graft and to allow early motion of the joint.

In many instances, intralesional osteophytes or sclerotic bone regions are encountered following re-

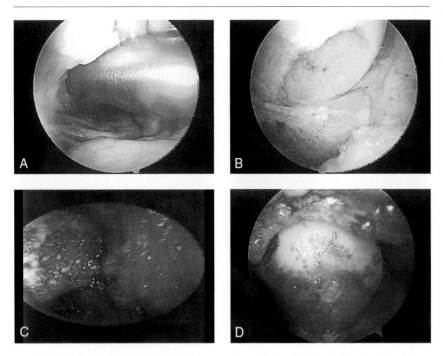

Figure 6   Bone grafting. **A,** Débridement of an osteochondritis dissecans lesion to bleeding healthy bone. **B,** The base of the lesion was drilled to create bleeding. **C,** Autologous bone graft was applied to the defect. **D,** Fibrin glue was applied over the defect to maintain the bone graft in place and to avoid extravasation into surrounding tissues.

moval of the calcified cartilage layer and/or fibrocartilage. Although it is ideal to avoid exposure of the cancellous bone, a high-speed burr should be used to remove the protuberant bone region and sclerotic bone layer. If that procedure is carefully performed, a thin layer of subchondral bone should remain, serving as an appropriate viable bed for chondrocyte attachment. After débridement, the tourniquet, if used, should be deflated and complete hemostasis should be obtained. Initial attempts at hemostasis should involve the use of cotton pledgets soaked in a 1:1000 epinephrine–normal saline solution mixture. The pledget is applied, and pressure is maintained during harvest of the periosteal graft. Thrombin spray has helped in cases of continued bleeding. Finally, if there are sites of excessive bleeding, particularly when

previous bone procedures such as microfracture have been performed, a needle-tip Bovie cautery unit (Bovie Medical Corporation, St. Petersburg, FL) on a low setting (20 to 25 coagulation setting) should be used judiciously.

When the bone deficiency is deeper than 6 to 8 mm, such as can occur with an osteochondral fracture, osteochondritis dissecans, or a failed osteochondral grafting procedure, concomitant or staged bone-grafting should be performed.[21] If it is performed in a staged manner, bone graft should be placed up to the level of the subchondral bone plate. Prior to bone grafting, it is important to remove all sclerotic bone; particularly in patients with osteochondritis dissecans, drilling through the bed following débridement allows appropriate blood flow into the defect, ensuring subsequent incorporation of

the bone graft (Figure 6). Fibrin glue, sutures, or resorbable membranes such as the Restore patch (DePuy, Warsaw, IN) can be used to maintain the bone graft in place. Postoperative continuous passive motion with touch-down to 25% partial weight bearing for 4 to 6 weeks is advised. The patient is then allowed to resume full weight bearing, but chondrocyte implantation is not done for another 5 to 8 months to allow reconstitution of a subchondral bone plate (Figure 7).

Alternatively, the "sandwich technique" can be used to treat a deep lesion.[20] With use of a high-speed burr, the sclerotic bone bed is removed down to bleeding cancellous bone and the base of the lesion is drilled as described previously. Following bone grafting to the level of the subchondral bone plate, a periosteal flap the size of the osseous defect is harvested and is anchored in place with the cambium layer facing up into the defect and the fibrous layer facing the bone graft. Leaving a small ridge of healthy subchondral bone can help to stabilize the placement of this initial periosteal flap. One of the authors (D.G.J.) has successfully used Microfix anchors to help anchor this first periosteal flap (Figure 8). Fibrin glue can be placed around the base of the defect at the periosteal edge to obtain hemostasis. Additionally, or as an alternative, simple compression of the bone graft and periosteal construct for 2 to 3 minutes can help stop the bleeding. A second periosteal flap is then applied, as will be described.

Harvest of Periosteal Graft

The defect should be measured with a sterile ruler to determine the appropriate graft size. Alternatively, a paper template of the defect site can be created by placing paper directly

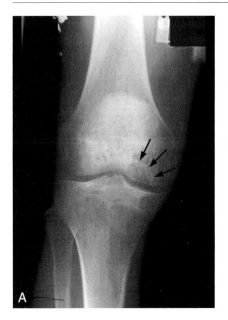 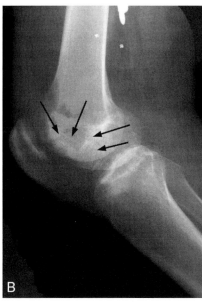

Figure 7 **A,** Postoperative anteroposterior radiograph made 4 months following application of bone graft to the defect. The arrows show the reconstitution of the subchondral bone contour following treatment with a continuous passive motion machine and no weight bearing for 4 weeks. **B,** Lateral radiograph demonstrating the normal subchondral contour (*arrows*).

over the site and tracing the defect on it with sequential dots with use of a surgical skin marker. One additional technique is to use a sterile knife-blade package as an aluminum template, pressing it directly into the defect to create an imprint of the lesion. The paper or aluminum template is created by cutting around the edge of the dots or imprint. The template should be 2 mm larger in diameter than the actual defect when the femoral condyle or tibial plateau surfaces are being treated. When the trochlear groove or patellar surfaces are being grafted, a template 3 mm larger in diameter than the actual lesion should be created to take into account the concave and convex surfaces, respectively.[21]

Several sites are available for harvest of a periosteal graft. The first option should be the proximal-medial aspect of the tibia distal to the pes anserinus insertion or distal to the semitendinosus tendon inser-

tion. This site typically has robust but thin enough periosteum, making it ideal for implantation. Normal periosteum is a thin membrane several cell layers thick consisting of an outer fibrogenic layer and an inner osteogenic cambium layer. An incision is made over the proximal part of the tibia through the subcutaneous fat and the thin fascial layer. Care should be taken to remove all overlying fascial and fatty layers before removal of the periosteum. This is typically best performed with use of sharp scissor dissection, revealing an underlying white, shiny periosteum. Attempts at periosteal débridement following harvest can cause button-holing through the graft surface with resultant sites of cell leakage at the time of implantation. Electrocautery should not be used around the periosteum before harvest as it will damage the periosteum and can kill cells in the cambium layer. Secondary sites of graft

harvest include the femoral meta-physeal-diaphyseal region, which can be exposed with retraction of the quadriceps musculature. Harvest of a periosteal graft from this location requires careful incision of the overlying synovium to expose the underlying periosteum. The synovium should be placed back into its normal anatomic location following graft harvest from the femur to prevent postoperative scarring. The femoral periosteum is typically thicker, and this theoretically may inhibit diffusion of synovial fluid and cell nutrition during the initial growth phase. Thicker periosteum may also predispose to increased rates of periosteal overgrowth. Finally, the required soft-tissue dissection in the suprapatellar region can lead to an increased prevalence of postoperative intra-articular adhesions. Therefore, femoral periosteum should be used only as a secondary source of periosteal graft during autologous chondrocyte implantation. After harvest, the periosteal graft should be kept moist. When multiple grafts are taken, each should be labeled to prevent confusion during implantation.

Resorbable membrane substitutes have become commercially available. Two examples are Chondrogide (Geistlich Biomaterials, Wolhusen, Switzerland) and Restore (DePuy). Haddo and associates[39] reported on 31 patients in whom Chondrogide had been used in place of periosteum. They reported no evidence of hypertrophy of the periosteal grafts and satisfactory clinical outcomes at 2 years. One of the authors (D.G.J.) used the Restore patch as a substitute for periosteum in 30 patients as well as in patients requiring autologous bone grafting. At the time of short-term follow-up (at 1 to 2 years), there were no ad-

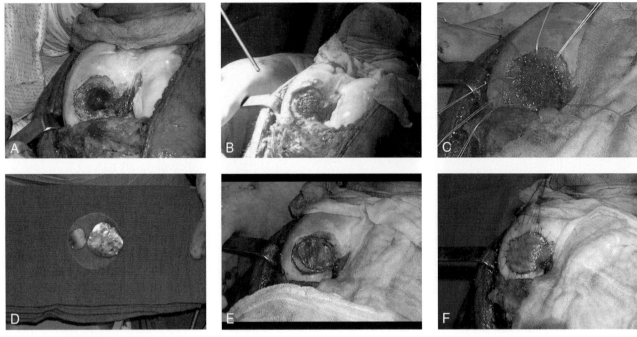

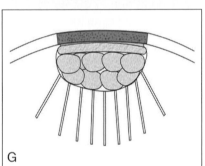

Figure 8 **A,** Bone lesion following débridement of sclerotic bone and drilling of the base of the lesion. Note the shelf of normal subchondral bone around the osseous defect. **B,** Bone graft application up to but not over the subchondral bone height. **C,** Application of Microfix anchors (Mitek) around the periphery of the bone defect. **D,** Restore patch (DePuy) with an aluminum template over the graft before preparation for suture fixation. **E,** Suture fixation of the Restore patch to the bone defect. **F,** Final suture fixation of the larger Restore patch and application of cells with use of the "sandwich" technique. **G,** Schematic of the "sandwich" technique, which includes drilling of the base of the lesion, application of bone graft, and placement of the bottom periosteal patch (with the cambium layer facing up) followed by cells and then the top periosteal patch (with the cambium layer facing down).

verse events or effects on clinical outcome. Bartlett and associates[40] reported similar results. The use of resorbable membranes as a defect cover, replacing the traditional autologous periosteum, has been termed collagen-associated autologous chondrocyte implantation.[41]

Graft Fixation

The periosteal graft is secured in place with 6-0 Vicryl suture with use of a P-1 cutting needle. Dyed suture is recommended as it is easy to see against the articular cartilage. Sterile mineral oil coating the suture helps to prevent binding between the suture and the periosteal graft. The

needle is passed first through the superficial surface of the periosteum about 2 mm from the graft edge and then into the cartilage margin, entering the vertical border perpendicular to the inside wall of the defect. The needle should enter the cartilage approximately 2 mm from the surface and extend peripherally, exiting the defect 4 mm from the edge of the defect. A simple instrument-tying technique is used with each throw. This localizes the knot over the periosteum rather than placing it on the articular surface, where it could be exposed to shear forces damaging fixation. All four quadrants of the graft should be tied ini-

tially to stabilize the graft. Additional sutures are then placed at 3-mm increments around the lesion, producing a watertight seal. An alternative method of suture placement is used during trochlear autologous chondrocyte implantation. In this procedure, the sutures are first placed along the medial margin and are then sequentially placed from medial to lateral, producing a convex surface to allow appropriate patellar tracking (Figure 9). Similarly, the contour of the graft should be considered when autologous chondrocyte implantation is performed in the patella, especially in a centrally based patellar lesion; the normal

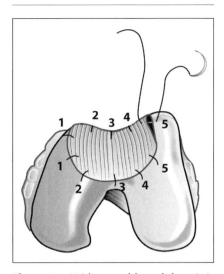

Figure 9 With a trochlear defect, it is important to create the normal trochlear configuration. The template must be oversized by approximately 3 mm. The periosteal patch is then sutured sequentially from medial to lateral, as denoted by the numbers 1 through 5, with care taken to recreate the normal convex surface, thus avoiding postoperative overload to the repair site. (Reprinted with permission from Minas T, Peterson L: Advanced techniques in autologous chondrocyte transplantation. *Clin Sports Med* 1999;18:13-44.)

Table 1
Normal Cartilage Maturation Process Following Autologous Chondrocyte Implantation

Stage	Time	Tissue
Proliferation	0 to 6 weeks	Soft, primitive repair tissue
Transition	7 weeks to 6 months	Expansion of matrix into putty-like consistency
Remodeling	6 to 18 months (changes can occur up to 3 years)	Matrix remodeling, tissue stiffens to normal hardness

convexity of the patella should be considered as should the height of graft placement along the defect, as shear forces in this area can lead to catching at the leading and trailing edges of the defect with knee motion.[21]

One region along the lesion should be left open to allow cell implantation. However, to prevent cell extrusion after implantation, the sutures are placed in the standard fashion but not tied immediately. Prior to cell implantation, the repair should be assessed to determine whether a watertight seal has been created. Normal saline solution without antibiotics should be placed into the planned area of cell implantation with use of a 1.5-inch (3.8-cm) 18-gauge angiocatheter and tu-

berculin syringe. The intra-articular portion of the knee is dried, and sites of leakage are noted. Additional sutures are placed into any leakage site, and testing is performed again. Once a watertight seal has been created, the cells can be implanted.

Cells, provided by Genzyme Biosurgery (Cambridge, MA), arrive in a small vial and should be maintained at 4°C until they are implanted. The typical concentration is 12 million cells/0.4 mL of serum-supplemented culture medium as described previously. Once again, one vial should cover a lesion of <6 cm². The cells have typically settled into a pellet at the bottom of the vial and must be gently resuspended into a solution form with use of an angiocatheter; cells are then injected into the defect. Sutures are tied over, and fibrin glue or Tisseel (as described below) is applied to the site of implantation. Only after a watertight seal has been verified should the wound edges be further sealed with fibrin glue.

Autologous fibrin glue is formed by taking the cryoprecipitate from 1 U of the patient's whole blood and combining it with a mixture of bovine thrombin and calcium chloride. An excellent alternative to this cumbersome technique is to use the commercially available fibrin glue called Tisseel (Baxter Healthcare, Glendale, CA). It is important to limit the amount of Tisseel or fibrin

glue placed into the joint as it has the potential to increase postoperative fibrous adhesions. Furthermore, Brittberg and associates[42] demonstrated potential deleterious effects of Tisseel on chondrocyte migration and healing potential in an in vivo rabbit model. As a result, care should be taken to limit the amount of Tisseel applied and to avoid exposing it to the chondrocytes.

In large, particularly long defects, the contour of the femur may not allow placement of the angiocatheter used for cell implantation far enough into the defect. This can limit the ability to create an even cell suspension at the base of the lesion. In these cases, leaving a more posterior, distal second site of cell implantation is helpful. Cells are implanted in this site first, the sutures are tied, and then cells are implanted into the more anterior, proximal site secondarily.

Postoperative Rehabilitation
Cartilage maturation occurs through several phases (Table 1), and this process must be considered during the critical rehabilitation process after surgery. The first phase, termed the proliferative phase, occurs during the first 6 weeks. Cells should be allowed to adhere to the subchondral bone plate, a process that can take from 12 to 18 hours. As a result, knee motion should be restricted for this period

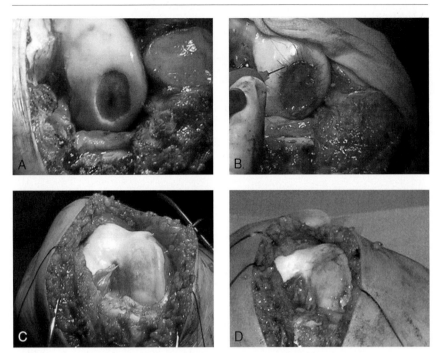

Figure 10 **A,** A well-contained lesion with normal articular cartilage borders. **B,** Following implantation, the repair site is protected from damage, and a more aggressive rehabilitation program can be initiated. **C,** A poorly contained lesion with limited normal articular cartilage margins. **D,** Following implantation, the repair site is not well protected by the surrounding cartilage. Thus, a slower rehabilitation program should be initiated, with full weight bearing allowed after 8 to 12 weeks.

of time following implantation, to allow cell adherence and early proliferation to occur. Continuous passive motion is initiated after 12 to 18 hours, to provide a chondrogenic stimulus as demonstrated by O'Driscoll and Salter.[43] The continuous passive motion machine should be used for 6 to 8 hours a day for the first 4 weeks after the surgery. A soft, primitive repair tissue forms during this initial phase.

The second phase of cartilage maturation, termed the transition phase, occurs during the next 4 to 6 months. This phase is characterized by expansion of the matrix released by the chondrocytes into a putty-like consistency. Weight bearing is begun after the first month. The size and location of the lesion influence the time at which to start weight bearing. Patients with a well-contained lesion that is protected by the surrounding native cartilage can start bearing weight as early as 4 weeks postoperatively (Figure 10, A and B). Patients with a poorly contained lesion should not bear full weight until 8 to 12 weeks after the surgery (Figure 10, C and D). Patients with multiple lesions should progress even more slowly. If there is varus or valgus knee malalignment of 3°, compared with the alignment on the contralateral side, in association with a medial or lateral-based lesion, respectively, an unloader brace should be used on initiation of weight bearing. If there is knee malalignment of >3°, performance of a concomitant or staged osteotomy, which would avoid the need for prolonged postoperative use of the unloader brace, should be seriously considered.

Patellofemoral lesions are not subjected to forces when the patient bears weight with the knee in full extension. Use of a hinged immobilizer locked in extension during walking allows such patients to bear weight during the initial 6 postoperative weeks. Open-chain exercises should be avoided during the first 4 to 6 months to reduce the shear forces that can occur across an implant on the patellofemoral articular surface. Continuous passive motion is initiated 1 month after surgery, but progression to >90° of flexion should occur more slowly than with a femoral lesion.

The final phase in cartilage maturation, termed the matrix remodeling phase, is characterized by progressive hardening of the cartilage tissue to the firm quality of the adjacent native cartilage. This process begins at about 6 months and continues over the ensuing 6 to 12 months. Although patients are allowed to resume regular activities at 1 year after the surgery, the graft continues to mature for up to 3 years. Factors that affect this process are lesion size and location as well as the patient's physiologic age and final desired activity level. Patients will continue to have some symptoms along the implant site as the activity level is increased during this period. However, as the graft matures, providing greater protection of the subchondral bone, preoperative symptoms should resolve slowly. Preoperative education of the patient regarding this biologic process and, in particular, the expected length of time until full recovery is critical. The informed patient is less likely to expose the graft to traumatic forces during the initial phases of cartilage maturation.

(DVD 41.1)

Discussion

MRI has become an increasingly important means of assessing articular cartilage and its repair.[44] It can be used to monitor the patient's progress after a biologic reconstructive procedure.[45,46] Henderson and associates[45] reviewed the results in 53 patients (72 lesions) for up to 2 years with clinical evaluation, MRI, second-look arthroscopy, and biopsy. MRI demonstrated that 75% of the defects had at least a 50% defect fill, 46% had a nearly normal signal, 68% had mild to no effusion, and 67% had mild to no underlying bone marrow edema at 3 months. These values improved to 94%, 87%, 91%, and 88%, respectively, at 12 months. At 24 months, there were additional improvements to 97%, 97%, 96%, and 93%, respectively. Improvement in clinical outcome correlated well with the information obtained from second-look arthroscopy and the core biopsies when that information was assessed along with the MRI findings at 12 months.[47] Brown and associates[48] evaluated the findings of 180 MRI examinations of 112 patients performed just over 1 year after cartilage-resurfacing procedures, including 86 microfractures and 35 autologous chondrocyte implantation procedures. The defects that had been treated with autologous chondrocyte implantation had, at all times, consistently better fill than the defects treated with the microfracture, but there was graft hypertrophy in 63% of the patients treated with autologous chondrocyte implantation. In contrast, the repair cartilage over the microfracture was depressed with respect to the level of the native cartilage and had a propensity for bone development and loss of adjacent cartilage with progressive follow-up.

Arthroscopic assessment remains the gold standard for postoperative evaluation. The repair is directly visualized, probe indention stiffness can be measured, and a biopsy can be done to allow histomorphologic assessment.[26] Arthroscopic probe indentation stiffness testing is useful. Vasara and associates[49] evaluated 30 patients arthroscopically, with measurement of indentation stiffness, and clinically following autologous chondrocyte implantation. The mean stiffness of the repair tissue was 62% of that of the adjacent cartilage. In six patients, the normalized stiffness was at least 80%, suggesting hyaline-like repair. The indentation stiffness following the repairs of osteochondritis dissecans lesions was less than that following repairs of lesions other than osteochondritis dissecans. Gadolinium-enhanced MRI of the cartilage during the follow-up of four patients suggested proteoglycan replenishment. The authors concluded that low stiffness values may indicate incomplete maturation or predominantly fibrous repair while increased stiffness correlated with improved clinical outcomes.

The initial experience with autologous chondrocyte implantation was reported by Brittberg and associates[23] in 1994. The cases of 23 patients were reviewed. Fourteen of 16 patients who had implants on the distal part of the femur had a good or excellent result, whereas only 2 of 7 patients who had implants on the patella had a satisfactory result. Second-look biopsies revealed hyaline-like cartilage in 11 of 15 distal femoral lesions but in only 1 of 7 patellar lesions. The biopsy results correlated well with the clinical outcomes, suggesting a direct correlation between hyaline-like repair tissue and good to excellent function 2 years after surgery.

In a later review, during the intermediate to long-term follow-up period (at 2 to 9 years), this initial trend was found to have continued.[24] This review was of the clinical, arthroscopic, and histologic results for the first 101 patients treated with an autologous chondrocyte implantation procedure. The results were better for patients who had been treated after the early series of patients, suggesting that there is a learning curve for the procedure. Graft failure occurred in 7 patients, with 4 of the failures seen in the first 23 patients but only three observed in the next 78 patients. Patient and physician-derived clinical rating scales; arthroscopic assessment of cartilage fill, integration, and surface hardness; biopsies; and standard histochemical techniques were used. Ninety-four patients underwent reevaluation, and a good or excellent clinical result was seen in 92% of those with an isolated femoral condylar lesion but in only 67% of those with multiple lesions. Patients with osteochondritis dissecans also did well, with 89% having a good or excellent result. In contrast to the findings in the initial series, patients with a patellar lesion did relatively well, with 65% having a good or excellent result. Strict attention to patellofemoral tracking and malalignment issues were found to be important, and concomitant advancement of the tibial tubercle and trochleoplasty procedures were believed to account for the improved clinical results in the patients with a patellar lesion. Of the patients who underwent implantation in the femoral condyle with concomitant reconstruction of the anterior cruciate ligament, 75% had a good or excellent result. Periosteal overgrowth as demonstrated arthroscopically was identified in 26 patients, but only 7 were symptomatic; the symptoms consistently resolved after arthroscopic trimming. Histologic analysis of the matrix in 37 biopsy specimens to assess for type II collagen showed a correlation between hyaline-like repair tissue and good to excellent clinical results.

An evaluation was performed on a subset, from the same series, of 61 patients who had been treated for an isolated cartilage defect on the femoral condyle or the patella.[26] The durability of the results was assessed by comparing the clinical status at 2 years with that at a mean of 7.4 years (range, 5 to 11 years) after transplantation. Fifty of the 61 patients had a good or excellent clinical result at 2 years, whereas 51 had a good or excellent result at 5 to 11 years. Hyaline-like repair tissue was demonstrated by 8 of 12 biopsies. An electromechanical indentation probe was used to assess the grafted areas in 11 patients during a second-look arthroscopy procedure (at a mean of 54.3 months [range, 33 to 84 months] postoperatively); 8 patients demonstrated stiffness measurements that were ≥90% of those of normal cartilage. The mean stiffness of grafted areas with hyaline-like repair tissue, as identified with histologic assessment, was 3.0 ± 1.1 N. In contrast, the mean stiffness of grafted areas with fibrous tissue was 1.5 ± 0.35 N. Once again, good or excellent clinical outcomes were directly correlated with the demonstration of a hyaline-like repair tissue at the implantation site, whereas fibrous fill was correlated with poorer clinical outcomes. More importantly, durability of the repair tissue was clearly demonstrated, with the results at 7 years equal to or better than the initial 2-year results.

In 1995, Genzyme Tissue Repair (Cambridge, MA) initiated an international registry to assess the clinical effectiveness of autologous chondrocyte implantation. Data from this registry were used to evaluate the first 50 patients treated in the United States.[17] The mean patient age was 36 years, and the mean defect size was 4.2 cm^2. Thirty-nine patients had undergone previous articular cartilage repair procedures on the affected knee during the previous 5 years. A marrow stimulation procedure had failed in nine patients. Outcomes were measured at a minimum of 3 years with the modified Cincinnati Knee Rating System, and graft failure was defined as replacement or removal of the graft due to mechanical symptoms or pain. Scores derived with the modified Cincinnati Knee Rating System range from 0 to 10 points, with lower scores representing poorer function and substantial pain with activities of daily living.[50] The median improvement in the score was four points for the clinician-based portion of the evaluation and five points for the patient-based portion. Neither previous treatment with marrow stimulation techniques nor the size of the defect had an impact on the results of the autologous chondrocyte implantation. The graft failed in three patients, and Kaplan-Meier analysis revealed an estimated rate of freedom from graft failure of 94% at 36 months.

The same registry was used to evaluate the results, at 6 years, in the first 76 patients treated with implantation in the United States (B Mosley, MD, LJ Micheli, MD, C Erggelet, MD, et al, New Orleans, LA, unpublished data presented at the American Academy of Orthopaedic Surgeons Annual Meeting, 2003).

The mean age of these patients was also 36 years. Fifty-seven patients had a single lesion, with a mean size of 4.4 cm^2. Nineteen patients had multiple lesions, with a mean total surface area of 10.8 cm^2. Nine treatment failures occurred within the first 24 months. Including the scores for these failures, the mean overall condition score improved from 3.1 points preoperatively to 6.0 points at 6 years ($P < 0.001$). Pain and swelling scores improved 2.7 and 2.6 points, respectively, compared with the baseline values.

Gillogly[51,52] (Keystone, CO, unpublished data presented at the American Orthopaedic Society for Sports Medicine Annual Meeting, 2001) evaluated 112 patients with a total of 139 defects treated with autologous chondrocyte implantation over a 5-year period. The average size of the defect was 5.7 cm^2, and >60% of the patients had had a failure of at least one prior procedure. Twenty-two of the patients had multiple defects. Forty-two patients had a patellofemoral lesion, 27 of which were trochlear and 15 of which were patellar. Outcomes were measured with use of the modified Cincinnati Knee Rating System and Knee Society Clinical Rating System.[53] There were three clinical failures, and three patients were lost to follow-up. The average duration of follow-up was 43 months. Ninety-three percent of the patients had a good or excellent outcome according to the clinician evaluation portion of the modified Cincinnati scale, whereas 89% had a good or excellent outcome according to the patient evaluation portion. There was no deterioration of the outcomes during the 2- to 5-year follow-up period. Workers' compensation claims had no effect on the clinical outcomes.

Seidner and Zaslav (San Francisco, CA, unpublished data presented at the American Academy of Orthopaedic Surgeons Annual Meeting, 2001) assessed the direct medical and nonmedical costs for, and the return-to-work status of, 24 patients (mean age, 35 years) treated with autologous chondrocyte implantation who used the same claims system of a single workers' compensation ensurer. The patients were followed until claim closure and were compared with a 3:1 matched control group of 76 patients treated with various other cartilage procedures. The patients' occupations ranged from light to heavy demand. The total medical costs for the patients treated with autologous chondrocyte implantation averaged $90,235, and the indemnity costs averaged $64,704. Seventeen patients returned to work. In comparison, the total medical costs in the control group averaged $80,407 and the indemnity costs averaged $89,226, with 20 patients returning to work. The authors concluded that autologous chondrocyte implantation results in a similar return-to-work rate at an average cost savings of $15,000 per patient in comparison with control patients.

Yates[54] performed a prospective longitudinal study of 24 patients with workers' compensation claims related to lesions of >2 cm^2 (mean lesion size, 4.7 cm^2; range, 2 to 10 cm^2). Five lesions were on the patella, and the remaining 19 lesions were on the distal part of the femur. Eighteen patients were followed at 1 year with use of the modified Cincinnati Knee Rating System. According to the clinician and patient evaluations of the modified Cincinnati Knee Rating System, the overall clinical scores improved from a mean of 3.2 points at baseline to 6.8

points at 1 year postoperatively. Fourteen patients had a good or excellent result. Of the 21 patients who were followed for more than 1 year, 13 returned to unrestricted work status at a mean of 7 months and an additional 4 returned to modified work status. This study demonstrated that autologous chondrocyte implantation can effectively enable patients in a workers' compensation population to return to their desired activity level.

Minas[55] evaluated the health economics of the autologous chondrocyte implantation procedure. He prospectively examined the efficacy of treatment and quality of life of 44 patients who had undergone the procedure and calculated the average cost per additional quality-adjusted life year. At 12 months after autologous chondrocyte implantation, there was improvement in patient function as measured with both the Knee Society Clinical Rating System (a mean improvement from 114.02 to 140.67 points, $P < 0.001$) and the Western Ontario and McMaster Universities Osteoarthritis Index (a mean improvement from 35.30 to 23.82 points, $P < 0.05$). Quality of life as measured with the Short Form-36 Physical Component Summary improved from a mean of 33.32 points before the biopsy to 41.48 points 12 months after implantation ($P < 0.05$). There was additional improvement in all three outcome measures during the following 12 to 24 months. As a result of these findings, Minas concluded that autologous chondrocyte implantation improved the quality of life of patients and was a cost-effective treatment of cartilage lesions.

There have been several studies comparing autologous chondrocyte implantation directly with other bi-

ologic reconstructive procedures. Horas and associates[56] compared autologous chondrocyte implantation with osteochondral cylinder transplantation in a prospective, single-center study of 40 patients assessed at 2 years. The mean lesion size and the mean age were 3.86 cm^2 and 31.4 years in the group treated with autologous chondrocyte implantation and 3.63 cm^2 and 35.4 years in the group treated with osteochondral cylinder transplantation. Seven of the 20 patients treated with autologous chondrocyte implantation had undergone a previous abrasion arthroplasty. Two patients treated with osteochondral cylinder transplantation had undergone a previous abrasion arthroplasty, and two had undergone microfracture. The recovery after the autologous chondrocyte implantation was slower than it was after the osteochondral cylinder transplantation as assessed on the basis of the Lysholm score at 6 months. Both groups had substantial improvement at 2 years as assessed with the Meyers score and the Tegner activity score. The one failure in the study was of an autologous chondrocyte implantation procedure, but it occurred in the only patient in either group who had treatment of a patellofemoral lesion. This patellofemoral lesion was large (5.6 cm^2), and failure was thought to be due to poor rehabilitation. Gross examination revealed complete, mechanically stable resurfacing of all of the defects treated with autologous chondrocyte implantation except for the one failure. Biopsies done in the autologous chondrocyte implantation group showed predominant areas of fibrocartilage with localized areas of hyaline-like regenerative tissue close to the subchondral bone. In the osteochondral cylinder transplantation group, all of the biopsies showed hyaline articular cartilage that was histomorphologically similar to the surrounding cartilage. All specimens from the patients treated with osteochondral cylinder transplantation had a persistent interface between the transplant and the surrounding cartilage, however. One important limitation of the study was the small number of patients in each treatment group, which raises questions about the effect of the learning curve, particularly in association with the autologous chondrocyte implantation procedure that occurred during the study period. This study also had a relatively short-term follow-up. With longer follow-up, the durability of the repair in both groups may be better delineated.

In a similar prospective, randomized study comparing autologous chondrocyte implantation and mosaicplasty, Bentley and associates[57] assessed 100 consecutive patients with a mean age of 31.3 years and a mean defect size of 4.66 cm^2. The mean duration of symptoms before the surgical repair was 7.2 years, and the mean number of previous surgical procedures (excluding arthroscopy) was 1.5. The mean duration of follow-up was 19 months. Fifty-eight patients underwent autologous chondrocyte implantation, and 42 patients underwent microfracture. According to the modified Cincinnati Knee Rating System, the Stanmore Functional Rating Scale, and objective clinical assessment, the result was excellent or good in 88% of the patients treated with autologous chondrocyte implantation compared with 69% of those treated with mosaicplasty.[53] Arthroscopic assessment of the lesions with the ICRS grading system at 1 year demonstrated a grade I or II appearance in 31 (84%) of the 37 patients treated with autologous chondrocyte implantation compared with only 8 (35%) of the 23 patients treated with microfracture. Biopsies were performed at 1 year after 19 autologous chondrocyte implantation procedures; 3 of the lesions were patellar, and 16 were femoral condylar. Seven patients had hyaline-like cartilage, seven had a mix of hyaline-like and fibrocartilaginous regions, and five had a fibrocartilaginous material that was well bonded to the subchondral bone. There were seven poor results in the mosaicplasty group, with poor graft incorporation at the interface in four, graft disintegration in three, and exposed subchondral bone at the margin in one.

Autologous chondrocyte implantation has been compared with the Steadman microfracture technique[59] in two studies. In a prospective, concurrently controlled study, Anderson and associates (Dallas, TX, unpublished data presented at the American Academy of Orthopaedic Surgeons Annual Meeting, 2002) compared the two techniques with 23 patients in each group. Defects of <2 cm^2 as well as patellar and tibial lesions were excluded. No difference between groups was noted with regard to the overall defect area, body mass index, number of prior procedures, or baseline scores. The improvements in overall scores from baseline measurements averaged 3.1 points in the group treated with autologous chondrocyte implantation compared with 1.3 points in the microfracture group. Two autologous chondrocyte implantation procedures and six microfracture procedures met the study criteria for failure. When the treatment failures were excluded from each group, those treated with autologous chondrocyte implantation had a mean improvement in the overall condition score of 4.7 points and those treated with microfracture had a mean improvement of 2.8 points. This difference was significant ($P = 0.023$).

In a separate study, Knutsen and associates[60] evaluated 80 patients in whom a single symptomatic cartilage defect of the femoral condyle had been treated with either autologous chondrocyte implantation or microfracture (40 in each group). Arthroscopic biopsy was done 2 years postoperatively, and histologic evaluation was performed by a pathologist and a clinical scientist, both blinded to the type of surgical treatment. At 2 years, both groups had significant clinical improvement. However, according to the SF-36 Physical Component score, the microfracture group had significantly more improvement than the group treated with autologous chondrocyte implantation ($P = 0.004$). Two failures occurred in the group treated with autologous chondrocyte implantation, and one occurred in the microfracture group. On review of the biopsy findings, the authors could not find a significant difference between the two groups, with the small numbers studied, with regard to the frequency with which hyaline or fibrocartilage was observed. No correlation between histologic appearance and clinical outcome was found in this study. One important question that arises is whether autologous chondrocyte implantation should have been used as a first-line treatment in many of these patients. The baseline clinical scores in the group treated with autologous chondrocyte implantation were somewhat higher than those in the microfracture group. This concern, combined with the relatively low mean lesion

Table 2
Recommended Surgical Treatment According to Lesion Size

Recommended Treatment	Lesion Size
Microfracture	1 to 2.5 cm^2; well-shouldered, protected edges
Osteochondral autograft	1 to 2.5 cm^2; grafts need to be perpendicular and flush to surface
Autologous chondrocyte implantation	>2 cm^2; background factors need to be addressed, patient must be compliant with rehabilitation
Osteochondral allograft	>4 cm^2; uncontained large lesion involving substantial osseous loss

size in both groups (5.1 cm^2 in the group treated with autologous chondrocyte implantation and 4.5 cm^2 in the microfracture group), suggests that many of these patients might have been more appropriately treated with a less invasive option. Unlike the microfracture technique, the autologous chondrocyte implantation procedure currently necessitates a concomitant arthrotomy, with its associated morbidity. As a result, most surgeons use the microfracture or mosaicplasty procedure for isolated lesions of <2 cm^2 and use autologous chondrocyte implantation for more extensive lesions causing greater functional deficits[61,62] (Table 2).

Summary
The experience with the traditional autologous chondrocyte implantation technique—that is, implantation of autologous chondrocytes with an autologous periosteal patch—is promising. Currently, minimally invasive procedures such as microfracture or mosaicplasty are probably best for lesions of <2 cm^2, but autologous chondrocyte implantation is recommended for lesions of ≥2 cm^2 or for patients with multiple lesions (Table 2). The repair process is a reproducible sequence of events that occur as the tissue matures. Proper patient selection and education are important for success. Potential long-term benefits of autologous chondrocyte implantation include durable repair tissue that functions in a manner similar to that of normal hyaline cartilage, withstanding the high shear and compressive loads applied during daily and sports activities. The intermediate-term results show that outcomes can improve after the first 2 years. A direct correlation between biopsies showing hyaline-like repair tissue and better clinical results has been found in several studies. The future of biologic regeneration and tissue engineering for the treatment of articular cartilage defects is promising. With further modifications of the techniques, arthroscopic or minimally invasive methods hopefully will be developed to repair these defects and allow patients to return to normal activity levels on a regular basis.

References
1. Curl WW, Krome J, Gordon ES, Rushing J, Smith BP, Poehling GG: Cartilage injuries: A review of 31,516 knee arthroscopies. *Arthroscopy* 1997;13:456-460.

2. Hjelle K, Solheim E, Strand T, Muri R, Brittberg M: Articular cartilage defects in 1,000 knee arthroscopies. *Arthroscopy* 2002;18:730-734.

3. Outerbridge RE: The etiology of chondromalacia patellae. *J Bone Joint Surg Br* 1961;43:752-757.

4. Brittberg M, Winalski CS: Evaluation of cartilage injuries and repair. *J Bone Joint Surg Am* 2003;85(Suppl 2):58-69.

5. Piasecki DP, Spindler KP, Warren TA, Andrish JT, Parker RD: Intraarticular injuries associated with anterior cruciate ligament tear: Findings at ligament reconstruction in high school and recreational athletes. An analysis of sex-based differences. *Am J Sports Med* 2003;31:601-605.

6. Shelbourne KD, Jari S, Gray T: Outcome of untreated traumatic articular cartilage defects of the knee: A natural history study. *J Bone Joint Surg Am* 2003;85(Suppl 2):8-16.

7. Mankin HJ: The response of articular cartilage to mechanical injury. *J Bone Joint Surg Am* 1982;64:460-466.

8. Nehrer S, Spector M, Minas T: Histologic analysis of tissue after failed cartilage repair procedures. *Clin Orthop Relat Res* 1999;365:149-162.

9. Robinson D, Nevo Z: Articular cartilage chondrocytes are more advantageous for generating hyalinelike cartilage than mesenchymal cells isolated from microfracture repairs. *Cell Tissue Bank* 2001;2:23-30.

10. Bulstra SK, Homminga GN, Buurman WA, Terwindt-Rouwenhorst E, van der Linden AJ: The potential of adult human perichondrium to form hyalin cartilage in vitro. *J Orthop Res* 1990;8:328-335.

11. Caplan AI, Elyaderani M, Mochizuki Y, Wakitani S, Goldberg VM: Principles of cartilage repair and regeneration. *Clin Orthop Relat Res* 1997;342:254-269.

12. Homminga GN, Bulstra SK, Bouwmeester PS, van der Linden AJ: Perichondral grafting for cartilage lesions of the knee. *J Bone Joint Surg Br* 1990;72:1003-1007.

13. Nakahara H, Dennis JE, Bruder SP, Haynesworth SE, Lennon DP, Caplan AI: In vitro differentiation of bone and hypertrophic cartilage from periosteal-derived cells. *Exp Cell Res* 1991;195:492-503.

14. Nakahara H, Goldberg VM, Caplan AI: Cultureexpanded human periosteal-derived cells exhibit osteochondral potential in vivo. *J Orthop Res* 1991;9:465-476.

15. Grande DA, Pitman MI, Peterson L, Menche D, Klein M: The repair of experimentally produced defects in rabbit articular cartilage by autologous chondrocyte transplantation. *J Orthop Res* 1989;7:208-218.

16. King PJ, Bryant T, Minas T: Autologous chondrocyte implantation for chondral

defects of the knee: Indications and technique. *J Knee Surg* 2002;15:177-184.

17. Micheli LJ, Browne JE, Erggelet C, et al: Autologous chondrocyte implantation of the knee: Multicenter experience and minimum 3-year follow-up. *Clin J Sport Med* 2001;11:223-228.

18. Hangody L, Fules P: Autologous osteo-chondral mosaicplasty for the treatment of full-thickness defects of weight-bearing joints: Ten years of experimental and clinical experience. *J Bone Joint Surg Am* 2003;85(Suppl 2):25-32.

19. Steadman JR, Rodkey WG, Briggs KK: Microfracture to treat full-thickness chondral defects: Surgical technique, rehabilitation, and outcomes. *J Knee Surg* 2002;15:170-176.

20. Peterson L, Minas T, Brittberg M, Lindahl A: Treatment of osteochondritis dissecans of the knee with autologous chondrocyte transplantation: Results at two to ten years. *J Bone Joint Surg Am* 2003;85(Suppl 2):17-24.

21. Minas T, Peterson L: Advanced techniques in autologous chondrocyte transplantation. *Clin Sports Med* 1999;18:13-44.

22. Minas T: Autologous chondrocyte implantation in the arthritic knee. *Orthopedics* 2003;26:945-947.

23. Brittberg M, Lindahl A, Nilsson A, Ohlsson C, Isaksson O, Peterson L: Treatment of deep cartilage defects in the knee with autologous chondrocyte transplantation. *N Engl J Med* 1994;331:889-895.

24. Peterson L, Minas T, Brittberg M, Nilsson A, Sjogren-Jansson E, Lindahl A: Two- to 9-year outcome after autologous chondrocyte transplantation of the knee. *Clin Orthop Relat Res* 2000;374:212-234.

25. Mithoefer K, Williams RJ III, Warren RF, et al: The microfracture technique for the treatment of articular cartilage lesions in the knee. A prospective cohort study. *J Bone Joint Surg Am* 2005;87:1911-1920.

26. Peterson L, Brittberg M, Kiviranta I, Akerlund EL, Lindahl A: Autologous chondrocyte transplantation: Biomechanics and long-term durability. *Am J Sports Med* 2002;30:2-12.

27. Maletius W, Messner K: The effect of partial meniscectomy on the long-term prognosis of knees with localized, severe chondral damage: A twelve- to fifteen-year followup. *Am J Sports Med* 1996;24:258-262.

28. Insall JN: Patella pain syndromes and chondromalacia patellae. *Instr Course Lect* 1981;30:342-356.

29. Laurin CA, Dussault R, Levesque HP: The tangential x-ray investigation of the patellofemoral joint: x-ray technique, diagnostic criteria and their interpretation. *Clin Orthop Relat Res* 1979;144:16-26.

30. Merchant AC: Classification of patellofemoral disorders. *Arthroscopy* 1988;4:235-240.

31. Rosenberg TD, Paulos LE, Parker RD, Coward DB, Scott SM: The forty-five-degree posteroanterior flexion weight-bearing radiograph of the knee. *J Bone Joint Surg Am* 1988;70:1479-1483.

32. Petersen TD, Rohr W Jr: Improved assessment of lower extremity alignment using new roentgenographic techniques. *Clin Orthop Relat Res* 1987;219:112-119.

33. Potter HG, Linklater JM, Allen AA, Hannafin JA, Haas SB: Magnetic resonance imaging of articular cartilage in the knee: An evaluation with use of fastspin-echo imaging. *J Bone Joint Surg Am* 1998;80:1276-1284.

34. Friemert B, Oberlander Y, Danz B, et al: [MRI vs. arthroscopy in the diagnosis of cartilage lesions in the knee: Can MRI take place of arthroscopy?]. *Zentralbl Chir* 2002;127:822-827.

35. Palosaari K, Ojala R, Blanco-Sequeiros R, Tervonen O: Fat suppression gradient-echo magnetic resonance imaging of experimental articular cartilage lesions: comparison between phase-contrast method at 0.23T and chemical shift selective method at 1.5T. *J Magn Reson Imaging* 2003;18:225-231.

36. Alonge TO, Rooney P, Oni OO: Osteophytes—an alternative source of chondrocytes for transplantation? *West Afr J Med* 2004;23:224-227.

37. Chaipinyo K, Oakes BW, Van Damme MP: The use of debrided human articular cartilage for autologous chondrocyte implantation: Maintenance of chondrocyte differentiation and proliferation in type I collagen gels. *J Orthop Res* 2004;22:446-455.

38. Minas T, Nehrer S: Current concepts in the treatment of articular cartilage defects. *Orthopedics* 1997;20:525-538.

39. Haddo O, Mahroof S, Higgs D, et al: The use of chondrogide membrane in autologous chondrocyte implantation. *Knee* 2004;11:51-55.

40. Bartlett W, Gooding CR, Carrington RW, Skinner JA, Briggs TW, Bentley G: Autologous chondrocyte implantation at the knee using a bilayer collagen membrane with bone graft: A preliminary report.

J Bone Joint Surg Br 2005;87:330-332.

41. Bartlett W, Skinner JA, Gooding CR, et al: Autologous chondrocyte implantation versus matrix-induced autologous chondrocyte implantation for osteochondral defects of the knee: A prospective, randomised study. *J Bone Joint Surg Br* 2005;87:640-645.

42. Brittberg M, Sjogren-Jansson E, Lindahl A, Peterson L: Influence of fibrin sealant (Tisseel) on osteochondral defect repair in the rabbit knee. *Biomaterials* 1997;18:235-242.

43. O'Driscoll SW, Salter RB: The repair of major osteochondral defects in joint surfaces by neochondrogenesis with autogenous osteoperiosteal grafts stimulated by continuous passive motion: An experimental investigation in the rabbit. *Clin Orthop Relat Res* 1986;208:131-140.

44. Watrin-Pinzano A, Ruaud JP, Cheli Y, et al: T2 mapping: An efficient MR quantitative technique to evaluate spontaneous cartilage repair in rat patella. *Osteoarthritis Cartilage* 2004;12:191-200.

45. Henderson I, Francisco R, Oakes B, Cameron J: Autologous chondrocyte implantation for treatment of focal chondral defects of the knee—a clinical, arthroscopic, MRI and histologic evaluation at 2 years. *Knee* 2005;12:209-216.

46. Polster J, Recht M: Postoperative MR evaluation of chondral repair in the knee. *Eur J Radiol* 2005;54:206-213.

47. Henderson IJ, Tuy B, Connell D, Oakes B, Hettwer WH: Prospective clinical study of autologous chondrocyte implantation and correlation with MRI at three and 12 months. *J Bone Joint Surg Br* 2003;85:1060-1066.

48. Brown WE, Potter HG, Marx RG, Wickiewicz TL, Warren RF: Magnetic resonance imaging appearance of cartilage repair in the knee. *Clin Orthop Relat Res* 2004;422:214-223.

49. Vasara AI, Nieminen MT, Jurvelin JS, Peterson L, Lindahl A, Kiviranta I: Indentation stiffness of repair tissue after autologous chondrocyte transplantation. *Clin Orthop Relat Res* 2005;433:233-242.

50. Noyes FR, Barber-Westin SD: Arthroscopic-assisted allograft anterior cruciate ligament reconstruction in patients with symptomatic arthrosis. *Arthroscopy* 1997;13:24-32.

51. Gillogly SD: Autologous chondrocyte implantation: Complex defects and combined procedures. *Op Tech Sports Med.* 2002;10:120-128.

52. Gillogly SD: Treatment of large

full-thickness chondral defects of the knee with autologous chondrocyte implantation. *Arthroscopy* 2003;19(Suppl 1):147-153.

53. Insall JN, Dorr LD, Scott RD, Scott WN: Rationale of the Knee Society clinical rating system. *Clin Orthop Relat Res* 1989;248:13-14.

54. Yates JW Jr: The effectiveness of autologous chondrocyte implantation for treatment of full-thickness articular cartilage lesions in workers' compensation patients. *Orthopedics* 2003;26:295-301.

55. Minas T: Chondrocyte implantation in the repair of chondral lesions of the knee: Economics and quality of life. *Am J Orthop* 1998;27:739-744.

56. Horas U, Pelinkovic D, Herr G, Aigner T, Schnettler R: Autologous chondrocyte implantation and osteochondral cylinder transplantation in cartilage repair of the knee joint: A prospective, comparative trial. *J Bone Joint Surg Am* 2003;85:185-192.

57. Bentley G, Biant LC, Carrington RW, et al: A prospective, randomised comparison of autologous chondrocyte implantation versus mosaicplasty for osteochondral defects in the knee. *J Bone Joint Surg Br* 2003;85:223-230.

58. Meister K, Cobb A, Bentley G: Treatment of painful articular cartilage defects of the patella by carbon-fibre implants. *J Bone Joint Surg Br* 1998;80:965-970.

59. Steadman JR, Briggs KK, Rodrigo JJ, Kocher MS, Gill TJ, Rodkey WG: Outcomes of microfracture for traumatic chondral defects of the knee: Average 11-year follow-up. *Arthroscopy* 2003;19:477-484.

60. Knutsen G, Engebretsen L, Ludvigsen TC, et al: Autologous chondrocyte implantation compared with microfracture in the knee: A randomized trial. *J Bone Joint Surg Am* 2004;86:455-464.

61. Farr J, Lewis P, Cole BJ: Patient evaluation and surgical decision making. *J Knee Surg* 2004;17:219-228.

62. Sgaglione NA, Miniaci A, Gillogly SD, Carter TR: Update on advanced surgical techniques in the treatment of traumatic focal articular cartilage lesions in the knee. *Arthroscopy* 2002;18(2, Suppl 1): 9-32.

Technical Aspects of Osteochondral Autograft Transplantation

Anthony Miniaci, MD, FRCSC
Paul A. Martineau, MD, FRCSC

Abstract

Osteochondral autograft transplantation is a well-established technique in the treatment of chondral and osteochondral defects. Cylindrical osteochondral plugs are harvested from areas of the articular surface with a lesser weight-bearing role and transferred to areas of osteochondral damage. Using a press-fit technique, the plugs are inserted to replace damaged or missing articular cartilage and to supply the chondral lesion with islands of viable and immediately functional hyaline cartilage. The presence of focal unipolar cartilage defects in the knee measuring 1 to 4 cm² is a current indication for osteochondral autograft transplantation. Excellent success also has been achieved with the use of this technique for fixation of lesions in patients with osteochondritis dissecans. Osteochondral autograft transplantation is a technically demanding but relatively inexpensive procedure that requires a single operation. Published results are favorable compared with those of other treatment techniques. However, optimal results depend on the location of the lesion, careful adherence to patient selection criteria, and the use of proper surgical techniques. Basic science research enables the continued refinement of surgical techniques and directs future advances in treatment augmentation.

Instr Course Lect 2007;56:447-455.

Articular cartilage plays an essential role in transferring loads across adjacent joint surfaces, reducing friction within the joint, and transferring stresses to the underlying subchondral bone.[1] Orthopaedic surgeons often treat patients with chondral injuries; however, the management of articulating surface injuries remains challenging.[2] Unlike many other tissues of the musculoskeletal system, cartilage is distinctive because it does not produce an adequate healing response.[3]

Most previous attempts at treating symptomatic cartilage lesions had limited success. Techniques such as abrasion chondroplasty and microfracture attempted to promote an adequate healing response by recruiting pluripotent mesenchymal cells from the bone marrow.[4] These procedures lead to the formation of fibrocartilage scar tissue with biochemical and biomechanical properties inferior to those of native hyaline cartilage.[5-12] Recent histologic and electron microscopy evaluation of biopsy specimens (obtained at follow-up arthroscopic procedures), showed that autologous chondrocyte transplantation, which was initially reported to form hyaline cartilage, actually forms a tissue with characteristics more comparable to fibrocartilage.[13-15]

Osteochondral autograft transplantation (OAT) is a well-established technique for the treatment of chondral and osteochondral defects. Also known as mosaicplasty, it was first described by Yamashita and associates,[16] and later popularized by Hangody and associates.[17] Basic science research and subsequent refinements in technique have continued over the years.[18,19]

OAT may be performed with either open or arthroscopic procedures. Cylindrical osteochondral plugs are harvested from areas of the articular surface with a lesser weight-bearing role and are transferred to the areas of osteochondral damage. The plugs, which are inserted using a press-fit technique, replace damaged or missing articular cartilage and supply the chondral lesion with islands of viable and immediately functional hyaline cartilage.

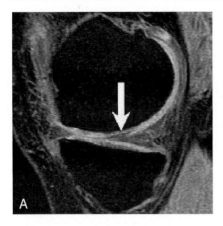 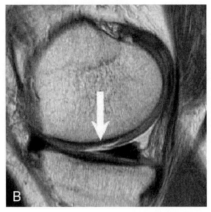 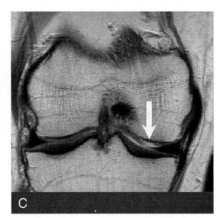

Figure 1   **A,** Sagittal fat-suppressed spoiled gradient echo, **B,** sagittal, and **C,** coronal fast spin-echo intermediate-weighted MRI scans showing focal full-thickness cartilage defect of the weight-bearing portion of the medial femoral condyle (*arrows*).

OAT is performed in one stage, and is relatively inexpensive. The main cost of OAT is the initial expenditure for specialized surgical instrumentation. Because it is an autologous transplant, the procedure carries no risk of disease transmission or HLA incompatibility. When used in carefully selected patients, the results of OATs are favorable compared with other currently available surgical alternatives for articular cartilage injuries.

Indications

OAT in the knee is currently indicated for patients with focal unipolar (one side of the joint only) cartilage defects measuring 1 to 4 cm^2. Lesions smaller than 1 cm^2 tend to be relatively asymptomatic. With lesions larger than 4 cm^2, the amount of donor tissue available for harvesting for an OAT becomes a limiting factor. Defects with bone loss up to 10 to 15 mm also can be reconstructed with this procedure.

Diagnosis and Clinical Evaluation

Patients with cartilage injuries often have a nonspecific clinical presentation. Patients may report pain, swelling, and/or episodes of locking and catching of the joint. Physical examination often shows joint effusion. The knee should be evaluated for other concurrent pathologies. An evaluation of patellofemoral tracking should be performed. A thorough assessment of lower limb alignment is mandatory, because malalignment should be corrected before or in conjunction with a mosaicplasty procedure. Greater than 3° of varus or valgus adjustment compared with the opposite normal side should be addressed; if adjustment is needed, a tibial valgus or femoral varus osteotomy can be performed at the same surgical procedure.

Imaging studies are an important factor in the preoperative workup. Weight-bearing radiographs including AP, lateral, and 45° flexion PA are initially obtained to evaluate the load-bearing areas of the femoral condyles.[20] Merchant axial patella views are used to assess the patellofemoral joint. A set of standing full-length lower extremity radiographs is also obtained to measure alignment.

MRI is useful for evaluating chondral injuries, and is helpful in preoperatively identifying the lo-

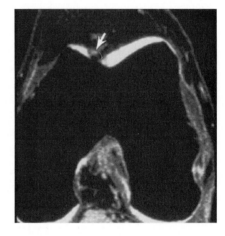

Figure 2   Axial fat-suppressed spoiled gradient-echo MRI scan shows a focal full-thickness defect of the femoral trochlea.

cation, size, depth, and extent of chondral lesions (Figure 1). T1-weighted, fat-suppressed, three-dimensional spoiled gradient echo sequences are sensitive for the assessment of cartilage injuries[21] (Figure 2). The appearance of lesions on MRI does not always correlate with symptoms. Only symptomatic lesions are treated. Previous studies have shown an 81% to 93% sensitivity, 94% to 97% specificity, and accuracy of 91% to 97% for the detection of chondral defects.[22-24] When imaged using this sequence, a chondral injury will appear as an altered contour in the articular surface rather than a change in signal intensity. Articular cartilage will display high signal intensity in contrast with the low signal intensity of the surrounding joint fluid.

Surgical Technique

MRI helps in preoperative planning with the size and location of the defect. Measurement of the size and depth of the defect is important to determine what is necessary for reconstruction of the defect and to determine whether the fragment is salvageable or not. The final determination is an intraoperative one.

Positioning

After anesthesia and routine preoperative antibiotics are administered, a tourniquet is applied to the upper thigh. It is important to inform the patient preoperatively of the potential need to harvest osteochondral plugs from the contralateral knee, especially when larger defects are involved. Therefore, both lower extremities are prepared and draped. OAT may be performed open through an arthrotomy or entirely arthroscopically. The patient also must be informed that even if an arthroscopic procedure is selected, a formal arthrotomy may be required to gain access to the lesion and harvest sites.

Arthroscopic Portals

Anterolateral and anteromedial portals are made 1 cm lateral and medial in relation to the patellar tendon. This portal positioning aids in accessing the lateral and medial borders of the trochlea for harvesting bone plugs. Judicious portal placement is of paramount importance for obtaining perpendicular access to the harvest and defect sites. Using a spinal needle to localize the lesion

and harvest sites may help in establishing an accurate portal position. Vertical portal incisions are preferred to facilitate maneuvering of the harvesting chisel so that it lies perpendicular to the bone. If an arthrotomy is needed, the vertical portal incisions are extensile. Approximately 9 plugs (depending on the size of the knee), 4.5 mm in size, may be harvested from each knee using these guidelines.

Graft Harvest

Initially, a thorough evaluation of the chondral lesion is performed arthroscopically. The defect is probed and its size, stability, and accessibility are assessed. The overlying damaged and loose cartilage is then débrided down to the calcified layer with an arthroscopic shaver.

The number, diameter, and position of the graft cylinders that will be required to fill the defect can be determined by placing the harvesting punch or the delivery chisel over the lesion. Using the sharpened end of the punch, superficial markings can be used to create a template of the lesion. Generally, plugs with a diameter of 3 to 5 mm are harvested. Smaller plugs have been shown to be too fragile, whereas larger plugs may be associated with degenerative changes at both the harvest site and on its opposing chondral surface.[25]

When resurfacing condylar defects, grafts should be harvested from the margins of the lateral and medial condyles above the sulcus terminalis.[26,27] To obtain a more anatomic reconstruction of lesions in the trochlear groove, this area can be resurfaced with bone plugs harvested from the intercondylar notch because both surfaces are concave. Harvest sites should be placed no closer than 2 to 3 mm apart. Donor sites placed too close together can

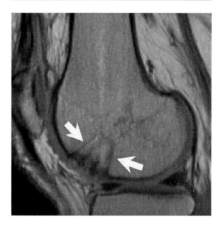

Figure 3 Sagittal spin-echo intermediate-weighted MRI scan shows osteochondral graft harvest site convergence (*arrows*).

cause the bone tunnels to intersect, which may cause collapse of the overlying bone or shortening of the harvested plugs (Figure 3). Manually driven harvesting punches are preferred. Power trephination may result in decreased chondrocyte survival rates because of thermal necrosis[18] (Figure 4).

The harvesting chisel is inserted perpendicular to the articular surface and is advanced with a mallet to the desired depth, approximately 15 to 20 mm. However, longer plugs may be harvested when attempting to reconstruct defects with bone loss greater than 10 mm in depth. Preoperative planning with MRI is important to determine the depth of the lesion and amount of bone loss present. To ensure stable plug implantation, at least half of the length of the plug needs to be buried in bone. Therefore, to reconstruct a 15-mm bone defect, a 30-mm plug is required. As the grafts are removed, they are measured and temporarily placed on a saline-soaked sponge.

Preparation and Implantation of the Recipient Site

After the exact location of the recipient plug is identified, the insertion

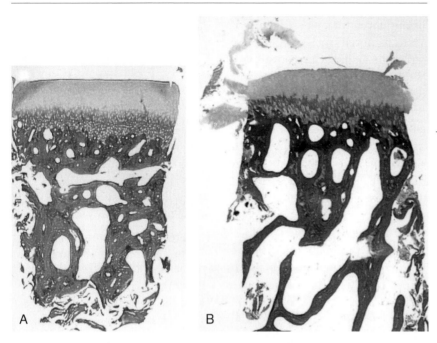

Figure 4 **A,** Manual punch-harvested 2.7-mm graft showing relatively little gross damage to the articular margins and underlying bone (light micrograph, Masson's trichrome, original ×100). **B,** Power trephine-harvested 2.7-mm graft showing significantly greater damage to both the articular margins and the entire articular surface (light micrograph, Masson's trichrome, original magnification ×100).

angle is determined using either a spinal needle or the graft insertion tool. This step is critical and ensures that the osteochondral plugs will be inserted perpendicular to the joint surface. The appropriately sized drill is advanced to the proper depth, which is the depth required to seat the graft fully but still allow the plug to sit at the level of the original articular cartilage surface. For example, if the transplant needs to sit 3 mm above the defect base to be at the level of the original surface and the plug is 20 mm long, then the hole should be drilled to 17 mm. The hole is then dilated with a tunnel dilator and the bone plug is placed into the insertion tool. If the cartilage on the harvested plug or the cartilage surrounding the recipient site is oblique, the graft should be properly oriented within the inserter before placement to best

match the contour of the surrounding cartilage and joint surface anatomy. Graft insertion should be performed with the inflow pump turned off because osteochondral grafts tend to swell in saline. Swelling can lead to a size mismatch between the harvested graft and the recipient tunnel, resulting in possible breakage of the graft during insertion. Turning off the inflow pump during insertion also prevents the graft from accidentally being expelled from the insertion tool because of fluid pressure.

The graft must be inserted using gentle manual pressure because excessive force can injure the chondrocytes. Mosaicplasty allows for the plug to be inserted to the exact depth. No hammer is necessary. Even low-impact pressures can cause damage to the chondrocytes in articular cartilage. Pressures greater

than 15 MPa in adults or 7.5 MPa in children have been shown to result in injury to the articular cartilage.[28] The use of a mallet is not recommended to place the osteochondral plug.

To better recreate the appropriate articular surface contour, peripheral plugs should be placed in the lesion before inserting the more central plugs (Figure 5). Central plugs are usually seated higher than the surrounding peripheral plugs. If the central plugs are inserted first, there is a tendency to place the plugs in a recessed position that creates a flattened contour; this placement eventually leads to fibrocartilage overgrowth on top of the plug that renders the transplanted hyaline cartilage ineffective (Figure 6).

The grafts should be seated with the base firmly set against the bottom of the drill hole, with good side-to-side contact. After all the grafts are placed, the knee is tested for range of motion and graft stability is assessed. Wounds are closed in a standard manner and a compressive dressing is applied. Grafts should be inspected prior to insertion. On occasion the graft is fractured upon removal from its donor site at the cartilage-bone interface. These plugs should not be used. If the plugs are good, careful insertion technique should avoid any further damage.

Open Procedures
At the present time, patellar osteochondral resurfacing cannot be performed arthroscopically. Surgical preference will dictate the location and size of the incision. A lateral parapatellar incision and approach is preferred by the authors because a concurrent tibial tubercle osteotomy can be performed to offload the patellofemoral joint and area of resur-

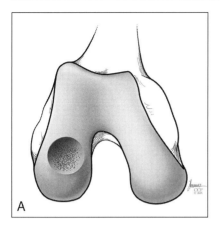
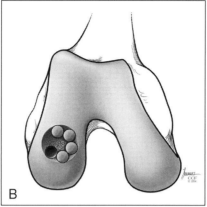
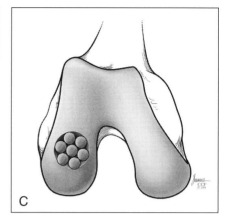

Figure 5   Osteochondral graft insertion sequence. **A,** Osteochondral defect on the femoral condyle. **B,** Peripheral plugs are first placed in the lesion. **C,** Central plugs are then placed after peripheral plugs are seated. (Reproduced with permission from Cleveland Clinic Foundation.)

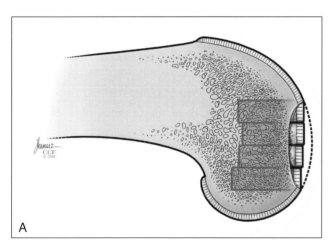
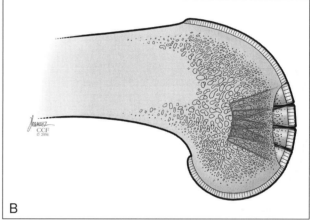

Figure 6   **A,** When central grafts are placed first, they tend to be placed in a recessed position creating a flattened contour **B,** Proper graft placement. (Reproduced with permission from Cleveland Clinic Foundation.)

facing. Estimations of graft size, harvesting, and insertion are performed using the same guidelines as described for the arthroscopic procedure. Graft placement should also follow the same criteria to maximize stable seating of the plugs and to recreate the articular contour as accurately as possible. The patellar articular surface is potentially more complex to reconstruct than the femoral condyles because of the presence of the central longitudinal ridge. The contour of the longitudinal ridge may be difficult to repro-

duce without some convergence of the graft plugs at each side of the ridge. Care must be taken to avoid plug intersection, which may lead to a short bony element of the graft, graft instability, displacement of the graft from the recipient site, or cyst formation.

A tibial tubercle osteotomy at the time of resurfacing of the patella is intended to realign the extensor mechanism to reduce the forces at the site of the resurfacing and to facilitate healing of the OAT; however, it is not always necessary.

Bipolar lesions of the patella and trochlea may be resurfaced using OAT techniques; however, the risk of graft displacement from the recipient site is increased because the transplanted plugs catch on opposing surfaces of the patellofemoral joint. These lesions are extremely difficult to reconstruct and the articular surface contour on each side must be accurately reconstituted to avoid graft dislodgment or breakage. The angulated surfaces of the trochlea also present a spatial challenge to reconstruction. Failure to appropri-

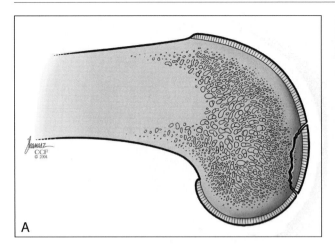
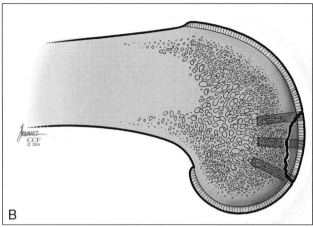

Figure 7   Illustration showing stabilization of OCD fragment with osteochondral plugs. **A,** Cross-sectional lateral view of in situ OCD fragment. **B,** Cross-sectional lateral view of OCD stabilized with osteochondral plugs. (Reproduced with permission from Cleveland Clinic Foundation.)

ately recreate the trochlear anatomy tends to result in the creation of a flat reconstructed trochlea, which can lead to excessive patellofemoral forces.

Osteochondritis Dissecans

Many different fixation techniques including bone pegs, wires, and metallic and bioabsorbable screws have been described for osteochondritis dissecans (OCD) fragments.[29-31] The goals of fixation are to restore articular congruity by anatomically reducing the fragment, and to provide satisfactory stabilization to enable healing. Metallic implants tend to provide superior compression and fixation strength but potentially require removal. Bioabsorbable implants may obviate the need for removal, but provide inferior compressive and fixation strength; patients may also have an adverse reaction to the implant's composition. The favored option for fixation of OCD is to press fit autologous osteochondral cylindrical grafts into the lesion (Figure 7). All of the fixation principles that are required for proper healing of an OCD fragment are provided by the osteochondral plugs.

The OAT techniques involve drilling across the fragment and into the base of the lesion, which stimulates a blood supply and provides stable fixation because of the interference fit. The grafts do not require removal. Appropriately sized plugs are strong enough to allow ease of handling and insertion, and provide adequate stability to the lesion for healing. Although the plugs breach the articular surface of the OCD, an intact cartilage surface is reconstructed. Surgery for OCD may be separated into two broad categories: fragment missing and fragment intact.

Fragment Missing

When the fragment is missing, the lesion is treated as if it were a traumatic osteochondral defect. The area is débrided and an autologous osteochondral transplantation resurfacing is performed. The cartilage and bony defects must be reconstructed while ensuring that the plugs are inserted at the proper level to restore the normal joint contour.

Fragment Intact

Stabilizing an OCD requires that the lesion be osteochondral (rather than purely chondral) and not fragmented. The osteochonodral nature of the injury is determined on preoperative imaging. Fragmented lesions or those without an osseous base cause difficulties in fixation and should possibly be débrided. Autologous plugs are harvested in the standard manner and transplanted into recipient holes strategically placed to stabilize the fragment. The lesion is stabilized using several peripheral plugs and a single central plug. The central plug must be of sufficient length to cross the entire diameter of the OCD and anchor solidly into the cancellous bone deep to the lesion. The depth of the lesion is best determined from the preoperative MRI. Initial compression can be provided by insertion of a central wire or screw, followed by peripheral fixation with osteochondral plugs, then replacement of the central fixation with an osteochondral plug. An accessory portal through the patellar tendon is a useful adjunct to provide an optimal angle of approach to an OCD on the lateral aspect of the medial femoral condyle. When using a technique in which the recipient site is dilated and the plugs are inserted in a press-fit manner, it is not possible to exchange the osteochondral plug obtained from the donor and recipient sites as described by Nakagawa and associates.[32]

Postoperative Protocol

Postoperatively, patients are placed in a hinged knee brace set at 0° to 90°. Therapy is initiated the next day and stresses range-of-motion exercises and isometric quadriceps strengthening. An emphasis is placed on regaining range of motion and reducing postoperative effusion. A graduated exercise program is advanced as the patient becomes more comfortable. Patients are permitted only touch-down weight bearing for the first 6 weeks. Although it is not proven whether the weight-bearing status affects the final results, basic science studies note that pistoning of unstable plugs can cause cyst formation beneath the plugs. Obtaining stable plugs at the time of implantation is of foremost importance; therefore, limiting the patient to touch-down weight bearing is an added precaution.

If the patient is relatively comfortable and radiographs are satisfactory (there should be no displacement of plugs or cyst formation) at the 6-week postoperative evaluation, the patient progresses to weight bearing as tolerated. Patients are permitted to return to participation in sport activities when there is minimal effusion, a near full range of motion is achieved, and the strength of the quadriceps is approximately 80% of that of the contralateral leg.

Postoperative radiographic assessment may be performed during the rehabilitation period and provides useful information on recipient-site cartilage thickness, contour, and graft congruence and

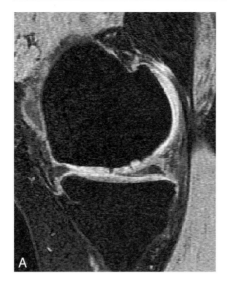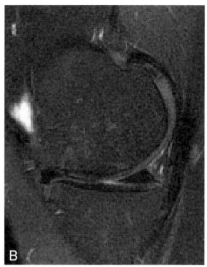

Figure 8   Normal contour and cartilage cover following OAT reconstruction of the medial femoral condyle. Sagittal spoiled gradient-echo MRI scan (**A**) and corresponding fast spin-echo T2-weighted MRI scan with fat saturation (**B**) show prior OAT reconstruction of a portion of the weight-bearing aspect of the medial femoral condyle. Irregularity can be seen on the subchondral cortical contour in the region of the prior reconstruction. Intact cartilage cover and well-recreated articular contour can be appreciated. Mature incorporation of the plugs is identified by resolution of marrow edema and loss of identification of discrete plug tracks.

incorporation, as well as allowing assessment of the graft harvest sites and evaluation of the potential complications of osteochondral transplantation.[33-37] MRI with fast spin-echo sequences rather than fat-suppressed spoiled gradient echo sequences offer advantages of increased sensitivity to subchondral osseous changes and decreased sensitivity to the artifacts secondary to the surgical debris typically present after OAT. These images help to assess healing of the fragments and continuity of the articular surface.

Magnetic resonance signal characteristics of recipient-site hyaline cartilage follow the imaging features of adjacent native articular cartilage (Figure 8). Over time, fibrocartilage-like tissue develops between transplanted plugs and even overgrows the hyaline cartilage of the transplanted plugs in locations where the joint contour is below the level of

the original height of the articular surface. This fibrocartilaginous tissue may show a mildly heterogenous increase in T2-weighted signal characteristics on fast spin-echo imaging, or mildly decreased signal intensity on spoiled gradient echo acquisitions when compared with adjacent articular cartilage.

Outcomes
Osteochondral Lesions

Many clinical studies show favorable outcomes to support the use of OAT for the treatment of osteochondral lesions. The report by Hangody and Fules[38] on 10 years of clinical experience using the mosaicplasty procedure detailed good to excellent results in 92% of patients treated with femoral condylar lesions, in 87% of those treated with tibia-sided resurfacing, and in 79% of patients with patellar or trochlear mosaicplasty. These results are similar to those published in previous studies and highlight the importance of the location of the defect on the patient's long-term prognosis.[33,39-41]

The locations best suited for treatment are the femoral condyles. Tibial plateau lesions are usually asymmetric arthritic lesions and rarely have a focal chondral or osteochondral defect. The authors have had limited experience in treating tibial plateau lesions with OATs. Several patients have been treated with OAT in the patellofemoral joint; this procedure is extremely technically demanding and can be expected to produce slightly inferior clinical results.

A prospective clinical trial comparing autologous chondrocyte implantation with OAT showed superior results in the group treated with OAT, particularly with regard to the presence of hyaline cartilage in the OAT group compared with the reparative fibrocartilage predominantly present in the group treated with autologous chondrocyte implantation.[15] The persistence of hyaline cartilage in patients treated with OATs had been previously observed in biopsy specimens from successfully treated patients.[17]

Another prospective trial showed the superiority of autologous chondrocyte implantation compared with OAT; however, this trial was subsequently criticized for the unorthodox rehabilitation protocol used for the OAT group and for the large mean size of the resurfaced lesions (a size that tended to be larger than that for which the OAT technique was known to be effective).[42-44]

Basic science research is improving the technical aspects of how grafts should be harvested, the care that needs to be taken when handling the plugs, and the means by which the recipient sites are prepared, and im-proving the understanding of the complex interrelationships that occur in both normal and transplanted cartilage, thus enabling the refinement of surgical techniques and directing future advances in treatment augmentation. The use of OAT and autologous chondrocyte implantation in combination may provide a promising surgical approach for treating larger osteochondral defects and for resolving the problem of gap retention between the transplanted osteochondral plugs and the native surrounding cartilage.[45] The treatment with visco-supplementation after OAT has recently been shown to improve chondrocyte survival after transplantation.[46]

Osteochondritis Dissecans Fixation

Reports of patients with OCD who were treated by fixation with OAT have shown 100% healing and return to full activity by 6 months after surgery.[33,39] Symptoms resolve and the defects heal following satisfactory stabilization. Assessment of International Knee Documentation Committee scores in this group of patients return to normal. These results hold true for treated OCD lesions in adults.

Summary

OAT for the treatment of symptomatic osteochondral defects and OCD is well established. OAT is a technically demanding but relatively inexpensive procedure and requires a single operation. The published results are favorable in comparison with other treatment techniques. However, optimal results are dependent on the location of the lesion, careful adherence to patient selection criteria, and the use of proper surgical techniques. Basic science research is enabling the continued refinement of surgical technique and is directing future advances in treatment augmentation.

References

1. Hasler EM, Herzog W, Wu JZ, Muller W, Wyss U: Articular cartilage biomechanics: Theoretical models, material properties, and biosynthetic response. *Crit Rev Biomed Eng* 1999;27:415-488.

2. Noyes FR, Bassett RW, Grood ES, Butler DL: Arthroscopy in acute traumatic hemarthrosis of the knee: Incidence of anterior cruciate tears and other injuries. *J Bone Joint Surg Am* 1980;62:687-695.

3. Hunter W: Of the structure and disease of articulating cartilages: 1743. *Clin Orthop Relat Res* 1995;317:3-6.

4. Kim HK, Moran ME, Salter RB: The potential for regeneration of articular cartilage in defects created by chondral shaving and subchondral abrasion: An experimental investigation in rabbits. *J Bone Joint Surg Am* 1991;73:1301-1315.

5. Campbell CJ: The healing of cartilage defects. *Clin Orthop Relat Res* 1969;64: 45-63.

6. Insall J: The Pridie debridement operation for osteoarthritis of the knee. *Clin Orthop Relat Res* 1974;101:61-67.

7. Pridie KH: A method of resurfacing osteoarthritic knee joints. *J Bone Joint Surg Br* 1959;41:618-619.

8. Buckwalter JA, Mankin HJ, Grodzinsky AJ: Articular cartilage and osteoarthritis. *Instr Course Lect* 2005;54:465-480.

9. Furukawa T, Eyre DR, Koide S, Glimcher MJ: Biochemical studies on repair cartilage resurfacing experimental defects in the rabbit knee. *J Bone Joint Surg Am* 1980;62:79-89.

10. Mandelbaum BR, Browne JE, Fu F, et al: Articular cartilage lesions of the knee. *Am J Sports Med* 1998;26:853-861.

11. Mankin HJ: The response of articular cartilage to mechanical injury. *J Bone Joint Surg Am* 1982;64:460-466.

12. Mitchell N, Shepard N: The resurfacing of adult rabbit articular cartilage by multiple perforations through the subchondral bone. *J Bone Joint Surg Am* 1976;58:230-233.

13. Brittberg M, Lindahl A, Nilsson A, Ohlsson C, Isaksson O, Peterson L: Treatment of deep cartilage defects in the knee with autologous chondrocyte transplantation. *N Engl J Med* 1994; 331:889-895.

14. Grande DA, Pitman MI, Peterson L, Menche D, Klein M: The repair of experimentally produced defects in rabbit articular cartilage by autologous chondrocyte transplantation. *J Orthop Res* 1989;7:208-218.

15. Horas U, Pelinkovic D, Herr G, Aigner T, Schnettler R: Autologous chondrocyte implantation and osteochondral cylinder transplantation in cartilage repair of the knee joint: A prospective, comparative trial. *J Bone Joint Surg Am* 2003;85:185-192.

16. Yamashita F, Sakakida K, Suzu F, Takai S: The transplantation of an autogeneic osteochondral fragment for osteochondritis dissecans of the knee. *Clin Orthop Relat Res* 1985;201:43-50.

17. Hangody L, Kish G, Karpati Z, Szerb I, Udvarhelyi I: Arthroscopic autogenous osteochondral mosaicplasty for the treatment of femoral condylar articular defects: A preliminary report. *Knee Surg Sports Traumatol Arthrosc* 1997;5:262-267.

18. Evans PJ, Miniaci A, Hurtig MB: Manual punch versus power harvesting of osteochondral grafts. *Arthroscopy* 2004;20:306-310.

19. Pearce SG, Hurtig MB, Clarnette R, Kalra M, Cowan B, Miniaci A: An investigation of 2 techniques for optimizing joint surface congruency using multiple cylindrical osteochondral autografts. *Arthroscopy* 2001;17:50-55.

20. Rosenberg TD, Paulos LE, Parker RD, Coward DB, Scott SM: The forty-five-degree posteroanterior flexion weight-bearing radiograph of the knee. *J Bone Joint Surg Am* 1988;70:1479-1483.

21. Chung CB, Frank LR, Resnick D: Cartilage imaging techniques: Current clinical applications and state of the art imaging. *Clin Orthop Relat Res* 2001;391:S370-S378.

22. Disler DG, McCauley TR, Wirth CR, Fuchs MD: Detection of knee hyaline cartilage defects using fat-suppressed three-dimensional spoiled gradient-echo MR imaging: Comparison with standard MR imaging and correlation with arthroscopy. *AJR Am J Roentgenol* 1995;165:377-382.

23. Disler DG, McCauley TR, Kelman CG, et al: Fat-suppressed three-dimensional spoiled gradient-echo MR imaging of hyaline cartilage defects in the knee: Comparison with standard MR imaging and arthroscopy. *AJR Am J Roentgenol* 1996;167:127-132.

24. Recht MP, Piraino DW, Paletta GA, Schils JP, Belhobek GH: Accuracy of fat-suppressed three-dimensional spoiled gradient-echo FLASH MR imaging in the detection of patellofemoral articular cartilage abnormalities. *Radiology* 1996;198:209-212.

25. Miniaci A: The effect of graft size and number on outcome of mosaic arthroplasty resurfacing: An experimental model in sheep. *Proceedings of the International Society of Arthroscopy, Knee Surgery, and Orthopaedic Sports Medicine.* 2001, p 169.

26. Ahmad CS, Cohen ZA, Levine WN, Ateshian GA, Mow VC: Biomechanical and topographic considerations for autologous osteochondral grafting in the knee. *Am J Sports Med* 2001;29:201-206.

27. Bartz RL, Kamaric E, Noble PC, Lintner D, Bocell J: Topographic matching of selected donor and recipient sites for osteochondral autografting of the articular surface of the femoral condyles. *Am J Sports Med* 2001;29:207-212.

28. Hand C, Lobo J, Miniaci A: Osteochondral autografting resurfacing. *Sports Med Arthros Rev* 2003, 11: 245-263.

29. Thomson NL: Osteochondritis dissecans and osteochondral fragments managed by Herbert compression screw fixation. *Clin Orthop Relat Res* 1987;224:71-78.

30. Rey Zuniga JJ, Sagastibelza J, Lopez Blasco JJ, Martinez GM: Arthroscopic use of the Herbert screw in osteochondritis dissecans of the knee. *Arthroscopy* 1993;9:668-670.

31. Slough JA, Noto AM, Schmidt TL: Tibial cortical bone peg fixation in osteochondritis dissecans of the knee. *Clin Orthop Relat Res* 1991;267:122-127.

32. Nakagawa Y, Matsusue Y, Nakamura T: A novel surgical procedure for osteochondritis dissecans of the lateral femoral condyle: Exchanging osteochondral plugs taken from donor and recipient sites. *Arthroscopy* 2002;18:E5.

33. Mainil-Varlet P, Rieser F, Grogan S, Mueller W, Saager C, Jakob RP: Articular cartilage repair using a tissue-engineered cartilage-like implant: An animal study. *Osteoarthritis Cartilage* 2001;9:S6-15.

34. Alparslan L, Winalski CS, Boutin RD, Minas T: Postoperative magnetic resonance imaging of articular cartilage repair. *Semin Musculoskelet Radiol* 2001;5:345-363.

35. Sanders TG, Mentzer KD, Miller MD, Morrison WB, Campbell SE, Penrod BJ: Autogenous osteochondral "plug" transfer for the treatment of focal chondral defects: Postoperative MR appearance with clinical correlation. *Skeletal Radiol* 2001;30:570-578.

36. Burkart A, Imhoff AB: Diagnostic imaging after autologous chondrocyte transplantation: Correlation of magnetic resonance tomography, histological and arthroscopic findings. *Orthopade* 2000;29:135-144.

37. Recht MP, Kramer J: MR imaging of the postoperative knee: A pictorial essay. *Radiographics* 2002;22:765-774.

38. Hangody L, Fules P: Autologous osteochondral mosaicplasty for the treatment of full-thickness defects of weight-bearing joints: Ten years of experimental and clinical experience. *J Bone Joint Surg Am* 2003;85(suppl 2):25-32.

39. Tytherleigh-Strong G, Hirahara A, Miniaci A: Arthroscopic autogenous osteochondral graft fixation (mosaicplasty) of unstable osteochondritis dissecans lesions of the knee. *Proceedings of the American Orthopaedic Society for Sports Medicine.* 2001, p 224.

40. Jakob RP, Franz T, Gautier E, Mainil-Varlet P: Autologous osteochondral grafting in the knee: Indication, results, and reflections. *Clin Orthop Relat Res* 2002;401:170-184.

41. Hangody L, Kish G, Karpati Z, Udvarhelyi I, Szigeti I, Bely M: Mosaicplasty for the treatment of articular cartilage defects: Application in clinical practice. *Orthopedics* 1998;21:751-756.

42. LaPrade RF: Autologous chondrocyte implantation was superior to mosaicplasty for repair of articular cartilage defects in the knee at one year. *J Bone Joint Surg Am* 2003;85:2259.

43. Kish G, Hangody L: A prospective, randomised comparison of autologous chondrocyte implantation versus mosaicplasty for osteochondral defects in the knee. *J Bone Joint Surg Br* 2004;86:619-620.

44. Bentley G, Biant LC, Carrington RW, et al: A prospective, randomised comparison of autologous chondrocyte implantation versus mosaicplasty for osteochondral defects in the knee. *J Bone Joint Surg Br* 2003;85:223-230.

45. Sharpe JR, Ahmed SU, Fleetcroft JP, Martin R: The treatment of osteochondral lesions using a combination of autologous chondrocyte implantation and autograft: Three-year follow-up. *J Bone Joint Surg Br* 2005;87:730-735.

46. Tytherleigh-Strong G, Hurtig M, Miniaci A: Intra-articular hyaluronan following autogenous osteochondral grafting of the knee. *Arthroscopy* 2005;21:999-1005.

Articular Cartilage Repair in Athletes

Kai Mithoefer, MD

Jason M. Scopp, MD

Bert R. Mandelbaum, MD

Abstract

Articular cartilage lesions in the athletic population commonly occur and result from the significant acute and chronic joint stress associated with high-impact sports. These lesions have poor intrinsic healing capacity, and the persistent defects in the joint surfaces cause pain, swelling, and mechanical symptoms that result in functional impairment and limitation of athletic participation. If untreated, articular cartilage lesions can lead to chronic joint degeneration and disability. Several techniques for articular cartilage repair have been recently developed with promising results. However, the significant joint stresses generated in athletes require an effective and durable cartilage surface restoration that can withstand the high mechanical demands in this population over time.

Instr Course Lect 2007;56:457-468.

Articular cartilage defects of the knee are a common occurrence. Curl and associates[1] described 53,569 hyaline cartilage lesions in 19,827 patients undergoing knee arthroscopy. Additionally, a recent prospective survey of 993 consecutive knee arthroscopies demonstrated evidence of articular cartilage pathology in 66% of patients.[2] Most lesions are single, high-grade lesions located on the femur. Levy and associates[3] noted an increasing frequency of chondral injuries in colle-

giate, professional, and world-class athletes. Along with this rising incidence in high-level competitive sports, increasing participation in organized recreational sports such as soccer, basketball, and football has been associated with a growing incidence of sports-related articular cartilage injuries.[4-6.] Articular cartilage lesions frequently occur in association with acute ligament or meniscal injuries, traumatic patellar dislocations, and osteochondral injuries, or they may develop from chronic ligamentous instability and malalignment.[6-8] Articular cartilage defects of the femoral condyles have been observed in up to 50% of athletes undergoing anterior cruciate ligament (ACL) reconstruction, with an increased propensity noted

in female athletes.[4,9] These injuries often limit participation in athletic activity and predispose the athlete to early joint degeneration.[10,11]

Because of the documented poor potential of articular cartilage defects to spontaneously repair, injuries to the articular cartilage surfaces present a therapeutic challenge, particularly in young and active individuals.[12-14]

The recent development of new surgical techniques has created considerable clinical and scientific interest in articular cartilage repair.[6,8,15-20] Because injuries to the articular cartilage of the knee have been shown to be one of the most common causes of permanent disability in athletes,[21,22] management of articular cartilage in this high-demand population has important long-term implications.[23,24] As a result of the documented detrimental effect of high-impact articular loading,[13,25] articular cartilage repair in the athletic population requires cartilage surface restoration that can withstand the significant mechanical joint stresses generated during high-impact, pivoting sports. In addition to reducing pain, increasing mobility, and improving knee function, the ability to return the patient to

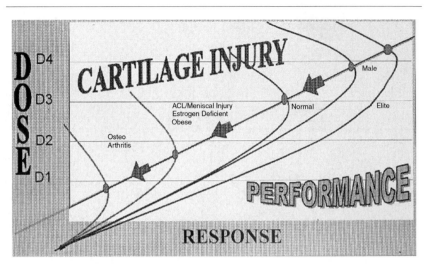

Figure 1 Diagram displaying the relationship between level of performance (response) and activity (dose; dosage 1 through 4) with performance and cartilage injury. (Reproduced with permission from Scopp JM, Mandelbaum BR: Osteochondral injury of the knee. *Hosp Phys* 2005;2:2-12.)

Natural History

The limited ability of articular cartilage to spontaneously repair has been well documented.[13,26] After acute injury and resultant tissue necrosis, the lack of vascularization of articular cartilage prevents the physiologic inflammatory response that is required for spontaneous healing. The limited intrinsic ability of mature chondrocytes to replicate and repair, and the lack of recruitment of extrinsic undifferentiated repair cells results in qualitatively and quantitatively insufficient repair cartilage. Repetitive loading of the injured articular cartilage results in additional cellular degeneration, with accumulation of degradative enzymes and cytokines, disruption of collagen ultrastructure, increased hydration, and fissuring of the articular surface. These biochemical and metabolic changes mimic the early changes observed in patients with osteoarthritis.[27]

Although laboratory studies have contributed a greater understanding about the progression of cartilage injury to osteoarthritis, prospective clinical information about the natural history of articular cartilage lesions is rare, particularly in athletes. This lack of long-term data can be largely attributed to the inability of clinicians to accurately diagnose and follow chondral lesions using noninvasive techniques. One recent study demonstrated that hyaline cartilage defects cause pain and swelling and predict severe changes in lifestyle and athletic activity in patients with ACL injuries.[28] Another study has shown that untreated articular cartilage defects in patients with ACL deficiency resulted in significantly worse outcome scores up to 19 years after the original injury compared with ACL injured knees without cartilage lesions.[29] A Swedish study reported on the long-term prognosis in 28 athletes with isolated severe chondral damage in the weight-bearing condyles.[30] Although 75% of athletes returned to athletic activity initially, a significant decline in athletic activity was observed 14 years after the initial injury, with radiographic evidence of osteoarthritis noted in 57% of these athletes. A prospective study of osteochondral lesions also reported poor results with strenuous athletic activity in 38% of patients and moderate to severe radiographic evidence of osteoarthritis in 45% at an average follow-up of 34 years.[31] This is consistent with the findings of a recent National Institutes of Health consensus conference on osteoarthritis that reported a relative risk of 4.4 to 5.3 for knee osteoarthritis in high-demand, pivoting athletes.[10] Despite these clinical results, the long-term outcomes of treated articular cartilage defects in athletes is still unclear.

Chondropenia

The increased risk for the development of knee osteoarthritis in athletes is well documented, particularly in those at the elite level.[10,11,21-24] Intact articular cartilage possesses optimal load-bearing characteristics and adjusts to the level of activity. Increasing weight-bearing activity in athletes and adolescents has been shown to increase the volume and thickness of articular cartilage.[32] In the healthy athlete, a positive linear dose-response relationship exists for repetitive loading activities and articular cartilage function. However, a recent study indicates that this dose-response curve reaches a threshold and that activity beyond this threshold can result in maladaptation and injury of articular cartilage[33] (Figure 1). High-impact joint loading above this threshold has been shown to decrease cartilage proteoglycan content, increase levels

Table 1
Chondropenia Severity Score

Patellofemoral		Medial Compartment		Lateral Compartment				
Cartilage:		Cartilage:		Cartilage:				
Patella		**Medial Femoral Condyle**		**Lateral Femoral Condyle**				
Normal	10	Normal	10	Normal	10			
Grade Ia	8	Grade Ia	8	Grade Ia	8			
Grade Ib	6	Grade Ib	6	Grade Ib	6			
Grade IIa	5	Grade IIa	5	Grade IIa	5			
Grade IIb	3	Grade IIb	3	Grade IIb	3			
Grade IIIa	2	Grade IIIa	2	Grade IIIa	2			
Grade IIIb	1	Grade IIIb	1	Grade IIIb	1			
Grade IV	0	Grade IV	0	Grade IV	0			
Trochlea		**Medial Tibial Plateau**		**Lateral Tibial Plateau**				
Normal	10	Normal	10	Normal	10			
Grade Ia	8	Grade Ia	8	Grade Ia	8			
Grade Ib	6	Grade Ib	6	Grade Ib	6			
Grade IIa	5	Grade IIa	5	Grade IIa	5			
Grade IIb	3	Grade IIb	3	Grade IIb	3			
Grade IIIa	2	Grade IIIa	2	Grade IIIa	2			
Grade IIIb	1	Grade IIIb	1	Grade IIIb	1			
Grade IV	0	Grade IV	0	Grade IV	0			
Meniscus	n/a	**Meniscus**		**Meniscus**				
		100% remaining	20	100% remaining	20			
		> 2/3 remaining	15	> 2/3 remaining	15			
		1/3 to 2/3 remaining	10	1/3 to 2/3 remaining	10			
		< 1/3 remaining	5	< 1/3 remaining	5			
		0% remaining	0	0% remaining	0			
Sums:	–		+		–	+	–	= Total CSS

n/a = not applicable, CSS = Chondropenia Severity Score

of degradative enzymes, and cause chondrocyte apoptosis.[25,27,34] If the integrity of the functional weight-bearing unit is lost, either as a result of acute injury or chronic microtrauma in the high-impact athlete, a chondropenic response is initiated that can include loss of articular cartilage volume and stiffness, elevation of contact pressures, and development or progression of articular cartilage defects. Concomitant pathologic factors such as ligamentous instability, malalignment, and meniscal injury or deficiency can further support progression of the chondropenic cascade. Without intervention, chondropenia leads to progressive deterioration of articular cartilage function and may ultimately progress to osteoarthritis (Tables 1 through 3).

Diagnosis

Diagnosis of articular cartilage lesions can be achieved by a combination of history, clinical examination, and radiographic evaluation. A high index of suspicion for an articular cartilage lesion is important in patients with acute hemarthrosis,[35] acute or chronic ligamentous instability, patellar dislocation or maltracking, or lower extremity mal-

Table 2
Chondropenia Severity Score (CSS) Patient Stratification

Severity	CSS Range
Normal	76 to 100
Mild	51 to 75
Moderate	26 to 50
Severe	< 26

alignment. Clinical symptoms of articular cartilage injury are not specific, but athletes will often report activity-related pain, effusion, catching, and locking of the knee. Plain radiographs, including weight-bearing AP and lateral views, Rosen-

Table 3
ICRS Arthroscopic Classification of Articular Cartilage Lesions

Articular Cartilage Lesions	ICRS Arthroscopic Classification
Normal	
Grade I	Superficial fissures
Grade II	< 1/2 cartilage depth
Grade III	> 1/2 cartilage depth to but not through subchondral plate
Grade IV	Osteochondral lesions through subchondral plate
a: < 2 cm²	
b: > 2 cm²	

ICRS = International Cartilage Repair Society

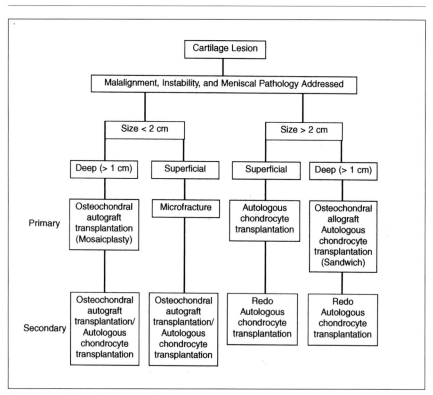

Figure 2 Clinical algorithm for the management of ACL lesions in athletes.

berg and tunnel views, long-leg films, and Merchant views, can help to identify osteochondral lesions, joint space narrowing, patellar maltracking, or lower extremity malalignment. Cartilage-sensitive MRI is a sensitive, specific, and accurate tool for noninvasive diagnosis of articular cartilage injuries. MRI scans should be obtained in three planes and using fast spin-echo imaging with a repetition time of 3,500 to 5,000 msec and a moderate echo time, which provides high-contrast resolution among articular cartilage, subchondral bone, and joint fluid.[36] In addition to its use for preoperative diagnosis of articular cartilage injuries, cartilage-sensitive MRI can be helpful for postoperative evaluation of cartilage repair.[37,38]

Treatment

Traditional treatment methods such as abrasion chondroplasty and subchondral bone drilling have not produced reliable and lasting cartilage repair, but newer techniques such as microfracture, mosaicplasty, autologous chondrocyte transplantation,

and osteochondral allograft transplantation have produced more encouraging results.[15-19] Prospective clinical results on these techniques, however, are limited.[39] Each of the new cartilage repair techniques is associated with unique advantages and limitations. Based on the available studies, an algorithm has been developed for the treatment of articular cartilage repair in athletes (Figure 2).

Microfracture
The microfracture technique described by Mithoefer and associates[16,17] presents an improvement of earlier marrow-stimulation techniques such as Pridie drilling. Microfracture includes débridement of the cartilage lesion to stable cartilage margins, careful removal of the calcified cartilage layer, and micropenetration of the subchondral bone using commercially available instrumentation. Subchondral bone

bridges (width, 4 mm) are maintained for preservation of the subchondral bone-plate integrity and function. Release of blood and marrow fat droplets from the microfracture holes results in the formation of a clot in the cartilage defect that contains pluripotent marrow-derived mesenchymal stem cells, which produce a mixed fibrocartilage repair tissue containing varying amounts of type II collagen[40-42] (Figure 3). Continuous passive motion and protected weight bearing are used for 6 weeks. Return to regular activities and sports can generally be achieved 6 to 8 months postoperatively.[16,17,38]

Because of its technical simplicity, limited invasiveness, low associated morbidity rate, and short postoperative rehabilitation period, microfracture has become a popular treatment option for articular cartilage lesions in athletes. Steadman

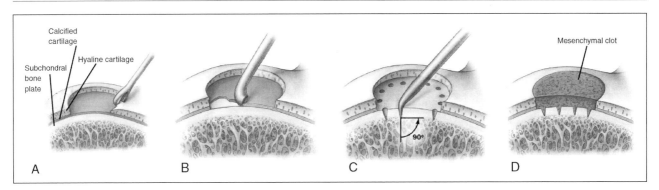

Figure 3 Microfracture technique for articular cartilage repair. **A,** Débridement to stable cartilage margins. **B,** Removal of the calcified cartilage layer. **C,** Micropenetration of the subchondral bone plate with microfracture awl. **D,** The resultant formation of a mesenchymal clot in the cartilage defects that contains pluripotent cells from the subchondral bone marrow. (Reproduced with permission from Mithoefer K, Williams RJ III, Warren RF, et al: Chondral resurfacing of articular cartilage defects in the knee with the microfracture technique. *J Bone Joint Surg Am* 2006;88(suppl 1):294-304.)

and associates[43] reported significant increases in the ability of patients to perform activities of daily living, strenuous work, and athletic activities after microfracture. Improved knee function has been reported in 58% to 95% of athletes after microfracture, with significantly increased activities of daily living, Marx knee activity rating, International Knee Documentation Committee Subjective Knee Evaluation, and Tegner scores.[42-44] In another study, Blevins and associates[45] demonstrated that 77% of elite athletes assessed were able to return to competition; however, these authors did not separately describe the rate of return to recreational athletic activity after undergoing microfracture. Steadman and associates[43] reported a return rate of 76% in National Football League players after undergoing microfracture. Blevins and associates[45] and Steadman and associates[44] reported that high-level athletes assessed who underwent microfracture returned to athletic activity at a mean of 9.3 and 10 months, respectively. Of the athletes who returned to athletic activity, 37% to 50% were still competing at a mean of 4.6 seasons or 37 months after their re-

turn.[44,45] Other studies have reported that 44% to 58% of athletes have been able to return to athletic activity after undergoing microfracture, 57% of them at the preinjury level of participation.[42,46]

Generally, the longer the interval between injury and microfracture, the lower the rate of return to high-impact athletic activity. Of athletes who have been symptomatic for less than 12 months before undergoing microfracture, 67% return to high-impact sports, whereas only 14% of those with symptoms of greater duration are able to return.[46] Inferior macroscopic grading and limited volume of the repaired cartilage after microfracture has been observed with prolonged intervals between the injury and the procedure and provides a plausible explanation for the less satisfactory clinical results.[45] Thus, early surgical treatment of articular cartilage lesions is critical for the return of the injured athlete to high-impact sports.

Although microfracture has been shown to be effective as a first-line procedure in athletes with articular cartilage lesions, the results of this technique in those who require adjuvant procedures are less predict-

able.[38] Among athletes who have undergone microfracture, 86% return to high-impact sports when it was the first-line procedure, whereas 67% who had surgery prior to microfracture fail to return to sports.

Athletes returning to high-impact sports after microfracture are typically younger than athletes who are unable to return.[43-46] Seventy-five percent of athletes who return to high-impact sports are younger than 40 years, whereas only 25% of athletes older than 40 years return.

Microfracture is generally most successful in the treatment of smaller lesions. Athletes with lesion size of 200 mm² or smaller have a significantly higher return rate (64%) than athletes with lesions larger than 200 mm² (22%).[46]

The most significant improvement after microfracture has been demonstrated within the first 2 postoperative years.[40,42,43,45] Following the initial functional improvement, deterioration of knee function has been reported after 2 years, with decreasing pain scores, Tegner scores, and International Knee Documentation Committee Subjective Knee Evaluation scores

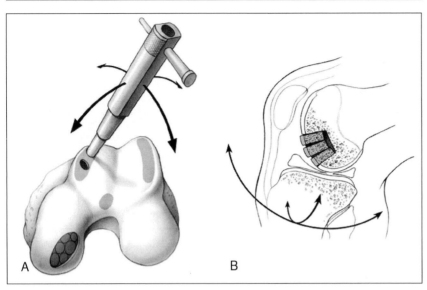

Figure 4 Illustration of mosaicplasty using osteochondral cylinder harvest from the peripheral trochlea **(A)** and press-fit insertion into the cartilage defect in a mosaic pattern with recreation of the condylar convexity **(B)**. The arrows indicate the planes of motion. (Reproduced with permission from Hangody L, Rathonyi GK, Duska Z, Vasarhelyi G, Fules P, Modis L: Autologous osteochondral mosaicplasty: Surgical technique. *J Bone Joint Surg Am* 2004;86(suppl 1):65-72).

in 47% to 80% of athletes.[38,42,45,46] The reason for this functional decline has not yet been identified.

Clinical evidence suggests that repair cartilage volume plays a critical role in the durability of functional improvement after microfracture because deterioration of knee function occurs primarily in patients who have been noted to have poor repair cartilage fill during second-look arthroscopy or on postoperative MRI scans.[37,38]

MRI evaluation after microfracture showed that most of the lesions still demonstrated depressed repair cartilage morphology. Incomplete peripheral integration with persistent gaps between the native and repair cartilage was observed in 53% to 96% of patients.[37,38] Lack of peripheral integration increases vertical shear stresses between repair and native cartilage and promotes repair cartilage degeneration. In addition, subchondral bony overgrowth has

been reported to occur in 25% to 40% of patients, resulting in a relative thinning of the overlying repair cartilage and biomechanical implications for the repair cartilage function and durability.[37,38] These factors may contribute to the observed functional deterioration in the athletes who participate in high-impact sports.

Microfracture provides the best functional improvement in young athletes with small articular cartilage lesions and short preoperative duration of symptoms. Current research is directed toward identifying and improving the factors that lead to insufficient repair cartilage volume after microfracture.

Osteochondral Autograft Transplantation (Mosaicplasty)

The use of osteochondral autografts for the repair of focal chondral and osteochondral lesions has been described by Bobic[47] and Kish and as-

sociates.[48] This technique provides a hyaline cartilage repair by harvesting cylindrical osteochondral grafts from areas of limited weight bearing, such as the peripheral trochlea, and transferring them into small to midsize (1 to 4 cm^2) defects of the weight-bearing cartilage using a press-fit technique. The technique, referred to as mosaicplasty, uses osteochondral plugs of different sizes to optimize the surface coverage of the resurfaced cartilage (Figure 4). Postoperative care includes restricted weight bearing for 4 weeks. Patients are typically allowed to return to athletic activity 6 to 9 months after the surgery. In a long-term study of 831 patients, Hangody and Fule[49] reported good or excellent results at 1- to 10-year follow-up in 79% to 92% of patients who underwent mosaicplasty; 69 of 83 patients assessed arthroscopically had congruent gliding surfaces, histologic evidence of the survival of the transplanted hyaline cartilage, and fibrocartilage filling of the donor sites. The effectiveness of osteochondral mosaicplasty has been specifically evaluated in athletes.[48,50] Kish and associates[48] described a mixed population (athletes and non-athletes) of 52 patients treated with mosaicplasty and observed for an average of 26 months. Return to full athletic activity was reported in 61% of patients. However, no skill level was reported in this study, and the average preoperative duration of symptoms of the athletes assessed was only 8 months. The authors noted that a longer duration of preoperative symptoms resulted in a delayed return to athletic activity after undergoing mosaicplasty.[48] Preoperative radiographic or clinical evidence of joint degeneration predicted a return to athletic activity at a lower level or even retirement from competitive sports altogether after mosaicplasty.[48] The athlete's age was demonstrated to be a significant predictive factor, with a return rate of 90% reported in athletes younger than 30 years, whereas only 23% of athletes older than 30 years returned to competition (70% of them at a lower level of athletic activity). The lower return rate in the older athletes was attributed to a slower overall recovery (slower progression of postoperative rehabilitation). A recent prospective, randomized trial of mosaicplasty and microfracture in athletes reported significantly better results with mosaicplasty at an average of 36 months.[50] In this study, 95% of patients treated with mosaicplasty showed good or excellent results, with significantly improved Hospital for Special Surgery knee scores and International Cartilage Repair Society (ICRS) scores. Ninety-three percent of patients were able to return to athletic activities at the preinjury level at an average of 6.5 months. Athletes younger than 30 years had significantly better results than older athletes. Macroscopic ICRS cartilage repair scores showed good to excellent results in 84% of athletes and MRI showed good to excellent results in 94%.

Despite the encouraging clinical results with this technique, some limitations still exist. Restoration of concave or convex articular cartilage surfaces can be technically demanding. Secure fixation of the plugs may be difficult to achieve, and load-bearing capacity may deteriorate early.[51] Incongruity and graft height mismatch can result in significant elevation of contact pressures.[52] Peripheral chondrocyte death from mechanical trauma at the graft and recipient edges can lead to lack of peripheral integration and persistent gap formation.[53,54] Donor site mor-

bidity has been described;[55] however, the rate of long-term morbidity appears to be low.[49,50] Donor site morbidity may be minimized by using smaller plugs from the medial trochlea or lateral trochlea distal to the sulcus terminalis.[56]

Mosaicplasty is an effective and durable technique for hyaline articular cartilage resurfacing of small to midsize chondral and osteochondral defects of the weight-bearing articular cartilage in young athletes with short intervals between injury and the procedure and without established degenerative changes.

Autologous Chondrocyte Transplantation

The successful repair of articular cartilage lesions of the human knee using autologous chondrocyte transplantation was first reported by Brittberg and associates.[15] Autologous chondrocytes are arthroscopically harvested from a less weight-bearing area, commercially extracted from the harvested cartilage, and multiplied in vitro (Carticel, Genzyme Biosurgery, Cambridge, MA). Elective reimplantation is performed 3 to 6 weeks after cartilage harvesting by débridement of the defect to an intact margin, carefully avoiding osseous bleeding from the bed of the defect. A size-matched periosteal flap is sutured to the cartilage margins and sealed with fibrin glue. The cultured chondrocytes are then injected under the periosteal flap covering the articular cartilage defect (Figure 5). In osteochondral defects deeper than 1 cm, implantation can be performed using a sandwich technique with the chondrocyte implant between two layers of periosteum with or without bone graft.[57] Postoperatively, protected weight bearing is maintained for 6 to 8 weeks, and return to participation

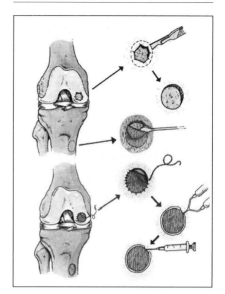

Figure 5 Stepwise technique of autologous chondrocyte transplantation using débridement to stable cartilage margins, harvesting and placement of the periosteal patch, and injection of autologous chondrocytes into the covered defect. Arrows indicate the steps in the procedure. (Reproduced with permission from Brittberg M, Peterson L, Sjogren-Jansson E, Tallheden T, Lindahl A: Articular cartilage engineering with autologous chondrocyte transplantation. A review of recent developments. *J Bone Joint Surg Am* 2003;85(suppl 3):109-115.)

in pivoting sports is usually allowed by 12 months.

Since this technique was first reported by Brittberg and associates, autologous chondrocyte transplantation has been described by several investigators as a successful technique for hyaline-like restoration of full-thickness articular cartilage lesions in the knee,[57-59] with long-term durability of the repair and improved knee function up to 11 years postoperatively.[60]

Two recent prospective multicenter studies have evaluated autologous chondrocyte transplantation in the high-demand athletic population.[61,62] Good to excellent results were reported in these studies in 72% to 96% of athletes, with im-

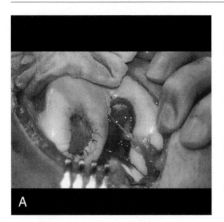 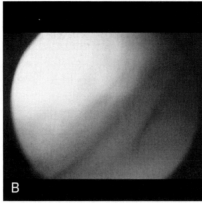 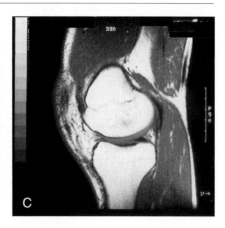

Figure 6 **A,** Intraoperative photograph of the knee of a high-impact athlete treated with autologous chondrocyte transplantation 4 months after injury for a full-thickness lesion of the weight-bearing femoral condyle. **B,** Second-look arthroscopy at 1 year postoperatively demonstrated complete restoration of the articular cartilage surface. **C,** MRI evaluation 7 years postoperatively after the patient returned to high-impact athletics at the preinjury level showed a maintained repair cartilage; the patient continued to participate in high-impact athletics.

Table 4
Factors Influencing Functional Outcome Articular Cartilage Repair in Athletes

Cartilage Repair	Age	Lesion Size	Duration of Symptoms	Athletic Skill Level
Microfracture	+	+	+	+
Mosaicplasty	+	+	+	+
Autologous chondrocyte transplantation	+	-	+	+
Allograft	+	n/a	n/a	n/a

+ = yes, - = no, n/a = not applicable

provement of Tegner scores ranging from 82% to 100%. The best results were obtained in athletes with single cartilage lesions of the medial femoral condyle; up to 96% returned to high-impact athletic activity, and up to 80% at the preinjury skill level. The rate of return to athletic activity in the two studies was higher in competitive athletes (83%) and adolescent athletes (96%), whereas the rate of return in recreational athletes was less predictable. The inferior return rate in recreational athletes was believed to result from chronic deconditioning caused by more prolonged morbidity and associated absence from participation in competitive sports with changing social demands.[2] The time to return to athletic activity was shorter in competitive, high-level athletes. Eighty-seven percent of returning athletes maintained the ability to participate in athletic activity 52 months after chondrocyte implantation. Some world-class athletes returned to professional high-impact athletics and maintained the level of play at 7 to 9 years after undergoing autologous chondrocyte transplantation (Figure 6). Eighty-six percent of athletes with single lesions returned to athletic activity, whereas 14% of athletes with multiple lesions returned. Younger age has been shown to predict improved functional outcome after autologous chondrocyte transplantation, with athletes younger than 25 years showing significantly better return rates to demanding athletic activities (Table 4).

Duration of symptoms also significantly affects the ability to return to athletic activity after undergoing autologous chondrocyte transplantation. Previous data showed an inverse correlation between preoperative duration of symptoms and return rate to competitive or recreational sport.[61,62] Although 66% to 100% of athletes who underwent autologous chondrocyte transplantation were symptomatic at less than 12 months of their return to athletic activity, only 15% who were symptomatic for more than 18 months were able to return. Prolonged periods without cartilage repair lead to chondropenia, early degenerative changes, and inferior results, which emphasizes the importance of early surgical treatment of articular cartilage lesions to maximize the postoperative level of function. Although the rate of return to athletic activity is better in athletes with fewer prior surgeries, return to athletic activity can be achieved in many athletes undergoing autologous cartilage transplantation as a secondary or salvage procedure.[16,17,46,61]

The limitations of autologous cartilage transplantation include its invasiveness and longer postoperative rehabilitation. Periosteal hypertrophy is a well-recognized complication that can lead to catching of the proud periosteum, and has been described in up to 26% of patients.[15,58-62] High joint loading forces and shear forces in athletes may lead to acute graft delamination (the graft of cartilage and periosteum detaches) from premature weight bearing or traumatic events. Careful monitoring for symptoms, restricted progression of joint loading, or prophylactic arthroscopic débridement of the proud periosteum may reduce the risk for traumatic delamination in athletes. Second-generation cell-based repair techniques using collagen membranes instead of periosteum, or matrix-associated chondrocyte implantation (chondrocytes embedded in a collagen or other scaffold/matrix) can reduce the risk for periosteal hypertrophy.[63,64] Although initial recovery with this technique is prolonged, autologous chondrocyte transplantation provides significant functional improvement with high rates of return to demanding athletic activities and excellent durability, even under high-impact athletic demands. The best results have been reported in young, competitive athletes with single femoral lesions and limited intervals between injury and the procedure.[61,62] The documented results of autologous chondrocyte transplantation in athletes

supports its role as an effective procedure in both primary and revision articular cartilage resurfacing.[61,62]

Osteochondral Allograft Transplantation

Osteochondral allografts have been successfully used for the treatment of large and deep chondral and osteochondral lesions from acute trauma, osteochondritis dissecans, osteonecrosis, and joint degeneration. The recipient site is initially prepared by débridement and removal of host bone from the area of the chondral or osteochondral lesion. A size- and depth-matched osteochondral allograft is then harvested and placed into the recipient bed and fixed either with screws or using a press-fit technique.[19,65] This technique provides a hyaline cartilage repair. Because chondrocyte viability, matrix composition, and mechanical properties of hypothermically stored cartilage grafts have been shown to deteriorate rapidly, implantation should be performed with a fresh graft within 28 days of graft harvest.[66] Several studies have shown that the transplanted bone is readily incorporated by the host, leading to good articular cartilage function. However, a recent survival analysis revealed deterioration over time, with a 95% survival rate at 5 years, 80% at 10 years, and 65% at 15 years.[67] Better outcomes have been reported in patients with unipolar lesions, without malalignment, rigid fixation, and age younger than 60 years.[68] Better outcomes are typically seen in young, active adults as well; however, no study has yet specifically investigated the use of this technique in the high-demand athletic population. Although some authors advocate the use of osteochondral allograft transplantation as a primary treatment for large and

deep lesions, fresh osteochondral allograft is primarily used as a salvage option for patients who are too young and active for joint arthroplasty with multiple failed cartilage procedures.

Concomitant Procedures

Combined pathology is frequently encountered by surgeons treating articular cartilage defects in the knees of athletes. Malalignment, ligamentous instability, or meniscal injury and deficiency are known to contribute to the development of articular cartilage lesions, and surgically addressing these concomitant pathologies is critical for an effective and durable articular cartilage repair.[8,15,20,58,60,67] A recent study demonstrated that isolated or combined adjuvant procedures, including ACL reconstruction, high tibial osteotomy, or meniscal allograft and repair, did not negatively affect the ability of patients to return to athletic activities after undergoing autologous chondrocyte transplantation.[61] Similarly, the treatment of associated injuries of the menisci or ACL did not influence the recovery time or level of athletic activity after undergoing mosaicplasty,[48] and better outcomes have been reported in patients undergoing simultaneous microfracture and ACL reconstruction.[43] Performing simultaneous adjuvant procedures in the athletic population avoids prolonged rehabilitation and absence from competition associated with staged procedures and increases the athlete's ability to return to demanding athletic activity.[45,48,51,62,67]

Summary

The goal of articular cartilage repair in athletes is to return the athlete to the preinjury level of athletic participation without increased risk for long-term arthritic degeneration. Several surgical techniques have been shown to improve function and athletic activity after articular cartilage injury in this population. The rate of improvement and ability to return to athletic activity is dependent on age, length of time between the injury and procedure, lesion size, and activity level. The choice of repair technique should be tailored to the individual patient and lesion characteristics using an established treatment algorithm (Figure 2). Each technique is associated with specific advantages and limitations, and second-generation techniques are being developed to improve the current shortcomings. Adjuvant procedures to correct concomitant pathology are critical for the success of the articular cartilage repair and do not seem to negatively affect the ability of athletes to return to high-demand sports. Long-term studies in this population are necessary to determine the efficacy of articular cartilage repair, to reverse chondropenia, and to prevent development of secondary arthritic degeneration.

References

1. Curl WW, Krome J, Gordon E, Rushing J, Smith BP, Poehling GG: Cartilage injuries: A review of 31,516 knee arthroscopies. *Arthroscopy* 1997;13:456-460.

2. Aroen A, Loken S, Heir S, et al: Articular cartilage lesions in 993 consecutive knee arthroscopies. *Am J Sports Med* 2004;32:211-215.

3. Levy AS, Lohnes J, Sculley S, et al: Chondral delamination of the knee in soccer players. *Am J Sports Med* 1996;24:634-639.

4. Arendt E, Dick R: Knee injury patterns among men and women in collegiate basketball and soccer: NCAA data and review of literature. *Am J Sports Med* 1995;23:694-701.

5. Jones SJ, Lyons RA, Sibert J, Evans R, Palmer SR: Changes in sports injuries to children between 1983 and 1998: Comparison of case series. *J Public Health Med* 2001;23:268-271.

6. Moti AW, Micheli LJ: Meniscal and articular cartilage injury in the skeletally immature knee. *Instr Course Lect* 2003;52:683-690.

7. Smith AD, Tao SS: Knee injuries in young athletes. *Clin Sports Med* 1995;14:629-650.

8. Mandelbaum BR, Browne JE, Fu F, et al: Articular cartilage lesions of the knee. *Am J Sports Med* 1998;26:853-861.

9. Piasecki DP, Spindler KP, Warren TA, Andrish JT, Parker RD: Intraarticular injuries associated with anterior cruciate ligament tear: Findings at ligament reconstruction in high school and recreational athletes. An analysis of sex-based differences. *Am J Sports Med* 2003;31:601-605.

10. Felson DT: Osteoarthritis: New Insights. Part 1. The disease and it's risk factors. *Ann Intern Med* 2000;133:635-646.

11. Kujala UM, Kettunen J, Paananen H, et al: Knee osteoarthritis in former runners, soccer players, weight lifters, and shooters. *Arthritis Rheum* 1995;38:539-546.

12. Jackson DW, Lalor PA, Aberman HM, Simon TM: Spontaneous repair of full-thickness defects of articular cartilage in a goat model. *J Bone Joint Surg Am* 2001;83:53-64.

13. Buckwalter JA, Mankin HJ: Articular cartilage: Part II. Degeneration and osteoarthrosis, repair, regeneration, and transplantation. *Instr Course Lect* 1998;47:487-504.

14. Buckwalter JA: Evaluating methods for restoring cartilaginous articular surfaces. *Clin Orthop Relat Res* 1999;367:S224-S238.

15. Brittberg M, Lindahl A, Nilsson A, et al: Treatment of deep cartilage defects in the knee with autologous chondrocyte transplantation. *N Engl J Med* 1994;331:889-895.

16. Mithoefer K, Steadman JR: The microfracture technique. *Tech Knee Surg* 2006;5:141-148.

17. Mithoefer K, Williams RJ III, Warren RF, et al: Chondral resurfacing of articular cartilage defects in the knee with the microfracture technique: Surgical technique. *J Bone Joint Surg Am* 2006;88(suppl 1):294-304.

18. Hangody L, Rathonyi GK, Duska Z, Vasarhelyi G, Fules P, Modis L: Autologous osteochondral mosaicplasty. Surgical technique. *J Bone Joint Surg Am* 2004;86(suppl 1):65-72.

19. Gross A: Fresh osteochondral allograft for posttraumatic knee defects: Surgical technique. *Oper Tech Orthop* 1997;7:334-339.

20. Minas T: The role of cartilage repair techniques, including chondrocyte transplantation, in focal chondral knee damage. *Instr Course Lect* 1999;48:629-643.

21. Drawer S, Fuller CW: Propensity for osteoarthritis and lower limb joint pain in retired professional soccer players. *Br J Sports Med* 2001;35:402-408.

22. Engstrom B, Forssblad M, Johansson C, et al: Does a major knee injury definitely sideline an elite soccer player? *Am J Sports Med* 1990;18:101-105.

23. Roos H: Are there long-term sequelae from soccer? *Clin Sports Med* 1998;17:819-883.

24. Roos H, Lindberg H, Ornell M: Soccer as a cause of hip and knee osteoarthritis. *Ann Rheum Dis* 1996;55:690-698.

25. Jackson DW, Lalor PA, Aberman HM, Simon TM: Spontaneous repair of full-thickness defects of articular cartilage in a goat model. *J Bone Joint Surg Am* 2001;83:53-64.

26. Vrahas MS, Mithoefer K, Joseph D: Long-term effects of articular impaction. *Clin Orthop Relat Res* 2004;423:40-43.

27. Lohmander LS, Roos H, Dahlberg L, Hoerrner LA, Lark MW: Temporal patterns of stromelysin, tissue inhibitor and proteoglycan fragments in synovial fluid after injury to the knee cruciate ligament or meniscus. *J Orthop Res* 1994;12:21-28.

28. Drongowski RA, Coran AG, Wojtys EM: Predictive value of meniscal and chondral injuries in conservatively treated anterior cruciate ligament injuries. *Arthroscopy* 1994;10:97-102.

29. Shelbourne KD, Jari S, Gray T: Outcome of untreated traumatic articular cartilage defects of the knee: A natural history study. *J Bone Joint Surg Am* 2003;85(suppl 2):8-16.

30. Maletius W, Messner K: The long-term prognosis for severe damage to the weightbearing cartilage in the knee: A 14-year clinical and radiographic follow-up in 28 young athletes. *Acta Orthop Scand* 1996;67:165-168.

31. Hefti F, Beguiristain J, Krauspe R, et al: Osteochondritis dissecans: A multicenter study of the European Pediatric Orthopedic Society. *J Pediatr Orthop B* 1999;8:231-245.

32. Jones G, Bennell K, Cicuttini FM: Effect

of physical activity on cartilage development in healthy kids. *Br J Sports Med* 2003;37:382-383.

33. Kiviranta I, Tammi M, Jurvelin J, et al: Articular cartilage thickness and glycosaminoglycan distribution in the canine knee joint after strenuous running exercise. *Clin Orthop Relat Res* 1992;283:302-308.

34. Arokoski J, Kiviranta I, Jurvelin J, Tammin M, Helminen HJ: Long-distance running causes site-dependent decrease of cartilage glycosaminoglycan content in the knee joint of beagle dogs. *Arthritis Rheum* 1993;36:1451-1459.

35. Kohn D: Arthroscopy in acute injuries of anterior cruciate-deficient knees: Fresh and old intraarticular lesions. *Arthroscopy* 1986;2:98-102.

36. Potter HG, Linklater JM, Allen AA, Hannafin JA, Haas SB: Magnetic resonance imaging of articular cartilage in the knee. *J Bone Joint Surg Am* 1998;80:1276-1284.

37. Brown WE, Potter HG, Marx RG, Wickiewicz TL, Warren RF: Magnetic resonance imaging appearance of cartilage repair in the knee. *Clin Orthop Relat Res* 2004;422:214-223.

38. Mithoefer K, Williams RJ, Warren RF, et al: The microfracture technique for treatment of articular cartilage lesions in the knee: A prospective cohort evaluation. *J Bone Joint Surg Am* 2005;87:1911-1920.

39. Jakobsen RB, Engebretsen L, Slauterbeck JR: An analysis of the quality of cartilage repair studies. *J Bone Joint Surg Am* 2005;87:2232-2239.

40. Frisbie DD, Trotter GW, Powers BE, et al: Arthroscopic subchondral bone plate microfracture technique augments healing of large chondral defects in the radial carpal bone and medial femoral condyle of horses. *Vet Surg* 1999;28:242-255.

41. Frisbie DD, Oxford JT, Southwood L, et al: Early events in cartilage repair after subchondral bone microfracture. *Clin Orthop Relat Res* 2003;407:215-227.

42. Gobbi A, Nunag P, Malinowski K: Treatment of chondral lesions of the knee with microfracture in a group of athletes. *Knee Surg Sports Traumatol Arthrosc* 2005;13:213-221.

43. Steadman JR, Briggs KK, Rodrigo JJ, Kocher MS, Gill TJ, Rodkey WG: Outcomes of microfracture for traumatic chondral defects of the knee: Average 11-year follow-up. *Arthroscopy* 2003;19:477-484.

44. Steadman JR, Miller BS, Karas SG, Schlegel TF, Briggs KK, Hawkins RJ: The microfracture technique in the treatment of full-thickness chondral lesions of the knee in National Football League players. *J Knee Surg* 2003;16:83-86.

45. Blevins FT, Steadman JR, Rodrigo JJ, Silliman J: Treatment of articular cartilage defects in athletes: An analysis of functional outcome and lesion appearance. *Orthopedics* 1998;21:761-768.

46. Mithoefer K, Williams RJ, Warren RF, Wickiewicz T, Marx RG: High-Impact athletics after knee articular cartilage repair: A prospective evaluation of the microfracture technique. *Am J Sports Med* 2006;34:1413-1418.

47. Bobic V: Arthroscopic osteochondral graft in ACL reconstruction: A preliminary clinical study. *Knee Surg Sports Traumatol Arthrosc* 1996;3:262-264.

48. Kish G, Modis L, Hangody L: Osteochondral mosaicplasty for the treatment of focal chondral and osteochondral lesions of the knee and talus in the athlete: Rationale, indications, technique, and results. *Clin Sports Med* 1999;18:45-66.

49. Hangody L, Fule P: Autologous osteochondral mosaicplasty for the treatment of full thickness defects of weight bearing joints: Ten years of experimental and clinical experience. *J Bone Joint Surg Am* 2003;85(suppl 2):25-32.

50. Gudas R, Kelesinskas RJ, Kimtys V, et al: A prospective randomized clinical study of mosaic osteochondral autologous transplantation versus microfracture for the treatment of osteochondral defects in the knee joint in young athletes. *Arthroscopy* 2005;21:1066-1075.

51. Whiteside RA, Bryant JT, Jakob RP, Mainil-Varlet P, Wyss UP: Short-term load bearing capacity of osteochondral autografts implanted by the mosaicplasty technique: An in vitro porcine model. *J Biomech* 2003;36:1203-1208.

52. Koh J, Wirsing K, Lautenschlager E, et al: The effect of graft height mismatch on contact pressures following osteochondral grafting. *Am J Sports Med* 2004;32:317-320.

53. Horas U, Pelinkovic D, Aigner T: Autologous chondrocyte implantation and osteochondral cylinder transplantation in cartilage repair of the knee joint: A prospective comparative trial. *J Bone Joint Surg Am* 2003;85:185-192.

54. Huntley J, Bush P, McBurnie J:

Chondrocyte death associated with human femoral osteochondral harvest as performed for mosaicplasty. *J Bone Joint Surg Am* 2005;87:351-360.

55. LaPrade RF, Botker JC: Donor-site morbidity after osteochondral autograft transfer procedures. *Arthroscopy* 2004;20:e69-e73.

56. Garretson R, Katolik L, Beck P, et al: Contact pressure at osteochondral donor sites in the patellofemoral joint. *Am J Sports Med* 2004;32:967-974.

57. Peterson L, Minas T, Brittberg M, et al: Treatment of osteochondritis dissecans of the knee with autologous chondrocyte transplantation. *J Bone Joint Surg Am* 2003;85(suppl 2):17-24.

58. Peterson L, Minas T, Brittberg M, Nilsson A, Sjogren-Jansson E, Lindahl A: Two- to 9-year outcome after autologous chondrocyte transplantation of the knee. *Clin Orthop Relat Res* 2000;374:212-234.

59. Knutsen G, Engebretsen L, Ludvigsen TC, et al: Autologous chondrocyte transplantation compared with microfracture in the knee: A randomized trial. *J Bone Joint Surg Am* 2004;86:455-464.

60. Peterson L, Brittberg M, Kiviranta I, Akerlund EL, Lindahl A: Autologous chondrocyte transplantation: Biomechanics and long-term durability. *Am J Sports Med* 2002;30:2-12.

61. Mithöfer K, Peterson L, Mandelbaum BR, Minas T: Articular cartilage repair in soccer players with autologous chondrocyte transplantation: Functional outcome and return to competition. *Am J Sports Med* 2005;33:1639-1646.

62. Mithöfer K, Minas T, Peterson L, Yeon H, Micheli LJ: Functional outcome of articular cartilage repair in adolescent athletes. *Am J Sports Med* 2005;33:1147-1153.

63. Bartlett W, Gooding CR, Carrington RW, Skinner JA, Briggs TW, Bentley G: Autologous chondrocyte implantation at the knee using bilayer collagen membrane with bone graft: A preliminary report. *J Bone Joint Surg Br* 2005;87:330-332.

64. Bartlett W, Skinner JA, Gooding CR, et al: Autologous chondrocyte implantation versus matrix-induced autologous chondrocyte implantation for osteochondral defects of the knee: A prospective, randomized study. *J Bone Joint Surg Br* 2005;87:640-645.

65. Jamali AA, Emmerson BC, Chung C, Convery FR, Bugbee WD: Fresh osteochondral allografts. *Clin Orthop Relat Res* 2005;437:176-185.

66. Williams RJ, Dreese JC, Chen CT: Chondrocyte survival and material properties of hypothermically stored cartilage: An evaluation of tissue used for osteochondral allograft transplantation. *Am J Sports Med* 2004;32:132-139.

67. Gross AE, Shahsa N, Aubin P: Long-term followup of the fresh osteochondral allografts for posttraumatic knee defects. *Clin Orthop Relat Res* 2005;435:79-87.

68. Shasha N, Aubin PP, Cheah HK, Davis AM, Agnidis Z, Gross AE: Long-term clinical experience with fresh osteochondral allografts for articular knee defects in high-demand patients. *Cell Tissue Bank* 2002;3:175-182.

Allografts in Articular Cartilage Repair

Simon Görtz, MD
William D. Bugbee, MD

Abstract

Hyaline articular cartilage is an avascular and insensate tissue with a distinct structural organization, which provides a low-friction and wear-resistant interface for weight-bearing surface articulation in diarthrodial joints. Ideally, articular cartilage is maintained in homeostasis over the lifetime of an individual, with its biomechanical properties inherently suited to transmit a variety of physiologic loads through a functional range of motion. However, in the skeletally mature individual, articular cartilage does not heal effectively when injured. Although several restorative options for biomimetic replacement in acquired articular cartilage defects do exist, fresh osteochondral allografting currently remains the only technique that restores anatomically appropriate, mature hyaline cartilage in large articular defects. The fundamental paradigm of fresh osteochondral allografting is the transplantation of mature orthotopic hyaline cartilage, with viable chondrocytes that survive hypothermic storage and subsequent transplantation while maintaining their metabolic activity and sustaining the surrounding collagen matrix. Fresh osteochondral allografts have application in the treatment of a wide spectrum of articular pathology, particularly conditions that include both an osseous and a chondral component. The surgical procedure for femoral condyle lesions is straightforward but demands precision to achieve reproducible results and to minimize early graft failures related to surgical technique. As with other cartilage-restorative procedures, the indications for use of fresh osteochondral allografts are still being expanded. Many clinical and basic scientific studies support the theoretical foundation and efficacy of small fragment allografting, although more scientific validation of empirical clinical practice is still needed.

Instr Course Lect 2007;56:469-481

The use of osteochondral transplants in biologic reconstruction of the knee joint has an extensive clinical history, dating back to Lexer's[1] pioneering work in the early 20th century. Transplantation of small-fragment fresh allografts evolved into a routine procedure of choice at certain institutions in North America in the 1970s[2-4] and has since undergone a renaissance as a result of renewed clinical interest and scientific investigation. Subsequently, refinements in transplantation protocols, increased availability of fresh donor tissue, as well as physician and patient demand have driven an emerging trend toward biologic resurfacing as an alternative to prosthetic joint arthroplasty and restoration in a select patient population. Although there are several reparative and restorative options for cartilage replacement,[5-9] osteochondral allografting remains the only biomimetic technique (emulating normal biology) that restores architecturally appropriate, mature hyaline cartilage in acquired articular cartilage defects.

Currently, fresh osteochondral allografts are used to treat a broad spectrum of articular and osteoarticular lesions,[10-12] ranging from focal chondral defects[13] to established osteoarthrosis.[14] Allografts also have been successfully used in the treatment of disease in the ankle joint[15,16] and, to a lesser extent, in the hip joint[17] and the shoulder.[18,19]

Background

The fundamental paradigm of fresh osteochondral allografting is the transplantation of mature orthotopic hyaline cartilage, with viable chondrocytes that survive hypothermic storage,[20-22] while maintaining the metabolic activity of the chondrocytes and sustaining the surrounding collagen matrix.[2,23-27] Hyaline cartilage possesses characteristics that make it ideal for transplantation. First, as an avascular tissue, it

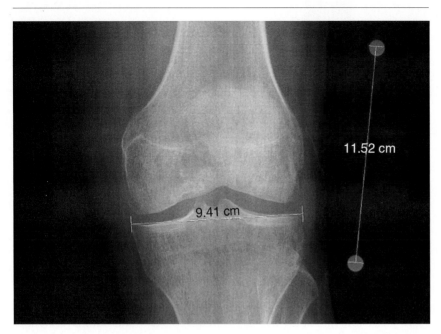

Figure 1 Anteroposterior radiograph of a left knee, displaying a tibial measurement and a radiographic magnification marker for allograft sizing.

does not require a blood supply; instead, its metabolic needs are met through diffusion from synovial fluid. Second, it is an aneural structure that does not require innervation to function. Third, articular cartilage is immunoprivileged because the chondrocytes are embedded in the acellular matrix; thus, it is relatively protected from host immune surveillance.[28]

The second component of the osteochondral allograft is the osseous portion. Conceptually, this component functions as the underlying support structure for the articular cartilage and is the means of attachment and fixation of the graft to the host. The osseous portion of the graft differs from the hyaline portion in that it was originally vascularized tissue and its cells are not thought to survive transplantation.[29] Rather, the osseous structure, like other types of bone graft,[30] functions as a scaffold for healing to the host by creeping substitution and can elicit an immune response.[31]

Generally, the osseous portion of the graft is limited to a few millimeters; however, depending on the clinical situation, the allograft may contain a more copious amount of bone, as required to restore injured or absent subchondral tissue. According to the aforementioned concepts, it is helpful to consider a fresh osteochondral allograft as a composite graft consisting of a living mature hyaline cartilage portion anchored to a nonliving subchondral bone portion, forming an intact structural and functional unit to replace a diseased or absent corresponding component in the recipient joint.

Graft Acquisition and Storage

Use of fresh osteochondral allografts is a unique treatment option with inherent issues mostly related to tissue acquisition, storage, and related logistics as well as safety concerns and immunologic ramifications. Understanding the processes of tissue recovery, testing, and storage of the allograft is critically im-

portant. Historically, the obstacles presented by these fundamental elements led to the development of fresh allograft programs only at specialized centers that both had a close association with an experienced and dedicated tissue bank and had invested substantial resources into initiating and incorporating specific protocols for safe and effective transplantation of fresh osteochondral tissue.[2,3,32]

Small-fragment osteochondral allografts are used while they are fresh to maximize chondrocyte viability; this makes the availability of suitable graft tissue the essential, and often limiting, factor in the transplantation algorithm. The age criterion for donors of fresh grafts is generally between 15 and 40 years. Also, the joint surface must pass a visual inspection for cartilage quality. Strict adherence to tissue-banking standards and quality control of protocols are important, and these criteria increase the likelihood, but do not guarantee, that the tissue will be acceptable for transplantation.[33]

Common to all fresh allograft procedures is the need to match the donor with the recipient. This match is done on the basis of size. To size allografts for the knee, an anteroposterior radiograph of the knee is made with a magnification marker and the medial-lateral dimension of the tibia is measured just distal to the joint surface (Figure 1). This measurement, corrected for magnification, is used, and the tissue bank makes a direct measurement of the donor tibial plateau. Alternatively, the affected condyle can be measured.[34] A match is considered acceptable if it is ±2 mm; however, it should be noted that there is substantial variability in anatomy, which is not reflected by size measurements. In particular, in patients with osteochondritis dissecans, the pathologically affected condyle typically is larger, wider, and flatter; therefore, a larger donor condyle generally should be used. It is imperative that the surgeon thoroughly inspect the tissue to be transplanted, optimally before beginning the actual procedure.

The use of fresh-frozen grafts improves graft availability, reduces immunogenicity, and may be appropriate for bulk allografting in major osseous reconstructions. However, freezing chondrocytes within their extracellular matrix effectively eliminates >95% of viable chondrocytes in the articular cartilage portion of osteochondral grafts.[35,36] Furthermore, clinical experience has indicated that the articular matrix in frozen allografts deteriorates over time, presumably because there are insufficient surviving cells within the matrix to maintain tissue homeostasis.[37]

Cryopreservation involves the freezing of whole tissue grafts in a nutritive medium, and cryopreserved grafts have shown variable degrees of residual, albeit drastically reduced, cell viability in different studies; the reasons for this variability are still the subject of debate and ongoing research.[38-40]

Conversely, it has been demonstrated, primarily in retrieval studies, that fresh cold-stored osteochondral allografts contain viable chondrocytes and that mechanical properties of the matrix are maintained many years after transplantation.[13,15,41] These experiences have generally supported the use of fresh rather than frozen tissue for small osteochondral allografts employed to reconstruct chondral and osteochondral defects. More recent studies have demonstrated that chondrocyte viability and the structural integrity of the matrix are preserved during hypothermal storage in nutritive culture medium containing amino acids, glucose, and inorganic salts.[21,42] Those studies showed that cell density, viability, and metabolic activity remained essentially unchanged for as many as 14 days after baseline, before deteriorating significantly ($P < 0.001$[21] and $P < 0.05$[42]) after 28 days while the hyaline matrix remained relatively intact. The clinical consequences of these storage-induced graft changes have yet to be determined.

Safety and Risk of Disease Transmission

The previously mentioned studies suggested that it is reasonable to store fresh allografts for more than 2 weeks after graft harvest, which is in contrast to the empirical practice of transplanting tissue within 7 days after recovery. The results of the more recent studies have coincided with a trend by tissue banks to hold tissue for 14 days, to await results of microbiologic testing, before releasing it for transplantation. Recovery, processing, and testing of donor tissue are performed according to guidelines established by the American Association of Tissue Banks,[33] which include the recording of a detailed donor history as well as serologic and bacteriologic testing.[43] As with transplantation of any allogeneic organ or tissue, there is a risk of transmission of infectious disease despite donor screening and testing.[44] Although advances in serologic testing for human immunovirus, hepatitis, and other pathogens have improved safety, a minute but measurable risk of transmission of serious disease remains. Both the surgeon and the patient should be aware of this risk of bacterial or viral disease transmission, and it must be discussed as part of the informed consent process. Unfortunately, no published data quantifying this risk are available.

Immunologic Ramifications

The immunologic ramifications of the use of fresh osteochondral allografts are another important consideration, and it should be noted that, in current practice, small-fragment allografts are not HLA or blood-type matched between the donor and recipient. Although it appears that hyaline cartilage is relatively immunoprivileged,[28] it is also evident that fresh unmatched osteochondral allografts elicit a variable immune response.[45] Human allograft retrieval studies have consistently shown that patients generally tolerate the transplant immunologically, with little or no histologic evidence of an immune-mediated pathologic response or frank transplant rejection.[26,30] However, in one study of fresh osteochondral allografts, 50% of individuals generated serum anti-HLA antibodies.[46] The presence of the anti-HLA antibodies correlated with an inferior appearance of the graft-host interface on MRI studies. Although this may suggest that humoral immunity plays a role in the outcome following the use of fresh allografts, the clinical relevance of this phenomenon is unknown.[47,48] The issue of immune behavior may ultimately become clinically relevant, and it is clearly an area where more knowledge is necessary to improve outcomes of the use of fresh osteochondral allografts.

Indications

As a result of their osteoarticular nature, fresh allografts are uniquely suited for the treatment of large compound osteochondral lesions. Primary allograft treatment can be

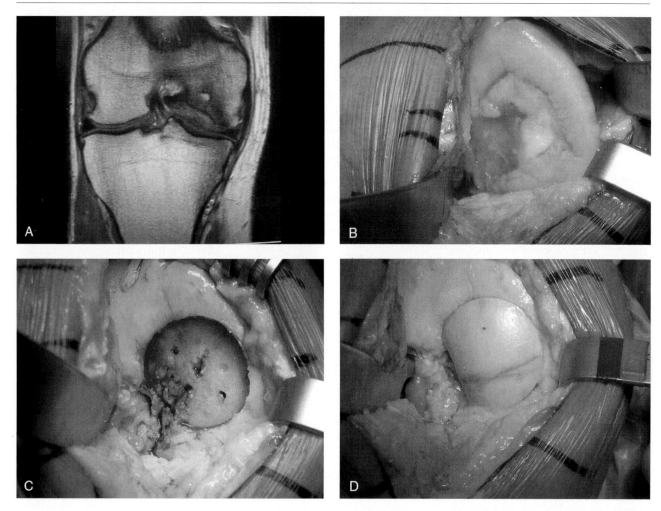

Figure 2 **A,** T1-weighted coronal MRI documenting an osteochondritis dissecans lesion in the right medial femoral condyle of a 33-year-old woman after prior microfracture and autologous chondrocyte implantation had failed. Note the extent of the subchondral signal abnormality, indicating marked osseous disease. **B,** Intraoperative appearance of the osteochondritis dissecans lesion of the medial femoral condyle. **C,** Intraoperative photograph after preparation of the graft bed by core reaming of the osteochondral defect and débridement down to bleeding bone. **D,** An osteochondral dowel plug in place and secured by several absorbable polydioxanone pins. Note the orthotopic appearance of the graft and its flush fit with the surrounding joint surface.

Table 1
Allograft Indications in 365 Knees Treated From 1985 to 2005 at the University of California, San Diego

Indication	Percent of Knees
Complex salvage: trauma, degenerative joint disease	29%
Osteochondritis dissecans	27%
Isolated femoral condylar lesion: degenerative or traumatic	22%
Patellofemoral conditions	14%
Osteonecrosis	8%

considered for large lesions (>2 cm^2) for which the surgeon believes other procedures may be inadequate, for purely chondral defects of a size that presents a relative contraindication to other treatments, and for cases in which bone involvement is greater than 6 to 10 mm deep (Figure 2, *A* , Table 1). Specific conditions that are most amenable to allografting in clinical practice include osteochondritis dissecans,[49,50] osteonecrosis,[49] and posttraumatic defects, such as those occurring after periarticular fractures about the knee.[41,51] Other indications for allografting of the knee include patellofemoral chondrosis or arthrosis[52] and certain instances of unicompartmental or multifocal posttraumatic and degenerative tibiofemoral arthrosis[14,32,53] (Table 2). Allografts have also proven valuable for the salvage of knees for which other cartilage resurfacing procedures, such as microfracture, implantation of autologous chondrocytes, and transfer of an osteochondral autologous plug, have failed (Figure 2, *B*).

Allografts have also been used successfully in the ankle joint. They are indicated for resurfacing of a tibiotalar joint with posttraumatic arthrosis,[15,16] for osteonecrosis of the talus, and for osteochondritis dissecans lesions not amenable to other restorative procedures.[54] The use of fresh allografts for bipolar resurfacing of the tibiotalar joint is unique in the ankle, as bipolar resurfacing with fresh allografts has not been proven to be successful in the knee. This approach also reflects the limited options for younger individuals with end-stage arthrosis of the tibiotalar joint.

In the hip, osteochondral allografts have been used in the treatment of osteonecrosis of the femoral head, with mixed results.[17] Current indications include symptomatic lesions with limited involvement of the head that have not responded to other treatments. In the shoulder, allograft reconstruction can be considered for large osteochondral lesions associated with glenohumeral dislocation and instability[18] as well as for osteochondritis dissecans and osteonecrosis of the humeral head.[19] It should be noted that the indications in the hip, shoulder, and conceivably other joints are evolving, al-

Table 2

Allograft Sites in 365 Knees treated from 1985 to 2005 at the University of California, San Diego

Site	Percent of Knees
Medial femoral condyle	36%
Lateral femoral condyle	18%
Medial tibial plateau	2%
Lateral tibial plateau	6%
Multifocal	20%
Trochlea	8%
Patella	5%
Bipolar patellofemoral	5%

though few published data on such applications are currently available.

Contraindications

Allografting in the knee should not be considered an alternative to prosthetic arthroplasty for an individual with symptoms and an acceptable age and activity level for prosthetic replacement. Bipolar and multicompartmental allografting procedures have been modestly successful in younger individuals; however, advanced multicompartment arthrosis, even in younger patients, is a relative contraindication to allografting. Other relative contraindications include uncorrected ligamentous instability, meniscal insufficiency, and axial malalignment of the limb. Thus, the biologic and mechanical status of the joint should be assessed preoperatively; all patients should be examined carefully for subtle or obvious instability, and the angular alignment of the limb should be evaluated. Any instability or malalignment should be addressed before allografting is considered or should be treated with a concomitant procedure to optimize the biomechanical environment and achieve a horizontal joint surface. If a realigning osteotomy is to be performed on the same articu-

lating side as the allografting is to be done, staging of the procedure is advised so as not to jeopardize the microvascularity of the recipient bone bed. Inflammatory disease or crystal-induced arthropathy is also considered a relative contraindication to allografting, as is any unexplained synovitis. The use of fresh osteochondral allografts in individuals with altered bone metabolism, such as is seen in association with chronic steroid use, smoking, or even the use of nonsteroidal anti-inflammatory agents, has not been studied extensively. Treatment of steroid-induced aseptic necrosis in the knee and hip has demonstrated mixed results, but this may represent the extent of the disease rather than the effect of steroid usage.

Surgical Technique
Femoral Condyle
The patient is positioned supine, and a proximal thigh tourniquet is applied. A leg or foot holder is valuable in this procedure, to position and maintain the leg in between 70° and 100° of flexion and thus gain access to the lesion. Implantation of a fresh osteochondral allograft generally necessitates an open procedure, including an arthrotomy of variable size (depending on the position and

dimension of the lesion). Eversion of the patella is not necessary for most femoral condylar lesions. Usually, diagnostic arthroscopy has been performed shortly before the allograft procedure and is not an imperative step in that procedure; however, if there are any unanswered questions regarding the status of the meniscus or of the other compartments of the knee, diagnostic arthroscopy can be performed before the allografting. The fresh graft, which has been placed in chilled saline solution on the back table, is inspected to confirm the adequacy of the size match and the quality of the tissue before the knee joint is opened.

A standard midline incision is made from the center of the patella to the tip of the tibial tubercle. This incision is elevated subcutaneously, either medial or lateral to the patellar tendon, depending on the location of the lesion (medial or lateral). A retinacular incision is then made from the superior aspect of the patella inferiorly. Great care is taken to enter the joint and incise the fat pad without disrupting the anterior horn of the meniscus or damaging the articular surface. Sometimes, when the lesion is posterior or very large, the meniscus must be detached and reflected, and generally this can be done safely, with a small cuff of tissue left adjacent to the anterior attachment of the meniscus for later reattachment and repair.

Once the joint capsule and synovium have been incised and the joint has been entered, retractors are placed medially and laterally. Care is taken to position the retractor within the notch to protect the cruciate ligaments and the articular cartilage. The knee is then flexed and/or extended until the degree of flexion that presents the lesion into

the arthrotomy site is achieved. Excessive flexion limits the ability to mobilize the patella. The lesion then is inspected and is palpated with a probe to determine its extent, margins, and maximum size. The two commonly used techniques for the preparation and implantation of osteochondral allografts include the press-fit plug (dowel) technique and the shell graft technique. Each technique has advantages and disadvantages. The press-fit plug technique is similar in principle to autologous osteochondral transfer systems. It is optimal for contained condylar lesions between 15 and 35 mm in diameter. Fixation is generally not required because of the stability achieved with the press-fit. Disadvantages include the fact that many lesions, such as very posterior femoral, tibial, patellar, and trochlear lesions, are not conducive to the use of a circular coring system. In addition, the more ovoid the lesion is in shape, the more normal cartilage that must be sacrificed at the recipient site to accommodate a circular donor plug. Shell grafts are technically more difficult to perform and typically require fixation. However, depending on the technique employed, less normal cartilage may need to be sacrificed. Also, certain lesions are more amenable to shell allografts because of their location.

Dowel Allograft
Several proprietary instrumentation systems are currently available for the preparation and implantation of press-fit dowel allografts up to 35 mm in diameter. Only one of the instrumentation systems will be discussed here; however, most systems are similar.

The symptomatic lesion is identified, and the size of the proposed graft is outlined and templated with

use of sizing dowels; it should be kept in mind that overlapping dowels may deliver the best area fit. After a size determination is made, a guidewire is driven into the center of the lesion, perpendicular to the curvature of the articular surface. The remaining articular cartilage is scored, and a core reamer is used to remove that cartilage and at least 3 to 4 mm of subchondral bone (Figure 2, C). When a patient has a deeper lesion, fibrous and sclerotic bone is removed to a healthy, bleeding osseous base. When a lesion is very deep, coring should not exceed 10 mm in depth, and packed morcellized autologous bone graft should be used to fill any deeper or more extensive osseous defects. The guidewire then is removed, and circumferential depth measurements of the prepared recipient site are made.

The corresponding anatomic location of the recipient site then is identified on the graft, which is placed into a graft holder or is held with bone-holding forceps. A saw guide then is placed in the appropriate position, again perpendicular to the articular surface, and an appropriately sized tube saw is used to core out the graft. Before the graft is removed from the condyle, an identifying mark is made to ensure proper orientation. Once the graft has been removed, the depth measurements that were determined from the recipient are transferred to the graft. This graft then is cut with an oscillating saw and is trimmed with a rasp to the appropriate thickness in all four quadrants, and the deep edges of the bone plug can be chamfered with a rongeur and bone rasp. Often, this procedure must be done multiple times to ensure precise thickness, preferably by refashioning the graft rather than the recipient site and optimally while keeping

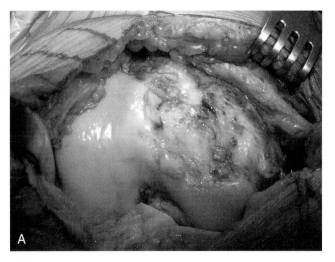

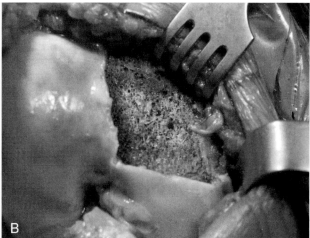

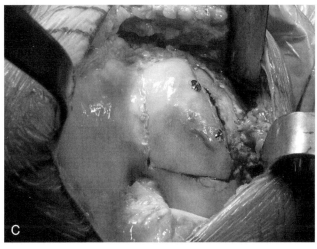

Figure 3 **A,** Intraoperative appearance of a posttraumatic defect, manifesting marked traumatic osteoarticular loss. **B,** Intraoperative photograph after freehand preparation of the graft bed for a shell allograft. **C,** An osteochondral shell graft in place, with additional screw fixation. The relief of the medial trochlear facet has been restored and is secured by compression screws placed outside of the articulating surface of the joint.

the graft moist throughout the procedure.

The graft is then irrigated copiously with high-pressure lavage to remove all marrow elements.[55] The recipient site can be dilated with use of a slightly oversized tamp to facilitate the insertion of the graft and prevent excessive impact loading of the articular surface when the graft is applied. At this point, bone graft is applied to any remaining osseous defects. The allograft is then inserted by hand in the appropriate rotation, and it is gently tamped in place until it is flush, again with minimization of mechanical insult to the articular surface of both the

native and the graft tissue.

Once the graft is seated, a determination is made regarding whether additional fixation is required. Typically, absorbable polydioxanone pins are used, particularly if the graft is large or has an exposed edge within the notch (Figure 2, *D*). Often, the graft needs to be trimmed in the notch region to prevent impingement. The knee is then brought through a complete range of motion to confirm that it is stable and there is no catching or soft-tissue obstruction. At this point, the wound is irrigated copiously, and, if no more adjunct procedures are planned, routine closure is performed. **(DVD 44.1)**

Shell Allograft

The defect (Figure 3, *A*) is identified by means of the described previously arthrotomy. The circumference of the lesion is marked with a surgical pen. An attempt is made to create a geometric shape that is amenable to hand-crafting of a shell graft; however, sacrifice of normal cartilage should be minimized. A number-15 blade is used to cut around the lesion. Sharp ring curets are used to remove all tissue inside this marked area. With use of both a motorized 4.0-mm burr and sharp curets, the defect is débrided to a depth of 4 to 5 mm (Figure 3,*B*). The graft is fashioned in a freehand manner by initially oversizing it slightly and then carefully removing excess bone and cartilage as necessary through multiple trial fittings. If there is deeper bone loss in the defect, more bone can be left on the graft and cancellous bone graft can be applied to the defect before insertion of the shell allograft. The shell allograft is placed flush with the articular surface, and the need for fixation is based on the degree of inherent stability. Bioabsorbable pins are typically used when fixation is required, but compression screws may be used as an alternative (Figure 3, *C*).

Postoperative Management

Early postoperative management includes the use of continuous passive motion while the patient is in the hospital. Patients generally are allowed a full range of motion unless they had undergone additional reconstructive procedures such as meniscal repair, anterior cruciate ligament reconstruction, or osteotomy that would alter the rehabilitation plan. Patients begin early range-of-motion exercises and quadriceps strengthening and maintain a toe-touch-only weight-bearing status for at least 8 weeks, and often 12 weeks, depending on the size of the graft, type of fixation, and ultimately radiographic evidence of incorporation.

At 4 weeks, patients are allowed to perform closed-chain exercises such as cycling. Progressive weight bearing as tolerated usually is permitted at 3 months, and if functional rehabilitation is complete, the patient is allowed to return to recreational and sports activities at approximately 6 months. Patients are generally cautioned about excessive impact loading of the allograft, particularly in the first year. As with any cartilage replacement procedure, long-term outcomes of osteochondral allograft-

ing are directly and inversely related to the time to treatment and the overall burden of disease in the affected joint. It is not unrealistic to expect a young patient with a focal lesion (traumatic or due to osteochondritis dissecans) to go back to normal impact-loading activities after 12 months and to return to preinjury function, whereas the goals in a salvage situation are usually to delay or even eliminate the need for prosthetic replacement by reducing pain and allowing a return to functional activities of daily living as well as low-impact leisure activities.

Typically, braces are not used unless the grafting involves the patellofemoral joint, in which case flexion is limited to <45° for the first 4 to 6 weeks, or unless bipolar tibial and femoral grafts are used, in which instance an unloader or range-of-motion brace is used to prevent excessive stress on the grafted surfaces.

Complications

The most unique issue regarding possible postoperative complications with fresh allografts relates to transmission of disease from the graft. Infection following the implantation of a fresh osteochondral allograft is rare, but its consequences can be devastating. Generally, all grafts are currently harvested and tested in accordance with American Association of Tissue Banks standards. However, allograft-associated bacterial infections have been reported.[56] Death during the immediate postoperative period has occurred as the result of implantation of a contaminated fresh osteochondral graft. As with most procedures, infection may become apparent in the days to weeks following surgery. Deep infection needs to be distinguished from superficial infection on the basis of the findings of physical

examination and joint aspiration. Deep infection involving the allograft should be addressed immediately with removal of the allograft because there is a risk that the fresh tissue is the source of the infection or is a nidus for recurrence. Patients need to be informed of this risk preoperatively and again counseled to look for signs of infection before and after discharge from the hospital.

The allograft procedure can fail as a result of nonunion or late fragmentation and graft collapse. Progression of disease (arthritis) may also lead to an inferior clinical outcome. Although healing of the graft-host interface occurs reliably, particularly with smaller grafts, the degree of revascularization appears to be variable. Fragmentation and collapse typically occur in areas of unvascularized allograft bone. Patients with this complication generally present with new-onset pain or mechanical symptoms. Radiographs may show joint space narrowing, cysts, or sclerotic regions. MRI can help to rule out contributory concomitant joint disease in the differential diagnosis of postoperative symptoms. In the event of mechanical allograft failure, MRI often shows areas of graft collapse. However, care must be taken in the interpretation of these images, as even normal well-functioning grafts demonstrate signal abnormalities. Depending on the status of the knee joint, the treatment options include observation, removal of the fragmented portion of the graft, repeat allografting, or conversion to an arthroplasty.

Results

Emmerson and associates[49] reported on a series of 66 knees in 64 patients in whom osteochondritis dissecans of the femoral condyle had been treated with fresh osteochondral al-

Table 3
Outcomes of Osteochondral Allografting in the Knee

Author	Site of Lesion	Diagnosis/Indication	No. of Cases	Mean Duration of Follow-up *(yr)*	Successful Outcome
Meyers et al[3]	Knee	Multiple	31	3.5	77%
Chu et al[11]	Knee	Multiple	55	6.2	76% good/exc. results
Ghazavi et al[13]	Knee	Trauma	126	7.5	85% survivorship
Aubin et al[60]	Femur	Trauma	60	10.0	85% survivorship
Görtz et al[57]	Femur	Trauma	43	4.5	88% good/exc. results
Garrett[50]	Femur	Osteochondritis dissecans	17	2-9	94% good/exc. results
Emmerson et al[49]	Femur	Osteochondritis dissecans	65	7.7	72% good/exc. results
Bugbee and Khadivi[59]	Knee	Osteonecrosis	21	5.3	88% good/exc. results
Park et al[58]	Knee	Osteoarthrosis	34	3.0	76% good/exc. results
Jamali et al[14]	Patellofemoral	Multiple	29	4.5	52% good/exc. results

lograft (Table 3, Figure 4). All patients were evaluated both preoperatively and postoperatively with a modified Merle d'Aubigné and Postel scale, which measures function, range of motion, and absence of pain, allotting 1 to 6 points to each, for a maximum of 18 points. There were 45 male and 19 female patients with a mean age of 28.6 years (range, 15 to 54 years). Forty-one lesions involved the medial femoral condyle, and 25 involved the lateral femoral condyle. All lesions were high-grade osteochondritis dissecans, and all had been treated previously with surgery. The mean allograft size was 7.5 cm². The mean duration of follow-up was 7.7 years (range, 2 to 22 years). One knee was lost to follow-up. Of the remaining 65 knees, 47 (72%) were rated good/ excellent, with a score of ≥15 points on the 18-point scale; 7(11%) were rated fair; and 1(2%) was rated poor. The mean clinical score improved from 13.0 points preoperatively to 16.3 points postoperatively (P < 0.01). Ten patients underwent a revision, with a mean time to the revision of 56 months. Fifty-nine of the 64 patients completed questionnaires. The mean subjective score for knee function improved from

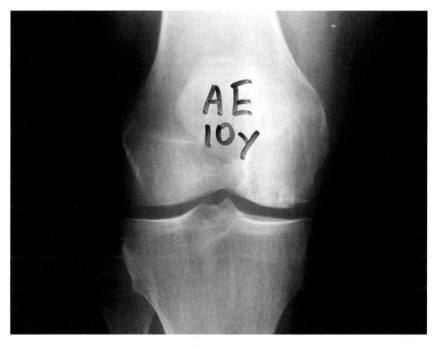

Figure 4 Anteroposterior radiograph of a right knee, made 10 years after placement of a shell allograft in the medial femoral condyle. The joint space has been maintained, without radiographic evidence of frank joint degeneration.

3.4 to 8.4 points on a 10-point scale (P < 0.01).

Garrett[50] reported his experience with the use of fresh osteochondral allografts as both press-fit plugs and large shell grafts in the treatment of osteochondritis dissecans. All patients had undergone previous surgery.[50] Sixteen of the 17 patients re-

ported relief of symptoms at 2 to 9 years postoperatively; the only failure was a particularly large graft that fragmented.

Between 1997 and 2004, 43 patients with an isolated cartilage lesion of the femoral condyle were treated with a fresh osteochondral allograft at the authors' institution.[57]

The study population included 23 male patients and 20 female patients with a mean age of 35 years. Twenty-nine patients had involvement of the medial femoral condyle; 13, the lateral femoral condyle; and 1, both condyles. All patients had undergone prior surgery. The mean allograft area was 5.88 cm^2. Thirty-eight (88%) of the 43 allograft procedures were considered to be successful (a score of ≥15 points on the 18-point modified Merle d'Aubigné and Postel scale) at a mean of 4.5 years postoperatively.

Park and associates[58] reported the results of osteochondral allografting in 34 patients with a clinically established and radiographically confirmed diagnosis of advanced knee arthrosis. Of these grafts, 19 were unipolar, 10 were bipolar, and 5 included multiple surfaces. The mean graft area was 10.5 cm^2. At the time of follow-up, at a mean of 3 years, 28 procedures were considered to be successes, with significant objective and subjective improvement ($P < 0.01$).

In a study on the use of allografts for the salvage of 21 knees (17 patients) with established severe osteonecrosis, 15 patients were satisfied with the result of the treatment and 14 believed that the overall condition of the knee was improved.[59] Furthermore, none of the knees had required conversion to total knee arthroplasty at a mean of 5.3 years following this challenging salvage procedure.

Chu and associates[11] reported on 55 consecutive knees treated with osteochondral allografting in patients with diagnoses such as traumatic chondral injury, osteonecrosis, osteochondritis dissecans, and patellofemoral disease. The mean age of this group was 35.6 years, and the duration of follow-up averaged 75 months (range, 11 to 147 months).

Of the 55 knees, 43 had a unipolar replacement and 12 had a bipolar resurfacing. On an 18-point scale, 42 (76%) of these 55 knees were rated as good to excellent and 3 were rated as fair. It is important to note that 36 of the 43 knees that had undergone unipolar femoral grafting had a good to excellent result and only 6 of the 12 knees treated with bipolar grafting had a good or excellent result.

McDermott and associates[12] reported on 100 patients in whom a fresh osteochondral graft had been implanted within 24 hours after harvest. Thirty-eight of 50 patients with a unifocal traumatic defect of the tibial plateau or femoral condyle were considered to have a successful result at an average of 3.8 years postoperatively. Patients with osteoarthritis and osteonecrosis fared much worse. Ghazavi and associates[13] reported on 126 knees in 123 patients who had been followed for an average of 7.5 years. Eighty-five percent of the procedures were rated as successful while the remainder had failed. Factors related to failure included an age older than 50 years, bipolar defects, malalignment, and a workers' compensation claim. Aubin and associates[60] later reported the long-term results for 60 patients in whom a fresh femoral graft had been implanted for the treatment of a posttraumatic lesion. Survivorship analysis showed the survival of 51 grafts at 10 years and 44 at 15 years. Forty-one of the patients had undergone a simultaneous realignment osteotomy, and 10 had undergone a concomitant meniscal transplantation. Radiographic analysis revealed moderate to severe arthritis in 31 of the knees at the time of the latest follow-up.

Summary

Fresh osteochondral allografts have a role in the treatment of a wide spectrum of articular pathological conditions, particularly those that include both an osseous and a chondral component. Many clinical and basic scientific studies have supported the theoretical foundation and efficacy of the use of small-fragment allografts, although more scientific validation of empirical clinical practice is still needed.

The surgical procedure for the treatment of femoral condylar lesions is straightforward but demands precision to achieve reproducible results and to minimize early graft failures related to surgical technique. As with other cartilage-restoration methods, the indications for the use of fresh osteochondral allografts are being expanded to include the primary treatment of focal femoral condylar lesions, use in joints with an advanced burden of disease, as well as use in other joints.

With respect to fresh grafts, tissue banking standards and techniques are still evolving with regard to enhancing graft quality and prolonging storage intervals, which will allow more surgeons and their patients to gain access to the procedure. Further understanding of the immunologic behavior of fresh allografts is clearly needed. Modulating the healing response by donor-recipient matching, use of bioactive growth factors, or other adjunct therapies may further improve short and long-term outcomes of procedures involving the use of fresh osteochondral allografts.

References

1. Lexer E: Substitution of whole or half joints from freshly amputated extremities by free plastic operations. *Surg Gynecol Obstet* 1908;6:601-607.

2. Czitrom AA, Langer F, McKee N, Gross AE: Bone and cartilage allotransplantation: A review of 14 years

of research and clinical studies. *Clin Orthop Relat Res* 1986;208:141-145.

3. Meyers MH, Akeson W, Convery FR: Resurfacing of the knee with fresh osteochondral allograft. *J Bone Joint Surg Am* 1989;71:704-713.

4. Shasha N, Aubin PP, Cheah HK, Davis AM, Agnidis Z, Gross AE: Long-term clinical experience with fresh osteochondral allografts for articular knee defects in high demand patients. *Cell Tissue Bank* 2002;3:175-182.

5. Bartlett W, Skinner JA, Gooding CR, et al: Autologous chondrocyte implantation versus matrix-induced autologous chondrocyte implantation for osteochondral defects of the knee: a prospective, randomised study. *J Bone Joint Surg Br* 2005;87:640-645.

6. Brittberg M, Lindahl A, Nilsson A, Ohlsson C, Isaksson O, Peterson L: Treatment of deep cartilage defects in the knee with autologous chondrocyte transplantation. *N Engl J Med* 1994;331:889-895.

7. Hangody L, Fules P: Autologous osteochondral mosaicplasty for the treatment of full-thickness defects of weight-bearing joints: ten years of experimental and clinical experience. *J Bone Joint Surg Am* 2003;85(Suppl 2):25-32.

8. Hubbard MJ: Arthroscopic surgery for chondral flaps in the knee. *J Bone Joint Surg Br* 1987;69:794-796.

9. Steadman JR, Briggs KK, Rodrigo JJ, Kocher MS, Gill TJ, Rodkey WG: Outcomes of microfracture for traumatic chondral defects of the knee: Average 11-year follow-up. *Arthroscopy* 2003;19:477-484.

10. Bugbee WD: Fresh osteochondral allografts. *J Knee Surg* 2002;15:191-195.

11. Chu CR, Convery FR, Akeson WH, Meyers M, Amiel D: Articular cartilage transplantation: Clinical results in the knee. *Clin Orthop Relat Res* 1999;360:159-168.

12. McDermott AG, Langer F, Pritzker KP, Gross AE: Fresh small-fragment osteochondral allografts: Long-term follow-up study on first 100 cases. *Clin Orthop Relat Res* 1985;197:96-102.

13. Ghazavi MT, Pritzker KP, Davis AM, Gross AE: Fresh osteochondral allografts for post-traumatic osteochondral defects of the knee. *J Bone Joint Surg Br* 1997;79:1008-1013.

14. Jamali A, Bugbee WD, Rabbani R, Convery FR: Fresh osteochondral

allografts for treatment of tibiofemoral arthrosis. Read at the Annual Meeting of the American Academy of Orthopaedic Surgeons; 2002 Feb 13-17; Dallas, TX.

15. Gross AE, Agnidis Z, Hutchison CR: Osteochondral defects of the talus treated with fresh osteochondral allograft transplantation. *Foot Ankle Int* 2001;22:385-391.

16. Meehan R, McFarlin S, Bugbee W, Brage M: Fresh ankle osteochondral allograft transplantation for tibiotalar joint arthritis. *Foot Ankle Int* 2005;26:793-802.

17. Meyers MH: Resurfacing of the femoral head with fresh osteochondral allografts. Long-term results. *Clin Orthop Relat Res* 1985;197:111-114.

18. Chapovsky F, Kelly JD IV: Osteochondral allograft transplantation for treatment of glenohumeral instability. *Arthroscopy* 2005;21:1007.

19. Johnson DL, Warner JJ: Osteochondritis dissecans of the humeral head: Treatment with a matched osteochondral allograft. *J Shoulder Elbow Surg* 1997;6:160-163.

20. Allen RT, Robertson CM, Pennock AT, et al: Analysis of stored osteochondral allografts at the time of surgical implantation. *Am J Sports Med* 2005;33:1479-1484.

21. Williams RJ III, Dreese JC, Chen CT: Chondrocyte survival and material properties of hypothermically stored cartilage: An evaluation of tissue used for osteochondral allograft transplantation. *Am J Sports Med* 2004;32:132-139.

22. Williams SK, Amiel D, Ball ST, et al: Prolonged storage effects on the articular cartilage of fresh human osteochondral allografts. *J Bone Joint Surg Am* 2003;85:2111-2120.

23. Convery FR, Akeson WH, Amiel D, Meyers MH, Monosov A: Long-term survival of chondrocytes in an osteochondral articular cartilage allograft: A case report. *J Bone Joint Surg Am* 1996;78:1082-1088.

24. Czitrom AA, Keating S, Gross AE: The viability of articular cartilage in fresh osteochondral allografts after clinical transplantation. *J Bone Joint Surg Am* 1990;72:574-581.

25. Kwan MK, Wayne JS, Woo SL, Field FP, Hoover J, Meyers M: Histological and biomechanical assessment of articular cartilage from stored osteochondral shell allografts. *J Orthop Res* 1989;7:637-644.

26. Oakeshott RD, Farine I, Pritzker KP, Langer F, Gross AE: A clinical and histologic analysis of failed fresh

osteochondral allografts. *Clin Orthop Relat Res* 1988;233:283-294.

27. Williams S, Amiel D, Ball S, et al: Fresh human osteochondral allograft retrievals: Reasons for failure. Presented as a poster exhibit at the Annual Meeting of the American Academy of Orthopaedic Surgeons; 2004 Mar 10-14; San Francisco, CA.

28. Langer F, Gross AE: Immunogenicity of allograft articular cartilage. *J Bone Joint Surg Am* 1974;56:297-304.

29. Rodrigo JJ, Thompson E, Travis C: Deep-freezing versus 4 degrees preservation of avascular osteocartilaginous shell allografts in rats. *Clin Orthop Relat Res* 1987;218:268-275.

30. Kandel RA, Gross AE, Ganel A, McDermott AG, Langer F, Pritzker KP: Histopathology of failed osteoarticular shell allografts. *Clin Orthop Relat Res* 1985;197:103-110.

31. Strong DM, Friedlaender GE, Tomford WW, et al: Immunologic responses in human recipients of osseous and osteochondral allografts. *Clin Orthop Relat Res* 1996;326:107-114.

32. Gross AE, Silverstein EA, Falk J, Falk R, Langer F: The allotransplantation of partial joints in the treatment of osteoarthritis of the knee. *Clin Orthop Relat Res* 1975;108:7-14.

33. American Association of Tissue Banks: Standards for tissue banking. Arlington, VA, American Association of Tissue Banks; 1987.

34. Highgenboten CL, Jackson A, Trudelle-Jackson E, Meske NB: Cross-validation of height and gender estimations of femoral condyle width in osteochondral allografts. *Clin Orthop Relat Res* 1994;298:246-249.

35. Enneking WF, Mindell ER: Observations on massive retrieved human allografts. *J Bone Joint Surg Am* 1991;73:1123-1142.

36. Ohlendorf C, Tomford WW, Mankin HJ: Chondrocyte survival in cryopreserved osteochondral articular cartilage. *J Orthop Res* 1996;14:413-416.

37. Enneking WF, Campanacci DA: Retrieved human allografts: A clinicopathological study. *J Bone Joint Surg Am* 2001;83:971-986.

38. Jomha NM, Lavoie G, Muldrew K, Schachar NS, McGann LE: Cryopreservation of intact human articular cartilage. *J Orthop Res* 2002;20:1253-1255.

39. Malinin TI, Wagner JL, Pita JC, Lo H:

Hypothermic storage and cryopreservation of cartilage: An experimental study. *Clin Orthop Relat Res* 1985;197:15-26.

40. Tomford WW, Fredericks GR, Mankin HJ: Studies on cryopreservation of articular cartilage chondrocytes. *J Bone Joint Surg Am* 1984;66:253-259.

41. Gross AE, Shasha N, Aubin P: Long-term followup of the use of fresh osteochondral allografts for posttraumatic knee defects. *Clin Orthop Relat Res* 2005;435:79-87.

42. Ball ST, Amiel D, Williams SK, et al: The effects of storage on fresh human osteochondral allografts. *Clin Orthop Relat Res* 2004;418:246-252.

43. Friedlaender GE: Appropriate screening for prevention of infection transmission by musculoskeletal allografts. *Instr Course Lect* 2000;49:615-619.

44. Tomford WW: Transmission of disease through transplantation of musculoskeletal allografts. *J Bone Joint Surg Am* 1995;77:1742-1754.

45. Stevenson S: The immune response to osteochondral allografts in dogs. *J Bone Joint Surg Am* 1987;69:573-582.

46. Sirlin CB, Brossmann J, Boutin RD, et al: Shell osteochondral allografts of the knee: Comparison of MR imaging findings and immunologic responses. *Radiology* 2001;219:35-43.

47. Friedlaender GE, Horowitz MC: Immune responses to osteochondral allografts: nature and significance.

Orthopedics 1992;15:1171-1175.

48. Phipatanakul WP, VandeVord PJ, Teitge RA, Wooley PH: Immune response in patients receiving fresh osteochondral allografts. *Am J Orthop* 2004;33:345-348.

49. Emmerson BC, Görtz S, Jamali AA, Chung C, Amiel D, Bugbee WD: Fresh osteochondral allografting in the treatment of osteochondritis dissecans of the femoral condyle. Read at the 2006 Symposium of the International Cartilage Repair Society; 2006 Jan 8-11; San Diego, CA.

50. Garrett JC: Fresh osteochondral allografts for treatment of articular defects in osteochondritis dissecans of the lateral femoral condyle in adults. *Clin Orthop Relat Res* 1994;303:33-37.

51. Shasha N, Krywulak S, Backstein D, Pressman A, Gross AE: Long-term follow-up of fresh tibial osteochondral allografts for failed tibial plateau fractures. *J Bone Joint Surg Am* 2003;85(Suppl 2):33-39.

52. Jamali AA, Emmerson BC, Chung C, Convery FR, Bugbee WD: Fresh osteochondral allografts. *Clin Orthop Relat Res* 2005;437:176-185.

53. Beaver RJ, Mahomed M, Backstein D, Davis A, Zukor DJ, Gross AE: Fresh osteochondral allografts for post-traumatic defects in the knee: A survivorship analysis. *J Bone Joint Surg Br* 1992;74:105-110.

54. Tasto JP, Ostrander R, Bugbee W, Brage M: The diagnosis and management of osteochondral lesions of the talus:

Osteochondral allograft update. *Arthroscopy* 2003;19(Suppl 1):138-141.

55. Lewandrowski KU, Rebmann V, Passler M, et al: Immune response to perforated and partially demineralized bone allografts. *J Orthop Sci* 2001;6:545-555.

56. United States Department of Health and Human Services, Centers for Disease Control and Prevention.: Update: Allograft associated bacterial infections. *MMWR Morb Mortal Wkly Rep* 2002;51:207-210.

57. Görtz S, Ho A, Bugbee W: Fresh osteochondral allograft transplantation for cartilage lesions in the knee. Read at the Annual Meeting of the American Academy of Orthopaedic Surgeons; 2006 Mar 22- 26; Chicago, IL.

58. Park DY, Chung CB, Bugbee WD: Fresh osteochondral allografts for younger, active individuals with osteoarthrosis of the knee. Read at the 2006 Symposium of the International Cartilage Repair Society; 2006 Jan 8-11; San Diego, CA.

59. Bugbee W, Khadivi B: Fresh osteochondral allografting in the treatment of osteonecrosis of the knee. Read at the Annual Meeting of the American Academy of Orthopaedic Surgeons; 2004 Mar 10- 14; San Francisco, CA.

60. Aubin PP, Cheah HK, Davis AM, Gross AE: Long- term followup of fresh femoral osteochondral allografts for posttraumatic knee defects. *Clin Orthop Relat Res* 2001;391(Suppl):S318-S327.

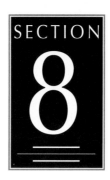

SECTION

8

Practice Management

Table 4	
Selected Sites With Images Useful for Orthopaedists	
www6.aaos.org/pemr/press.htm	Members-only section contains free downloadable PowerPoint presentations for AAOS member use
www.primalpictures.com	Web access to orthopaedic anatomy images by subscription
www.visiblehumanexperience.com	From the Center for Human Simulation at the University of Colorado; free PowerPoint presentations with selected anatomic images
www.orthopaediclist.com	Free source for orthopaedic products, including a section on radiographic identification of implants
www.brisbio.ac.uk/	Bristol BioMed Image Archive. Categorized archive of 20,000 images for teaching. Requires free registration
www.merckmedicus.com	Interactive Website sponsored by Merck with options for creating images for presentations
www.orthopaedicweblinks.com	
www.bartleby.com	Images from *Gray's Anatomy*
www.nlm.nih.gov/nlmhome.html	NLM image database containing >60,000 images
www.images.md/users/index.asp	Online encyclopedia of medical images
www.orthogate.com/gallery/main.php	Orthogate image gallery
www.uwec.edu/kin/majors/AT/aidil/index.htm	Athletic injury digital image library
www.eatonhand.com/handbase/images.htm	Hand list photo archives

45 Orthopaedic Information: How to Find It Fast on the Internet

Orthopaedic Information: How to Find It Fast on the Internet

J. Sybil Biermann, MD
Gregory J. Golladay, MD
J.F. Myles Clough, MD
Steven R. Schelkun, MD
A. Herbert Alexander, MD

Abstract

The Internet is a rapidly expanding source of information that has gained a valued place in the knowledge armamentarium of the orthopaedic surgeon. Access to current knowledge, published literature, and a vast array of academic, federal, and commercial information has changed the information landscape for both orthopaedic surgeons and their patients.

It is valuable to highlight readily available information for orthopaedic surgeons to use for continuing medical education, literature updates, patient education materials, and presentations. There are multiple techniques for accessing and organizing orthopaedic information as well as for identifying and using specific, high-quality, frequently updated Internet sources of information.

Instr Course Lect 2007;56:483-489

The traditional source of medical information was the medical library. Although traditional brick and mortar libraries still clearly play a role, the expansion of the Internet has allowed most library resources to be accessed online from the desktop computer (Table 1). Additionally, the union of electronic communications with the vastness of the Internet has engendered several unique mechanisms for information delivery and exchange.

MEDLINE Searching

Perhaps the oldest generally used Internet source for obtaining medical information is the National Library of Medicine's MEDLINE database.[1] One component of this database is PubMed (www.pubmed.gov), which is the National Library of Medicine's journal literature search system. PubMed is freely available through the World Wide Web. MEDLINE, accessed through PubMed, is primarily useful for searching English-language journals; it contains more than 4000 searchable publications and more than 15 million records dating back to the mid-1960s. Updated weekly, it is the most commonly used database for the search of scientific papers and abstracts.

PubMed contains the MEDLINE database as well as some additional material, including selected citations from before 1966 and some nonmedical scientific literature (general science, chemistry, and physics).[2] PubMed also contains links (segments of text or graphical items that serve as a cross reference between parts of a hypertext document or between files or hypertext documents) to many sites providing full-text articles and other related resources, a clinical queries search filter, a single citation matcher, the ability to save and automatically update searches, a spell checker, and filters that enable the user to group search results.

Certain features of PubMed bear special mention. A brief online tutorial, targeted primarily at the novice user, is accessible on the site, and taking this tutorial is an excellent time investment as it can markedly increase the rate of retrieval of useful articles. A medical librarian is another valuable resource for obtaining help in using PubMed in general or

Table 1
Comparison of Library and Internet Resources

Library	Internet
Textbooks	Textbook sites
Catalogs	Index sites
Journals	Journal sites and electronic journals
Index Medicus	PubMed
Librarian	Search engines
MEDLINE search	Image search
	Organizations— eg, AAOS
	Discussion groups
	Push sites that deliver specified information
	Patient information sites—eg, AAOS

for obtaining assistance with a specific search. The Orthogate Website also contains a three-part tutorial that provides step-by-step explanations of how searches can be optimized. This tutorial details the importance of utilization of accepted terms as well as understanding the logic that PubMed uses in generating search matches (www.orthogate.com/ clough/pubmed_1.htm).

One feature of particular interest to orthopaedic surgeons is the ability to identify and link to "related articles." Once a particularly germane article is identified, clicking on the associated link will lead directly to that citation. There is also the ability to save searches for later review.

The MEDLINE database can be accessed through several Websites besides PubMed. These sites all use the same database, but the search interface is tailored to the specific site. Examples include Medscape (www.medscape.com) and myMedline (www.mymedline.com). These sites offer a different type of user interface, usually with some functions available for saving or customizing searches. Because these sites use the PubMed searching capabilities, they do not actually add searching or sorting capabilities or citations.

Internet Searching

The Internet is not only disorganized, but it resists organization. A massive amount of orthopaedic information is posted. A high proportion of this mass has a commercial message and is therefore suspect with regard to the objectivity of the information. Search engines may be the best tool for sorting information, but they have unique idiosyncrasies. Using them takes little time or talent, but using them effectively requires learning and practice. There is no effective mechanism for ensuring, or even screening for, the quality of information on the Internet. Several studies have shown the variability in content and completeness of Internet-derived information.[3,4]

Search Engines and Directories

The two most common means with which to find information on the Internet are "directories" and "search engines." Directories are lists of resources, usually in the form of links directing the user to the Internet addresses of useful sites. Institutions or individuals have collected these lists.

Search engines are the most commonly used methods for finding information on the Web. However, there is considerable variability in how search engines work, and consequently the quality and validity of the information returned by the search vary as well. The rate of technological advances is such that the search parameters change from year to year. Search engines, unlike directories, are robotic devices that search a database to find pages that contain the "search string," the words that the user presents to the search engine. The databases searched by the search engines vary enormously. Some engines search only one Website, whereas others search a substantial fraction of the entire Internet. The most commonly used search engine, Google (www.google.com), searches the largest number of sites on the Internet.

Depending on the type of information being searched, an alternative is to use a "web directory" such as Yahoo (www.yahoo.com), in which sites are generally viewed by a human and classified into groups of interest. However, with the advance of technology and the exponential proliferation of Web material, the importance of directories as a solution to the problem of facilitating good searches is likely to wane.

Most search engines use software programs known as "robots," "spiders," or "crawlers." This technology accesses new pages, categorizes it, and sends information back to the parent database without a human ever seeing it. Commercial webmasters design their sites to be attractive to search engines by inserting relevant "keywords" in the title and metadata pages, and as a result the engines "find" commercial sites preferentially. Framing search strings to find orthopaedic content requires use of as many jargon, or specific medical, terms as the searcher thinks might be on the target site. Doing so will help to restrict the search results to valuable orthopaedic content. For example, searching for "hip arthroplasty" rather than "hip replacement" will likely yield more content of interest to the medical professional. In another example, in January 2006, a search on www.google.com for "cartilage tear"

Table 2
Advanced Search Features

Subject	Intent	Search String	Advanced Feature
1. Shaft	Find all synonyms	Shaft diaphysis	"At least one"
2. Nonunion femoral shaft	Find "Nonunion femoral diaphysis"	Nonunion femoral shaft	"All of the words"
3. Bone grafting	Find "Bone grafting"	Bone grafting	"Exact phrase"
4. Femoral shaft	Avoid other femoral fracture types	Supracondylar hip neck	"Without the word"

yielded in excess of 395,000 pages. Nineteen of the first 20 pages were directed at informing patients or attracting patients to a particular clinician. Using the more specific term "meniscus tear" yielded 270,000 pages. Three of the first 20 pages were directed at professionals, and the rest were patient-information pages. The search string "meniscus tear portal" still yielded 11,000 pages, but 13 of the first 20 were directed at physicians. Defining exactly what information is to be found is the most important and most difficult skill in searching the Internet.

In the early years of searching the World Wide Web, it was critical to use exact search terms such as AND, OR, and NOT to include or exclude search parameters. Currently, most search engines have sufficient sophistication to allow information to be entered into a query field with use of common language terms. When a general search engine is used to look for medical information for professionals, it is generally best to use the "advanced search" function that most search engines offer. Whereas the standard search assumes that the user requires "all of the words" of the search string to be present on the target page, the advanced search allows one to define "the exact phrase," "at least one of the words," or "without the words" (Table 2). Other features of the Google ad-

vanced search (www.google.com/advanced_search?hl=en) restrict the results by language, file format, date of updating, and domain. It is also possible to search for pages that link to a specific page.

If one wanted to frame a search for the subject *bone-grafting* in the *treatment of ununited femoral shaft fractures,* one might want to combine all four subjects of Table 2. It is much easier to do this with the advanced search feature rather than by constructing the search string (nonunion femoral shaft OR diaphysis "bone-grafting"-supracondylar-hip-neck) oneself. Incidentally, this search yielded 293 pages in January 2006.

Quality of Information

Even with a successful search, one needs to be careful about accepting Internet-derived information.

In general, a health information site should be evaluated on the basis of several critical factors. The first factor is authorship—the credibility of the individual who wrote the material, or posted the information. The second is currency. Old information is often more dangerous than no information. The third is the presence of advertising on the site; whether for a product, goods, or a specific method of care, advertising should alert the reader to potential bias in the article. The completeness of an article—that is,

whether it presents all relevant information on a particular subject—is important. Obviously, the accuracy of the information is also of importance.

Some sites rate health information. One such site, Health on the Net (HON) (www.hon.ch/), is maintained by a nonprofit organization that provides a search mechanism that can help ensure that searches are limited to credible sites. However, HON cannot realistically hope to evaluate every potential site or to ensure that updates to a given site will comply with HON standards after the site has received the HON rating.

It is recommended that physicians maintain a list of credible sites to give to patients, and the list may be customized according to practice type and physician preference. Examples of credible sites include those provided by the American Academy of Orthopaedic Surgeons (www.aaos.org), the Arthritis Foundation (www.arthritis.org), and Orthopaedic Web Links (www.orthopaedicweblinks.com/Patient_Information).

Textbook Sites

Textbook sites can be ideal for users seeking fairly general orthopaedic information about a broad range of topics. The best of these sites are documents covering the whole of a subject, laid out with the overarch-

Table 3
Selected Orthopaedic Online Textbooks

Wheeless' Textbook of Orthopaedics (Duke University Website)

Stryker Orthopaedics Hyperguide (requires free registration)

Orthopaedic Knowledge Online (free to AAOS members, or pay per view)

Orthoteers (requires annual registration fee)

Flinders Orthopaedic Registrars' Notebook (free)

Southern Orthopaedic Association Orthopaedic Care Textbook (good quality but incomplete coverage)

eMedicine (Orthopaedics) (full-text articles, requires free registration)

Book of Orthopaedics and Traumatology (written from the perspective of the developing world)

Medscape WorldOrtho

ing idea of a textbook in mind. Many textbook sites are more superficial, some are revision notes from trainees, and some are "book dumps," meaning that a document originally designed for paper has been transferred unaltered to the Internet, often leading to navigation and formatting difficulties. Some, however, are well thought out and planned for the Internet and examples are listed in Table 3.

Of the sites listed in Table 3, Wheeless' Textbook of Orthopaedics (www.wheelessonline.com) is the most comprehensive and the best illustrated, cross-referenced, and organized. It was assembled during the author's residency at Duke University and has been taken over by that institution and updated regularly. It is one of the most outstanding examples of the use of hypertext in a reference work in the whole of medicine. The eMedicine collection of orthopaedic subjects (www.emedicine.com/orthoped/index.shtml) is not as complete and is less intensively cross-referenced, but its individual articles are clear, up-to-date reviews written by experts. Medscape (www.medscape.com) also provides very full treatment of orthopaedic subjects with full-text articles

adapted from recent published work.

Orthopaedic Directory Sites
(Link Pages)

Orthopaedic directory sites are lists of links to topics that have been selected as germane to the subject. Orthopaedic Web Links (OWL) (www.orthopaedicweblinks.com) is the largest directory of links to sites of orthopaedic interest. The sites are selected and validated by orthopaedic surgeons. OWL is large enough, with more than 5000 links, to have been set up as a searchable database. Alternatively, one can browse through the subdivisions (eg, Orthopaedic Topics > Trauma > Femur).

Directories are most useful when the need is to find an entry to a subject, not necessarily everything there is to find. They are most helpful if one repeatedly refers to a particular area; the directory can be bookmarked for future use. The most valuable aspect of many directory sites is that a human, not a robot, selected the resources. Although these types of sites can be quite helpful, as new material is added constantly on the Web, they are necessarily incomplete, and they may also suffer from "link-rot" as the sites that they origi-

nally collected are withdrawn or change addresses.

Patient Information Sites

The advent of the Internet has accelerated what was a gradual progression from a physician-centered culture to a patient-centered culture, enabling the process of shared decision-making. In many orthopaedic practices, surgeons are finding that patients are frequently using the Internet to obtain information about their diagnoses and treatment.[5-7]

Fortunately, there are many excellent sources of patient information on the Internet. Peer-reviewed, current information is maintained on Your Orthopaedic Connection (www.orthoinfo.org), the patient information arm of the American Academy of Orthopaedic Surgeons (AAOS) Website. MedlinePlus, the public information arm of the National Library of Medicine Website, contains material and links to patient information in medicine. The orthopaedic arm of this is found as "Bones, Joints and Muscles Topics" (www.nlmnih.gov/medlineplus/bonesjointsandmuscles.html). Finally, Orthopaedic Web Links maintains a site with extensive links to a wide variety of patient education materials (www.orthopaedicweblinks.com/Patient_Information/index.html).

Imaging and the Web
Acquiring Images

The Internet is a rich source of orthopaedics-related images, which current search engines allow one to search and access with relative ease. Google and Yahoo are two of the most popular general search engines that allow one to specify "images" as a search item and type in search terms. The images that are returned from the search are viewed originally as thumbnails but are actually links to the original source. Double-clicking on the thumbnail takes one to the original site on which the image appeared. If an image is to be saved for educational purposes, this can usually be done by right-clicking over the image (for PC users) and then clicking on the "save as" feature in the dialog box. Keep in mind that most images on Internet sites are low resolution, designed for fast web-page-loading, and they do not enlarge well. However, they are suitable for electronic presentations.

Most Windows operating systems have an option to save and print the entire active screen with the "Print Screen" key on the keyboard, which saves the entire screen image to the computer clipboard. However, images saved in this way contain excess material such as menu bars and headers and may require electronic cropping before use. If only an image, chart, or graph needs to be saved, a stand-alone screen capture program may be considered. Using the web browser to search for "screen capture" or "screen print programs" will reveal a long list of available programs from which to choose, and many have free trial downloads.

Most professional journals are offered online. Portable document format (PDF) files are becoming a universal format for viewing documents on any computer. These documents can be found and downloaded from the Internet. Most familiar to the orthopaedist will be *The Journal of Bone and Joint Surgery* (JBJS) and the *Journal of the American Academy of Orthopaedic Surgeons* (JAAOS) articles and subspecialty journals such as the *Journal of Orthopaedic Trauma* that are available to subscribers. These are relatively high-quality files that contain not

only the text, but also the images, charts, and graphs from articles that may be of use to an orthopaedist preparing for a presentation. Usually, these files open in the free application Adobe Acrobat Reader (Adobe Systems, San Jose, California). However, as indicated by the name, these files may be read only. Images or charts cannot be selected and saved, and text cannot be modified with this version of Adobe Acrobat. With the full version of Adobe Acrobat, any of the images, graphs, or charts can be selected and saved. In addition, many new programs with which to create and manipulate PDF files are available. The search engine in the web browser will provide a list of the newest programs from which to choose. As mentioned above, stand-alone screen

Table 4
Selected Sites With Images Useful for Orthopaedists

www6.aaos.org/pemr/press.htm	Members-only section contains free downloadable PowerPoint presentations for AAOS member use
www.primalpictures.com	Web access to orthopaedic anatomy images by subscription
www.visiblehumanexperience.com	From the Center for Human Simulation at the University of Colorado; free PowerPoint presentations with selected anatomic images
www.orthopaediclist.com	Free source for orthopaedic products, including a section on radiographic identification of implants
www.brisbio.ac.uk/	Bristol BioMed Image Archive. Categorized archive of 20,000 images for teaching. Requires free registration
www.merckmedicus.com	Interactive Website sponsored by Merck with options for creating images for presentations
www.orthopaedicweblinks.com	
www.bartleby.com	Images from *Gray's Anatomy*
www.nlm.nih.gov/nlmhome.html	NLM image database containing >60,000 images
www.images.md/users/index.asp	Online encyclopedia of medical images
www.orthogate.com/gallery/main.php	Orthogate image gallery
www.uwec.edu/kin/majors/AT/aidil/index.htm	Athletic injury digital image library
www.eatonhand.com/handbase/images.htm	Hand list photo archives

capture programs may also be used to select and copy these images.

Online Sources of Images Related to Orthopaedics
Several Internet sites have free or available-by-subscription images. A brief listing is presented in Table 4.

Image Archiving and Retrieving
There are dozens of image archiving and retrieval applications on the market. How to organize images on a home or office computer is a personal choice based on organizational preferences, the nature of the images being saved, and how they are to be retrieved for use. In many orthopaedic practices, images are saved either according to the pathologic condition (for example, ankle or hip fractures, or knee arthroscopy

images) or specific patients. The features that are most important for medical image retrieval include the name and medical record number of the patient; the date of injury, surgery, or follow-up; and the diagnosis. All images of a specific patient can be saved within a single folder on the computer. Each folder should have a unique identifier (name) to aid in retrieval. Within each folder, the individual images for each patient are often arranged chronologically by date of injury, surgery, or follow-up. An understanding of how the computer organizes files will aid in organization. Dates are usually written by year, month, and day, from left to right (for example, 2006/01/21), and only image files starting with this date format will be displayed chronologically.

Once images of a patient have been organized, it may be desirable for another physician to view them. For example, images may be sent to the referring physician for follow-up, then to a colleague for a second opinion, or loaned to a friend for a presentation. Keep in mind that the privacy rules that apply to protection of confidential patient information also apply to images and information transferred by means of the Internet. Patient identification information may not be included on or with the images. Internet resources will help in this regard. Commercial services allow storage of medical images on a secure server, where they can be viewed by others by invitation and password only. MyView-Box (www.myviewbox.com) is a service for physicians that allows, for a small fee, secure server storage, storage of multiple images in a separate folder for each patient, and transmission of e-mails to an invited reviewer with a password for view-

ing, allowing images to be immediately available to consultants. Commercial e-mail programs such as America Online (AOL), Yahoo, and Microsoft Online (MSN) are unsuitable for transmission of patient images because of both the lack of security and restrictions on the size of transmitted images. Recently, several secured e-mail services have become available. These transmit "encrypted" messages, including images, and usually require password verification. Because of the encryption, many may be compliant with Health Insurance Portability and Accountability Act (HIPAA) guidelines and suitable for transmittal of patient information to colleagues. To search for these applications, enter "secured email" as the search term in the web browser and look specifically for the ones that state that they are HIPAA-compliant.

Copyright and Fair Use

Any work that is published on paper or on the Internet must be assumed to fall under the protection of the Copyright Act (Title 17, US Code), and permission obtained from the author or publisher to use all or any portion of that material unless it can be determined that the material is no longer covered by copyright protection and now belongs in the "public domain." All works published in the United States before 1923 are in the "public domain." After that date, the copyright status may be difficult to determine. The absence of a copyright symbol or notice is not sufficient to establish the lack of copyright protection. For example, works published after March 1, 1989, do not need to display a copyright notice or symbol to be protected.

The only exception to the copy-

right rule, and the one most important to orthopaedic surgeons, pertains to materials that are used under the "fair use" rule as outlined in section 107 of the Copyright Act. This rule recognizes that society may benefit from the unauthorized use of copyrighted material only if the purpose is for criticism, comment, news reporting, teaching, scholarship, or research.

Section 107 stipulates that four factors be considered when determining whether a particular use is "fair":

1. The purpose and character of the use, including commercial or noncommercial nature or nonprofit educational use.

2. The nature of the copyrighted work.

3. The amount of the copyrighted material used.

4. The effect of the use on the potential market for or value of the copyrighted work.

Certainly, many intended purposes for "borrowing" material, images, charts, and graphs from published works fall under this exception. As a general rule, if a small portion of somebody else's work is used, such as an image, graph, or chart, in a noncommercial way and the purpose of the use is for education, research, or teaching, then this could be considered fair use.

It is still a good idea to make every attempt to identify the author of the image or material and ask for permission for use. Even if it is decided that the work falls under the "fair use" category, credit still must be given to the author by naming the source as a reference.

Additional information can be found at fairuse.stanford.edu/ Copyright_and_Fair_Use_Overview/ chapter0/0-b.html#3 and at www. copyright.gov/title17/.

AAOS Website

Arguably the most comprehensive resource for the orthopaedic practitioner, the AAOS Website contains a multitude of information related to the practice and knowledge of orthopaedic surgery.

Professional education resources include access, review, and search of the Journal of the American Academy of Orthopaedic Surgeons and the American volume of the Journal of Bone and Joint Surgery. Orthopaedic Knowledge Online is a peer-reviewed source of topically organized medically related information available to AAOS members and, on a fee basis, to nonmembers. Use of video in this section for procedurally oriented material is particularly helpful. Extensive continuing medical education (CME) materials on the AAOS site are listed topically and include the AAOS-produced Self-Assessment Examinations.

Practice tools on the AAOS Website include prefabricated, customizable PowerPoint presentations (Community Orthopaedic Awareness Program) on a variety of general orthopaedic topics, Current Procedural Terminology (CPT) coding articles and monographs, practice management information and advice center, the Orthopaedic Medical Legal Advisor (OMLA), a publication with hints on risk management, the "Pitfalls and Pearls" section, and the opportunity for participation by AAOS fellows.

Finally, the AAOS supports free web-hosting of members' Websites, for individual and group practices,

with use of a template-guided, customizable site. AAOS fellows may log onto "Create Your Own Website" under "Member Services" using their AAOS password (available by calling the AAOS). Once the fellow is there, an overview introduces him or her to the process of creating a Website, and this is followed by directions for creating the site, including design examples, help screens, and examples of suggested text. This is all done online, and additional e-mail assistance is available from AAOS Member Services. One particularly useful element of the "Create Your Own Website" process is a feature that shows one how to link the AAOS patient information topics so that the selected ones appear on the fellow's individual or group practice Website. These patient information topics may also be printed by patients visiting the Website, or by the fellow for use as patient-information handouts. Each printout includes the logo for the individual Website as well as the AAOS logo. Return visits to "Create Your Own Website" are possible at any time to update and/or change information.

Another important feature of the AAOS Website is "Your Orthopaedic Connection." There, a direct link to patient-based orthopaedic information written and peer-reviewed by AAOS members is readily available for review and download. Additionally, AAOS press releases and other public media productions, including streaming videotapes and public service announcements, are available

there. As mentioned above, all articles can be linked directly to the AAOS member's individual and group Websites. The "Your Orthopaedic Connection" Website has grown rapidly, with more than 450 articles on a wide variety of patient-education-related topics and the recent development of in-depth "informed choice" modules.

References

1. United States National Library of Medicine, National Institutes of Health: Fact sheet: The National Library of Medicine. www.nlm.nih.gov/pubs/factsheets/nlm.html. 2005.

2. United States National Library of Medicine, National Institutes of Health fact sheet: What's the difference between MEDLINE and PubMed? www.nlm.nih.gov.library.unl.edu/pubs/factsheets/ dif_med_pub.html. 2005.

3. Bichakjian CK, Schwartz JL, Wang TS, Hall JM, Johnson TM, Biermann JS: Melanoma information on the Internet: often incomplete—a public health opportunity? *J Clin Oncol* 2002;20:134-141.

4. Lee CT, Smith CA, Hall JM, Waters WB, Biermann JS: Bladder cancer facts: Accuracy of information on the Internet. *J Urol* 2003;170:1756-1760.

5. Krempec J, Hall J, Biermann JS: Internet use by patients in orthopaedic surgery. *Iowa Orthop J* 2003;23:80-82.

6. Beall MS III, Golladay GJ, Greenfield ML, Hensinger RN, Biermann JS: Use of the Internet by pediatric orthopaedic outpatients. *J Pediatr Orthop* 2002;22:261-264.

7. Beall MS III, Beall MS Jr, Greenfield ML, Biermann JS: Patient Internet use in a community outpatient orthopaedic practice. *Iowa Orthop J* 2002;22:103-107.

Index